CT and MRI of the Abdomen and Pelvis

A Teaching File

Second Edition

CT and MRI of the Abdomen and Pelvis
A Teaching File

Second Edition

Editors

Pablo R. Ros, MD, MPH, FACR
Professor of Radiology,
Harvard Medical School
Executive Vice Chairman and Associate Radiologist-in-Chief
Department of Radiology
Brigham and Women's Hospital
Chief, Division of Radiology
Dana-Farber Cancer Institute
Boston, Massachusetts

Koenraad J. Mortele, MD
Associate Professor of Radiology,
Harvard Medical School
Associate Director, Division of Abdominal Imaging &
    Intervention
Director, Abdominal and Pelvic MRI
Director, CME
Department of Radiology
Brigham and Women's Hospital
Boston, Massachusetts

Associate Editors

Vincent Pelsser, MD
Clinical Fellow
Division of Abdominal Imaging Intervention
Department of Radiology
Brigham and Women's Hospital
Boston, Massachusetts
Assistant Professor of Radiology
Department of Radiology
McGill University
Jewish General Hospital
Montreal, Quebec, Canada

Sylvester Lee, MD
Greenville Radiology, PA
Greenville Memorial Hospital
Greenville, SC

Wolters Kluwer | Lippincott Williams & Wilkins
Health

Acquisitions Editor: Lisa McAllister
Managing Editor: Kerry Barrett
Project Manager: Alicia Jackson
Senior Manufacturing Manager: Benjamin Rivera
Marketing Manager: Angela Panetta
Creative Director: Doug Smock
Cover Designer: Larry Didona
Production Service: GGS Book Services
Printer: Maple Press

© 2007 by LIPPINCOTT WILLIAMS & WILKINS, a WOLTERS KLUWER business
530 Walnut Street
Philadelphia, PA 19106 USA
LWW.com

1st Edition © 1997 Williams & Wilkins

Printed in the USA

Library of Congress Cataloging-in-Publication Data
CT and MRI of the abdomen and pelvis : a teaching file / editors, Pablo
    R. Ros, Koenraad J. Mortele; associate editors, Vincent Pelsser,
    Sylvester Lee. — 2nd ed.
        p.; cm.
    Rev. ed. of: CT and MRI of the abdomen and pelvis / Pablo R. Ros.
c1997.
    Includes bibliographical references and index.
    ISBN 13 978-0-7817-7237-2
    ISBN 0-7817-7237-0
    1. Abdomen—Tomography—Case studies.   2. Abdomen—Magnetic resonance imaging—
Case studies.   3. Pelvis—Tomography—Case studies.   4. Pelvis—Magnetic resonance
imaging—Case studies.   I. Ros, Pablo R.   II. Mortele, Koenraad J.   III. Ros, Pablo R. CT
and MRI of the abdomen and pelvis.
    [DNLM: 1. Abdomen—pathology—Atlases.   2. Diagnosis, Differential—Atlases.
3. Digestive System Diseases—diagnosis—Atlases.   4. Magnetic   Resonance Imaging—
Atlases.   5. Pelvis—pathology—Atlases.   6. Tomography, X-Ray Computed—Atlases.
WI 17 C959 2007]
RC944.R674 2007
617.5'507548—dc22

To purchase additional copies of this book, call our customer service department at (800) 638-3030 or fax orders to (301) 223-2320. International customers should call (301) 223-2300.

Visit Lippincott Williams & Wilkins on the Internet: at LWW.com. Lippincott Williams & Wilkins customer service representatives are available from 8:30 am to 6 pm, EST.

10 9 8 7 6 5 4 3 2 1

DEDICATION

To Sylvia, my wife.

PABLO ROS, MD

To my daughter Charlotte, the apple of my eye, and my son Christophe, the boy of my dreams. I hope this book will inspire both of them in their quest for knowledge.

To my parents, my brothers Bart and Piet, and lifelong friends whose love and efforts molded me into the satisfied person I am.

To my colleagues and mentors, for their inspiration and relentless love for teaching and learning.

To all the residents and fellows I have had the privilege to teach, since they are the daily source of joy in my professional life.

KOENRAAD J. MORTELE, MD

To my parents, Albert and Odile, for their continuous support.

To my brother, Bernard, for his invaluable advice.

To Chantal, for her love.

VINCENT PELSSER, MD

To the medical students and residents
who inspired me through the years,

To my friends, parents and colleagues
who were always present with words of encouragement,

To my wife, Donna,
whose love, patience, and understanding made this long journey possible.

SYLVESTOR LEE

PUBLISHER'S FOREWORD

Teaching Files are one of the hallmarks of education in radiology. There has long been a need for a comprehensive series of books, using the Teaching File format, that would provide the kind of personal consultation with the experts normally found only in the setting of a teaching hospital. Lippincott Williams & Wilkins is proud to have created such a series; our goal is to provide the resident and practicing radiologist with a useful resource that answers this need.

Actual cases have been culled from extensive teaching files in major medical centers. The discussions presented mimic those performed on a daily basis between residents and faculty members in all radiology departments.

The format of this series is designed so that each case can be studied as an unknown, if desired. A consistent format is used to present each case. A brief clinical history is given, followed by several images. Then, relevant findings, differential diagnosis, and final diagnosis are given, followed by a discussion of the case. The authors thereby guide the reader through the interpretation of each case.

We hope that this series will become a valuable and trusted teaching tool for radiologists at any stage of training or practice, and that it will also be a benefit to clinicians whose patients undergo these imaging studies.

THE PUBLISHER

PREFACE TO THE SECOND EDITION

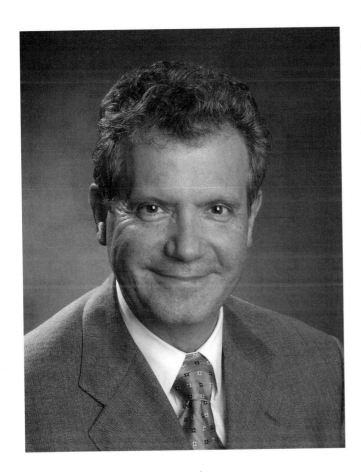

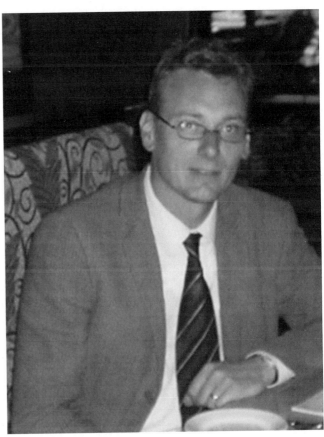

Although it is said that sequels rarely improve on the original movie, we hope our readers will agree that this second edition of our book, *CT and MRI of the Abdomen and Pelvis: A Teaching File*, is clearly better than its predecessor. The images are technically better; there is an increased number of cases illustrating more entities; it includes advanced technology, such as three-dimensional reformatted images; and it has more collaborators with specialized expertise than the first edition.

This project started a few years ago when we kept receiving emails and verbal comments from radiologists asking if they could get a copy of the first edition since it was out of print. Because we did not have additional copies of the book on hand, we started to think about writing a second edition. Because we had a professional relationship of over 10 years and understood each other very well, it was natural to decide to pool our efforts and talents to tackle this second edition.

We initially thought we could keep 80% of the old cases, add 20% of new ones, and update a few of the older images. Doing that would have taken only a few months. We really underestimated the amount of work to be done. Because we wanted to offer to our readers a complete, modern collection of outstanding cases, we ended up adding many more cases, changing almost all of the images, and making this second edition a more robust and complete teaching atlas. We selected the best possible cases out of our daily practice at the Brigham and Women's Hospital and Dana-Farber Cancer Institute in Boston, Massachusetts, and put them in an unknown case format, as we would present them in our routine case conferences. We also tried to incorporate cases that one of us has had the chance to see during our visits to other departments, particularly the Armed Forces Institute of Pathology in Washington, DC, and the University Hospital in Ghent, Belgium, or received in consultation from the United States and abroad. We have kept the best material from the first edition because we realized that some cases were so unique that we could not replace them.

At the end, we had trouble limiting the number of cases we wanted to include from our pool and staying within the space allowed by this single volume. We enjoyed meeting weekly with Vincent and trying to convince each other to include "just one more case" in a particular section, constantly updating differential diagnoses and making sure we had the best and most updated discussions and references for each case.

The structure of the book is similar to the first edition. We have divided the cases according to the traditional abdominal sections: Liver and Biliary System; Pancreas; Gastrointestinal Tract; Spleen; Mesentery, Omentum, and Peritoneum; Kidney, Ureter, and Bladder; Pelvis; Retroperitoneum and Adrenal Glands; and Abdominal Wall. For each case, after a

brief history, up to four images follow, which by definition are CT and/or MRI images. A brief description of the findings, the differential diagnosis, the final diagnosis, and a short discussion complete the case. This format allows the readers to take these cases as unknowns, thereby simulating the daily clinical practice of a radiologist.

We hope our readers will have fun with the second edition of *CT and MRI of the Abdomen and Pelvis: A Teaching File* and sense the enthusiasm of the authors for teaching abdominal imaging using a case format. If our readers gain even a small nugget of additional knowledge, we will feel satisfied that the educational goal of this book has been achieved.

PABLO R. ROS, MD, MPH, FACR
KOENRAAD J. MORTELE, MD

PREFACE TO THE FIRST EDITION

This book is the fruit of our collaboration that spans at least 6 years, when both of us were in the Department of Radiology at the University of Florida College of Medicine, Gainesville. Although the point-of-view of one of us (Sly) changed from medical student to radiology resident, fellow, and finally attending, we tried to duplicate the experience of reviewing interesting cases presented in the Abdominal Imaging divisional conferences, in "hot seat" sessions for the senior residents, and most importantly, in daily read-out sessions.

Our goal was to select the "best in show" material out of an archive of over 5,000 teaching file cases and put it in book format. The Abdominal Imaging teaching file at the University of Florida College of Medicine contains primarily cases that have been performed at Shands Hospital at the University of Florida and also cases originating from the Armed Forces Institute of Pathology, Washington, D.C. It also includes cases collected in visiting professorships in the United States and Canada, as well as other countries in Europe, Central and South America, and Asia, cases that have been presented in film-reading panels in national and international meetings, and cases that have been brought by visitors to the department. All cases entered into the teaching file have to be proven by either surgery, biopsy, laboratory data, or clinical and/or radiologic follow-up. Cases with an obvious pathognomonic imaging diagnosis (e.g., pneumoperitoneum) are also included. From this pool, we selected the best ones and divided them into chapters according to the traditional abdominal sections: liver and biliary tree, pancreas, spleen, gastrointestinal tract, kidney, retroperitoneum and adrenal, mesentery and omentum, and pelvis. We also added a chapter called "Unknowns and Aunt Minnies," which contains a potpourri of cases with a short differential diagnosis.

The format for each case is the same. A brief clinical history is followed by two to four images, which by definition are either computed tomography, magnetic resonance imaging scans, or a combination of both. Then, pertinent findings, differential diagnosis, final diagnosis, and a brief discussion follow.

This format is designed so that cases can be taken as unknowns. A simple piece of paper will cover the entire information given on each case. If the reader wants to know the findings or the differential diagnosis before knowing the final diagnosis, this can be easily accomplished by removing the paper.

To make this book reflect real life, we took actual cases from an extensive teaching file and recreated the discussions performed on a daily basis in hundreds of departments of radiology between residents and faculty members. We duplicated our discussions at the viewbox, emphasizing a practical approach. The cases in each chapter are not presented with traditional divisions (congenital, inflammatory, neoplastic, vascular, etc.), but are all mixed up, again mimicking real life. The end result, we hope, is that radiologists at any stage in their training or careers will benefit from reading this book.

We had fun selecting the cases, going over differential diagnosis lists, and trying to summarize a pertinent discussion for each case. We hope the reader will also enjoy going over them and learning more about diseases of the abdomen and pelvis using computed tomography and magnetic resonance imaging as diagnostic tools.

PABLO R. ROS, MD, FACR
SYLVESTER LEE, MD

ACKNOWLEDGMENTS

The second edition of this book would not have been possible without the efforts of several contributors. First, we would like to acknowledge the residents, fellows, and staff of the Division of Abdominal Imaging and Intervention at Brigham and Women's Hospital. All of them directly or indirectly contributed to this book by either donating cases or by presenting the differential diagnosis when these cases were initially read. Special thanks go to Drs. Jeffrey Girshman and Cheryl A. Sadow for providing us with particularly illustrative cases, and to Dr. Stuart G. Silverman for his continuous support and encouragement.

We also wish to extend our gratitude to the many clinical colleagues around the world who provided outstanding cases: Drs. Giovanni Artho, Caroline Reinhold, Dean Baird, George A. Taylor, Jeannette M. Perez-Rossello, Susan A. Connolly, Angela D. Levy, Manuel Fernandez, Adelard De Backer, and Luis Ros. Without their help, this book would not be as enriched.

We must recognize two people who helped us out when the need was the highest: Drs. Mehmet S. Erturk and Liesbeth J. Meylaerts, both research fellows in our department who allowed us to accomplish this task in a timely manner by co-authoring the Hepatobiliary and Pelvis chapters.

We would like to thank the technologists who obtained the images, and the ones specialized in post-processing, especially Jean M. Allen and Mark T. Delano, for creating many of the post-processed images used in this book.

We thank the staff at Lippincott Williams & Wilkins, particularly Kerry Barrett and Lisa McAllister, for the opportunity to write this second edition as well as their endless patience and support for this project.

Special appreciation also goes to Rob J. Mabe and Mildred D. Dewire, our administrative assistants, not only for preparing and sending the materials to the publisher, but also for making our days go smoothly.

Last but not least, we would like to thank Dr. Vincent Pelsser, Clinical Fellow in our Division, for his tremendous spirit, dedication, and efforts to get this project completed before the end of his fellowship. As we truthfully expressed to him several times during the year: this book would have never seen the light without his help.

PABLO R. ROS, MD, MPH, FACR
KOENRAAD J. MORTELE, MD

TABLE OF CONTENTS

CHAPTER TWO   PANCREAS   101

CHAPTER THREE GASTROINTESTINAL TRACT 154

CHAPTER FOUR   SPLEEN   217

CHAPTER FIVE   MESENTERY, OMENTUM, AND PERITONEUM   259

CHAPTER SIX   KIDNEYS, URETER, AND BLADDER   291

CHAPTER SEVEN   PELVIS   354

CHAPTER NINE ABDOMINAL WALL 465

CT and MRI of the Abdomen and Pelvis

A Teaching File

Second Edition

CHAPTER ONE

LIVER AND BILIARY SYSTEM

MEHMET S. ERTURK,
KOENRAAD J. MORTELE,
VINCENT PELSSER,
AND PABLO R. ROS

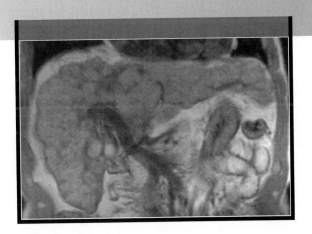

Clinical History: 69-year-old woman presenting with right upper quadrant pain, nausea, and vomiting.

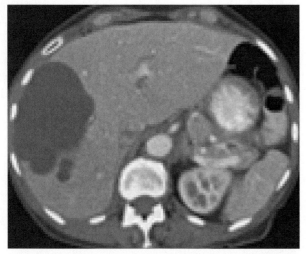

Figure 1.1   A

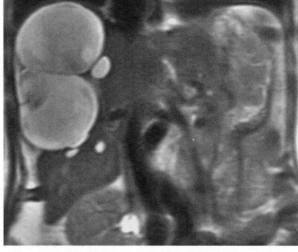

Figure 1.1   B

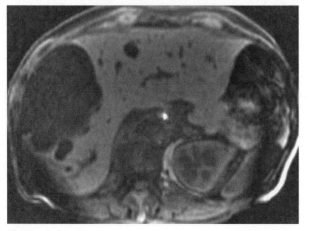

Figure 1.1   C

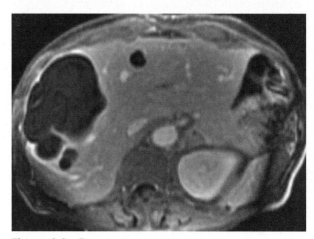

Figure 1.1   D

Findings: Axial nonenhanced computed tomography (NECT) image (A) demonstrates a large cystic lesion in the right lobe of the liver measuring 10 × 7.2 cm in its largest dimension. Coronal T2-weighted image (WI) (B) shows the cystic nature of the lesion and the presence of some septations. Unenhanced (C) and gadolinium-enhanced (D) fat-suppressed axial T1-WI demonstrate the peripheral capsular enhancement of the lesion.

Differential Diagnosis: Bile duct cyst, echinococcal cyst, hepatic abscess, necrotic neoplasm.

Diagnosis: Biliary cystadenoma.

Discussion: Biliary cystadenoma is a rare slow-growing cystic neoplasm occurring predominantly in middle-aged women. It can be complicated by hemorrhage, infection, rupture, and malignant transformation into cystadenocarci-

nomas. Typically, biliary cystadenoma is almost entirely cystic with very little solid component present; the presence of septations in most cases allows differentiation from simple bile duct cysts. These septated cystic neoplasms may also be indistinguishable from echinococcal cysts. Appropriate history is often necessary to distinguish the two entities; in this case, echinococcal cyst would be a good second choice if there were a history of travel to an endemic area with exposure to sheep and dogs. Calcifications can occur in the wall of the biliary cystadenoma. The presence of thick calcifications and a large solid component should raise the possibility of a cystadenocarcinoma. Both hepatic abscesses and necrotic metastases have a different CT appearance than a typical biliary cystadenoma with a thick irregular enhancing wall rather than thin well-defined septated cysts.

CASE 1-2

Clinical History: 43-year-old woman with abdominal discomfort.

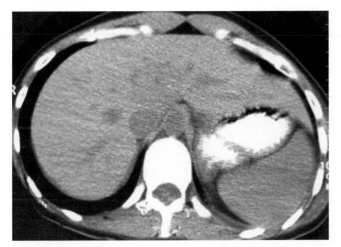

Figure 1.2   A

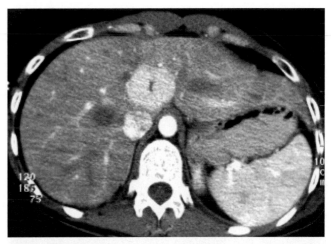

Figure 1.2   B

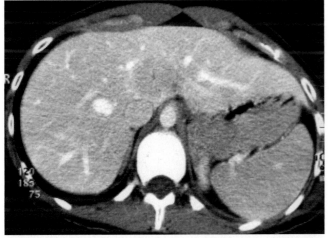

Figure 1.2   C

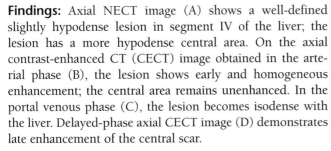

Figure 1.2   D

Findings: Axial NECT image (A) shows a well-defined slightly hypodense lesion in segment IV of the liver; the lesion has a more hypodense central area. On the axial contrast-enhanced CT (CECT) image obtained in the arterial phase (B), the lesion shows early and homogeneous enhancement; the central area remains unenhanced. In the portal venous phase (C), the lesion becomes isodense with the liver. Delayed-phase axial CECT image (D) demonstrates late enhancement of the central scar.

Differential Diagnosis: Hepatocellular carcinoma, hepatocellular adenoma.

Diagnosis: Focal nodular hyperplasia.

Discussion: Pathologically, focal nodular hyperplasia (FNH) is defined as a benign condition characterized by a central fibrous scar with surrounding nodules of hyperplastic hepatocytes and small bile ductules. On unenhanced CT studies, FNH is typically a homogeneous, hypodense mass. In a third of cases, a low-density central area corresponding to the central scar is seen. On contrast-enhanced studies, FNH enhances rapidly and homogeneously during the arterial phase and becomes hyperdense relative to normal liver. The nonenhancing low attenuation scar appears conspicuous against the hyperdense lesion. Foci of enhancement within the scar may be seen and represent hypertrophic arteries. In the portal venous phase and delayed phases of contrast enhancement, the difference in attenuation between FNH and normal liver decreases, and the FNH becomes iso- or hypodense compared to normal liver. Delayed images can show increased contrast uptake in the central scar, as seen in this case. The presence of an enhancing central scar is the most important CT feature that allows one to differentiate FNH from hepatocellular adenomas and carcinomas. Also, the latter tend to enhance more heterogeneously than FNH and are often surrounded by a capsule.

CASE 1-3

Clinical History: 29-year-old woman presenting with vague abdominal pain.

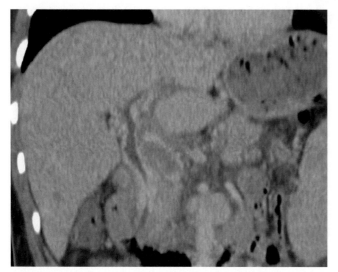

Figure 1.3   A

Figure 1.3   B

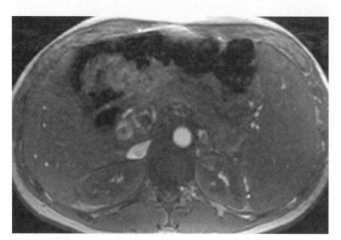

Figure 1.3   C

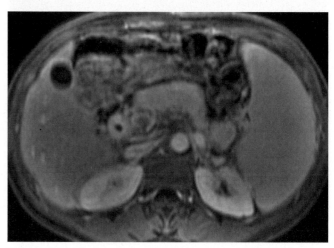

Figure 1.3   D

Findings: Coronal reformatted CECT image (A) demonstrates a hypodense thrombus in the extrahepatic portal vein and obvious enhancement of the wall of the extrahepatic bile duct. Axial T2-WI (B) shows multiple serpiginous structures with flow-void surrounding the common bile duct. Flow-sensitive axial MRI (C) and axial gadolinium-enhanced fat-suppressed T1-WI (D) show bright signal within the rim of tissue surrounding the common bile duct; this indicates the presence of blood flow.

Differential Diagnosis: Extrahepatic cholangiocarcinoma.

Diagnosis: Cavernous transformation of the portal vein with pericholedochal varices.

Discussion: Portal vein thrombosis can be secondary to multiple causes including malignancies (hepatocellular carcinoma, cholangiocarcinoma, metastases, and pancreatic neoplasms), trauma, hematologic disorders, and thrombophlebitis from sepsis, diverticulitis, or appendicitis. In up to 50% of the cases, however, the etiology is unknown. Portal vein thrombosis can either be intrahepatic or extrahepatic, with cirrhosis being the most common cause for intrahepatic thrombosis. Cavernous transformation of the portal vein is the formation of multiple periportal collaterals in the expected location of the portal vein. This can often alter the enhancement pattern of the liver because of compensatory arterial blood flow to the liver. The collateral vessels are thought to represent the hypertrophic vasa vasorum in the wall of the portal vein rather than true recanalization of the thrombosed portal vein. Other collateral vessels can often extend to the wall of the gallbladder and bile ducts, as seen in this example.

CASE 1-4

Clinical History: 76-year-old man with hepatic mass incidentally discovered at the time of an echocardiogram.

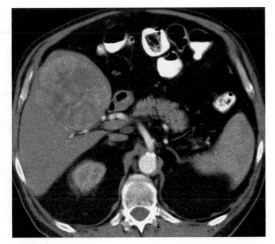

Figure 1.4 A

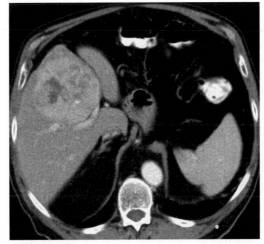

Figure 1.4 B

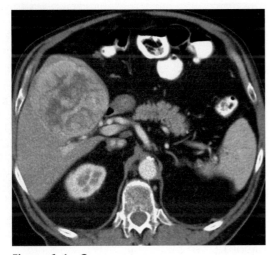

Figure 1.4 C

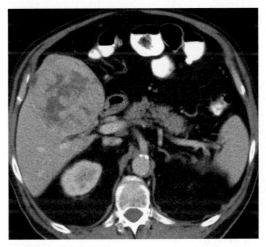

Figure 1.4 D

Findings: Axial early (A) and late (B and C) arterial phase CECT images show a 10-cm, well-defined, heterogeneously enhancing lesion in segment V of the liver. The lesion shows rapid washout of contrast on the portal venous phase axial CECT image (D).

Differential Diagnosis: Metastasis, cholangiocarcinoma.

Diagnosis: Hepatocellular carcinoma.

Discussion: Hepatocellular carcinoma (HCC) is thought to arise from at least two different pathways. The first, and least common, is in patients without any underlying liver disease. In one series, 40% of non-Asian patients with HCC did not have any underlying liver disease. The second is in patients who have a background of chronic liver disease. It is thought that the regenerating nodule is the first lesion in a spectrum of lesions leading to hepatocellular carcinoma. The multistep progression ranges from regenerating nodules, to low-grade dysplastic nodules, to high-grade dysplastic nodules, and finally, to HCC. HCC can present in three different ways on imaging studies: (a) a single solitary lesion (expansile HCC), which is often very large; (b) multifocal HCC, which is comprised of multiple separate nodules; and (c) cirrhotomimetic or diffuse HCC, which is composed of multiple tiny indistinct nodules. This case is an example of the expansile form of hepatocellular carcinoma. This case is unusual in that there is no radiographic or laboratory evidence for cirrhosis in this patient. The heterogeneous hypervascular appearance of the lesion in a male patient is nevertheless suggestive for an HCC. Cholangiocarcinomas would be less likely because they show an early rimlike enhancement and cause contraction of the liver capsule secondary to desmoplastic reaction. Metastasis would be a good choice for this case, although metastasis tends to be multiple instead of solitary.

Clinical History: 56-year-old man with history of chronic hepatitis B virus infection.

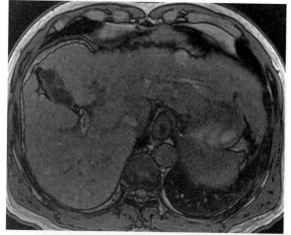

Figure 1.5   A

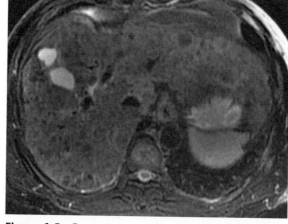

Figure 1.5   B

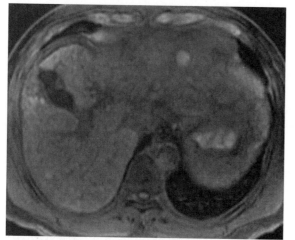

Figure 1.5   C

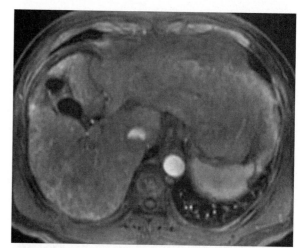

Figure 1.5   D

Findings: Out-of-phase axial T1-WI (A) demonstrates a 1 cm round nodule of increased signal intensity in the left lobe of the liver. Fat-suppressed axial T2-WI (B) demonstrates the same lesion to be of decreased signal intensity. Unenhanced (C) and gadolinium-enhanced arterial phase fat-suppressed T1-WI (D) show lack of early enhancement of the lesion.

Differential Diagnosis: Focal fat, hemorrhage, or hemorrhagic metastasis.

Diagnosis: Dysplastic nodule.

Discussion: Few tissue components will appear bright on T1-WIs, such as fat, glycogen, blood, protein, and melanin. Therefore, any lesion that contains any of these components can appear bright on a T1-WI. Focal fat, hepatocellular carcinoma, hepatocellular adenoma, focal nodular hyperplasia, and metastatic liposarcoma can potentially contain fat pathologically; however, in this case, the lesion is still bright on out-of-phase T1-WI and fat-suppressed T1-WI. Also, these lesions are usually bright on T2-WI. Blood products in hematomas or hemorrhagic metastases can have a variety of magnetic resonance (MR) signal characteristics based on the stage of evolution of the blood. Most regenerative nodules are isointense to surrounding liver on T1- and T2-WI. Dysplastic nodules are typically of low signal intensity on T2-WI due to the presence of iron and of slight increased signal intensity on T1-WI due to the presence of abundant glycogen. This is the opposite of the typical signal characteristics of a hepatocellular carcinoma. Also, note the lack of early arterial enhancement of a typical dysplastic nodule.

Case images courtesy of Dr. Giovanni Artho, McGill University Health Center, Montreal, Canada.

CASE 1-6

Clinical History: 81-year-old woman presenting with generalized abdominal pain.

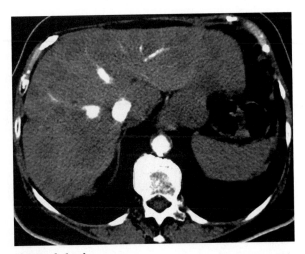

Figure 1.6 **A**

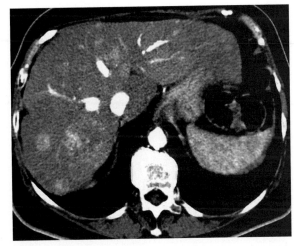

Figure 1.6 **B**

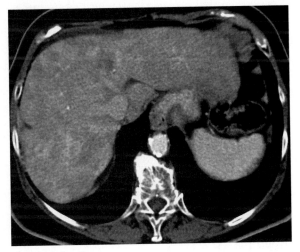

Figure 1.6 **C**

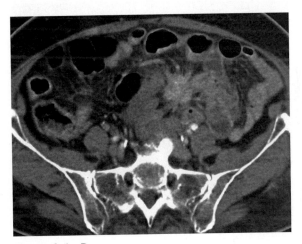

Figure 1.6 **D**

Findings: Axial early arterial (A), late arterial (B), and portal venous phase (C) CECT images demonstrate numerous lesions in the liver that are enhancing homogenously in the late arterial phase and washout during the portal venous phase. Axial CECT image (D) through the mid abdomen shows a spiculated left-sided mesenteric mass.

Differential Diagnosis: Multifocal hepatocellular carcinoma.

Diagnosis: Multiple liver metastases from carcinoid tumor.

Discussion: Metastatic disease is almost always multiple, with solitary metastasis occurring in only 2% of cases. The structure of the endothelial lining plays a role in making the liver susceptible to metastatic disease. The endothelial cells of the sinusoids have small perforations that measure 0.1 μm in diameter. No basal lamina is present at the sites of these perforations. Therefore, the normal barriers to metastatic disease are not present in the liver, allowing metastases to enter from the sinusoids into the extracellular matrix of the space of Disse. Most hepatic metastases are hypovascular and, therefore, will be hypodense on CECT. This is especially true for colorectal adenocarcinoma metastases. Scanning for these metastases is best performed during the portal phase of contrast injection. Detection of hypervascular metastases is excellent with dynamic CT scanning, especially during the late arterial phase, as seen in this case. Primary tumors that cause hypervascular liver metastases include renal cell carcinoma, endocrine tumors, carcinoid, sarcomas, thyroid carcinoma, and some subtypes of breast, lung, and pancreas carcinoma. Hepatocellular carcinoma in a noncirrhotic liver typically presents as a large heterogeneous mass and not as multiple small lesions.

Clinical History: 47-year-old woman with abnormal liver function tests and abdominal pain.

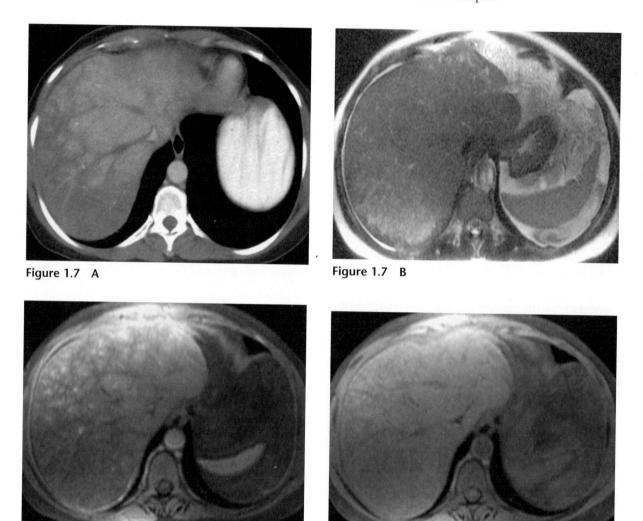

Figure 1.7   A

Figure 1.7   B

Figure 1.7   D

Figure 1.7   C

Findings: Axial CECT image (A) shows hepatomegaly, ascites, and heterogeneous enhancement of the liver. Note lack of enhancement of the right and middle hepatic veins. Axial T2-WI (B) and fat-suppressed T1-WI (C) images show congestion of the liver, decreased signal intensity on T1-WI, and increased signal intensity on T2-WI. Gadolinium-enhanced fat-suppressed axial T1-WI (D) confirms the thrombosis of the middle and right hepatic veins.

Differential Diagnosis: Passive hepatic congestion, veno-occlusive disease.

Diagnosis: Acute Budd-Chiari syndrome.

Discussion: Budd-Chiari syndrome results from the occlusion of the hepatic veins, the inferior vena cava (IVC), or both. Various conditions have been associated with the obstruction of hepatic venous drainage including idiopathic causes, hypercoagulable states from pregnancy, oral contraceptives, polycythemia vera, trauma, tumors involving or obstructing the IVC or hepatic veins, and webs in the IVC. This leads to stasis and increased postsinusoidal pressure in the liver, which decreases portal blood flow. The reduced hepatic venous flow causes ascites, hepatomegaly, collateral vessel formation, and splenomegaly. The poorly enhanced portions of the liver are due to decreased portal flow, venous congestion, and rarely infarcts. MR is very useful to detect Budd-Chiari syndrome. The typical findings on CT of mosaiclike enhancement, ascites, and hepatomegaly are readily seen on MR. MR also adds the ability to image in multiple planes, and MR angiography (MRA) can evaluate the hepatic veins and IVC. In this example, there was no evidence of flow in the hepatic veins. Thrombolysis and anticoagulant therapy has limited success in Budd-Chiari syndrome; portosystemic shunting or liver transplantation are therapeutic alternatives.

CASE 1-8

Clinical History: 58-year-old woman presenting with weight loss and abdominal distention.

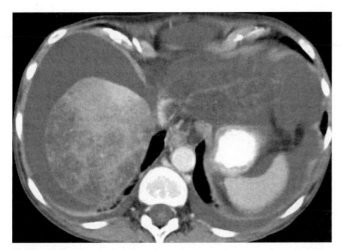

Figure 1.8 A

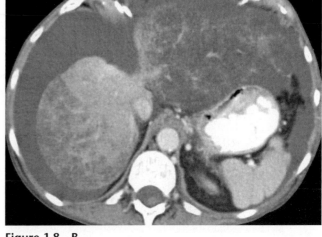

Figure 1.8 B

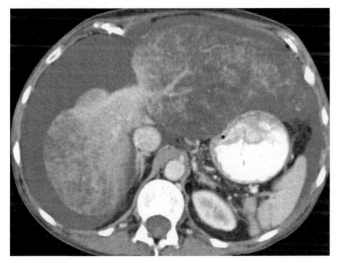

Figure 1.8 C

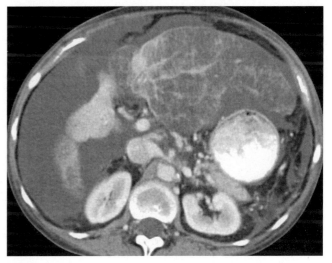

Figure 1.8 D

Findings: Axial CECT images demonstrate dysmorphic changes in the liver and the presence of patchy areas of lower attenuation, especially in the left hepatic lobe.

Differential Diagnosis: Uneven fatty change of the liver, hepatocellular carcinoma.

Diagnosis: Cirrhosis with fatty liver.

Discussion: Cirrhosis can produce many findings by CT. These include morphologic changes, such as an enlarged caudate lobe or enlarged left lateral segment, atrophy of the left medial segment and right anterior segments, a nodular contour, fatty change, portal hypertension (with ascites, collaterals, and splenomegaly), increased density of the mesenteric fat due to congestion, and the presence of regenerating nodules and hepatic fibrosis. Fatty liver is a common early finding of cirrhosis and often precedes other CT findings. As atrophy and fibrosis occur in conjunction with the formation of regenerating nodules, the contour of the liver becomes nodular and retracted. In this example, there is heterogeneous low density to the liver, which could be confused with an uneven fatty change or a diffuse neoplastic process, such as hepatocellular carcinoma. The key to the differentiation is the lack of mass effect by these low areas of attenuation. The vessels are seen to have a normal course through the liver without displacement. In unclear cases, MRI, with the use of in- and out-of-phase T1-WI, may bring clarification. Areas that contain fat will show significant drop in signal on the out-off phase images.

Clinical History: 65-year-old man presenting with hematuria.

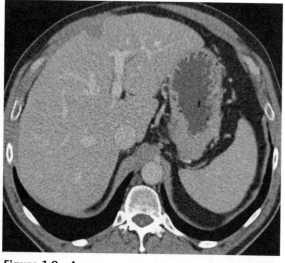

Figure 1.9   A

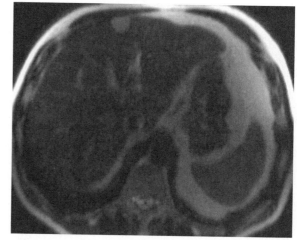

Figure 1.9   B

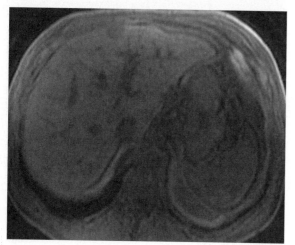

Figure 1.9   C

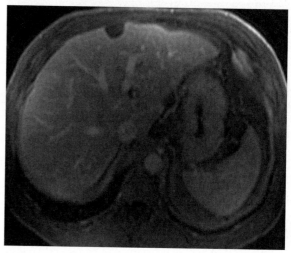

Figure 1.9   D

Findings: Axial CECT image (A) shows a slightly hypoattenuating lesion in the segment IVa, beneath the hepatic capsule. On axial T2-WI (B) and T1-WI (C), the lesion appears hyperintense and slightly hypointense, respectively. The lesion shows no enhancement on gadolinium-enhanced fat-suppressed axial T1-WI (D).

Differential Diagnosis: Biliary cystadenoma, bile duct cyst, cystic metastasis.

Diagnosis: Ciliated hepatic foregut cyst.

Discussion: Ciliated hepatic foregut cyst is a rare cystic lesion of the liver; its histogenesis is still unclear, but most authors consider that it arises from budding of the embryonic foregut in the liver. Ciliated hepatic foregut cyst is a benign, solitary cyst composed of a ciliated pseudostratified columnar epithelium, a subepithelial connective tissue layer, a smooth muscle layer, and an outer fibrous capsule. The lesion is almost always single and situated in the medial segment of the left lobe (segment IV), beneath the Glisson's capsule. On CT images, the density of ciliated hepatic foregut cyst may vary since it may contain various elements ranging from serous to mucoid material. Thus, on unenhanced CT, the lesion can be hypoattenuating or isoattenuating to normal liver parenchyma. On MRI, all ciliated hepatic foregut cysts are hyperintense on T2-WI. On T1-WI, however, the lesion may be hypo-, iso-, or hyperintense depending on its content. When a ciliated hepatic foregut cyst appears isodense relative to liver on CT images, it might be difficult to differentiate it from a solid hepatic lesion; in such cases, T2-WI is found to be useful to reach an accurate diagnosis.

Clinical History: 36-year-old woman with history of oral contraceptive use presents with abdominal pain and hypotension.

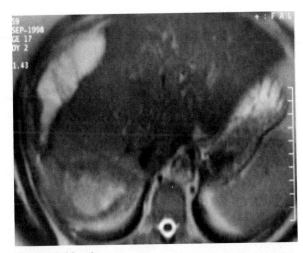

Figure 1.10   A

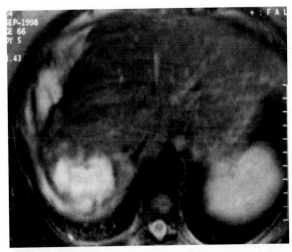

Figure 1.10   B

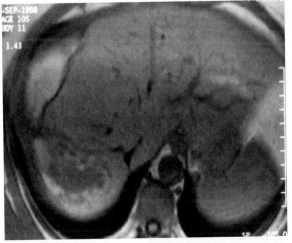

Figure 1.10   C

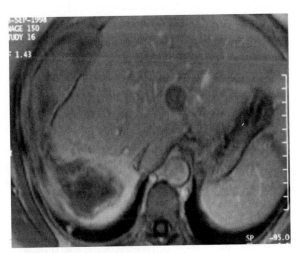

Figure 1.10   D

Findings: Axial T2-WI (A) demonstrates a slightly hyperintense lesion in segment VII of the liver, with central areas of hyperintensity. There is an associated subcapsular fluid collection. Heavily weighed axial T2-WI (B) shows the central area to be hyperintense, suggesting necrosis. Axial T1-WI (C) shows the subcapsular collection and the intratumoral collection to be hyperintense. Gadolinium-enhanced T1-WI (D) shows a hypervascular appearance of the hepatic lesion and lack of enhancement of the subcapsular collection.

Differential Diagnosis: Metastasis, hepatocellular carcinomas, abscess.

Diagnosis: Hepatocellular adenoma with rupture and subcapsular hematoma.

Discussion: Large hepatocellular adenomas will often rupture, and this can lead to massive and often fatal hemoperitoneum. Because of this possible grave complication, large hepatocellular carcinomas are often surgically removed prophylactically. In this example, the rim of increased signal intensity in the lesion on the T1-WI represents hemorrhage; the presence of methemoglobin shortens the T1 signal. The large size of the lesion, the presence of internal hemorrhage and a subcapsular hematoma, the hypervascular aspect of the lesion, the age of the patient, and history of oral contraceptive use makes hepatocellular adenoma the best diagnosis. In the setting of cirrhosis, a ruptured hepatocellular carcinoma would be a good diagnosis. Melanin-containing metastases and protein-containing abscesses can also appear bright on T1-WI.

Clinical History: 37-year-old woman with liver lesion detected on sonography.

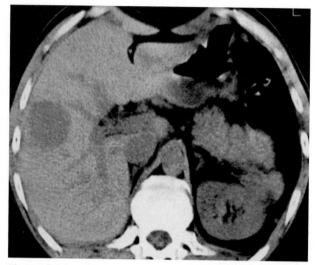

Figure 1.11   A

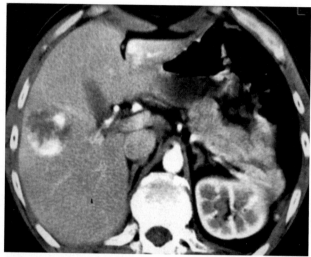

Figure 1.11   B

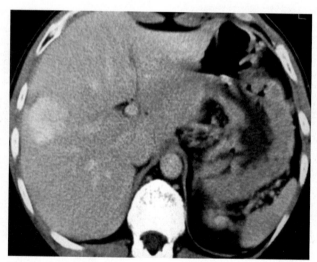

Figure 1.11   C

Findings: Unenhanced (A), arterial phase (B), and delayed-phase (C) CECT images show a well-defined homogeneous hypodense lesion in the right lobe of the liver that shows early peripheral nodular incomplete enhancement with delayed fill-in of the lesion.

Differential Diagnosis: Metastasis.

Diagnosis: Hemangioma.

Discussion: Hemangiomas are the most common benign liver tumors. They are more commonly seen in women than men (5:1 ratio). They are typically asymptomatic and found incidentally. Hemangiomas tend to be stable lesions; however, growth of hemangiomas during pregnancy has been reported. They tend to be small and are multiple in about 10% of cases. Punctate and coarse calcifications, fibrosis, and central cystic

degeneration can occur, especially in giant hemangiomas. Dynamic contrast administration demonstrates dense peripheral nodular incomplete enhancement of the lesion with sequential filling in of the lesion over time. This can take minutes to hours to occur. This enhancement is typically isodense to the aorta on all phases. The contrast will wash out of the liver but at a much faster rate than the hemangioma, which will be hyperdense relative to the liver. The enhancement pattern of hypervascular metastasis tends to be ringlike rather than globular. Puddling of contrast in the periphery of the lesion is very characteristic for a hemangioma and is only seen in a minority of metastases, especially treated breast cancer metastases. Also, without a history of a primary malignancy, a solitary metastasis is unlikely in this case, making a hemangioma the best diagnosis.

CASE 1-12

Clinical History: 66-year-old woman with leukemia presenting with abnormal liver function tests.

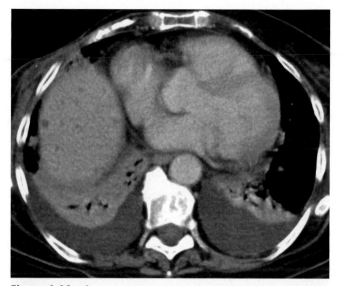

Figure 1.12   A

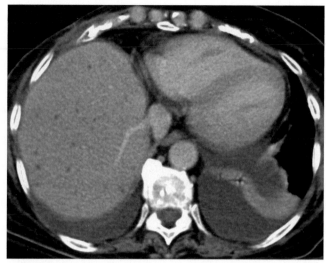

Figure 1.12   B

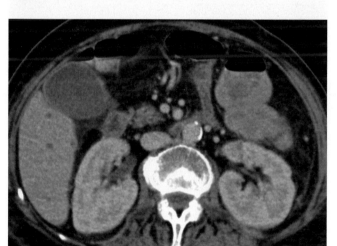

Figure 1.12   D

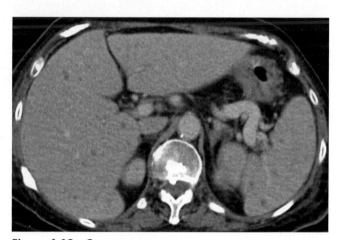

Figure 1.12   C

Findings: Axial CECT images demonstrate multiple, small, low-attenuation lesions seen throughout the liver and spleen. Splenomegaly and bilateral pleural effusions are also present.

Differential Diagnosis: Metastatic disease, septic emboli, von Meyenburg complexes (biliary hamartomas).

Diagnosis: Hepatic candidiasis.

Discussion: Candidiasis is the most common fungal infection encountered in immunocompromised hosts, and with the increase in incidence of human immunodeficiency virus (HIV)/acquired immunodeficiency syndrome (AIDS), it is becoming even more prevalent. In autopsy series, hepatic candidiasis is found in approximately 50% of patients with acute leukemia and lymphoma. The diagnosis is often difficult clinically, secondary to the nonspecific signs and symptoms of fever, abdominal pain, and hepatomegaly. The CT appearance of hepatic candidiasis varies depending on the phase of the infection. During the acute phase, there are multiple, small, low-attenuation lesions throughout the liver and spleen. After treatment with antifungal therapy, there can be calcifications within the lesions as well as areas of high attenuation on the unenhanced images due to the fibrosis. Other fungal infections such as *Aspergillus*, *Cryptococcus*, and *Pneumocystis carinii* can mimic the healing phase of hepatic candidiasis with multiple hepatic and visceral calcifications. This case demonstrates the acute phase of hepatic candidiasis with multiple low-attenuation lesions within the liver and spleen.

Clinical History: 68-year-old woman presenting with abdominal pain and melena.

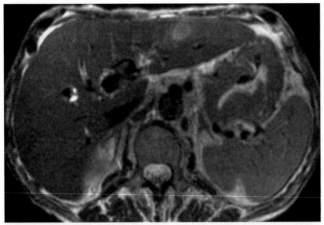

Figure 1.13   A

Figure 1.13   B

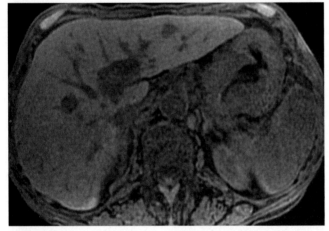

Figure 1.13   C

Figure 1.13   D

Findings: Axial T2-WI (A) demonstrates a 2 cm round, slightly hyperintense lesion within the left lobe of the liver. Note the presence of gastric wall thickening. Heavily weighted axial T2-WI (B) shows drop in signal of the lesion, suggesting it is solid. Unenhanced (C) and gadolinium-enhanced (D) fat-suppressed axial T1-WI show that the lesion is hypointense precontrast and has a peripheral rimlike enhancement pattern.

Differential Diagnosis: Hepatocellular carcinoma, lymphoma.

Diagnosis: Liver metastasis from gastric adenocarcinoma.

Discussion: Assessing the liver for metastatic disease is crucial for the staging and prognosis of patients with malignancies. Approximately 24% to 36% of patients who die of a malignancy will demonstrate liver metastatic disease at autopsy. Neoplasms arising from the gastrointestinal tract, in particular, have a propensity to metastasize to the liver secondary to the drainage through the portal vein. Approximately 45% of patients with gastric carcinoma have metastasis to the liver at the time of diagnosis. The appearance of multiple, round, mildly hyperintense lesions in the liver on T2-WI is most commonly due to metastatic disease. Hepatocellular carcinoma is a possibility, but the enhancement pattern, and lack of cirrhosis would make this diagnosis less likely. Lymphoma can involve the liver both primarily or secondarily. However, primary hepatic lymphoma is exceedingly rare. Associated lymphadenopathy and coexistent splenic involvement are typically seen in disseminated lymphoma.

Clinical History: 46-year-old woman with acute right upper quadrant pain and fever.

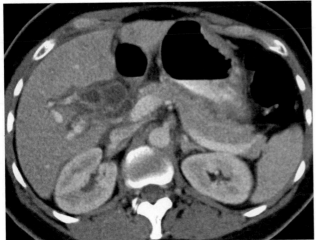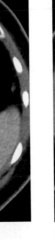

Figure 1.14 A

Figure 1.14 B

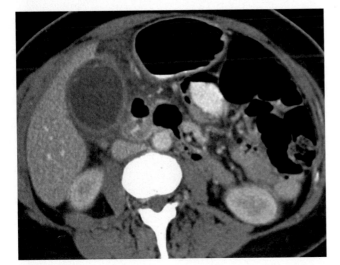

Figure 1.14 C

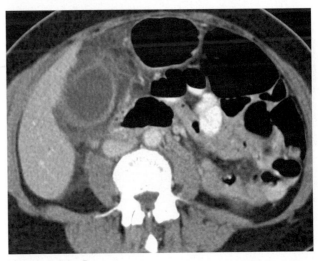

Figure 1.14 D

Findings: Axial CECT images demonstrate the dilated gallbladder, thickened gallbladder wall, subhepatic fat stranding, and low-attenuation periportal cuffing. Also note poor enhancement of the gallbladder wall with sloughing of the wall at the level of the fundus.

Differential Diagnosis: None.

Diagnosis: Acute cholecystitis.

Discussion: Acute cholecystitis is the fourth most common cause of hospital admissions for patients with acute abdomen pain. It typically results from obstruction of the cystic duct or gallbladder neck due to cholelithiasis with resulting inflammation of the gallbladder wall. Acute cholecystitis is caused by gallstones in most patients, with acalculous cholecystitis occurring in approximately 5% to 10%. In a patient with suspected acute cholecystitis, ultrasonography is typically the imaging procedure of choice. Although CT plays a small role in the evaluation of patients with acute cholecystitis, it is important to carefully evaluate the gallbladder in abdominal CT scans, since CT is commonly used as the initial exam in most patients with acute abdominal pain. The typical CT findings in acute cholecystitis include gallstones, gallbladder distention (>5 cm in anteroposterior diameter), mural thickening (>3 mm), pericholecystic fluid, poor definition of the gallbladder wall at the interface with the liver, inflammatory stranding in the pericholecystic fat, and hyperemia of the adjacent liver parenchyma. Of all these findings, the presence of pericholecystic inflammatory change is assumed to be the most specific because other findings, such as gallbladder wall thickening and distention, do not necessarily indicate cholecystitis.

Clinical History: 14-month-old boy presents with increasing abdominal girth.

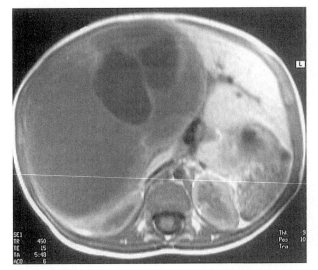

Figure 1.15 A

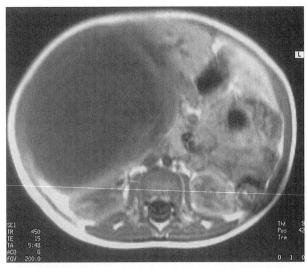

Figure 1.15 B

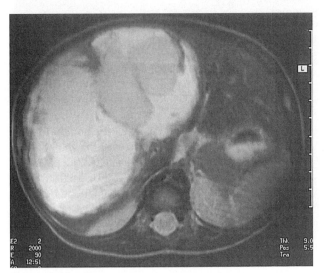

Figure 1.15 C

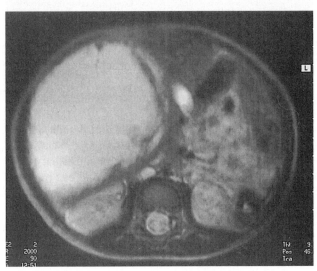

Figure 1.15 D

Findings: Axial T1-WI (A and B) demonstrate a low signal intensity lesion replacing the right lobe of the liver. Note the normal gallbladder. Axial T2-WI (C and D) demonstrate these same lesions to be hyperintense following the signal characteristics of simple fluid.

Differential Diagnosis: Undifferentiated embryonal sarcoma, infantile hemangioendothelioma, hepatoblastoma, metastasis.

Diagnosis: Mesenchymal hamartoma.

Discussion: Mesenchymal hamartoma is a cystic mass of the liver thought to be developmental in origin. It usually grows slowly to a very large size before discovery. Rapid growth can occur as fluid accumulates in the hamartoma's lobules. The

MR signal characteristics of mesenchymal hamartoma reflect its cystic nature. The signal follows that of fluid with varied appearance of the cysts in a given patient, indicating the variable accumulation of proteinaceous material in the cysts. In this age group, other hepatic masses would include an infantile hemangioendothelioma, hepatoblastoma, metastases (most commonly from neuroblastoma), and undifferentiated embryonal sarcoma (UES). Mesenchymal hamartoma is typically a cystic mass, whereas the other lesions tend to be solid except for occasional areas of necrosis. UES is commonly cystic from necrosis due to its rapid growth and aggressive nature. However, UES usually occurs in late childhood. A large cystic lesion in an infant is most likely to be a mesenchymal hamartoma.

Clinical History: 79-year-old woman presenting with right upper quadrant pain post endoscopic retrograde cholangiopancreatography (ERCP).

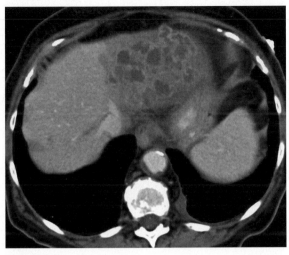

Figure 1.16   A

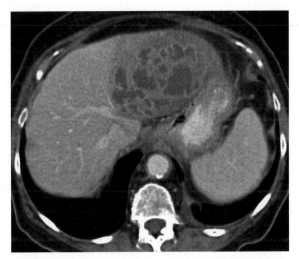

Figure 1.16   B

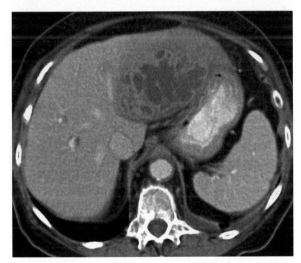

Figure 1.16   C

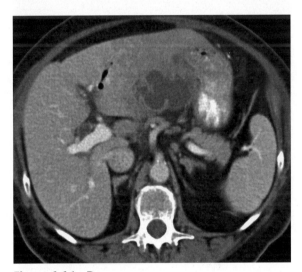

Figure 1.16   D

Findings: Axial CECT images demonstrate several rim-enhancing low-attenuation lesions within the left lobe of the liver. The surrounding parenchyma demonstrates decreased attenuation. Note presence of pneumobilia post ERCP (D).

Differential Diagnosis: Metastases.

Diagnosis: Pyogenic abscesses of the liver.

Discussion: Most hepatic abscesses in the United States are pyogenic in origin, but with the increase in immunocompromised patients from chemotherapy, organ transplants, and AIDS, fungal abscesses are also increasing. Pyogenic abscesses are most commonly due to gram-negative bacilli, with *Escherichia coli* most commonly cultured in adults. Approximately 50% of pyogenic abscesses are due to anaerobic or a mixture of aerobic and anaerobic organisms. The infection can reach the liver by several routes: (a) via the portal vein (appendicitis, diverticulitis, or infected colon cancer); (b) via the biliary system (cholangitis, iatrogenic); (c) via direct extension (peptic ulcer disease or pyelonephritis); (d) via the hepatic artery (endocarditis or arterial catheters); and (e) trauma. Pyogenic abscesses tend to be multiple in 50% to 60% of the cases, with a predilection for the right lobe of the liver. This is thought to be secondary to the preferential flow of blood from the superior mesenteric vein into the portal vein and into the right lobe. Typically, abscesses are low in attenuation on CECT and show peripheral rim enhancement. Perilesional edema is the cause of the decreased attenuation of the surrounding parenchyma. Diagnosing these lesions is crucial because antibiotic therapy is often not sufficient for treatment, and aspiration and drainage is necessary for total resolution. In this case, multiple aspirations and drainages were performed using CT guidance.

Clinical History: 37-year-old woman with liver mass seen on ultrasound (US) done for recurrent epigastric pain.

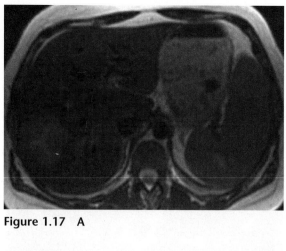

Figure 1.17   A

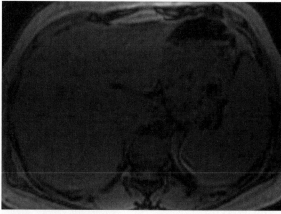

Figure 1.17   B

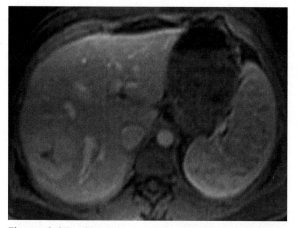

Figure 1.17   C

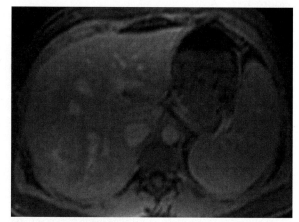

Figure 1.17   D

Findings: Axial T2-WI (A) demonstrates a slightly hyperintense lesion that is also slightly hyperintense on the T1-WI (B). There is increased signal seen in the central scar on the T2-WI. Gadolinium-enhanced fat-suppressed axial T1-WI in the arterial (C) and late phases (D) show early homogeneous enhancement of the lesion with rapid washout and delayed enhancement of the central scar.

Differential Diagnosis: Metastasis, hepatocellular adenoma, hepatocellular carcinoma.

Diagnosis: Focal nodular hyperplasia.

Discussion: Focal nodular hyperplasia (FNH) is a benign tumorlike condition in the liver that is composed of abnormally arranged nodules of normal liver separated by fibrous septa. Bile ductules are often present within the fibrous septa or between the hepatocytes. These lesions are unencapsulated and lack the presence of central veins and portal triads. Because of the nature of FNH, one third of these lesions tend to be isointense and similar in appearance to the normal liver parenchyma on T1-WI and T2-WI, often making it difficult to detect. Approximately two thirds of FNH are slightly bright on the T2 images, slightly dark on the T1 images, or both. The presence of the central scar makes the diagnosis of FNH most likely. The central scar can often aid in the diagnosis because it will be hypointense on the T1-WI and hyperintense on the T2-WI relative to the liver. In addition, the central scar enhances on the postgadolinium images. This is in distinction to the central scar seen in fibrolamellar carcinoma, which tends to be hypointense on both the T1- and T2-weighted sequences and enhances late. The increased signal of the central scar in the FNH may be related to the high fluid content of the loose myxomatous fibrous tissue in the central scar. In fibrolamellar hepatocellular carcinoma, however, the central scar is poorly vascularized, and the fibrosis is dense; therefore, its MR characteristics are more typical of those of collagen. The central scar, lack of cirrhosis, and age of the patient makes FNH the best diagnosis.

CASE 1-18

Clinical History: 4-month-old boy with elevated alpha-fetoprotein (AFP) and irritability.

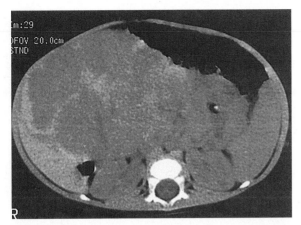

Figure 1.18 A

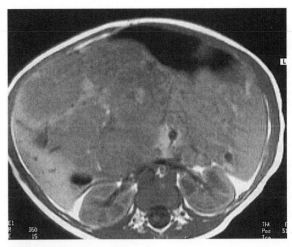

Figure 1.18 B

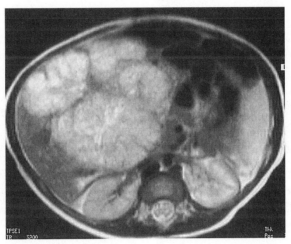

Figure 1.18 C

Findings: Axial NECT image (A) demonstrates a 10-cm lesion in the liver with septations. Axial T1-WI (B) demonstrates a hypointense mass with linear areas of increased signal intensity. Axial T2-WI (C) demonstrates this lesion to be hyperintense. The linear areas noted on T1 are hypointense on the T2 image. Round areas of hemorrhage are present.

Differential Diagnosis: Infantile hemangioendothelioma, metastatic neuroblastoma, mesenchymal hamartoma, hepatocellular carcinoma.

Diagnosis: Hepatoblastoma.

Discussion: Hepatoblastoma is the third most common abdominal malignancy in children following Wilms tumor and neuroblastoma. They are typically found in children less than 3 years of age, with the peak age being less than 18 months. Histologically, hepatoblastomas may be composed of epithelial cells or be of mixed cellularity (epithelial and mesenchymal components). Mixed hepatoblastomas frequently have coarse calcifications due to osseous or cartilaginous mesenchymal elements. An elevated AFP almost ensures the diagnosis of hepatoblastoma. On CT, hepatoblastomas are usually low in attenuation on both CECT and NECT. The MRI findings of hepatoblastoma are similar to those seen in a hepatocellular carcinoma. Like hepatocellular carcinoma, hepatoblastomas will be hypointense on T1-WI and hyperintense on the T2-WI. The linear areas seen in this example represent fibrous septa found in mixed hepatoblastomas. Although hemorrhage and necrosis are rare in small hepatoblastomas, they can occasionally occur in very large lesions. These areas of hemorrhage and necrosis are not nearly as large as those typically seen in undifferentiated embryonal sarcoma and mesenchymal hamartoma. Both infantile hemangioendothelioma and metastatic neuroblastoma will not produce an elevated AFP. Metastatic neuroblastomas, like most metastases, tend to be multiple.

Clinical History: 69-year-old woman with history of Crohn disease presenting with fatigue, fever, and chills.

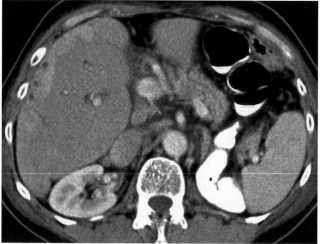

Figure 1.19 A

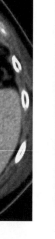

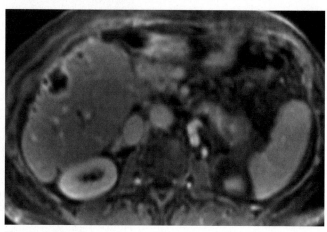

Figure 1.19 B

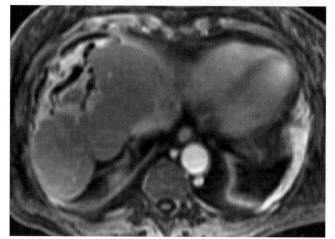

Figure 1.19 C

Figure 1.19 D

Findings: Axial CECT image (A) shows heterogeneous enhancement of the liver parenchyma and dilated bile ducts in the periphery. Axial T2-WI (B) shows increased signal intensity areas corresponding to dilated bile ducts and subcapsular fluid. On the gadolinium-enhanced fat-suppressed T1-WI, there is faint enhancement of the bile ducts and of the peripheral liver parenchyma (C) and a 2-cm cystic lesion in the right hepatic lobe with peripheral enhancement (D).

Differential Diagnosis: Intrahepatic cholangiocarcinoma.

Diagnosis: Ascending cholangitis and liver abscess in a patient with primary sclerosing cholangitis.

Discussion: Primary sclerosing cholangitis (PSC) is an uncommon disease of unknown etiology that is character-ized by fibrotic strictures of intrahepatic and extrahepatic bile ducts. It is associated with inflammatory bowel disease in 71% of cases. Ascending cholangitis is an important complication of PSC, usually occurring in patients with tight strictures or bile duct stones or after endoscopic procedures. Ascending cholangitis predisposes patients with PSC to hepatic abscess formation. As in this case, a heterogeneous enhancement of liver may be seen in the early phase on CECT studies in patients with acute cholangitis. Biliary ductal dilatation and mural contrast enhancement of the bile ducts is often seen on CECT or MRI studies. The morphologic changes observed in the liver are caused by liver cirrhosis induced by the longstanding PSC.

Clinical History: 37-year-old woman presenting with sudden onset of right upper quadrant pain.

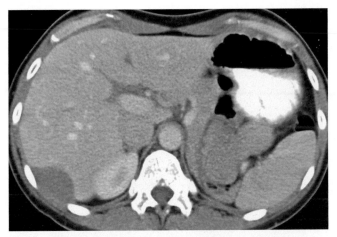

Figure 1.20   A

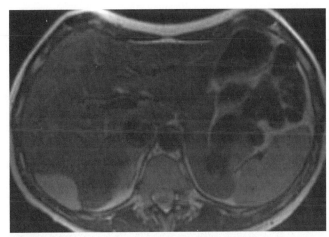

Figure 1.20   B

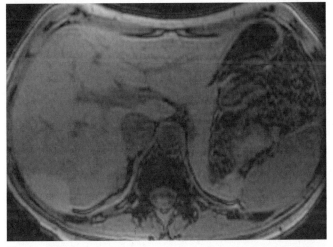

Figure 1.20   C

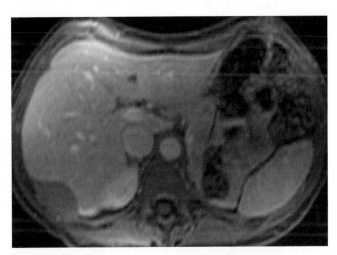

Figure 1.20   D

Findings: Axial CECT image (A) shows a 2.5 × 5.0 cm, nonenhancing, subdiaphragmatic mass that is located posterior to the right lobe of the liver. On MRI, the lesion is homogeneously hyperintense on both axial T2-WI (B) and T1-WI (C) and shows no enhancement after administration of gadolinium (D).

Differential Diagnosis: Peritoneal metastasis.

Diagnosis: Subcapsular hematoma of the liver.

Discussion: Possible causes of subcapsular hematoma include trauma, bleeding disorders, and rupture of a hepatic tumor, cyst, or abscess. Preeclampsia and "HELLP" syndrome (hemolysis, elevated liver enzymes, and low platelet count) have a particular predilection to cause a subhepatic hematoma. On CT, the appearance of a hematoma depends on its age. In an acute or subacute setting, hematomas have a higher Hounsfield unit (HU) value than water due to the presence of aggregated fibrin components; in chronic cases, a hematoma has an HU value equal to that of water. Liver and perihepatic hematomas demonstrate the MRI characteristics of blood and of the breakdown products of hemoglobin. A subacute hematoma appears as a hyperintense mass on T1-WI and has intermediate signal intensity on T2-WI. Chronic hematomas are usually dark on T1-WI and T2-WI due to the presence of hemosiderin. Some hematomas may show rim enhancement following intravenous gadolinium administration.

Clinical History: 39-year-old man with large mesenteric mass. Preoperative workup showed intrahepatic bile duct dilatation.

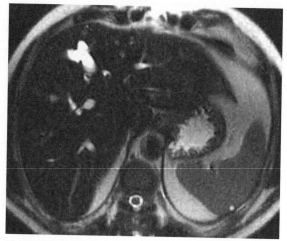

Figure 1.21   A

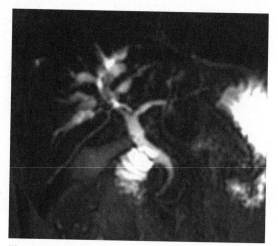

Figure 1.21   B

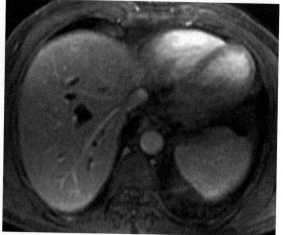

Figure 1.21   C

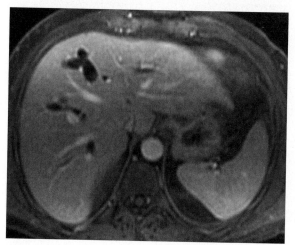

Figure 1.21   D

Findings: Axial T2-WI (A) and oblique coronal thick-slab magnetic resonance cholangiopancreatography (MRCP) image (B) show segmental fusiform dilation of the bile ducts in segment IV of the liver. Gadolinium-enhanced fat-suppressed axial T1-WI (C and D) shows enhancement of portal radicles in the walls of the dilated bile ducts.

Differential Diagnosis: Biliary stricture, recurrent pyogenic cholangitis, cholangiocarcinoma.

Diagnosis: Focal Caroli disease.

Discussion: Caroli disease can be either localized (most commonly) or diffuse in its presentation. When localized, it tends to involve the left lobe more often than the right. Bile inspissation in Caroli disease results in cholelithiasis and biliary stasis, which can lead to ascending cholangitis and cholecystitis. Recurrent episodes of cholangitis are common and can lead to stenosis of the ducts, requiring percutaneous drainage and antibiotics. Cholangiocarcinomas can complicate Caroli disease, foreshortening its course. Because of the possible association with congenital fibrosis (i.e., Caroli syndrome), portal hypertension is often found in these patients, which can lead to gastrointestinal hemorrhage. Surgical resection of the involved segment can be of benefit and is often curative. As one would expect, the MR findings of Caroli disease parallels that of CT. There are multiple cystic spaces that are saccular or fusiform shaped and communicate with the biliary tree, which is not obstructed. The involvement is only intrahepatic. The dilated bile ductules radiate toward the porta hepatis and follow the portal branches. The "central dot" sign refers to the presence of dilated bile ductules surrounding a portal radicle; this sign is characteristic for Caroli disease.

Case images courtesy of Dr. Giovanni Artho, McGill University Health Center, Montreal, Canada.

Clinical History: 34-year-old man presenting with fever, chills, and right upper quadrant pain.

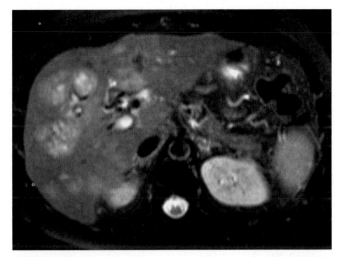

Figure 1.22   A

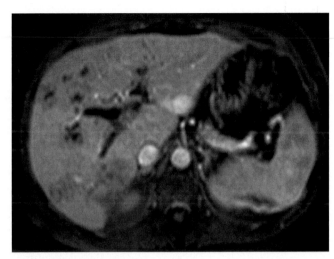

Figure 1.22   B

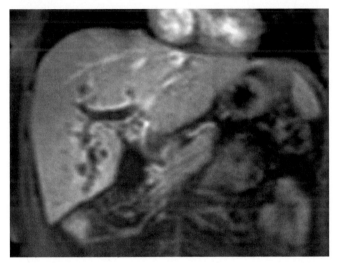

Figure 1.22   C

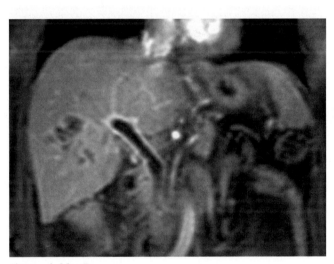

Figure 1.22   D

Findings: Fat-suppressed axial T2-WI (A) shows multiple, ill-defined lesions with heterogeneous hyperintensity. On gadolinium-enhanced, fat-suppressed axial (B) and coronal (C and D) T1-WI, the lesions show rim enhancement, and there is lack of signal in the main portal vein and its branches.

Differential Diagnosis: None.

Diagnosis: Portal vein thrombosis and hepatic abscesses.

Discussion: Portal vein thrombosis may be primary or secondary to other systemic or local disease. Liver cirrhosis is the most common cause of secondary portal vein thrombosis. Other secondary causes include tumor invasion (particularly hepatocellular carcinoma), trauma, blood dyscrasia, and intra-abdominal sepsis. Complete or partial obstruction of the regional portal vein branches is frequently observed around a hepatic abscess. Moreover, marked periportal inflammation and stenosis of the portal venules surrounding a hepatic abscess and associated thrombosis of the portal branches have also been reported. In this case, there is complete thrombosis of the portal vein and its multiple branches. Flow-sensitive gradient-echo MRI can be helpful to depict the absent portal vein flow as an area of hypointensity. The signal intensity of the clot at MRI depends on its age: acute thrombus (<5 weeks old) is hyperintense relative to muscle and liver on both T1-WI and T2-WI; older thrombus (2–18 months old) is hyperintense relative to liver only on T2-WI, as seen in this case. In the setting of a bland thrombus, gadolinium-enhanced T1-WI shows no enhancement of the thrombus.

Clinical History: 29-year-old woman presenting with pelvic pain. She has lost weight in the last 6 months with the help of herbal supplements.

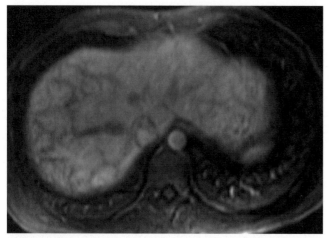

Figure 1.23   A

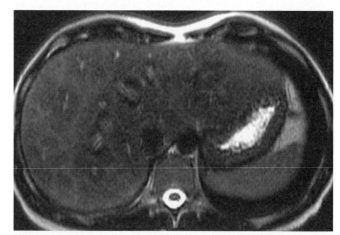

Figure 1.23   B

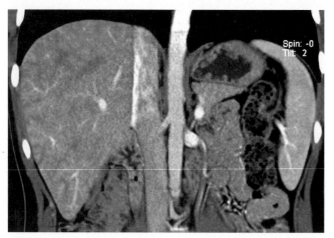

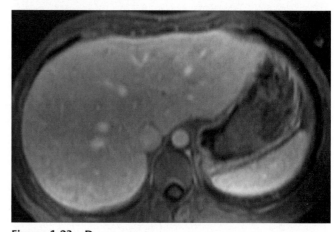

Figure 1.23   C

Figure 1.23   D

Findings: Coronal CECT image (A) demonstrates a mosaiclike enhancement within the periphery of the liver. Axial T2-WI (B) shows periportal cuffing and low signal intensity areas around the patent hepatic vein branches. Gadolinium-enhanced, fat-suppressed axial T1-WI during the arterial phase (C) confirms the CT findings by demonstrating mosaiclike enhancement of the liver parenchyma. Note normalization of the parenchymal enhancement on the portal venous phase, fat-suppressed axial T1-WI (D).

Differential Diagnosis: Budd-Chiari syndrome, passive hepatic congestion.

Diagnosis: Hepatic veno-occlusive disease.

Discussion: Hepatic veno-occlusive disease (VOD) is an uncommon disorder of hepatic venous outflow obstruction that occurs at the level of the small postsinusoidal venules. The disease was originally described in 1954 as "bush-tea" disease in Jamaica. Today, it is well known that hepatic VOD is associated with a vast array of causes and reported in context of chemotherapy, radiation therapy, immunosuppression, and intake of herbal teas. Reported CT features of VOD include ascites, hepatomegaly, gallbladder wall thickening, and narrowed but patent hepatic veins. MRI features of VOD consist of hepatomegaly, hepatic vein narrowing, periportal cuffing, gallbladder wall thickening, marked hyperintensity of the gallbladder wall on T2-WI, and ascites. In Budd-Chiari syndrome, the IVC or hepatic veins are thrombosed; passive hepatic congestion dilates the IVC and hepatic veins due to backflow of blood from the right heart.

CASE 1-24

Clinical History: 52-year-old woman with cirrhosis.

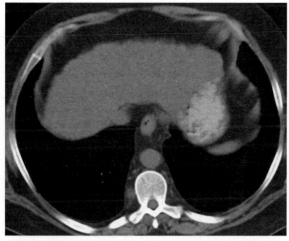

Figure 1.24 A

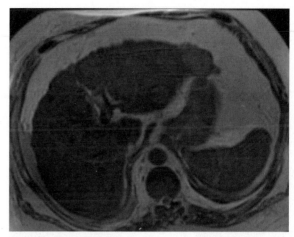

Figure 1.24 B

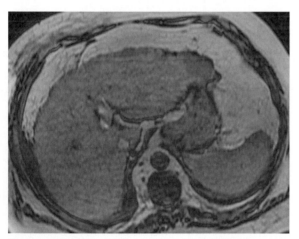

Figure 1.24 C

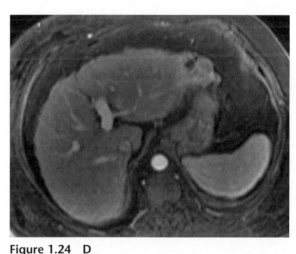

Figure 1.24 D

Findings: Axial NECT image (A) shows a well-defined, slightly hyperdense mass in the left lobe of the liver and a small, shrunken, nodular liver. Axial T2-WI (B) and opposed-phase T1-WI (C) demonstrate the nodule to be of moderate high and low signal intensity, respectively. Gadolinium-enhanced, fat-suppressed axial T1-WI during the arterial phase (D) shows early heterogeneous enhancement of the lesion.

Differential Diagnosis: Metastasis.

Diagnosis: Hepatocellular carcinoma in a cirrhotic liver.

Discussion: There are many different etiologies for hepatocellular carcinoma (HCC), which can be divided into three main categories: chronic hepatitis B, cirrhosis, and carcinogens. Cirrhosis in the United States is most commonly due to alcoholism, and HCCs occur in approximately 3% of these patients. Other causes of cirrhosis that can lead to HCC include hemochromatosis and, less commonly, inborn errors of metabolism such Wilson disease, glycogen storage disease, and alpha-1-antitrypsin deficiency. Carcinogens found to be associated with HCC include aflatoxins produced by the fungus *Aspergillus fumigates*, siderosis from high dietary iron, and Thorotrast. MRI characteristics for HCC vary depending on the amount of fibrosis, fat, necrosis, and hemorrhage present within the lesion. HCC is most commonly hypointense on the T1-WI but can be isointense or hyperintense as well. This is due in part to the amount of fat, hemorrhage, and glycogen present in the tumor, which will have increased signal on the T1-WI. HCC is predominantly hyperintense on the T2-WI and demonstrates early heterogeneous enhancement with gadolinium administration.

Clinical History: 41-year-old woman presenting with epigastric pain.

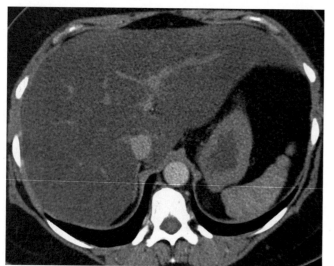

Figure 1.25   A

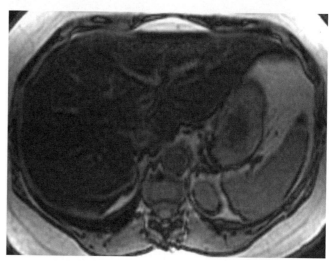

Figure 1.25   B

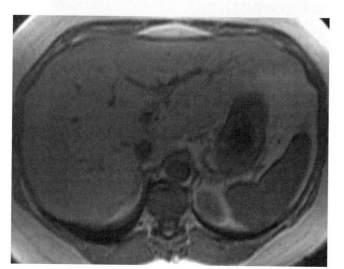

Figure 1.25   C

Figure 1.25   D

Findings: Axial CECT image (A) demonstrates diffuse low attenuation of the liver without displacement of the hepatic vessels. Axial T2-WI (B) shows abnormally increased signal of the liver parenchyma and the liver to be diffusely hyperintense relative to the spleen. In- (C) and out-of-phase (D) T1-WI show significant signal drop in the liver on the out-of-phase images.

Differential Diagnosis: None.

Diagnosis: Diffuse fatty liver.

Discussion: There is a multitude of disorders that can lead to fatty liver. The most common cause in the United States is alcoholic liver disease. Other causes include nonalcoholic steatohepatitis, cirrhosis, diabetes, parenteral nutrition, steroids, obesity, and chemotherapeutic drugs. Fatty liver can produce hepatomegaly and rarely causes significant elevation of liver function tests. The diagnosis is usually made incidentally. The diagnosis of fatty liver is easily made on CT scans. The spleen is normally 8 to 10 HU lower in attenuation than the liver on an NECT. A reversal of this relationship leads to the diagnosis of fatty liver. Because of the variability in enhancement of the liver and spleen, mild fatty change may be difficult to detect on a CECT. On CECT, a difference of 25 HU suggests fatty liver. The fatty liver causes no mass effect, so the vessels are normal in appearance. MRI demonstrates the liver to be of increased signal intensity on T2-WI. Dual-echo T1-WI (in and out of phase) or chemical shift imaging should be performed to confirm the diagnosis in subtle cases.

CASE 1-26

Clinical History: 53-year-old woman presenting with gross hematuria.

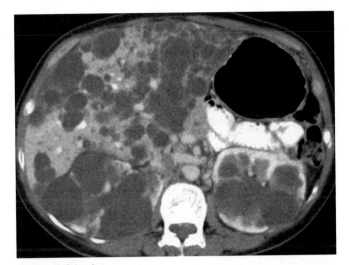

Figure 1.26   A

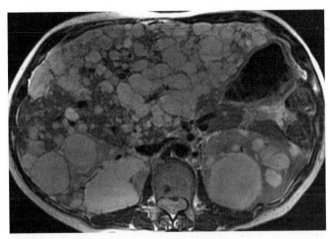

Figure 1.26   B

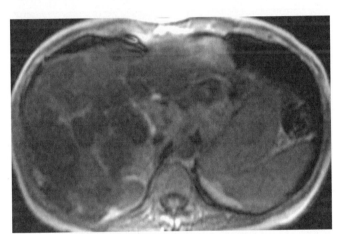

Figure 1.26   C

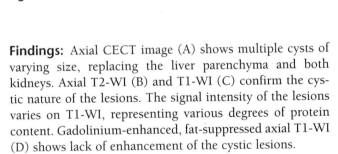

Figure 1.26   D

Findings: Axial CECT image (A) shows multiple cysts of varying size, replacing the liver parenchyma and both kidneys. Axial T2-WI (B) and T1-WI (C) confirm the cystic nature of the lesions. The signal intensity of the lesions varies on T1-WI, representing various degrees of protein content. Gadolinium-enhanced, fat-suppressed axial T1-WI (D) shows lack of enhancement of the cystic lesions.

Differential Diagnosis: Caroli disease, multiple hepatic abscesses, cystic metastases.

Diagnosis: Autosomal dominant polycystic disease.

Discussion: Autosomal dominant polycystic liver disease is often found in association with renal polycystic disease and is thought to result from progressive dilation of abnormal ducts as part of a ductal plate malformation at the level of the small intrahepatic bile ducts. These small bile ducts

do not have continuity with the remaining biliary tree, which explains the noncommunicating nature of the cysts in polycystic liver disease. Patients are usually asymptomatic, and liver dysfunction occurs only sporadically. On unenhanced CT scans, polycystic liver disease typically appears as multiple homogenous and hypodense cystic lesions; cysts do not show wall or content enhancement on contrast-enhanced images. At MRI, hepatic cysts in polycystic liver disease typically demonstrate very low signal intensity on T1-WI and homogenous high signal intensity on T2-WI. The signal intensity of the lesions can vary on T1-WI, representing various degrees of protein content. Cysts do not enhance after administration of intravenous gadolinium. Although the diagnosis of polycystic liver disease is easily made with both CT and MRI, MRI is more sensitive for the detection of complicated cysts.

Clinical History: 55-year-old woman with left lower quadrant pain.

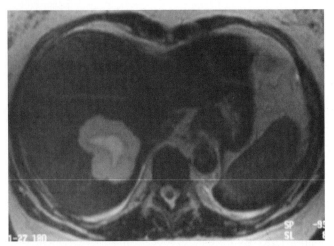

Figure 1.27   A

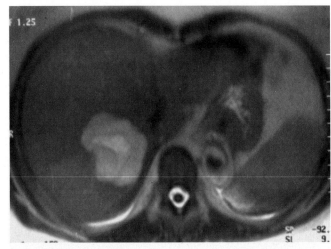

Figure 1.27   B

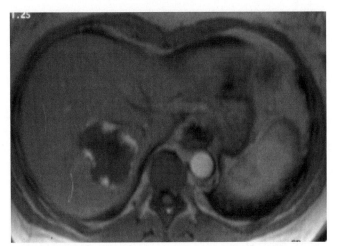

Figure 1.27   C

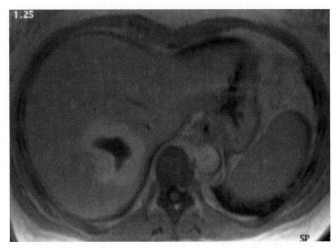

Figure 1.27   D

Findings: Axial T2-WI (A) and heavily weighted T2-WI (B) show a large, hyperintense, well-defined lesion with a more hyperintense central area. On early-phase, gadolinium-enhanced, fat-suppressed axial T1-WI (C), a peripheral, incomplete nodular enhancement pattern is seen. On delayed-phase image (D), the central area of the lesion remains unenhanced.

Differential Diagnosis: Metastasis, hepatocellular carcinoma.

Diagnosis: Atypical hemangioma with cystic degeneration.

Discussion: Large, heterogeneous hemangioma is a type of an atypical hemangioma, a category that consists of lesions, such as rapidly filling hemangiomas, calcified hemangiomas, hyalinized hemangiomas, cystic or multilocular hemangiomas, hemangiomas with fluid-fluid levels, and pedunculated hemangiomas. Large hemangiomas are often heterogeneous, and they are termed giant hemangiomas when they exceed 10 cm in diameter. On unenhanced CT scans, large, heterogeneous hemangiomas appear hypodense and heterogeneous with marked central areas of lower density. After intravenous administration of contrast material, the typical peripheral nodular enhancement pattern is still observed. Nevertheless, the progressive central enhancement may not lead to complete filling on delayed images. At MRI, on T1-WI, hemangiomas with cystic degeneration appear sharply marginated and hypointense with a cleftlike area of lower intensity. Accordingly, T2-WI shows a markedly hyperintense cleftlike area. The enhancement pattern is similar to that seen at CT; the cleftlike area remains hypointense, and therefore, the lesion shows incomplete filling.

Clinical History: 91-year-old man presenting with failure to thrive.

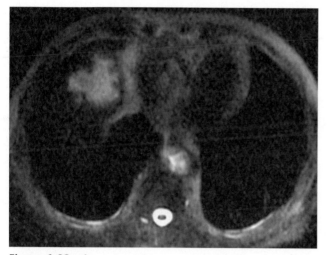

Figure 1.28   A

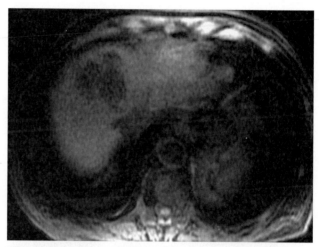

Figure 1.28   B

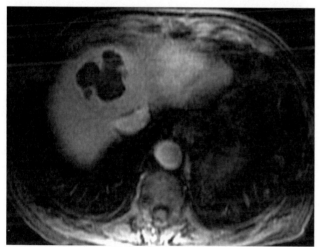

Figure 1.28   C

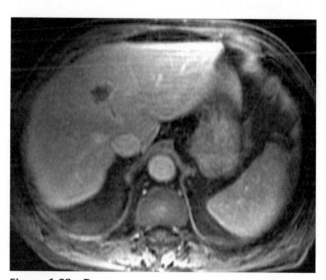

Figure 1.28   D

Findings: Axial T2-WI (A) shows a hyperintense lesion within the right hepatic lobe. The lesion is hypointense on fat-suppressed axial T1-WI (B) and shows, on the gadolinium-enhanced, fat-suppressed axial T1-WI (C), early arterial wall enhancement. Gadolinium-enhanced, fat-suppressed axial T1-WI (D) at a lower level shows thrombus in the middle hepatic vein.

Differential Diagnosis: Cystic metastasis of the liver, amebic abscess.

Diagnosis: Pyogenic liver abscess.

Discussion: Hepatic abscesses, like most other focal hepatic processes, prolong T1 and T2 relaxation times and appear hyperintense on T2-WI and hypointense on T1-WI. In one series, approximately 60% of the abscesses were hypointense on the T1-WI, and 72% were hyperintense on the T2-WI; 35% of the abscesses demonstrated increased signal intensity on the T2-WI around the lesion, which is thought to represent perilesional edema. After administration of gadolinium, abscesses typically show rim enhancement, which is secondary to increased capillary permeability in the surrounding liver parenchyma. Small lesions (<1 cm) may enhance homogeneously, mimicking hemangiomas. The abscess wall enhancement on dynamic postgadolinium images may be considered as a distinctive feature of pyogenic liver abscesses. The abscess wall shows a fast and intense enhancement that persists on portal venous and late-phase images. Some of the lesions may contain internal septations, which also reveal persistent enhancement on late-phase images. Although less likely, a solitary, infected, necrotic metastasis or primary liver tumor could also have this appearance.

Clinical History: 45-year-old woman with long history of sickle cell anemia requiring multiple transfusions.

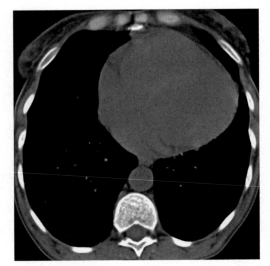

Figure 1.29 A

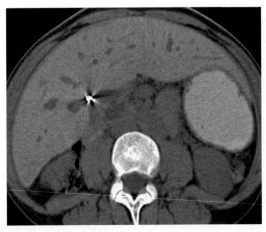

Figure 1.29 B

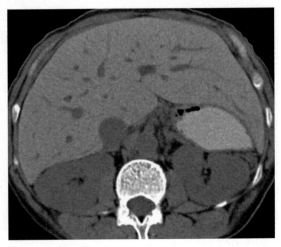

Figure 1.29 C

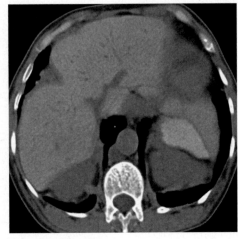

Figure 1.29 D

Findings: Axial NECT images demonstrate increased attenuation of the liver. Note cardiomegaly, absent spleen, and prior cholecystectomy.

Differential Diagnosis: Primary hemochromatosis, Thorotrast exposure.

Diagnosis: Hemosiderosis in a patient with sickle cell anemia.

Discussion: Hemosiderosis, which is typically related to iron overload due to multiple transfusions or hematologic diseases, affects the reticuloendothelial system (RES). This leads to the deposition of iron in the liver and spleen and bone marrow, causing them to be hyperdense on NECT. The normal density of the liver is 30 to 60 HU, reaching 75 to 130 HU with hemosiderosis. Other causes of increased liver density include primary hemochromatosis, glycogen storage disease, drugs (e.g., amiodarone, methotrexate, gold), and occasionally Wilson disease. These diseases, however, usually do not affect the spleen, since the iron gets stored in the hepatocytes. Thorotrast, however, does affect the spleen. Thorotrast was a contrast agent introduced in 1928, but its use was discontinued in the mid 1950s when it was found to lead to the development of angiosarcomas and other visceral neoplasms. It would be unlikely that a patient of this age would have been exposed to this agent. Patients with hemosiderosis do not need surveillance for cirrhosis or hepatocellular carcinoma unless the iron saturation level of the RES is reached; at that time, iron will be stored in hepatocytes leading to fibrosis and cirrhosis. This is called secondary hemochromatosis.

CASE 1-30

Clinical History: 34-year-old woman with hepatomegaly and abdominal pain.

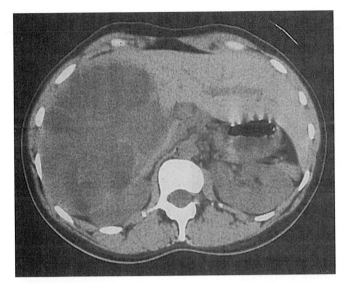

Figure 1.30   A

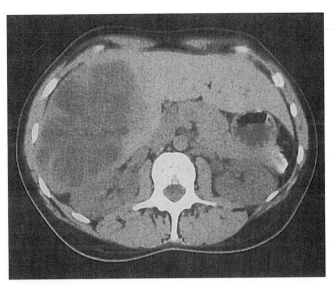

Figure 1.30   B

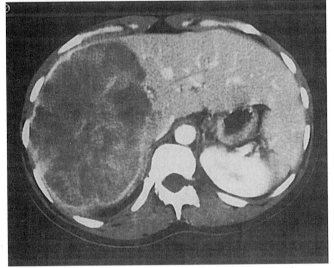

Figure 1.30   C

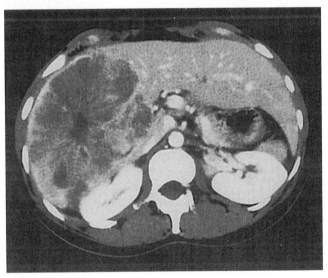

Figure 1.30   D

Findings: Axial NECT images (A and B) demonstrate a 10-cm, low-attenuation mass in the right lobe of the liver. Axial CECT images (C and D) reveal this lesion to have heterogeneous enhancement with a central area without enhancement.

Differential Diagnosis: Hepatic adenoma, focal nodular hyperplasia.

Diagnosis: Fibrolamellar hepatocellular carcinoma.

Discussion: Fibrolamellar hepatocellular carcinoma (HCC) differs from a typical HCC in that there is no underlying liver disease (cirrhosis), the alpha-fetoprotein level is usually normal, and the age of onset is typically under 40 years of age.

Fibrolamellar HCC equally affects males and females. The prognosis for fibrolamellar HCC is better than typical HCC. CT findings include a large heterogeneously enhancing mass with a nonenhancing fibrous central scar, which is well seen in this example. The lesion is typically solitary and can have calcifications centrally within the lesion. A hepatic adenoma could have a similar appearance by CT. However, hepatic adenomas do not usually have a scar, and a history of oral contraceptive use is usually present. Fibrolamellar HCC will often have gallium uptake, which can aid in the diagnostic workup. Heterogeneous enhancement and lack of enhancement of the central scar allow differentiation between fibrolamellar HCC and focal nodular hyperplasia on CECT.

Clinical History: 41-year-old man presenting with abdominal bloating.

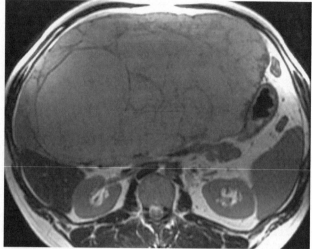

Figure 1.31   A

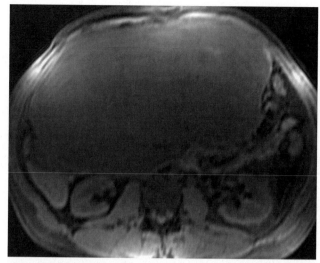

Figure 1.31   B

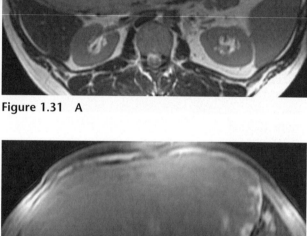

Figure 1.31   C

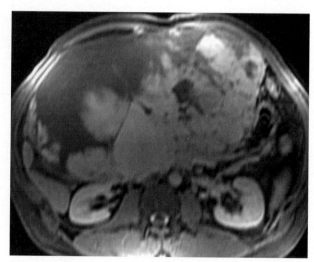

Figure 1.31   D

Findings: Axial MRI show a very large well-defined hepatic mass showing hyperintensity on the T2-WI (A) and hypointensity on the fat-suppressed T1-WI (B). There are multiple internal septations within the lesion, seen as hypointense bands on the T2-WI. On the dynamic gadolinium-enhanced, fat-suppressed axial T1-WI (C-D), the lesion shows nodular peripheral incomplete enhancement during the early phase with gradual fill-in of the lesion on the delayed image.

Differential Diagnosis: Hypervascular metastasis.

Diagnosis: Giant hemangioma of the liver.

Discussion: Giant hemangioma may present as a symptomatic abdominal mass and thus may come to medical and surgical attention. Symptoms may vary from slight abdominal discomfort to spontaneous rupture, a life-threatening complication. Giant hemangiomas may reach impressive dimensions and occasionally cause significant mass effect on vascular and biliary structures and adjacent organs. Giant hemangiomas have a typical heterogeneous appearance on T1-WI and T2-WI. In most patients, the central area of giant hemangiomas is hypointense on T1-WI and hyperintense on T2-WI due to the cystic degeneration. Pathology usually shows thrombosis, hyalinization, and fibrosis in the lesion. Fibrous septations are commonly encountered within the giant hemangiomas and correspond at pathology to strands of cellular fibrous tissue. On dynamic gadolinium-enhanced MRI, complete filling of the lesion is rarely shown.

CASE 1-32

Clinical History: 15-year-old girl with right upper quadrant pain and elevated liver enzymes.

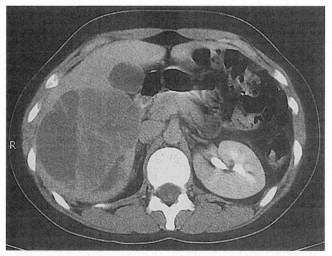

Figure 1.32 A

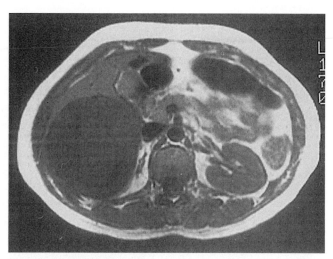

Figure 1.32 B

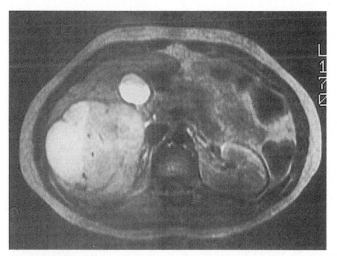

Figure 1.32 C

Findings: Axial CECT image (A) demonstrates a complex cystic lesion in the right lobe of the liver. Axial T1-WI (B) demonstrates the lesion to be hypointense. Note the subtle area of lower signal intensity seen on the right side of the lesion. This same lesion is hyperintense on the axial T2-WI (C). Note the area of increased signal intensity on the right side of the lesion representing necrosis.

Differential Diagnosis: Mesenchymal hamartoma, hepatocellular carcinoma, hepatic adenoma, necrotic metastasis.

Diagnosis: Undifferentiated embryonal sarcoma.

Discussion: Undifferentiated embryonal sarcoma (UES) is an uncommon malignant neoplasm of mesenchymal origin composed of spindle-shaped sarcomatous cells. About 90% of these lesions occur before the age of 15 years, with most occurring in older children (6–12 years). Even with surgery, chemotherapy, and radiotherapy, the prognosis is poor, with a life expectancy of less than 12 months. UES is typically a large mass with areas of hemorrhage and necrosis. Therefore, the lesion will appear as a combination of large cystic and solid areas. The only good differential diagnosis for this appearance in the pediatric patient is the benign mesenchymal hamartoma. Other possibilities, such as hepatocellular carcinoma and adenoma, are much less likely in the pediatric patient. UESs are typically hypointense on T1-WI and hyperintense on T2-WI, with the areas of necrosis having the signal characteristics of water. The solid component of UES enhances after gadolinium administration.

Clinical History: 69-year-old man with weight loss and discoloration of his skin.

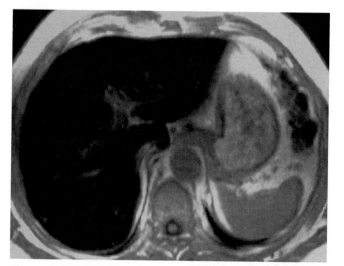
Figure 1.33   A

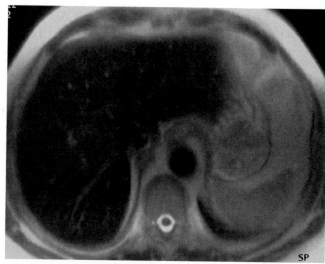
Figure 1.33   B

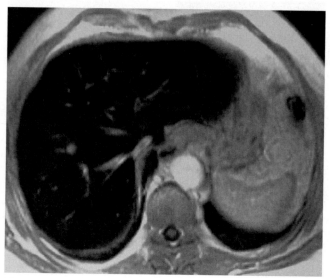
Figure 1.33   C

Findings: Axial T1-WI (A) and T2-WI (B) demonstrate diffuse decreased signal intensity of the liver compared to the dorsal spinal muscles. The signal intensity of the spleen is normal. Gadolinium-enhanced axial T1-WI (C) shows the persistent low signal intensity of the liver.

Differential Diagnosis: Hemosiderosis.

Diagnosis: Primary hemochromatosis.

Discussion: Hepatic iron overload can be divided into primary idiopathic hemochromatosis versus iron overload states from multiple blood transfusions. Primary hemochromatosis is induced by an abnormal uptake of iron in the gut. The iron is transported towards the liver by the portal vein where it gets stored. Other organs that can be involved in primary hemochromatosis include the heart, pancreas, endocrine glands, and skin (bronze diabetes). Deposition of iron in the hepatocytes seen in primary hemochromatosis causes, because of the metallic susceptibility of iron, decreased signal in the liver on both T1-WI and T2-WI, as is seen in this case. This decreased signal can be measured against the signal seen in adjacent skeletal muscles. T2* and gradient-echo images are the most sensitive sequences to detect iron. Transfusional hemosiderosis, on the other hand, which involves the reticuloendothelial system, causes decreased signal within the liver and spleen with sparing of the pancreas. Patients with primary hemochromatosis will develop cirrhosis if untreated and have an increased incidence of hepatocellular carcinoma.

CASE 1-34

Clinical History: 77-year-old man with history of lymphoma presenting with lethargy after chemotherapy.

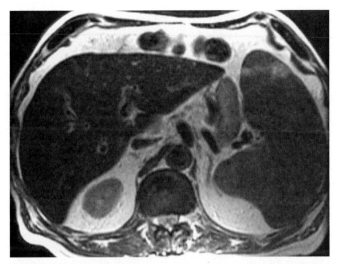

Figure 1.34   A

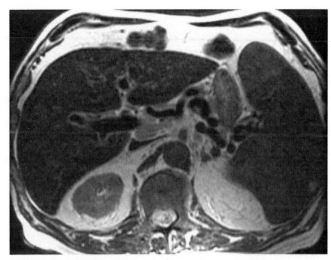

Figure 1.34   B

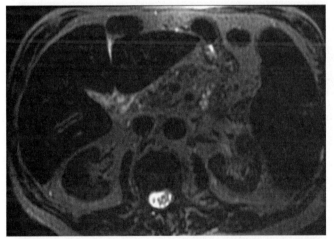

Figure 1.34   C

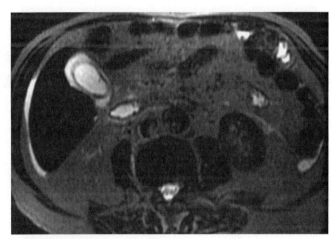

Figure 1.34   D

Findings: Axial T2-WI (A and B) and heavily weighted axial T2-WI (C and D) demonstrate periportal edema, mild hepatomegaly, and edematous gallbladder wall. Note presence of splenomegaly.

Differential Diagnosis: Congestive heart failure, liver transplant rejection, HIV/AIDS.

Diagnosis: Drug-induced acute hepatitis.

Discussion: Hepatitis can be infectious (viral, bacterial, or fungal) or inflammatory (drug-induced or autoimmune) in origin. In most cases, hepatitis refers to viral hepatitis, which accounts for the majority of the fulminant hepatic failures from hepatitis. It can be acute or chronic in nature. If the inflammatory changes last for more than 6 months, the patient is thought to have chronic hepatitis. The findings of acute hepatitis on CT and MRI are nonspecific. These include hepatomegaly, which can lead to abdominal pain, portal lymphadenopathy, and gallbladder wall thickening. Periportal edema can be seen as lucency or hyperintensity surrounding the portal branches. Other causes for periportal edema include AIDS, trauma, congestive heart failure (CHF), and liver transplant rejection. In this patient, there was no history of trauma or a liver transplant, and the patient had no symptoms of CHF. AIDS is a possibility, especially in a younger patient, but the other abdominal findings for AIDS, such as lymphadenopathy, AIDS nephritis, and AIDS cholangitis, were not present in this case.

CASE 1-35

Clinical History: 23-year-old woman with right upper quadrant pain and fever. Patient has a history of foreign travel.

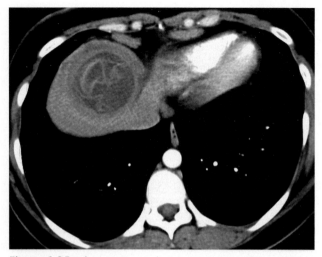

Figure 1.35   A

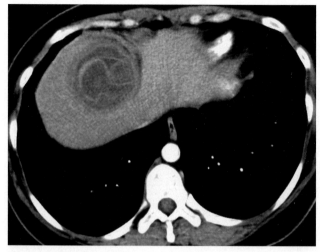

Figure 1.35   B

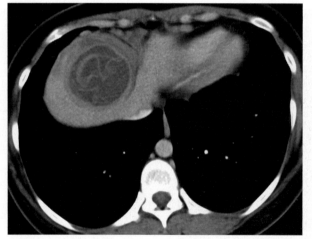

Figure 1.35   C

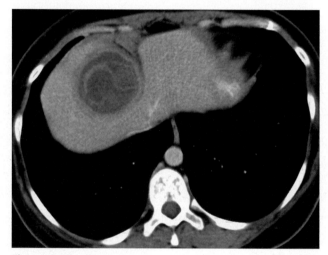

Figure 1.35   D

Findings: Axial CECT images in the arterial (A and B) and portal venous (C and D) phase show a 7-cm, low-density lesion in segment VIII of the liver with multiple septations and a thick wall.

Differential Diagnosis: Old hematoma, pyogenic abscess, biliary cystadenoma/carcinoma.

Diagnosis: Echinococcal cyst (hydatid cyst).

Discussion: Hydatid disease is endemic to many parts of the world where sheep are raised such as Australia, Africa, South America, and the Middle East. The United States is also seeing an increase in the number of cases most likely due to the influx of immigrants and travelers from these endemic countries. Patients usually present with symptoms that mimic choledocholithiasis such as recurrent jaundice, colicky right upper quadrant pain, and fevers. *Echinococcus granulosus* is the most common of the various forms of *Echinococcus* infections. Human disease follows the ingestion of the ova by humans in regions where people herd sheep and have close contact with dogs. Hepatic echinococcosis can have complications, such as intracystic infection, rupture of the cyst, bile duct communication, and pleural effusion. Because these lesions can be large, they can compress adjacent vascular structures and cause portal hypertension or IVC occlusion. This case is typical of an echinococcal cyst with presence of a thick wall and septations. Biliary cystadenoma and hematoma would not account for the patient's fever and pain unless the lesion was superinfected. Pyogenic abscesses would be an excellent diagnostic consideration. However, the history of traveling to an endemic area makes echinococcal cyst the most likely diagnosis.

Clinical History: 59-year-old woman with weight loss.

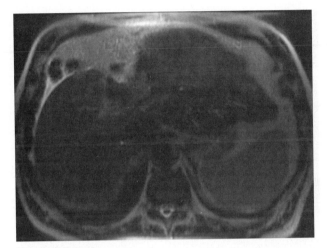

Figure 1.36   A

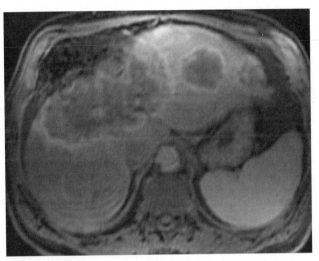

Figure 1.36   B

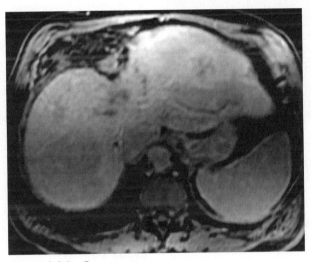

Figure 1.36   C

Findings: Axial T2-WI (A) shows a slightly hyperintense lesion in the left hepatic lobe with dilated intrahepatic bile ducts. Note the presence of central hypointense area in the mass. On gadolinium-enhanced, fat-suppressed axial T1-WI obtained in the arterial phase (B), the lesion shows peripheral rimlike enhancement. On delayed-phase image (C), a complete fill-in of the lesion, which appears hyperintense to liver, is observed.

Differential Diagnosis: Hepatocellular carcinoma, metastasis.

Diagnosis: Intrahepatic cholangiocarcinoma.

Discussion: Intrahepatic or peripheral cholangiocarcinoma (ICAC), an adenocarcinoma of biliary duct origin, originates in the small intrahepatic ducts; it represents 10% of all cholangiocarcinomas. On MRI, ICAC appears as a large mass of decreased signal intensity on T1-WI and shows mildly increased signal intensity on T2-WI. In some cases, a central hypointense area might be seen on T2-WI, which corresponds to the presence of central fibrosis. The pattern of enhancement on gadolinium-enhanced images depends largely on the size of the lesion. Whereas large ICACs (>4 cm) show an early peripheral rimlike enhancement with progressive centripetal fill-in and delayed enhancement of the central area of fibrosis, smaller lesions (2–4 cm) may enhance homogeneously. Although a similar pattern of enhancement may also be seen in hemangioma, the degree of enhancement is typically greater in hemangiomas. Other features of ICAC include presence of satellite nodules, encasement of the portal vein without invasion, capsular retraction, and dilatation of intrahepatic bile ducts distal to the lesion.

Clinical History: 31-year-old woman with longstanding history of ulcerative colitis presenting with jaundice and malaise.

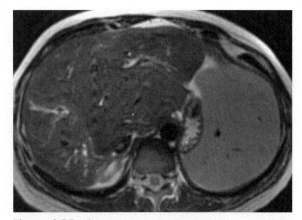

Figure 1.37   A

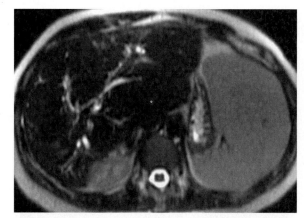

Figure 1.37   B

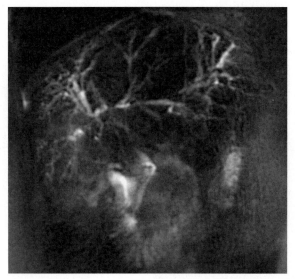

Figure 1.37   C

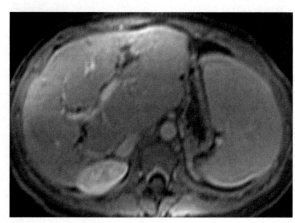

Figure 1.37   D

Findings: Axial T2-WI (A) and heavily weighted axial T2–WI (B) demonstrate hypertrophy of left and caudate lobes, splenomegaly, and segmental mild dilatation of the intrahepatic bile ducts. There is a mild prominence and irregularity with multiple strictures of the intrahepatic and proximal extrahepatic bile ducts on the thick-slab MRCP image (C). Gadolinium-enhanced, fat-suppressed axial T1-WI (D) confirms the ductal dilatation. No enhancing mass is seen.

Differential Diagnosis: Oriental cholangiohepatitis, acute cholangitis.

Diagnosis: Primary sclerosing cholangitis.

Discussion: Primary sclerosing cholangitis is an autoimmune disorder characterized by obliterative fibrotic inflammation of the bile ducts that eventually leads to cholestasis and biliary cirrhosis. It usually presents in patients younger than 40 years old and is more common in males. Typically, intra- and extrahepatic bile ducts are involved simultaneously (80%). A strong association with inflammatory bowel disease, especially ulcerative colitis, is noted (70%). Although patients may be asymptomatic, 75% have progressive fatigue, intermittent obstructive jaundice, and pruritus. On MRI, the characteristic appearance of the disease is multiple stenoses, minor dilatations, and beaded appearance of the bile ducts. In patients with cirrhosis, associated imaging findings, such as splenomegaly and especially caudate lobe hypertrophy, are present. On MRCP, by using heavily T2-WI sequences, the signal of static or slow-moving fluid-filled structures, such as the bile ducts, is greatly increased, resulting in increased duct-to-background contrast and confidence in diagnosis.

Clinical History: 66-year-old man with longstanding cirrhosis and elevated alpha-fetoprotein.

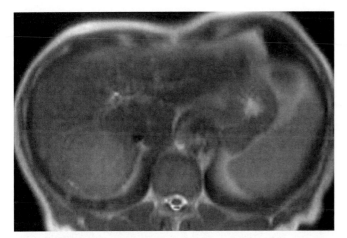

Figure 1.38   A

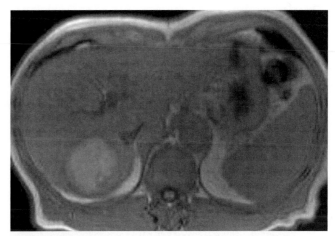

Figure 1.38   B

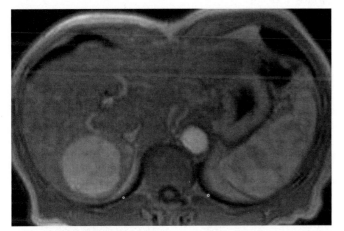

Figure 1.38   C

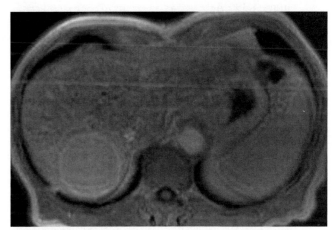

Figure 1.38   D

Findings: Axial T2-WI (A) and T1-WI (B) show a well-defined hyperintense lesion in the right lobe of the liver. Note the peripheral band of low signal intensity surrounding the lesion. Early- (C) and delayed-phase (D) gadolinium-enhanced axial T1-WI show early homogeneous enhancement with washout and delayed capsular enhancement.

Differential Diagnosis: Melanoma metastasis, hepatocellular adenoma.

Diagnosis: Encapsulated hepatocellular carcinoma.

Discussion: Hepatocellular carcinoma (HCC) has a variable incidence based on geographic location. In low-incidence areas, such as the United States, this lesion is seen most commonly in the elderly population with cirrhosis related to alcohol consumption. The onset is usually slow and insidious, with symptoms of abdominal pain and occasionally fever and malaise. In high-incidence areas, such as Asia and sub-Saharan Africa, HCC is seen in middle-aged patients and tends to have a more rapid onset with abdominal pain, fever, and weight loss. The etiology in the high-incidence areas is thought to be secondary to viral hepatitis (types B and C). This case demonstrates the encapsulated form of HCC. These lesions tend to have a better prognosis because of the greater ease in resection than the nonencapsulated form. The fibrous capsule tends to be hyperintense on the delayed contrast-enhanced images, as seen in this example. The enhancing center of the lesion makes the diagnosis of an abscess unlikely. A melanoma metastasis, however, is a possibility, although metastases are more commonly multiple and do not have capsular enhancement. The patient's age and gender would make a hepatic adenoma unlikely.

Clinical History: 72-year-old woman presenting with abdominal pain.

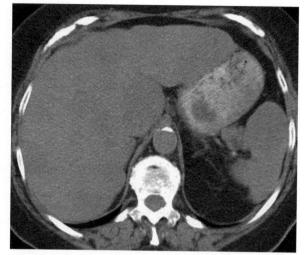

Figure 1.39   A

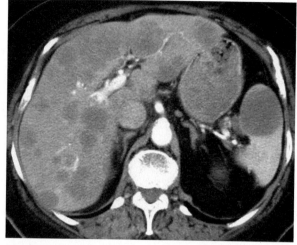

Figure 1.39   B

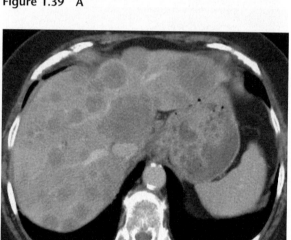

Figure 1.39   C

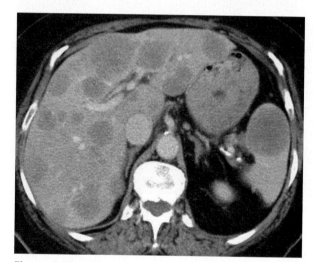

Figure 1.39   D

Findings: Axial NECT image (A) shows multiple rounded hypodense lesions in the liver. Axial CECT images in the arterial (B) and portal venous phase (C and D) demonstrate numerous hypovascular masses in the liver and spleen.

Differential Diagnosis: Metastases, hepatocellular carcinoma, multiple abscesses.

Diagnosis: Lymphoma of the liver.

Discussion: Lymphoma of the liver can be either primary or secondary. Secondary involvement with lymphoma is fairly common, being seen in 50% to 60% of patients with Hodgkin and especially non-Hodgkin disease at autopsy. Nevertheless, hepatic involvement by lymphoma is detected in only 15% to 25% of the cases by imaging. Secondary lymphoma of the liver is especially common in patients with AIDS. Primary lymphoma is rare and is usually of the large-cell type. It presents most often as a large multilobulated mass, often with areas of necrosis and hemorrhage. There is usually minimal enhancement with intravenous contrast. This case demonstrates not a single large mass of lymphoma but, instead, multiple small nodules scattered throughout the liver and spleen. This pattern is nonspecific and could be secondary to metastases, abscesses, and multifocal primary neoplasms [e.g., hepatocellular carcinoma (HCC), angiosarcoma]. A search for a primary cancer would be warranted in the workup of this patient. Multiple HCCs would be less likely because no evidence of cirrhosis is seen and splenic involvement is rare in HCC. Moreover, the hypovascular appearance would be unusual for HCC.

Clinical History: 46-year-old man with right upper quadrant pain.

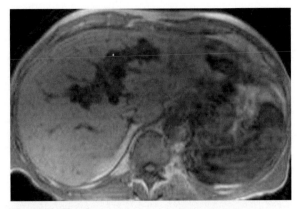

Figure 1.40 A

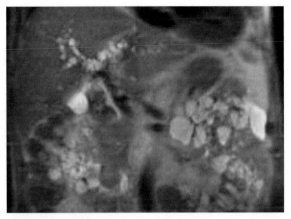

Figure 1.40 B

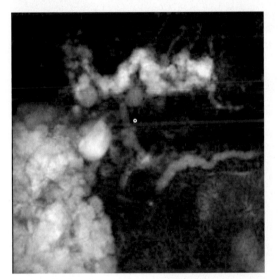

Figure 1.40 C

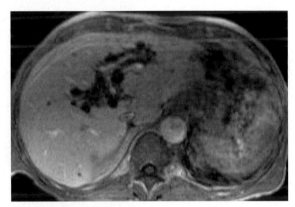

Figure 1.40 D

Findings: Axial T1-WI (A) shows dilation of intrahepatic bile ducts. Coronal T2-WI (B) shows saccular dilatation of the central intrahepatic bile ducts. Oblique coronal thick-slab MRCP image (C) shows dilated bile ducts communicating with the biliary tree. No strictures are seen. Also note presence of numerous cysts in the kidneys. Gadolinium-enhanced axial T1-WI (D) shows enhancement of portal vein radicles surrounded by dilated bile ducts.

Differential Diagnosis: Polycystic liver disease, primary sclerosing cholangitis, recurrent pyogenic cholangitis.

Diagnosis: Caroli disease (diffuse form).

Discussion: Caroli disease is defined as congenital nonobstructive cystic dilatation of the intrahepatic biliary tree. It can be diffuse or localized. It is believed that Caroli disease is part of the spectrum of fibrocystic diseases that range from congenital hepatic fibrosis to choledochal cysts. Caroli disease can be associated with medullary sponge kidney and autosomal recessive polycystic kidney disease or present as an isolated phenomenon and not associated with other entities. The key to the diagnosis of Caroli disease is recognizing that the saccular dilatations are in communication with the biliary tree. The saccular dilatations in Caroli disease tend to radiate toward the porta hepatis following the path of the portal vein branches. This is in contradistinction to polycystic liver disease, which is randomly dispersed in the liver. The saccular dilatations in Caroli disease tend to be irregularly shaped, a feature that also helps to distinguish it from polycystic liver disease; the saccular dilatations in polycystic liver disease tend to be spherical and vary in size. Recurrent pyogenic cholangitis and primary sclerosing cholangitis usually do not produce saccular dilatation, as in this case, and involvement is frequently extrahepatic and characterized by the presence of strictures.

Clinical History: 35-year-old man with elevated liver enzymes.

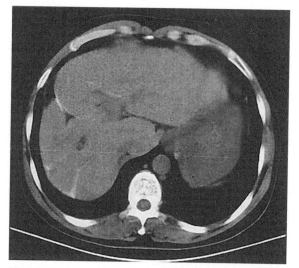

Figure 1.41 A

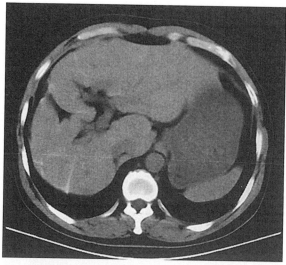

Figure 1.41 B

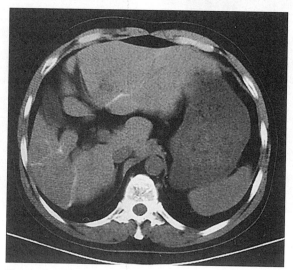

Figure 1.41 C

Findings: Axial NECT images demonstrate morphologic changes in the liver and calcifications extending from the liver capsule toward the center of the liver.

Differential Diagnosis: None.

Diagnosis: Hepatic schistosomiasis.

Discussion: Schistosomiasis is one of the most common parasites affecting humans in the world. Various types of schistosomiasis are found including *Schistosoma japonicum*, which is prevalent in Asia. The schistosomes live in the bowel lumen and lay eggs in the mesenteric veins. The eggs then embolize to the portal vein, where they cause an inflammatory reaction with a granulomatous response, eventual fibrosis, and presinusoidal hypertension. The eggs themselves do not survive and subsequently calcify. Chronic infection with *S. japonicum*

results in the formation of cirrhosis and risk of development of hepatocellular carcinoma. *S. japonicum* has a classic CT appearance in the liver. The most pathognomonic pattern is the presence of calcified septae usually aligned perpendicular to the liver capsule; this typical feature is known as the "tortoise shell" or "turtleback" appearance. Other recognized CT features include capsular calcification, junctional notches or depressions, irregularity of hepatic contour, and extension of periportal fat deep into the liver substance as a result of fibrosis and parenchymal retraction. MRI is unable to identify these characteristic calcifications accurately. The fibrous septae show an abnormal decreased and increased signal intensity on T1-WI and T2-WI, respectively.

Case images courtesy of Dean Baird, Tripler Army Medical Center, Honolulu, HI.

Clinical History: 44-year-old woman undergoing treatment for breast cancer.

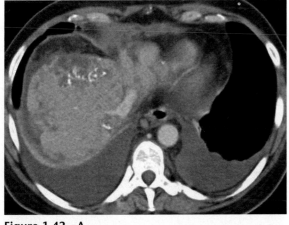

Figure 1.42   A

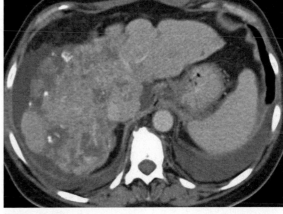

Figure 1.42   B

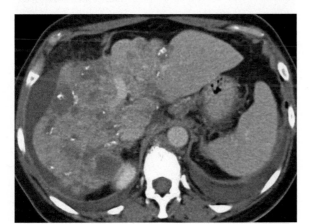

Figure 1.42   C

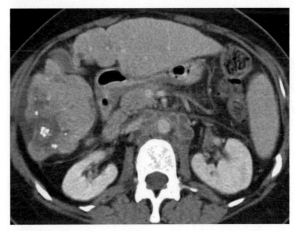

Figure 1.42   D

Findings: Axial CECT images show multiple low-attenuation lesions seen diffusely throughout the liver. These lesions are associated with capsular retraction and presence of multiple small calcifications. Note necrotic retroperitoneal lymphadenopathy.

Differential Diagnosis: Untreated calcified mucinous metastases, granulomatous disease, oriental cholangiohepatitis, *Echinococcosis multilocularis*, *Pneumocystis carinii* pneumonia (PCP).

Diagnosis: Calcified metastases of breast carcinoma after chemotherapy.

Discussion: Some liver metastases are spontaneously calcified. These include metastases from primary tumors, such as mucinous carcinoma of the gastrointestinal (GI) tract, osteosarcoma, leiomyosarcoma, papillary serous ovarian cystadenocarcinoma, medullary carcinoma of the thyroid, and breast carcinoma. Treated metastases from nearly any

primary tumor, granulomatous disease (tuberculosis and histoplasmosis), *Echinococcosis alveolaris*, oriental cholangiohepatitis, and PCP are also in the differential diagnosis of calcified hepatic lesions. However, granulomatous disease and PCP would not have accounted for the low-attenuation lesions with capsular retraction in the liver, and there were no dilated ducts to consider oriental cholangiohepatitis. In *E. multilocularis*, CT and MRI typically display multiple, irregular, ill-defined lesions scattered throughout the involved liver, generally hypodense on CT and with high signal intensity on MRI T2-WI. This radiologic pattern may mimic either metastases or pyogenic abscesses. However, there is poor or no enhancement after bolus administration of contrast medium, emphasizing poor vascularization of the parasitic lesion. In advanced stages, typical irregular calcifications, within the areas of central necrosis, are found in 90% of infected patients.

Clinical History: 78-year-old man presenting with rectal bleeding is evaluated with abdominal CECT imaging; the patient was found to have rectal cancer.

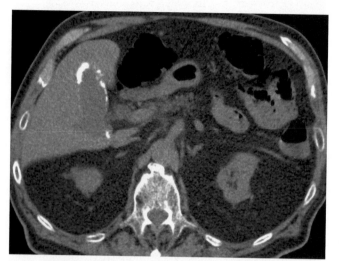

Figure 1.43   A

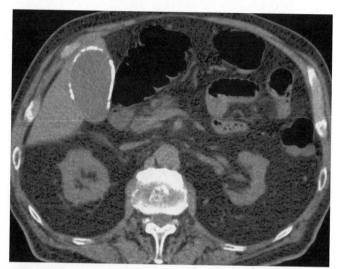

Figure 1.43   B

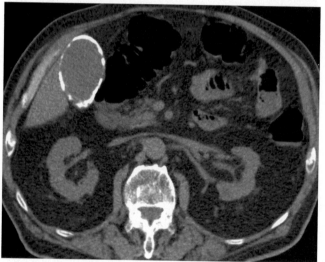

Figure 1.43   C

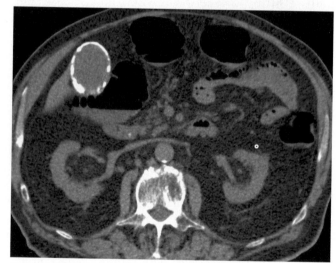

Figure 1.43   D

Findings: Axial NECT images demonstrate extensive calcification within the wall of the gallbladder.

Differential Diagnosis: Echinococcal cyst, calcified hematoma.

Diagnosis: Porcelain gallbladder.

Discussion: Porcelain gallbladder is due to the extensive deposition of calcium in a chronically inflamed gallbladder wall. Porcelain gallbladder is five times more frequent in women than in men and almost always associated with cholelithiasis. Some patients may present with symptoms including abdominal pain, nausea, vomiting, and fever; others may be asymptomatic. Because of the high incidence of gallbladder carcinoma in patients with porcelain gallbladder (11–33%), prophylactic cholecystectomy is advocated for patients even in the absence of clinical symptoms. Calcification of the wall occurs in two different patterns: broad, continuous calcification of the muscularis propria, as seen in this case, or multiple, punctate calcifications scattered throughout the mucosa and submucosa. A reliable diagnosis can be achieved with abdominal CT imaging by showing the characteristic calcification patterns of the gallbladder wall.

CASE 1-44

Clinical History: 77-year-old man presenting with jaundice.

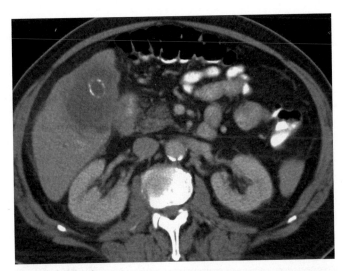

Figure 1.44 A

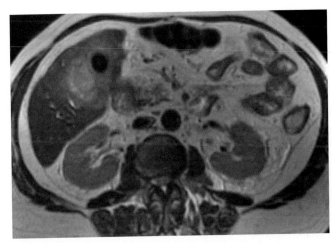

Figure 1.44 B

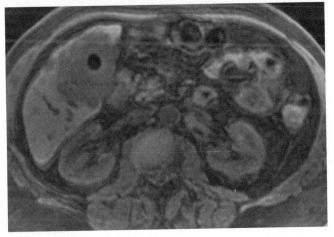

Figure 1.44 C

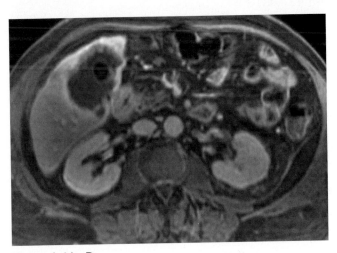

Figure 1.44 D

Findings: Axial CECT image (A) demonstrates a large low-attenuation lesion involving the posterior portion of the gallbladder with extension into the liver. Note the presence of a calcified stone in the presumed location of the gallbladder. Axial T2-WI (B) and fat-suppressed T1-WI (C) demonstrate the mass to be moderately hyperintense and hypointense, respectively. The stone appears as a signal void. Gadolinium-enhanced, fat-suppressed axial T1-WI (D) shows enhancement of the thick irregular wall of the mass.

Differential Diagnosis: Metastasis, acute cholecystitis.

Diagnosis: Gallbladder adenocarcinoma with liver invasion.

Discussion: Gallbladder cancer is an uncommon malignancy. Histologically, gallbladder cancer is usually an adenocarcinoma, although other cell types such as squamous cell carcinoma, anaplastic carcinoma, and sarcomas have been reported. Gallstones are present in more than 70% of the cases of gallbladder cancer; there is a slight female predominance. Gallbladder adenocarcinoma can present as a focal or diffuse thickening of the gallbladder wall, a polypoid lesion, or a mass replacing the gallbladder. Metastases are present at the time of diagnosis in approximately 75% of cases. This case demonstrates many findings of gallbladder carcinoma. There is typically an ill-defined, low-attenuation mass involving the gallbladder wall and invading the liver parenchyma (segment IV). Although not seen in this case, multiple liver metastases are often present and account for the poor prognosis. Acute cholecystitis can also invade the liver; however, the wall is typically not thickened irregularly, and clinical symptoms are more severe.

Clinical History: 31-year-old woman with weight loss.

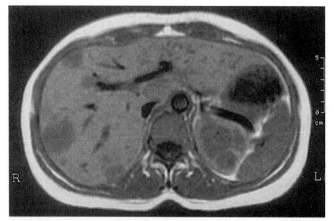

Figure 1.45   A

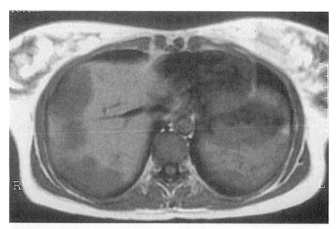

Figure 1.45   B

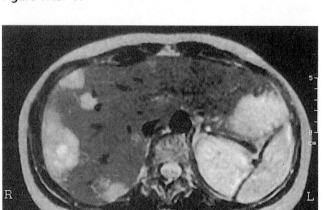

Figure 1.45   C

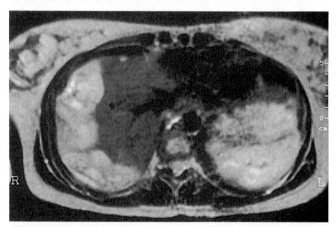

Figure 1.45   D

Findings: Axial T1-WI (A and B) demonstrate multiple large peripherally located hypointense masses in the right lobe of the liver. Axial T2-WI (C and D) show these same lesions to be of high signal intensity with bright centers. Also note the capsular retraction induced by some of the lesions.

Differential Diagnosis: Metastases.

Diagnosis: Hepatic epithelioid hemangioendothelioma (diffuse form).

Discussion: Epithelioid hemangioendothelioma (EHE) is a slow-growing vascular malignancy that can arise in other parts of the body including the lung. The prognosis varies from 2 to 20 years. They have a slight female predominance and present in the fourth through sixth decades of life.

There are two forms of EHE: nodular and diffuse. The two forms can coexist because the nodules can enlarge and coalesce, simulating the diffuse form. The nodular form is hard to distinguish from multiple metastases and can be both central and peripheral inlocation. The diffuse form, as in this case, is typically peripheral in location and will not usually deform the liver contour but rather retract the overlying liver capsule. The peripheral location is thought to be due to the spread of the neoplasm through the portal and hepatic veins. The liver will classically appear to have a rind of tumor along its periphery and hypertrophy of the uninvolved segments due to shunted blood.

Case images courtesy of Dr. Luis Ros, MD, Zargoza, Spain.

CASE 1-46

Clinical History: 58-year-old woman with recent resection of colon cancer presenting with right lower quadrant pain and fever.

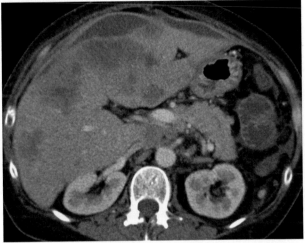

Figure 1.46   A

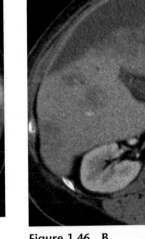

Figure 1.46   B

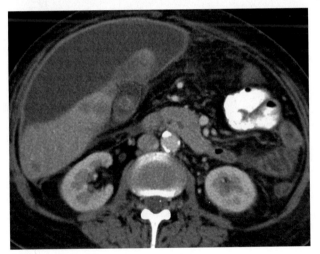

Figure 1.46   C

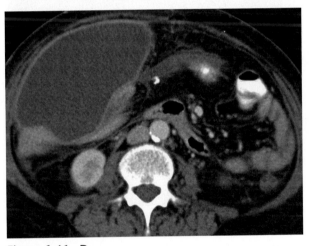

Figure 1.46   D

Findings: Axial CECT images demonstrate multiple low-density lesions in the liver and a well-defined, low-attenuation elliptical subcapsular fluid collection. Note presence of enhancing rim surrounding the collection.

Differential Diagnosis: Hematoma, infected necrotic neoplasm.

Diagnosis: Hepatic metastases and subcapsular pyogenic abscess.

Discussion: The epidemiology of pyogenic abscess has changed significantly in the modern antibiotic era. Pyogenic abscesses, particularly when multiple, may be caused by hematogenous dissemination (either via the portal vein from gastrointestinal infection or disseminated sepsis via the hepatic artery), ascending cholangitis, or superinfection of necrotic tissue. A solitary hepatic abscess is often crypto-genic and has no clear-cut predisposing etiology. Over half of liver abscesses are polymicrobial. *Escherichia coli* is the most common bacterium, but other anaerobic and aerobic organisms can be involved. There is no gender difference regarding incidence of pyogenic abscesses; middle-age patients are most frequently involved. On contrast-enhanced CT scan, large abscesses are generally hypodense and well defined; they may be unilocular with smooth margins or complex with internal septations and irregular contour. Rim enhancement is relatively uncommon, as is presence of gas. On MRI, pyogenic abscesses show variable signal intensity on T1-WI and T2-WI, depending on their protein content. Perilesional edema, characterized by subtle increased signal intensity, can be seen on T2-WI.

Clinical History: 53-year-old man presenting with abdominal distention.

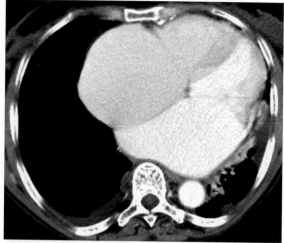

Figure 1.47 A

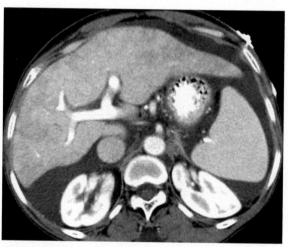

Figure 1.47 B

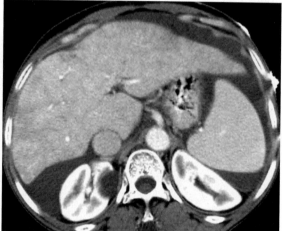

Figure 1.47 C

Figure 1.47 D

Findings: Axial CECT images demonstrate heterogeneous enhancement of the liver with areas of low and high attenuation. Note the dilated IVC and hepatic veins as well as cardiomegaly.

Differential Diagnosis: Fatty liver, diffusely infiltrating neoplasm, Budd-Chiari syndrome.

Diagnosis: Hepatic congestion from right-sided heart failure.

Discussion: Patients who have right-sided cardiac dysfunction from a myocardial infarction or cardiomyopathy will develop right-sided congestive failure. As blood begins to pool in the IVC and hepatic veins from vascular stasis, these vessels will begin to dilate. This will, in turn, cause heterogeneous enhancement of the liver because of the inability of the blood and contrast from the portal vein and hepatic artery to pass through the liver and back to the heart. Grossly, hepatic congestion secondary to cardiac failure has a characteristic mottled appearance referred to as a "nutmeg liver" since it resembles the appearance of a sectioned nutmeg. This case demonstrates the typical findings in hepatic congestion. There is dilatation of both the IVC and hepatic veins and heterogeneous enhancement of the liver. A diffusely infiltrating neoplasm, such as hepatocellular carcinoma, would be unlikely because there is no mass effect. A heterogeneous fatty liver is a possibility because there is no displacement of the vessels found in this entity. The history of a cardiomyopathy as well as the dilated IVC and hepatic veins makes hepatic congestion the best diagnosis.

Case images courtesy of Dr. Giovanni Artho, McGill University Health Center, Montreal, Canada.

Clinical History: 43-year-old Asian woman presenting with jaundice and fever.

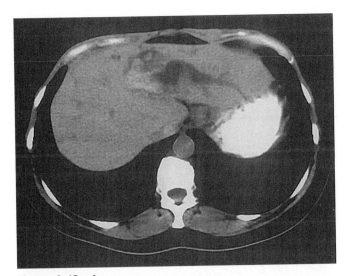

Figure 1.48   A

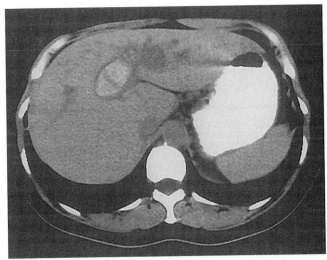

Figure 1.48   B

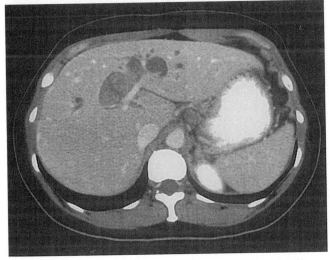

Figure 1.48   C

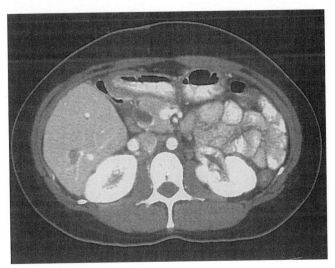

Figure 1.48   D

Findings: Axial NECT images (A and B) demonstrate intrahepatic biliary dilatation with calcified foci within the dilated ducts. Axial CECT images (C and D) again demonstrate the dilated ducts and the calcified foci. Note the dilated common bile duct.

Differential Diagnosis: Caroli disease.

Diagnosis: Oriental cholangiohepatitis (recurrent pyogenic cholangitis).

Discussion: Recurrent pyogenic cholangitis is a disease that is endemic to the Far East and is thought to be secondary to infestation by the parasite *Clonorchis sinensis* due to ingestion of raw fish. The parasite is thought to either cause direct damage to the biliary ducts or act as a focus for the formation of stones. This results in biliary dilatation and cholangitis. Patients present with intermittent bouts of jaundice, fever, and right upper quadrant pain. Radiologically, recurrent pyogenic cholangitis presents with intrahepatic and often extrahepatic biliary dilatation. The intrahepatic dilatation is often found centrally, and multiple areas of strictures are seen on cholangiograms. Stone formation and sludge is commonly seen in these patients. This case demonstrates intrahepatic and extrahepatic biliary dilatation, stone formation, and a clinical history that helps to make the diagnosis almost certain. Caroli disease with abscess formation is another diagnostic possibility, but the extrahepatic biliary dilatation is not seen in Caroli disease.

Clinical History: 45-year-old man with history of longstanding cirrhosis.

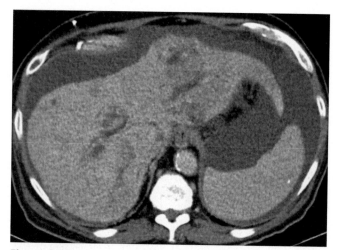

Figure 1.49   A

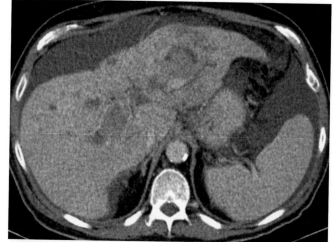

Figure 1.49   B

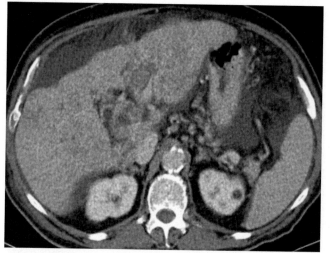

Figure 1.49   C

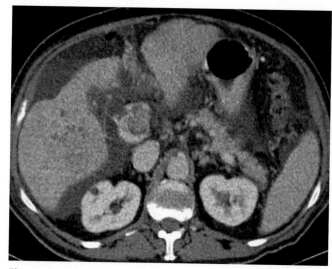

Figure 1.49   D

Findings: Axial NECT images (A and B) demonstrate irregular liver contour and multiple nodular lesions in the liver; some of the lesions contain hypodense areas consistent with intratumoral necrosis. The portal veins are enlarged and heterogeneous. Axial CECT images (C and D) obtained in the portal venous phase demonstrate enhancement of the thrombus within the enlarged portal veins.

Differential Diagnosis: Bland portal vein thrombosis.

Diagnosis: Multifocal hepatocellular carcinoma with extension into portal vein.

Discussion: Hepatocellular carcinoma (HCC) may invade the portal and hepatic veins. In patients with gross direct extension of HCC into the portal vein, the diagnosis of malignant portal vein thrombus is not challenging; dramatic expansion of the main and lobar portal vein branches is a relatively reliable imaging feature for malignant portal vein thrombus. Vein expansion typically does not occur with benign thrombi. Another specific characteristic of malignant portal vein thrombus is the presence of neovascularity within it. The enhancement of the thrombus during arterial phase of a contrast-enhanced dynamic CT study is highly specific for the diagnosis. Other findings of a malignant portal vein thrombosis include obvious generalized enhancement of the thrombus and contiguity of the thrombus with a parenchymal HCC.

Clinical History: 74-year-old woman with history of colon cancer resected 13 years ago.

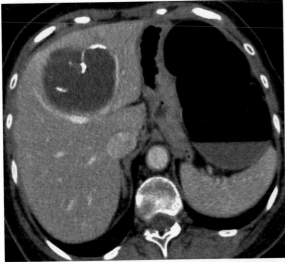

Figure 1.50   A

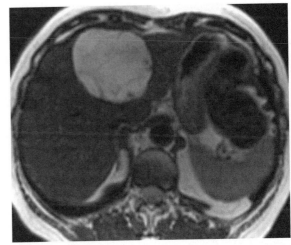

Figure 1.50   B

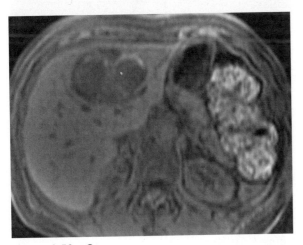

Figure 1.50   C

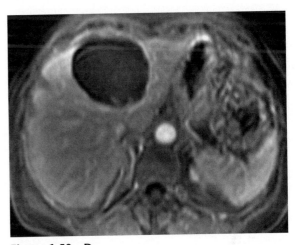

Figure 1.50   D

Findings: Axial CECT image (A) shows a large and predominantly cystic lesion in segment IV of the liver. There are several areas of calcifications associated with the lesion. The lesion is heterogeneously high in signal on the axial T2-WI (B). The calcifications appear as focal areas of low signal intensity. The lesion is heterogeneous on the fat-suppressed axial T1-WI (C); the high signal intensity material within the lesion is caused by the presence of ionic calcium in the calcifications. On gadolinium-enhanced, fat-suppressed axial T1-WI (D), thin peripheral enhancement is present.

Differential Diagnosis: Echinococcal cyst, hematoma, biliary cystadenoma, abscess.

Diagnosis: Cystic liver metastasis from mucinous adenocarcinoma of the colon.

Discussion: Most hepatic metastases are solid, but some have a complete or partially cystic appearance. Metastases that are cystic can mimic abscesses, hemorrhagic infarcts, hematomas, simple cysts, and hydatid cysts. Cystic metastases usually display a degree of complexity with mural nodules, thickened walls, septations, and fluid/debris levels. A detailed clinical history may help to exclude hematomas, hydatid cysts, and abscesses from consideration. Cystic metastases may be especially seen with mucinous adenocarcinomas, such as colorectal or ovarian carcinoma. Calcification is frequently encountered in metastases from primary mucinous adenocarcinomas. The calcification is either produced by the tumor itself or represents dystrophic calcification due to necrosis and/or hemorrhage within the tumor before or during chemotherapy.

Clinical History: 45-year-old man presenting with enlarging abdominal girth and abnormal liver function tests.

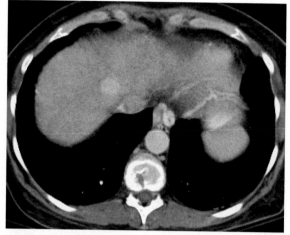

Figure 1.51   A

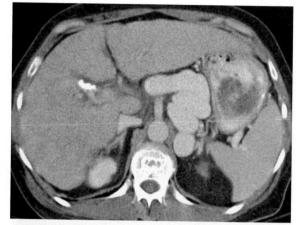

Figure 1.51   B

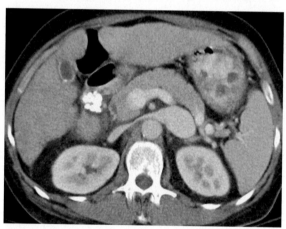

Figure 1.51   C

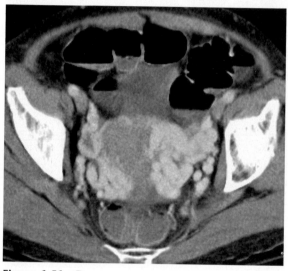

Figure 1.51   D

Findings: Axial CECT images demonstrate a nodular contour of the liver with the presence of a hypervascular liver lesion (A). Also note enlarged vessels near the gastric fundus (B) and enlargement of the left renal vein (C). There are also early enhancing engorged vessels in the pelvis (D).

Differential Diagnosis: Collateral vessels mimicking opacified bowel.

Diagnosis: Cirrhosis with hepatocellular carcinoma and portal hypertension leading to massive collateral vessel formation including gastric and pelvic varices and a splenorenal shunt.

Discussion: There are multiple causes for portal hypertension, the most common being cirrhosis. These causes can be divided into three categories: intrahepatic, extrahepatic presinusoidal, and extrahepatic postsinusoidal. Intrahepatic causes are more common and include cirrhosis, schistosomiasis, hepatitis, and neoplasms. Extrahepatic presinusoidal causes include portal vein thrombosis, and extrahepatic postsinusoidal causes include pericarditis, congestive heart failure, and Budd-Chiari syndrome. Portal hypertension leads to the formation of spontaneous portosystemic shunts to bypass the liver, as is seen in this case. There is enlargement of the coronary vein and short gastric veins as the blood gets directed from the portal vein through these vessels into the azygous vein and finally the superior vena cava (SVC). This case demonstrates how large these collaterals can become and how they can impress on the fundus of the stomach and simulate a mass on upper GI series. A large splenorenal shunt is also present that could be confused with normal opacified bowel if the entire scan is not viewed carefully.

Clinical History: 59-year-old woman presenting with pancytopenia.

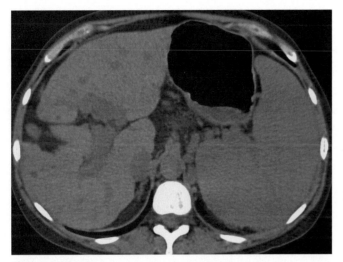

Figure 1.52   A

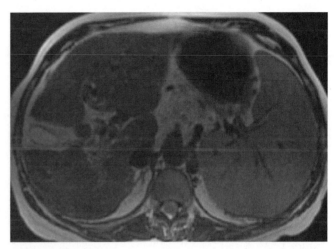

Figure 1.52   B

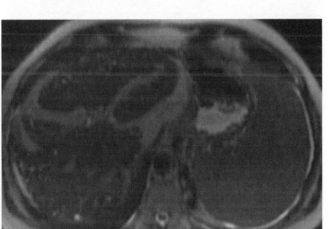

Figure 1.52   C

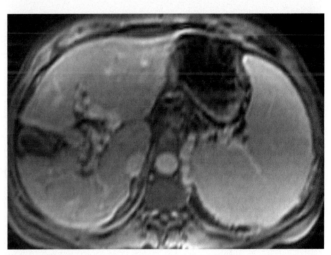

Figure 1.52   D

Findings: Axial NECT image (A) demonstrates a dysmorphic liver with atrophy of the right hepatic lobe. Also note the presence of splenomegaly. Axial T2-WI (B) and heavily weighted T2-WI (C) show edema of the gallbladder wall. Gadolinium-enhanced, fat-suppressed axial T1-WI (D) shows attenuation of the intrahepatic portal radicles and perisplenic varices.

Differential Diagnosis: Hepatitis, viral hepatitis induced cirrhosis, hepatic schistosomiasis.

Diagnosis: Congenital hepatic fibrosis.

Discussion: Congenital hepatic fibrosis is induced by a ductal plate abnormality and can be associated with autosomal recessive polycystic kidney disease. These patients will present with liver failure and symptoms of portal hypertension, such as bleedings from esophageal varices. Congenital hepatic fibrosis can also be an isolated phenomenon or be associated with other entities, such as Caroli disease and medullary sponge kidney. Some of the common CT findings of congenital hepatic fibrosis include hepatomegaly with areas of fibrosis that appear as linear low-attenuation areas on CT. The periportal fibrosis causes the vessels to be markedly attenuated, leading to portal hypertension and splenomegaly, as seen in this case. Periportal fibrosis may mimic periportal edema, a nonspecific CT finding seen in acute hepatitis.

Clinical History: 58-year-old woman with history of breast cancer, screening for metastasis.

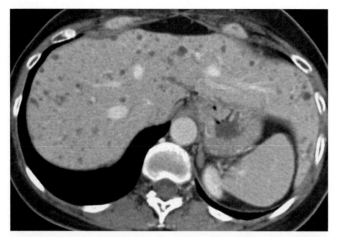

Figure 1.53 A

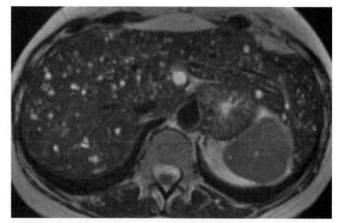

Figure 1.53 B

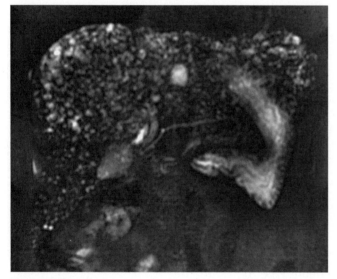

Figure 1.53 C

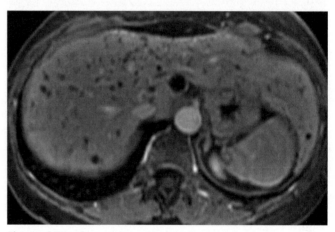

Figure 1.53 D

Findings: Axial CECT image (A) demonstrates multiple, small, nonenhancing, low-density lesions throughout the liver. Axial T2-WI (B) and thick-slab coronal-oblique MRCP image (C) show the lesions to be markedly hyperintense. No enhancement is seen on the gadolinium-enhanced, fat-suppressed axial T1-WI (D).

Differential Diagnosis: Metastases, infection (fungal), multiple bile duct cysts.

Diagnosis: Bile duct hamartomas.

Discussion: Bile duct hamartomas (von Meyenburg complexes) are dilated clusters of biliary ducts that are lined by a single layer of cuboidal epithelium within a fibrous stroma. These clusters are filled with proteinaceous material and biliary fluid. They can be single or multiple in their presentation. They are part of the spectrum of fibropolycystic hepa-torenal diseases and are, therefore, sometimes associated with polycystic liver disease, polycystic kidney disease, congenital hepatic fibrosis, and Caroli disease. As is seen in this case, the lesions are usually small (<1–1.5 cm) and have low attenuation. Typically, they are adjacent to the portal area or subcapsular in location. Because of their fluid content, they are markedly hyperintense on T2-WI. They are typically more irregular in shape than bile duct cysts. Unlike Caroli disease, the cysts do not communicate with the biliary tree. Because they can be multiple, they can be confused with metastatic disease or disseminated infections; however, the latter typically demonstrate peripheral enhancement on postcontrast CT and MRI images.

Clinical History: 41-year-old woman who felt a lump in her left breast.

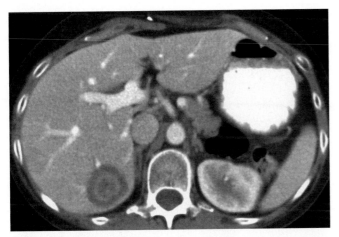

Figure 1.54 A

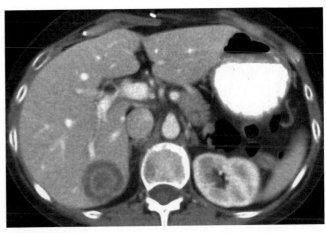

Figure 1.54 B

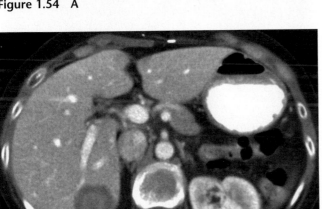

Figure 1.54 C

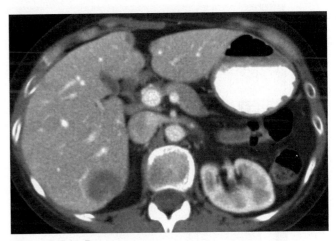

Figure 1.54 D

Findings: Axial CECT images show a hypodense lesion in segment VII of the liver. The lesion causes retraction of the overlying liver capsule.

Differential Diagnosis: Hepatic abscess, lymphoma.

Diagnosis: Metastasis from breast cancer.

Discussion: Hepatic capsular retraction, defined as focal flattening or concavity of the normal convex hepatic contour, can be associated with a spectrum of benign and, more commonly, malignant primary and secondary hepatic neoplasms. In patients with breast carcinoma, capsular retraction occurs adjacent to subcapsular hepatic metastases and is usually seen after treatment with chemotherapy. Although the underlying pathophysiology for this phenomenon is poorly understood, it is thought to be a chemotherapeutic response due to shrinkage of tumor with subsequent scarring and nodular regeneration of uninvolved areas. Nevertheless, untreated breast carcinoma metastases tend to be associated with capsular retraction as well. CT allows recognition and evaluation of capsular retraction. Hepatic metastases from breast cancer are typically hypovascular and most commonly hypoattenuating to normal hepatic parenchyma on both unenhanced and contrast-enhanced CT images.

CASE 1-55

Clinical History: 1½-year-old girl with abdominal distension and congestive heart failure (CHF). Patient has normal alpha-fetoprotein levels.

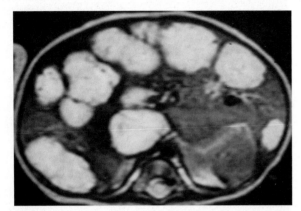

Figure 1.55 A

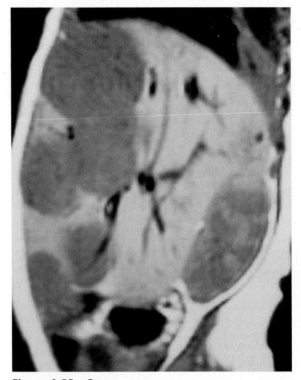

Figure 1.55 C

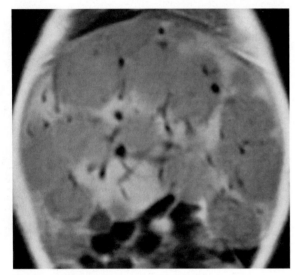

Figure 1.55 B

Findings: Axial T2-WI (A) shows numerous well-defined homogeneous hyperintense lesions scattered throughout the liver. Note hepatomegaly. Coronal (B) and sagittal (C) T1-WI demonstrate homogeneous low signal within the lesions.

Differential Diagnosis: Hepatoblastoma, metastases, mesenchymal hamartoma.

Diagnosis: Infantile hemangioendothelioma.

Discussion: Infantile hemangioendotheliomas are vascular tumors derived from endothelial cells. They are considered benign but can occasionally show aggressive features and distant metastasis. They become clinically evident when large due to platelet sequestration, CHF, and Kassabach-Merrit syndrome. The majority present in children younger than 6 months of age (90% less than 1 year); they tend to spontaneously regress after 18 months. Some have been reported to persist into adulthood. The lesions can range in size from a few millimeters to up to 10 to 15 cm and are usually multiple. Calcifications, when they occur, tend to be fine and granular rather than coarse. Infantile hemangio-endotheliomas tend to be intensely bright on T2-WI, like hemangiomas. However, they can also be heterogeneous on both T1-WI and T2-WI due to the areas of hemorrhage, necrosis, and scarring. Their enhancement pattern is similar to that of cavernous hemangiomas. Mesenchymal hamar-tomas are typically not multiple and rarely have a large solid component. The multiple lesions and history of CHF make infantile hemangioendothelioma the best diagnosis.

Case images courtesy of Dr. Susan A. Connolly, Children's Hospital Boston, Boston, MA.

Clinical History: 53-year-old man presenting with intermittent right upper quadrant pain for 6 years.

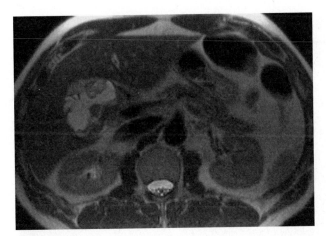

Figure 1.56 A

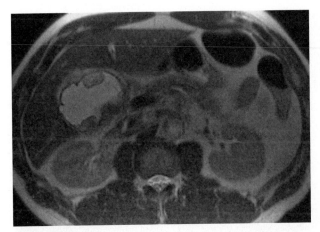

Figure 1.56 B

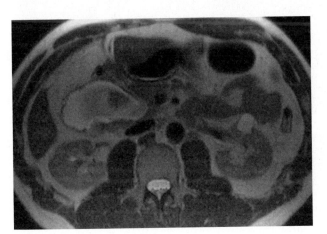

Figure 1.56 C

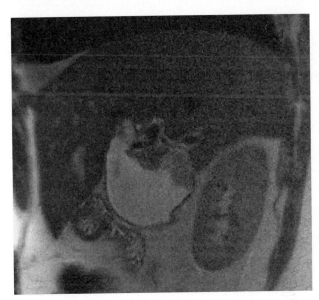

Figure 1.56 D

Findings: Axial (A–C) and coronal (D) T2-WI show a cystically dilated common bile duct with irregular filling defects arising from the duct wall.

Differential Diagnosis: None.

Diagnosis: Bile duct carcinoma in a type I choledochal cyst.

Discussion: Choledochal cyst is a rare congenital malformation with a female-to-male ratio of 3:1. It is much more common in Asia. Formation of a choledochal cyst is thought to be related to reflux of pancreatic secretions into the bile duct as a consequence of an anomalous junction of the common bile duct and pancreatic duct, the so-called "long common channel." The diagnosis is typically made in the childhood due to the presence of one or more symptoms of the classical triad of obstructive jaundice, right upper quadrant pain, and a palpable mass. Todani's classification of

choledochal cysts comprises five types of cysts: saccular or fusiform dilatation of the extrahepatic duct (type I), diverticulum of the extrahepatic duct (type II), choledochocele (type III), multiple cysts or involvement of both the intra- or extrahepatic ducts (type IV), and intrahepatic bile duct cysts only (type V or Caroli disease). Choledochal cyst frequently causes malignant change in the epithelial lining; bile duct carcinoma arising in a choledochal cyst has been reported in up to 15% of cases. On T2-WI, the tumor is visualized as solitary or multiple filling defects in the hyperintense choledochal cyst. Gadolinium-enhanced T1-WI in different planes can be used to demonstrate enhancement and extraluminal extension of the tumor.

Case images courtesy of Dr. Angela D. Levy, Armed Forces Institute of Pathology, Washington, DC.

Clinical History: 30-year-old man with recent trip to India presenting with fever and diarrhea.

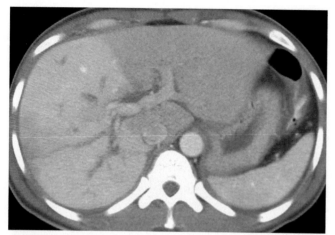

Figure 1.57 **A**

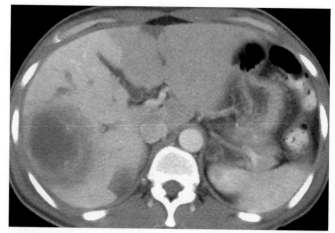

Figure 1.57 **B**

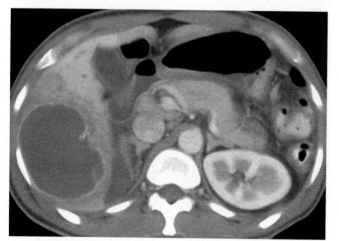

Figure 1.57 **C**

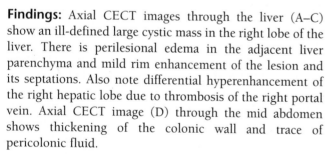

Figure 1.57 **D**

Findings: Axial CECT images through the liver (A–C) show an ill-defined large cystic mass in the right lobe of the liver. There is perilesional edema in the adjacent liver parenchyma and mild rim enhancement of the lesion and its septations. Also note differential hyperenhancement of the right hepatic lobe due to thrombosis of the right portal vein. Axial CECT image (D) through the mid abdomen shows thickening of the colonic wall and trace of pericolonic fluid.

Differential Diagnosis: Pyogenic or fungal abscess, necrotic metastasis, hepatocellular carcinoma.

Diagnosis: Amebic abscess.

Discussion: Amebic abscesses are caused by the parasite *Entamoeba histolytica*. Amebiasis is more commonly seen in the GI tract (amebic colitis) rather than the liver. Spread to the liver occurs through the portal system and, therefore, involves the right lobe more than the left lobe secondary to preferential blood flow to the right lobe. The liver is the most common extraintestinal organ involved by amebiasis followed by lung and brain. Amebic abscesses tend to occur in the dome of the liver and can be complicated by intraperitoneal rupture with subsequent peritonitis. Conservative treatment with metronidazole and chloroquine is effective in most cases, with percutaneous drainage reserved for larger abscesses and for those adjacent to the heart. The finding on CT of a rim-enhancing lesion is nonspecific and can be seen with any type of abscess or necrotic tumor. Enhancing septations, however, are less commonly seen with necrotic tumors and suggest an abscess. The lack of evidence for cirrhosis would make hepatocellular carcinoma less likely. An abscess of a different etiology or cystic metastases cannot be excluded in this case; nevertheless, the associated colonic wall thickening suggests amebiasis.

Case images courtesy of Dr. Giovanni Artho, McGill University Health Center, Montreal, Canada.

CASE 1-58

Clinical History: 22-year-old man with multiple subcutaneous soft tissue nodules.

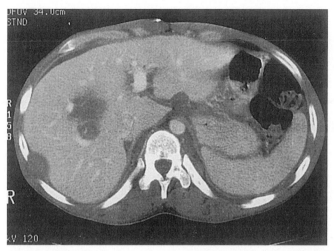

Figure 1.58 A

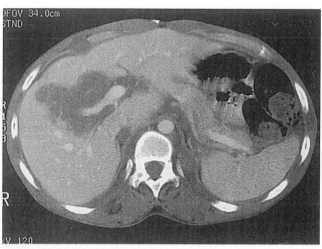

Figure 1.58 B

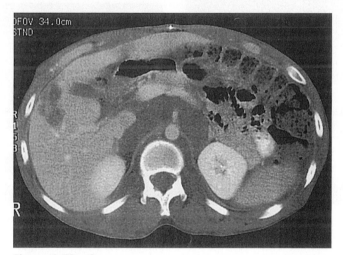

Figure 1.58 C

Findings: Axial CECT images demonstrate a low-attenuation soft tissue mass surrounding the portal vein and other soft tissue masses involving the retroperitoneum and chest wall.

Differential Diagnosis: Lymphoma, metastases.

Diagnosis: Plexiform neurofibromatosis involving the liver.

Discussion: Von Recklinghausen disease or neurofibromatosis type 1 is the most common form of neurofibromatosis. It is often referred to as peripheral neurofibromatosis because many of the most striking findings include lesions outside the intracranial central nervous system. These include café-au-lait spots, neurofibromas, and skeletal anomalies. The neurofibromas are typically round or spherical. Plexiform neurofibromas, on the other hand, are tortuous masses of enlarged peripheral nerves. The autonomic innervation of the

biliary system arises from the celiac plexus and travels with the biliary tract. Therefore, hepatic neurofibromas will often be located along the path of the portal vein. Neurofibromas and plexiform neurofibromas are usually low in attenuation and tend to surround adjacent vessels and organs without significant obstruction or invasion. In this case, the portal vein is completely encased by the mass, and yet there is no obstruction of the vessel or signs of portal hypertension. This mass is not causing biliary dilatation either. The key to the diagnosis is the coexistence of the neurofibroma in the retroperitoneum and intercostal space causing rib notching. The typical location of these masses in the periportal region, retroperitoneum, and inferior surface of the rib without obstruction of the portal vein and biliary system makes neurofibromatosis the most likely diagnosis.

Clinical History: 50-year-old man presenting with longstanding abdominal pain.

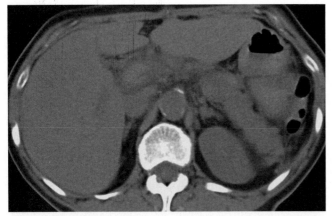

Figure 1.59   A

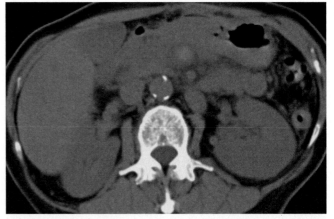

Figure 1.59   B

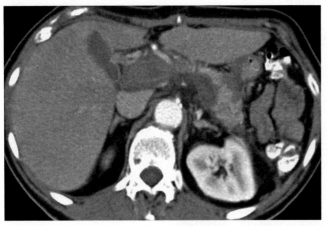

Figure 1.59   C

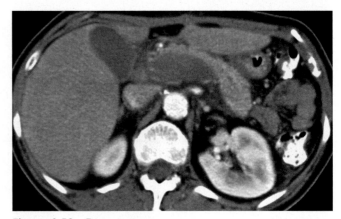

Figure 1.59   D

Findings: Axial NECT images (A and B) demonstrate the enlarged superior mesenteric and portal veins with presence of high-density material in their lumen. On the axial CECT images (C and D), the filling defects in the enlarged portal and splenic veins are evident.

Differential Diagnosis: None.

Diagnosis: Acute portal vein thrombosis.

Discussion: Portal vein thrombosis occurs in various clinical settings, with the most common being liver cirrhosis. Other reasons include infectious diseases (such as sepsis, cholangitis, or pancreatitis), neoplasms, hypercoagulable states, myeloproliferative disorders, surgery, and embolism from the superior mesenteric or splenic vein. Unenhanced CT images, as seen in this case, may show focal high attenuation in the portal, superior mesenteric, or splenic veins and venous enlargement when thrombosis is acute. Chronic venous thrombosis can manifest as linear areas of calcification within the thrombus. CECT images demonstrate a filling defect partially or totally occluding the lumen of the portal vein. Indirect signs of portal vein thrombosis are the presence of cavernous transformation of the portal vein, the presence of portosystemic collateral vessels and arterioportal shunts, and transient hepatic attenuation differences (THAD) in the liver.

CASE 1-60

Clinical History: 37-year-old woman with known steatohepatitis and alcohol abuse.

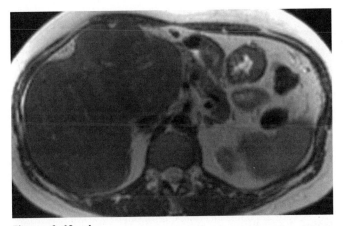

Figure 1.60   A

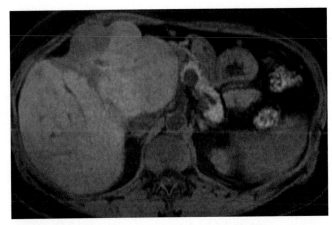

Figure 1.60   B

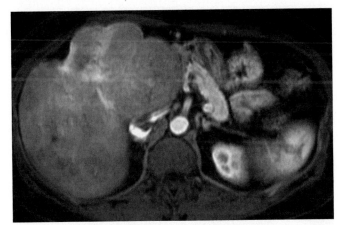

Figure 1.60   C

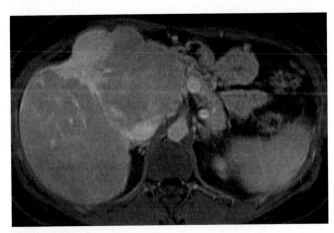

Figure 1.60   D

Findings: Axial MRI demonstrate marked enlargement of the lateral segment of the left lobe of the liver and concomitant decrease in the size of the right liver lobe. An ill-defined wedge-shaped area within the medial segment of the left liver lobe shows increased signal intensity on the axial T2-WI (A), decreased signal intensity on the fat-suppressed axial T1-WI (B), and delayed enhancement on gadolinium-enhanced, fat-suppressed axial T1-WI (C and D). Hepatic vessels are seen traversing through this region without evidence of distortion. Also note capsular retraction adjacent to the abnormal area.

Differential Diagnosis: Hepatocellular carcinoma, intrahepatic cholangiocarcinoma.

Diagnosis: Confluent hepatic fibrosis.

Discussion: Confluent hepatic fibrosis can present as a masslike area (14%) in patients with underlying cirrhosis, especially primary sclerosing cholangitis. It typically affects the anterior segments of the right lobe and medial segments of the left lobe. Confluent hepatic fibrosis usually has a wedge-shaped appearance, but in some patients, the entire segment might be involved. The typical appearance of confluent hepatic fibrosis is an area of low signal intensity on T1-WI and high signal intensity on T2-WI. It usually demonstrates delayed enhancement on gadolinium-enhanced images. The typical geographic pattern of involvement and retraction of the overlying hepatic capsule can be helpful in diagnosing this condition. Possible explanations for the hyperintense appearance of confluent fibrosis on T2-WI are a relative reduction in the signal of the remaining liver parenchyma due to increased iron deposition, edema due to venous thrombosis, or most likely, inflammatory changes within the fibrosis.

Clinical History: 2-year-old boy presents with a palpable abdominal mass.

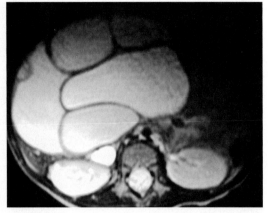

Figure 1.61   A

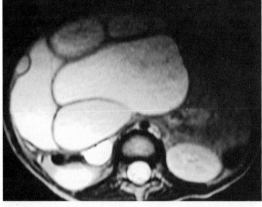

Figure 1.61   B

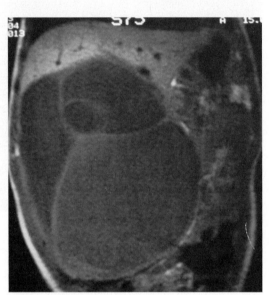

Figure 1.61   C

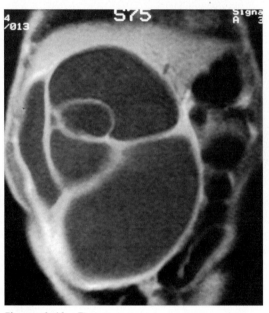

Figure 1.61   D

Findings: Axial T2-WI (A and B) demonstrates a large 9-cm cystic mass in the right lobe of the liver. Note the presence of numerous septations. Unenhanced (C) and gadolinium-enhanced (D) coronal T1-WI demonstrate the low signal intensity appearance of the lesion and enhancement of the wall and septations following gadolinium administration.

Differential Diagnosis: Undifferentiated embryonal sarcoma, infantile hemangioendothelioma, hepatoblastoma, and metastasis.

Diagnosis: Mesenchymal hamartoma.

Discussion: Mesenchymal hamartoma is a benign cystic lesion of the liver that is thought to arise from the mesenchymal tissue surrounding the portal tracts. The patients typically are between 1 and 2 years of age, but some cases have been reported in older patients up to their teen years. The lesions are typically large, located in the right lobe of the liver, and composed of multiple cysts. There is a variable amount of solid component, but the cystic component usually predominates. Typically, mesenchymal hamartomas appear more solid in younger patients; occasionally, the cysts are small, and the lesion can appear solid. Both infantile hemangioendotheliomas and hepatoblastomas rarely have a large cystic component, and the age of the patient makes undifferentiated embryonal sarcoma unlikely. Metastases from neuroblastoma tend to be multiple and solid rather than cystic.

Case images courtesy of Dr. Susan A. Connolly, Children's Hospital Boston, Boston, MA.

Clinical History: 40-year-old man presenting with obstructive jaundice.

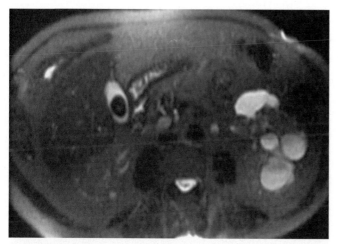

Figure 1.62   A

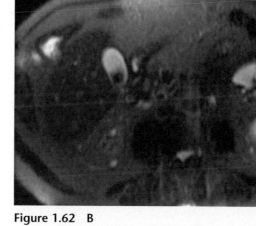

Figure 1.62   B

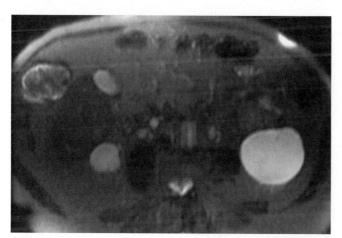

Figure 1.62   C

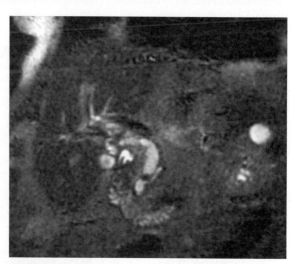

Figure 1.62   D

Findings: Heavily weighted axial T2-WI (A–C) and thin-slab MRCP image (D) show a large stone in the gallbladder and a dilated common bile duct with a dependent filling defect inside. Note renal cysts.

Differential Diagnosis: Blood clot, cholangiocarcinoma, pneumobilia.

Diagnosis: Choledocholithiasis.

Discussion: Gallstones in the common bile duct (CBD) are the most common cause of biliary obstruction. They are found in approximately 15% of patients undergoing chole-cystectomy; they typically result from migration out of the gallbladder into the CBD. Clinical symptoms include right upper quadrant pain, obstructive jaundice, and fever (in the presence of ascending cholangitis). MRI is highly accurate in the detection of CBD stones, with a reported accuracy of up to 97%. CBD stones are typically hypointense on both T1-WI and T2-WI and surrounded by bile. On axial images, the stone is typically located in a dependent position in the duct. This position differentiates CBD stones from pneumo-bilia (filling defect in the nondependent position) and bile flow artifacts (typically central in location). MRCP is the imaging test of choice to evaluate patients who have a low to moderate probability of having a CBD stone. In patients with a high probability, ERCP is recommended because this tech-nique allows immediate therapeutic intervention.

Clinical History: 28-year-old man with right upper quadrant pain.

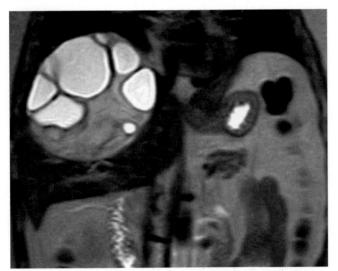

Figure 1.63 A

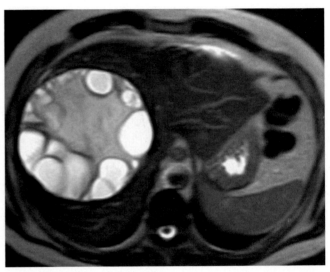

Figure 1.63 B

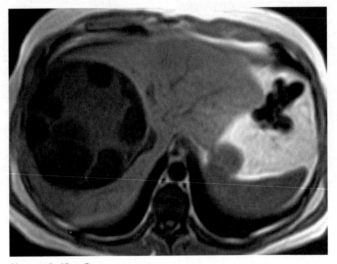

Figure 1.63 C

Findings: Coronal (A) and axial (B) T2-WI demonstrate a large cystic mass in the right lobe of the liver that is surrounded by a hypointense rim and contains more hyperintense smaller cysts in its periphery. On the axial T1-WI (C), the hypointense rim is well visualized, and the peripheral cysts are hypointense relative to the center of the lesion.

Differential Diagnosis: Pyogenic abscess, amebic abscess, biliary cystadenoma.

Diagnosis: Hydatid cyst.

Discussion: Hepatic echinococcosis is an endemic disease in the Mediterranean basin and other sheep-raising countries. Humans become infected by ingestion of eggs of the tapeworm *Echinococcus granulosus*, either by eating contaminated food or from contact with dogs. On MRI, hepatic hydatid cysts usually have a hypointense rim on both T1-WI and T2-WI, which represents the fibrous and sometimes calcific pericyst. The hydatid matrix or "sand" appears hyperintense on T1-WI and hypointense on T2-WI. When present, daughter cysts are seen as cystic structures attached to the peripheral germinal layer. Relative to the intracystic fluid, they are hypointense on T1-WI and hyperintense on T2-WI. Calcifications can be present in the periphery of hydatid cysts; on MRI, however, they are less well seen than with CT, and if present, appear as linear areas of signal void.

Clinical History: 21-year-old woman presenting with left flank pain and a palpable mass.

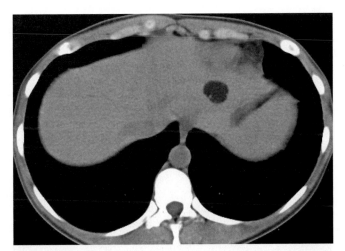

Figure 1.64   A

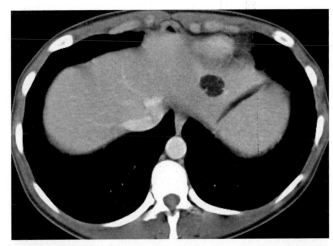

Figure 1.64   B

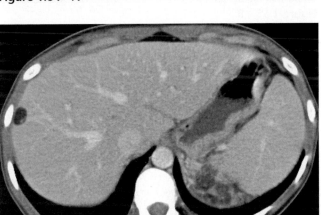

Figure 1.64   C

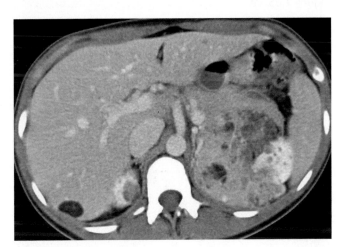

Figure 1.64   D

Findings: Axial NECT image (A) shows a very low-density lesion in the left lobe of the liver. Axial CECT images (B–D) demonstrate other low-attenuation lesions that are of fat density in the liver. In addition, fat-containing lesions are identified in both kidneys.

Differential Diagnosis: Lipomas, myelolipomas, metastatic liposarcoma, focal fatty change.

Diagnosis: Multiple hepatic angiomyolipomas in a patient with tuberous sclerosis.

Discussion: Lipomatous tumors of the liver include simple lipomas that are purely fat and lesions that contain fat and soft tissues, such as adenolipomas, angiomyolipomas,

and angiolipomas. Angiomyolipomas of the liver are often associated with renal angiomyolipomas and tuberous sclerosis. They can be solitary or multiple. Lipomas of the liver are of fat density measuring about –30 HU. They do not typically demonstrate contrast enhancement. In this case, the septations seen in the left lobe lesion have contrast enhancement, ruling out a simple lipoma. Other lesions in the liver that contain fat include liposarcoma metastases, hepatocellular carcinoma, and hepatic adenoma. Metastases from malignant teratomas will frequently contain fat but almost always contain calcium as well. The presence of fatty lesions in the liver and kidneys is diagnostic of multiple angiomyolipomas associated with tuberous sclerosis.

Clinical History: 29-year-old woman presenting with multiple palpable peripheral lymph nodes.

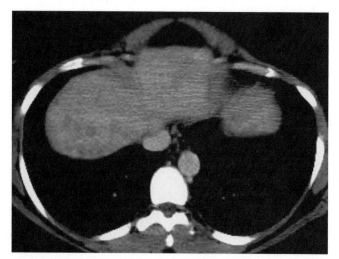

Figure 1.65   A

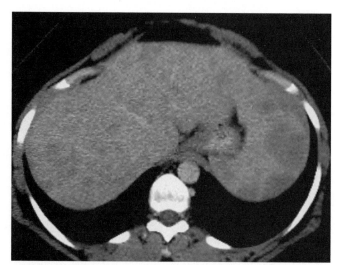

Figure 1.65   B

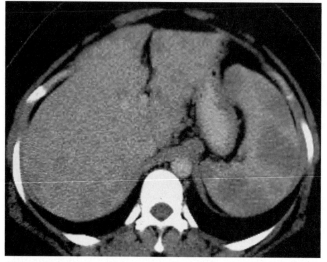

Figure 1.65   C

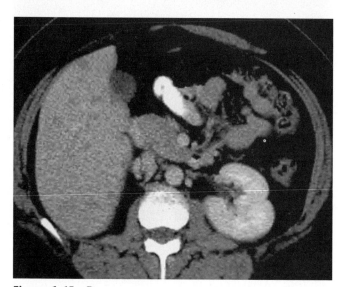

Figure 1.65   D

Findings: Axial CECT images (A–D) demonstrate ill-defined hypodense nodules scattered throughout the liver and spleen. The lesions show no enhancement after the administration of contrast material.

Differential Diagnosis: Lymphoma, diffuse metastatic disease, fungal microabscesses.

Diagnosis: Sarcoidosis.

Discussion: Sarcoidosis is a granulomatous systemic disease of unknown etiology that can involve numerous organs including the liver and spleen. Although histologic evidence of sarcoidosis involving the liver is seen in 50% to 80% of autopsy specimens, liver dysfunction is uncommon. On CT, hepatic sarcoidosis manifests with minimal organomegaly. In only 5% to 15% of patients, coalescing granulomas become apparent as multiple hypoattenuating nodules. Compared to the hepatic nodules, splenic nodules are larger and more common, as seen in this case. Affected patients frequently have abdominal or systemic symptoms and elevated angiotensin-converting enzyme (ACE) levels. Multiple nodules seen in hepatic sarcoidosis might be mistaken for more common diseases, such as metastases and lymphoma. Simultaneous involvement of the spleen favors a diagnosis of sarcoidosis and lymphoma, and metastatic disease can be ruled out in the absence of a known primary tumor. Nevertheless, a thorough investigation of laboratory data, including tumor markers or soluble interleukin-2 receptors, is still needed for differentiating sarcoidosis from malignant lymphoma or other malignancies.

Clinical History: 59-year-old woman with progressive jaundice and weight loss.

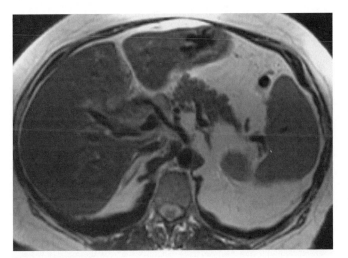

Figure 1.66   A

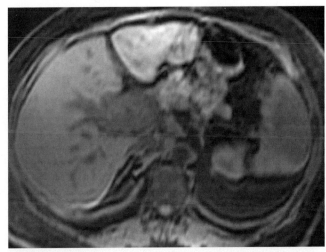

Figure 1.66   B

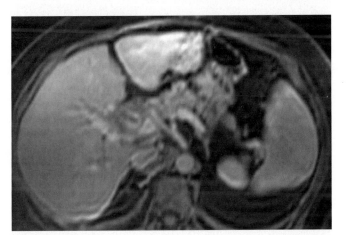

Figure 1.66   C

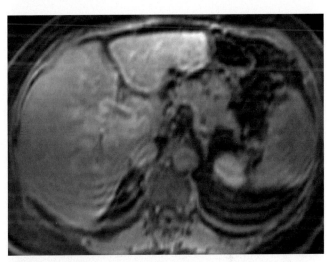

Figure 1.66   D

Findings: Axial T2-WI (A) demonstrates an ill-defined slightly hyperintense mass in the porta hepatis. The lesion appears hypointense on the fat-suppressed axial T1-WI (B). Following gadolinium administration, the lesion shows progressive enhancement on the gadolinium-enhanced, fat-suppressed T1-WI (C and D). Also, note the abnormal hyperenhancement of the common hepatic duct, which is encased by the mass.

Differential Diagnosis: Hepatocellular carcinoma, metastasis.

Diagnosis: Cholangiocarcinoma (Klatskin tumor).

Discussion: Cholangiocarcinoma (CAC) is a malignant neoplasm of the bile ducts that has an increased incidence in patients with sclerosing cholangitis, inflammatory bowel disease, and gallstones. CACs occur most commonly in the larger extrahepatic ducts, with more than 90% occurring at the confluence of the ducts or more distally. Although extrahepatic CACs often present early with jaundice secondary to biliary obstruction, the prognosis is still very poor. A Klatskin tumor is a CAC at the bifurcation of the left and right hepatic ducts. This will cause biliary dilatation in both lobes of the liver. Because the bile ducts are small, a tumor mass is often not seen by imaging when the patients present with jaundice. This case, on the other hand, demonstrates the tumor mass invading into the liver. When a tumor mass is seen, it typically enhances late on CT and MRI and demonstrates mildly increased signal on T2-WI, as seen in this example. Neither hepatocellular carcinomas nor metastases frequently cause biliary dilatation or are associated with abnormal hyperenhancement of the bile duct wall.

Clinical History: 50-year-old woman with history of breast cancer. MRI was performed to exclude metastatic disease.

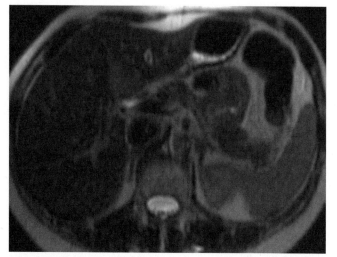

Figure 1.67   A

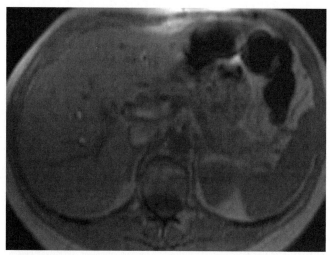

Figure 1.67   B

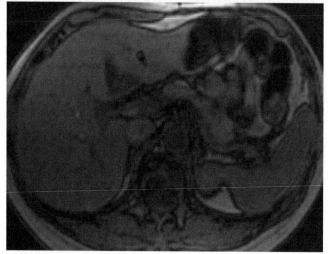

Figure 1.67   C

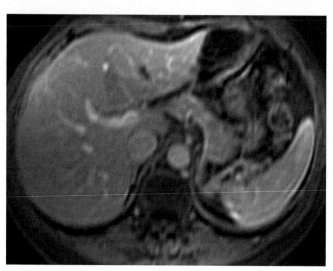

Figure 1.67   D

Findings: Axial T2-WI (A) shows an area of high signal intensity adjacent to porta hepatis. On axial in-phase T1-WI (B), the area is isointense with the adjacent liver parenchyma and shows signal drop on out-of-phase T1-WI (C). On gadolinium-enhanced, fat-suppressed axial T1-WI (D), the area is slightly hypointense compared to surrounding liver parenchyma.

Differential Diagnosis: Metastasis.

Diagnosis: Focal fatty change.

Discussion: Hepatic steatosis can be either diffuse or focal. Focal steatosis can be recognized on the basis of the typical distribution within the liver (adjacent to the gallbladder fossa, the falciform ligament, the porta hepatis, or in the subcapsular region). Absence of mass effect and the presence of nondistorted blood vessels traversing the mass are key CT imaging findings. Nevertheless, atypical distribution patterns have been described, and especially when fatty change has a nodular configuration, it may be difficult to exclude a metastatic lesion on the basis of US and CT findings alone. In this context, chemical shift MRI is extremely useful; the combination of in-phase and opposed-phase gradient-echo imaging, with signal dropout seen in focal fatty change, allows a reliable differentiation of solitary or multifocal nodular steatosis from metastatic disease. As seen in this case, focal fat is mildly hyperintense on fast-spin echo T2-WI and is usually not detectable on in-phase T1-WI.

Clinical History: 84-year-old woman patient with longstanding Crohn disease presenting with nausea and vomiting.

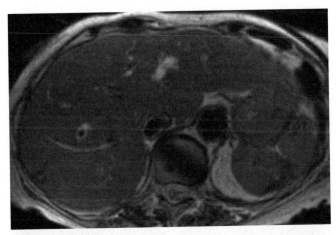

Figure 1.68   A

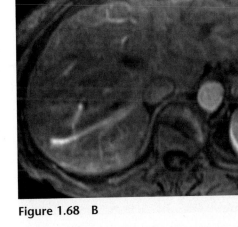

Figure 1.68   B

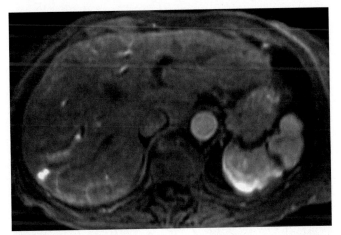

Figure 1.68   C

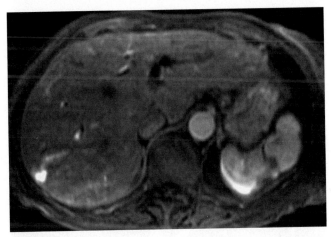

Figure 1.68   D

Findings: Axial T2-WI (A) demonstrates a hypointense lesion at the posterior aspect of the right hepatic lobe. On gadolinium-enhanced, fat-suppressed axial T1-WI (B–D) in the arterial phase, the right hepatic vein enhances rapidly, and there is a strongly enhancing lesion located within the posterior aspect of the right hepatic lobe.

Differential Diagnosis: Hypervascular liver neoplasm, peliosis hepatis.

Diagnosis: Intrahepatic portosystemic shunt (hepatic varix).

Discussion: Several appearances of intrahepatic portosystemic shunts have been described. The most frequently reported intrahepatic portosystemic shunt is between the right portal vein and the IVC. This type of portosystemic shunt typically occurs in the clinical setting of portal hypertension. Other appearances of intrahepatic portosystemic shunts include multiple diffuse communications between peripheral portal and hepatic veins, a single communication between a portal vein branch and a hepatic vein in one hepatic segment, and a single communication between a portal vein branch and a hepatic vein through an aneurysm. Both congenital and acquired causes, such as development of intrahepatic portosystemic collaterals vessels in cirrhotic patients and trauma, have been postulated for intrahepatic portosystemic shunts, but their origin is still not fully understood. On gadolinium-enhanced MRI obtained during the portal venous phase, the communication between a portal vein branch and the hepatic vein can be demonstrated. Another imaging finding is an early and asymmetrical enhancement of a hepatic vein in the late arterial phase, as seen in this case.

Clinical History: 43-year-old woman treated for metastatic breast cancer.

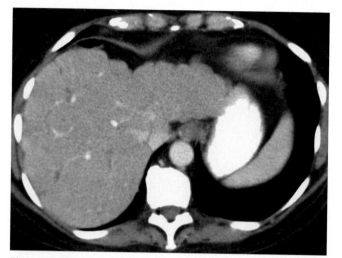

Figure 1.69   A

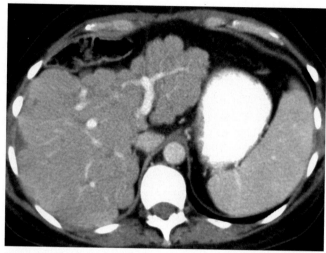

Figure 1.69   B

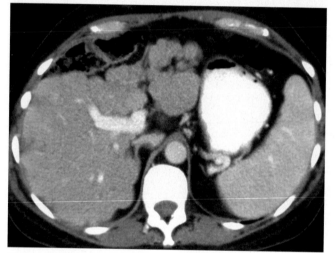

Figure 1.69   C

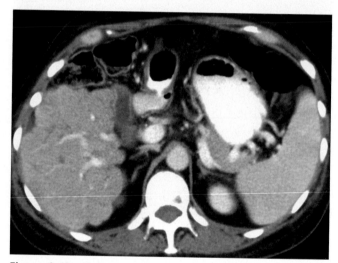

Figure 1.69   D

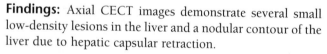

Findings: Axial CECT images demonstrate several small low-density lesions in the liver and a nodular contour of the liver due to hepatic capsular retraction.

Differential Diagnosis: Cirrhosis.

Diagnosis: Pseudocirrhosis in metastatic breast cancer.

Discussion: In patients with hepatic metastases from breast cancer, hepatic capsular retraction occurs adjacent to subcapsular hepatic metastases and is typically seen after treatment with chemotherapy. Although this appearance mimics cirrhosis, most of these patients do not experience the sequelae of portal hypertension, such as variceal bleeding, ascites, and cytopenia. In fact, the pathogenesis of this pseudocirrhotic appearance is not clearly understood; it may result from hepatic infiltration by the metastatic tumor and/or hepatotoxic effects of chemotherapy. Since cirrhosis and pseudocirrhosis due to diffuse metastatic disease of the liver require different clinical management strategies, it is crucial to correlate imaging findings with clinical history to reach an accurate diagnosis.

CASE 1-70

Clinical History: 67-year-old woman who had spinal surgery now presenting with leukocytosis, diarrhea, and elevated alkaline phosphatase level.

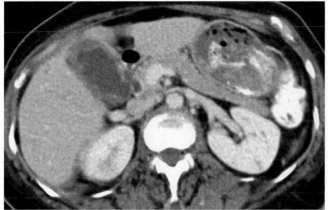

Figure 1.70   A

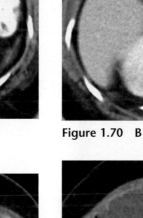

Figure 1.70   B

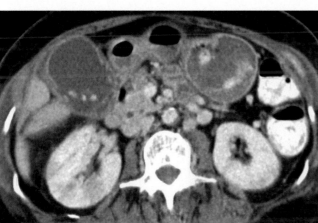

Figure 1.70   C

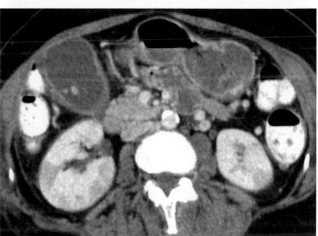

Figure 1.70   D

Findings: Axial CECT images show a thickened and edematous gallbladder wall. There are multiple stones in the gallbladder.

Differential Diagnosis: Gallbladder carcinoma, acute cholecystitis.

Diagnosis: Chronic cholecystitis with cholelithiasis.

Discussion: Chronic cholecystitis has the same causes as the acute form, but why and how cholecystitis becomes chronic has not been fully explained yet. It is believed that when a patient with silent cholelithiasis becomes symptomatic, intermittent cystic duct obstruction and superimposed acute inflammation trigger the chronic changes. Patients with chronic cholecystitis may be asymptomatic or may present with acute cholecystitis episodes. Chronic cholecystitis is a difficult diagnosis to make on imaging, regardless of the technique used. Findings include gallstones and thickening of the gallbladder wall; however, correlation with the clinical findings is critical. An edematous appearance is suggestive for acute exacerbation. Surrounding inflammatory changes in the pericholecystic fat may be absent, and the gallbladder may be normal in size.

Clinical History: 40-year-old woman with alpha-fetoprotein level of 300,000 ng/mL.

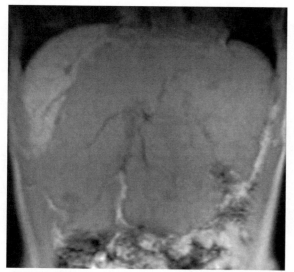

Figure 1.71 A

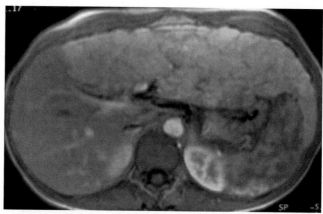

Figure 1.71 B

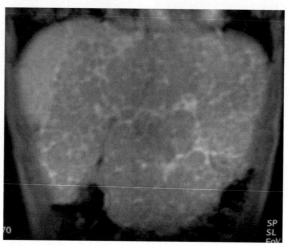

Figure 1.71 C

Findings: Coronal T1-WI (A) shows a large mildly hypointense mass replacing the entire left hepatic lobe. Gadolinium-enhanced axial T1-WI (B) obtained in the arterial phase demonstrates the rapid enhancement of the numerous lesions in the left hepatic lobe. Gadolinium-enhanced coronal T1-WI (C) obtained in the delayed phase shows the washout of the lesions and enhancement of interspersed liver parenchyma.

Differential Diagnosis: Cirrhosis.

Diagnosis: Cirrhotomimetic hepatocellular carcinoma.

Discussion: Cirrhotomimetic or diffuse type hepatocellular carcinoma (HCC) is a subtype of HCC that is composed of multiple tiny indistinct nodules. The prominent clinical feature of patients with cirrhotomimetic HCC is rapid dete-rioration of the general condition terminating in hepatic failure. The liver has a tendency to rapidly enlarge, and this is often accompanied by abdominal pain. It is also known that, in most cases with cirrhotomimetic HCC, the disease is associated with extensive portal venous thrombosis and substantial elevation of alpha-fetoprotein (AFP) level. On unenhanced MRI, the tumor appears as an ill-defined area of abnormal signal intensity compared to the normal liver parenchyma. On T1-WI and T2-WI, cirrhotomimetic HCC is mild to moderately hypointense and hyperintense, respectively. Cirrhotomimetic HCC typically shows a rapid enhancement in arterial phase and a heterogeneous washout on delayed-phase images on gadolinium-enhanced T1-WI, as seen in this case.

Clinical History: 55-year-old woman presenting with progressive abdominal discomfort.

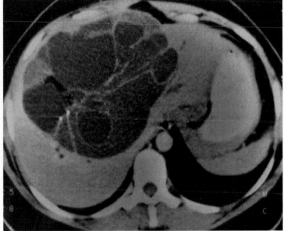

Figure 1.72   A

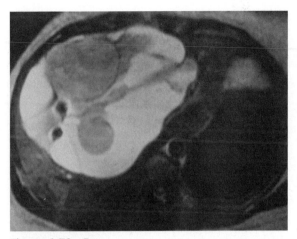

Figure 1.72   B

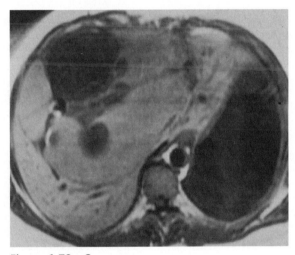

Figure 1.72   C

Findings: Axial CECT image (A) demonstrates a large heterogeneous cystic lesion with enhancing solid parts and internal septations within the liver. The lesion demonstrates predominantly high signal intensity on the axial T2-WI (B) and heterogeneous signal intensity on the axial T1-WI (C).

Differential Diagnosis: Necrotic neoplasm, hepatic abscess, echinococcal cyst.

Diagnosis: Biliary cystadenocarcinoma.

Discussion: Biliary cystadenoma and cystadenocarcinoma are currently considered forms of the same disease, with cystadenocarcinoma being overtly malignant and cystadenoma having malignant potential. Biliary cystadenomas/carcinomas are typically large lesions, which may become up to 30 cm in size; they occur predominantly in middle-aged women. Symptoms are usually related to the mass effect of the lesion and consist of intermittent pain or biliary obstruction. At microscopy, a single layer of mucin-secreting cells lines the cyst wall. The fluid within the tumor can be proteinaceous, mucinous, and occasionally gelatinous, purulent, or hemorrhagic due to trauma. The MRI characteristics of an uncomplicated biliary cystadenoma/cystadenocarcinoma correlate well with the pathologic features. The appearance of the content is typical for a fluid-containing multilocular mass, with homogeneous low signal intensity on T1-WI and homogeneous high signal intensity on T2-WI. A variable signal intensity within the locules of biliary cystadenoma/cystadenocarcinoma, due to differences in protein content, on both T1-WI and T2-WI is reported as an important sign that can be useful in the characterization of a multiseptated hepatic lesion.

Clinical History: 61-year-old woman with acute myelogenous leukemia presenting with fever and neutropenia.

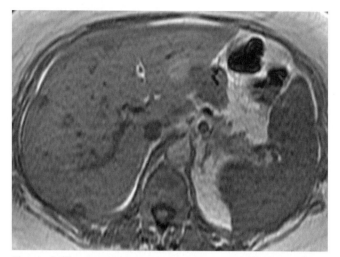

Figure 1.73   A

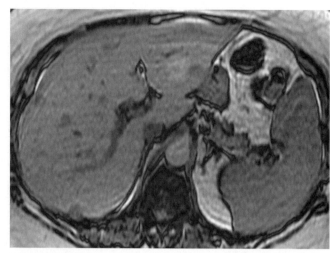

Figure 1.73   B

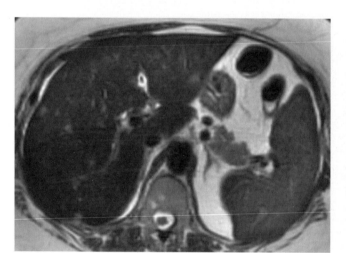

Figure 1.73   C

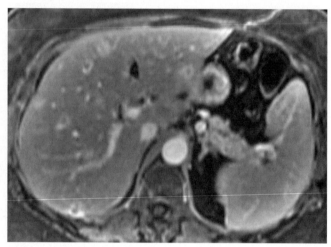

Figure 1.73   D

Findings: Axial T1-WI in-phase (A) and out-of-phase (B) demonstrate multiple hypointense lesions within the liver. On the axial T2-WI (C), the lesions appear hyperintense. On the gadolinium-enhanced, fat-suppressed axial T1-WI (D), the lesions show rimlike or complete enhancement.

Differential Diagnosis: Metastases, leukemia.

Diagnosis: Hepatic candidiasis.

Discussion: Fungal hepatic abscesses typically occur in immunocompromised patients as opportunistic infections; AIDS, leukemia, lymphoma, and intense chemotherapy are among the predisposing conditions. The cause of hepatic manifestation is the hematogenous dissemination of the infectious organism that results in small miliary microabscesses scattered throughout the liver parenchyma. Most hepatic fungal abscesses are caused by *Candida albicans*.

Recent studies have shown that MRI is superior to CT scanning in depicting hepatic fungal involvement. Hepatic fungal lesions have different appearances depending on their presentations. The untreated abscesses are rounded lesions, less than 1 cm in diameter, that are minimally hypointense on T1-WI and gadolinium-enhanced images and markedly hyperintense on T2-WI. In the subacute presentation after treatment, lesions appear mildly to moderately hyperintense on T1-WI and T2-WI and demonstrate enhancement on gadolinium-enhanced images. A dark ring is usually seen around these lesions with all sequences. Completely treated lesions are minimally hypointense on T1-WI, isointense to mildly hyperintense on T2-WI, moderately hypointense on early gadolinium-enhanced images, and minimally hypointense on delayed gadolinium-enhanced images.

CASE 1-74

Clinical History: 49-year-old man with acute myelogenous leukemia and neutropenia.

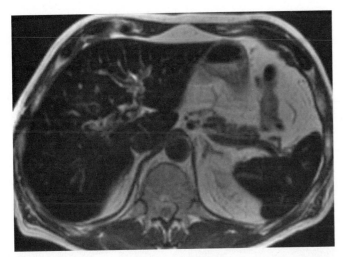

Figure 1.74   A

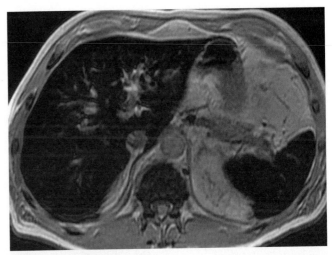

Figure 1.74   B

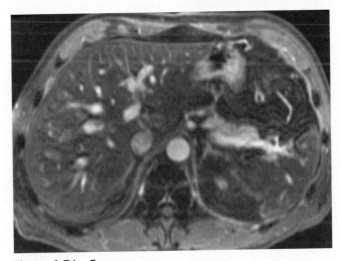

Figure 1.74   C

Findings: The liver, spleen, and bone marrow demonstrate diffuse hypointensity on the axial T2-WI (A) and T1-WI (B). Gadolinium-enhanced, fat-suppressed axial T1-WI (C) shows the decreased signal intensity of the liver and spleen. Note normal signal in the pancreas.

Differential Diagnosis: Primary hemochromatosis.

Diagnosis: Hemosiderosis.

Discussion: Chronic iron overload is characterized by increased focal or generalized deposition of iron within the tissues. On tissue examination, this has been commonly termed hemosiderosis. Primary hemochromatosis is a genetic disorder where the liver is the main organ for abnormal iron deposition (in the hepatocytes), consisting of ferritin and hemosiderin. Patients with hemolytic anemias or who receive multiple blood transfusions also develop iron overload, termed hemosiderosis. Iron from the transfused erythrocytes is deposited in the reticuloendothelial system (RES) in the liver, spleen, and bone marrow. Because the pancreas does not contain an RES, iron is not deposited in this organ in hemosiderosis, as seen in this case. MRI shows a reduction in signal intensity of the affected organs due to the paramagnetic susceptibility of ferritin and ferric ions, which profoundly shorten the T1 and T2 relaxation times of adjacent protons. Signal intensity loss is detected most readily on gradient-echo images.

Clinical History: 72-year-old man with coronary artery disease.

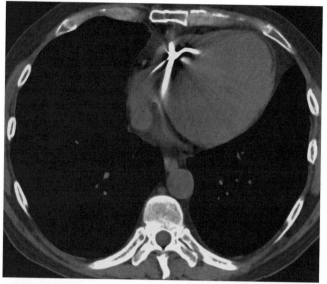

Figure 1.75 A

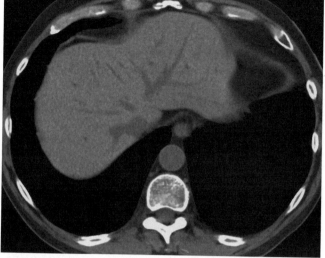

Figure 1.75 B

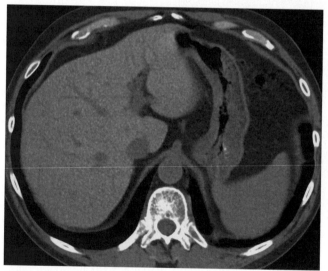

Figure 1.75 C

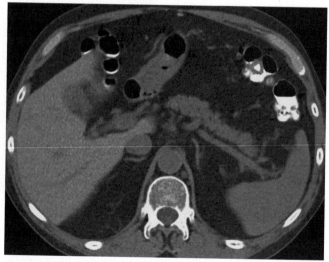

Figure 1.75 D

Findings: Thoracic axial NECT image (A) demonstrates a cardiac pacemaker lead. On hepatic axial NECT images (B–D), the density of the liver is homogeneously increased.

Differential Diagnosis: Primary hemochromatosis, Wilson disease, Thorotrast, methotrexate, gold.

Diagnosis: Hyperdense liver due to amiodarone.

Discussion: The normal liver attenuation on NECT is very similar to spleen, typically less than 10 HU more. Homogeneous increased density of the liver may be due to a variety of different causes including drug toxicity, pri-mary hemochromatosis, hemosiderosis, and cirrhosis. Pharmaceuticals that may cause an increase in liver density on CT include Thorotrast, thallium, gold, methotrexate, and amiodarone. Amiodarone is an antiarrhythmic drug with an iodine content of approximately 40%. During long-term therapy, both the drug and its major metabolite, desethylamiodarone, are deposited in the liver. The accu-mulation of iodine within the liver causes a homogenous increased density of the organ on NECT images. Increased liver density may occur with therapeutic levels of the drug and does not necessarily correlate with amiodarone toxicity.

Clinical History: 73-year-old man with weight loss and abdominal pain.

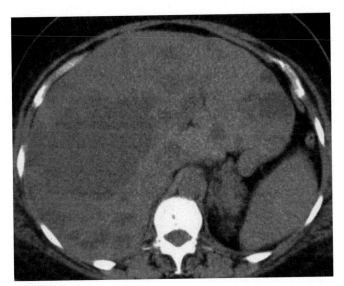

Figure 1.76 A

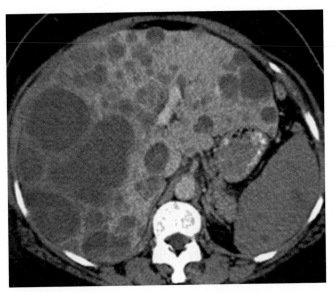

Figure 1.76 B

Findings: Axial NECT image (A) shows multiple hypodense lesions throughout the liver. On the axial CECT image (B), the lesions show ring-shaped peripheral enhancement. There are multiple lesions in the spleen as well.

Differential Diagnosis: Hemangiomatosis, hepatocellular carcinoma, metastases, lymphoma.

Diagnosis: Diffuse angiosarcoma.

Discussion: Angiosarcoma is a rare neoplasm that occurs most frequently in males in the seventh decade of life. Angiosarcoma is 30 times less common than HCC and is associated with previous exposure to toxins, such as Thorotrast, vinyl chloride, arsenicals, and steroids. Clinically, patients frequently present with generalized weakness, weight loss, abdominal pain, hepatomegaly, and ascites. There are two gross patterns of growth: multifocal or multinodular lesions (71%) or a large solitary mass. Nodules typically range in size from a few millimeters to over 5 cm. When there is no evidence of Thorotrast deposition, angiosarcomas present with single or multiple masses that are hypodense on unenhanced CT scans except for hyperdense areas of fresh hemorrhage. In case of rupture of a hepatic angiosarcoma, the diagnosis is made by demonstrating free intraperitoneal fluid and a focal high-density area adjacent to the tumor, the latter representing acute blood clot. Although centripetal enhancement with contrast material can be seen mimicking a hemangioma, in most cases, angiosarcomas have imaging features that are atypical for hemangiomas, such as peripheral ring-shaped enhancement or focal areas of enhancement that show less attenuation than the aorta.

Clinical History: 65-year-old man with history of cirrhosis.

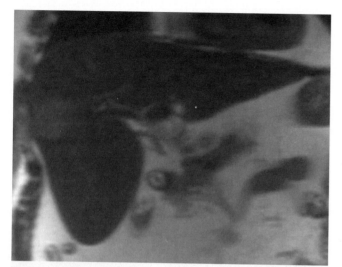

Figure 1.77 A

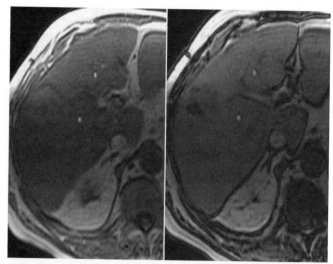

Figure 1.77 B

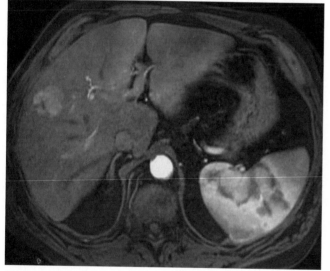

Figure 1.77 C

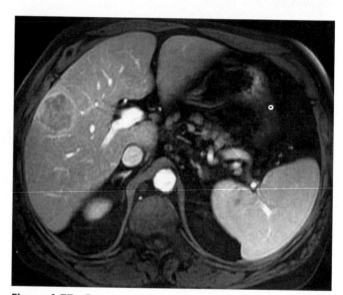

Figure 1.77 D

Findings: Coronal T2-WI (A) shows a mildly hyperintense lesion in right hepatic lobe. The lesion is slightly hyperintense on the in-phase T1-WI (B, left). On the out-of-phase T1-WI, the lesion shows a drop in signal (B, right). After the administration of gadolinium, the lesion shows rapid enhancement in the arterial-phase, gadolinium-enhanced, fat-suppressed axial T1-WI (C) and washout with rim enhancement on the delayed enhanced images (D).

Differential Diagnosis: Metastasis.

Diagnosis: HCC with fatty metamorphosis.

Discussion: Fatty change is frequently seen in histologic specimens of hepatocellular carcinoma (HCC). In fact, fatty metamorphosis can be seen in up to 35% of small HCCs (<1.5 cm) fatty change seen in small HCCs is usually diffuse. HCCs larger than 1.5 cm typically demonstrate a patchy fatty change pattern. HCCs containing fat appear hyperintense on in-phase T1-WI. Nevertheless, hyperintensity of HCC on T1-WI is due not exclusively to fat content of the tumor but also to other causes such as hemorrhage and excessive copper accumulation. Chemical shift imaging has been found useful to detect the presence of fat in HCCs. Fat-containing HCCs exhibit high signal intensity on in-phase T1-WI, and signals drop on out-of-phase T1-WI, as seen in this case.

CASE 1-78

Clinical History: 45-year-old man with colorectal carcinoma.

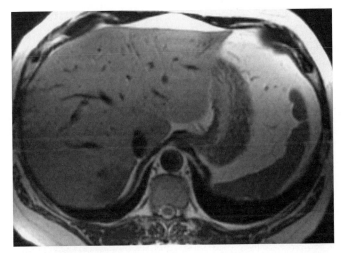

Figure 1.78   A

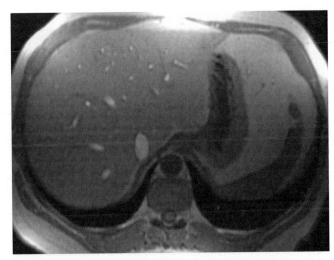

Figure 1.78   B

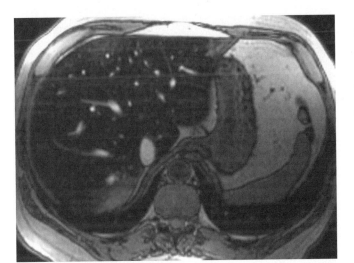

Figure 1.78   C

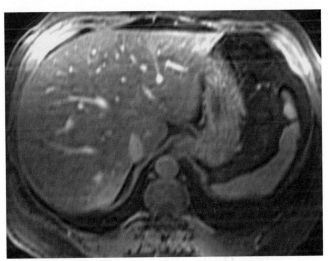

Figure 1.78   D

Findings: Axial T2-WI (A) shows two slightly hyperintense areas within the posterior aspect of the right lobe and left lobe of the liver. These areas are isointense with the liver parenchyma on in-phase T1-WI (B). On the out-of-phase T1-WI (C) and gadolinium-enhanced, fat-suppressed axial T1-WI (D), these areas appear hyperintense in comparison with the liver parenchyma.

Differential Diagnosis: Hypervascular liver lesions.

Diagnosis: Focal fatty sparing within a steatotic liver.

Discussion: Focal fatty change of the liver is a well-recognized entity that usually occurs in segments IV and V,

adjacent to the porta hepatis, adjacent the fissure for the falciform ligament, in the gallbladder fossa, or in the subcapsular region. Occasionally, focal fatty sparing has a nodular configuration and occurs outside of these typical locations. In such cases and especially in a liver with diffuse steatosis, areas of focal fatty sparing can be misinterpreted as focal tumoral lesions. Gradient-echo in-phase T1-WI shows hyperintense liver parenchyma due to fatty change with a hypointense area representing focal fatty sparing. On out-of-phase gradient-echo images, steatotic liver parenchyma loses signal, and focal fatty sparing remains hyperintense.

Clinical History: 77-year-old man, with a history of colon cancer and cirrhosis, who underwent treatment with radio-frequency ablation for a liver mass histopathologically diagnosed as hepatocellular carcinoma.

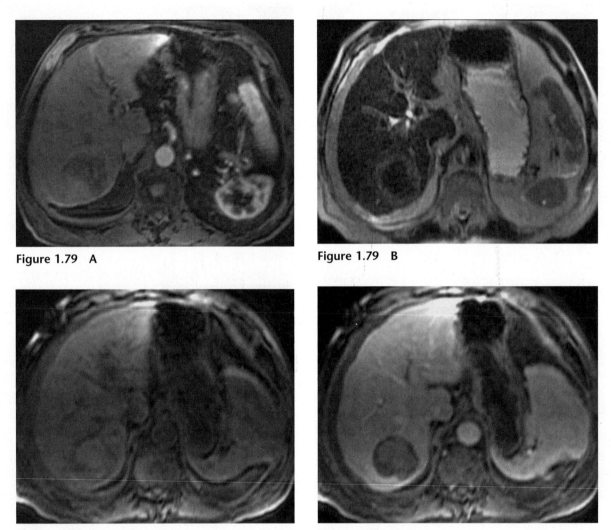

Figure 1.79 A

Figure 1.79 B

Figure 1.79 C

Figure 1.79 D

Findings: Pretreatment, gadolinium-enhanced, fat-suppressed axial T1-WI (A) shows an enhancing mass in the posterior aspect of the right lobe of the liver. On posttreatment axial T2-WI (B), the ablation area is hypointense and has a surrounding hyperintense rim. On the fat-suppressed axial T1-WI (C), the ablation area appears hyperintense with a hypointense surrounding rim. On the gadolinium-enhanced, fat-suppressed axial T1-WI (D), there is no evidence for residual enhancing viable tumor.

Differential Diagnosis: None.

Diagnosis: Coagulation necrosis in a hepatocellular carcinoma secondary to radiofrequency ablation.

Discussion: Radiofrequency ablation causes coagulation necrosis that typically has an intermediate to high signal intensity relative to the liver parenchyma on T1-WI and low signal intensity on T2-WI. Edema due to the thermal injury appears as a hyperintense rim around the ablation area on T2-WI and as a hypointense rim on T1-WI. In fact, a recently ablated area may demonstrate an atypical signal intensity pattern on T1-WI and T2-WI because of the presence of hemorrhage and necrosis. In general, any area of hypointensity on T1-WI or hyperintensity on T2-WI is suspicious for residual or recurrent tumor and should be further investigated with gadolinium-enhanced MRI. On gadolinium-enhanced MRI, the ablated area remains unenhanced except for an enhancing thin rim that represents peripheral hyperemia. Residual or recurrent tumor tissue appears as an enhancing nodular area.

Clinical History: 56-year-old woman with breast cancer imaged with CT for follow-up.

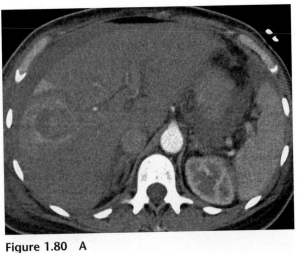

Figure 1.80   A

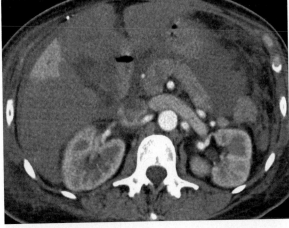

Figure 1.80   B

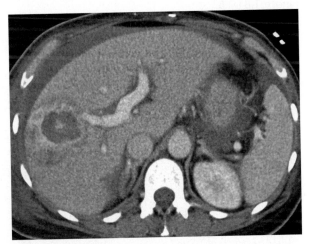

Figure 1.80   C

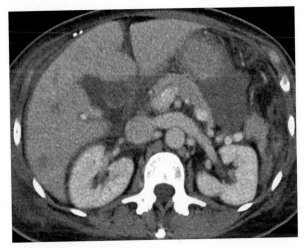

Figure 1.80   D

Findings: Axial CECT images obtained during the arterial phase (A and B) show a heterogeneously enhancing lesion in the right lobe of the liver. Note the triangular area of hyperenhancement peripherally to the tumor; this area has straight, nonspherical boundaries, and a linear nonenhancing structure is seen centrally. On the portal venous phase CECT images (C and D), the triangular area showing arterial enhancement becomes isodense with the rest of the liver parenchyma.

Differential Diagnosis: None.

Diagnosis: Transient hepatic attenuation difference due to breast cancer metastasis.

Discussion: It is well known that malignant liver tumors tend to invade the portal venous system and, to a lesser extent, the hepatic veins. Portal vein thrombosis (PVT) associated with a malignant liver tumor occurs when the tumor extends into the portal vein branches that supply the

involved hepatic segments or lobe. PVT is associated with two kinds of hepatic perfusion anomalies. First, a transient hepatic attenuation difference (THAD) during the late hepatic arterial phase might be present. The reason for this anomaly is thought to be an increase in the attenuation of segments with a dominant arterial flow due to their poor perfusion by the thrombosed portal vein branches. The hyperattenuated areas have straight boundaries, and lack of masslike margins can often be seen during the arterial phase of dynamic contrast-enhanced CT or MRI. Typically, the perfusion anomaly disappears during the portal venous phase. In some cases, depiction of the thrombosed peripheral portal branch is possible in the center of the THAD area. A second type of perfusion anomaly seen with peripheral portal vein thrombosis includes a diminished enhancement of the involved liver segments during the portal venous phase due to locally decreased portal vein perfusion.

Clinical History: 30-year-old man presenting with elevated liver enzymes.

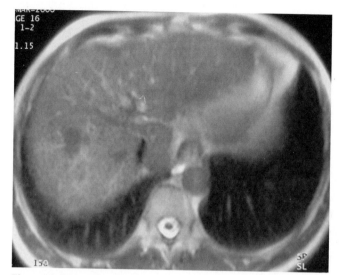

Figure 1.81 A

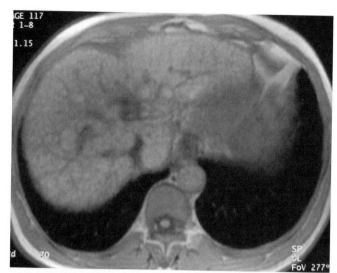

Figure 1.81 B

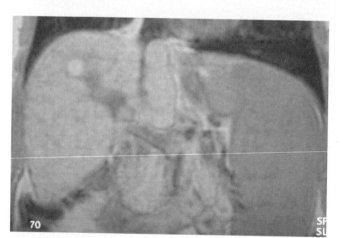

Figure 1.81 C

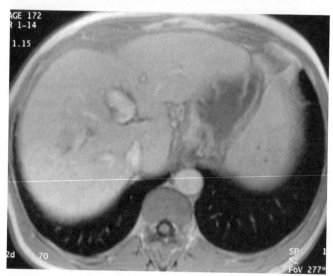

Figure 1.81 D

Findings: On axial T2-WI (A), there is a hypointense lesion within the right hepatic lobe. On the axial (B) and coronal (C) T1-WI, the lesion appears hyperintense. On gadolinium-enhanced axial T1-WI (D), the lesion shows no predominant arterial enhancement.

Differential Diagnosis: Alcoholic cirrhosis, hepatitis-induced cirrhosis.

Diagnosis: Wilson disease.

Discussion: Wilson disease, or hepatolenticular degeneration, is an autosomal recessive disorder of copper metabolism. In Wilson disease, impaired biliary excretion of copper results in accumulation of toxic levels of copper in the liver, cornea (in the form of Kayser-Fleischer rings), and brain. In the liver, copper deposition occurs in the periportal regions and along the hepatic sinusoids and triggers an inflammatory reaction. The inflammatory reaction causes episodes of acute hepatitis and associated fatty change and periportal inflammation. Chronic active hepatitis occurs subsequently, with cyclic changes invoking fibrosis and eventual cirrhosis. On one hand, CT may show fatty changes that are, in fact, indistinguishable from those of cirrhosis or other pathologic conditions. On the other hand, the copper deposition may result in diffuse increased attenuation values on CT due to high atomic number of copper. Ionic copper deposition appears hypointense on T2-WI and hyperintense on T1-WI, as seen in this case.

Clinical History: 44-year-old woman with history of carcinoid tumor presenting with right upper quadrant pain following hepatic chemoembolization.

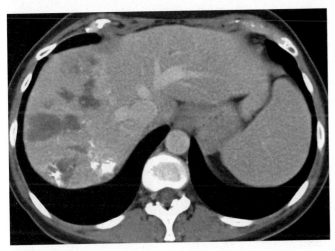

Figure 1.82   A

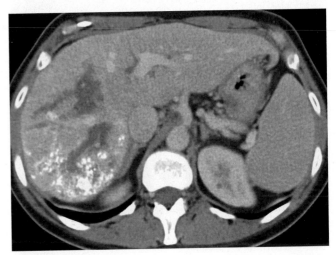

Figure 1.82   B

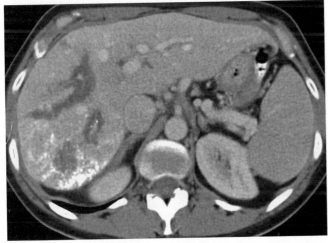

Figure 1.82   C

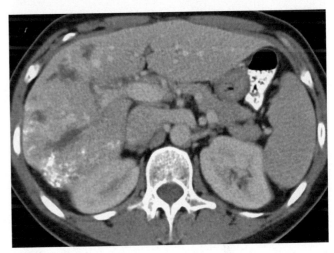

Figure 1.82   D

Findings: Axial CECT images demonstrate multiple hyperdense metastases that were treated with lipiodol-based solution during chemoembolization. In addition, there are tubular low-density areas along the portal vein branches in the right hepatic lobe.

Differential Diagnosis: Bile duct obstruction.

Diagnosis: Bile duct necrosis.

Discussion: Transcatheter arterial chemoembolization (TACE) has been frequently used to treat malignant tumors of the liver. Bile duct injury is one of the complications of TACE. It has been suggested that repeated TACE procedures may induce ischemic bile duct injuries. In contrast to the normal liver parenchyma, the intrahepatic bile ducts do not have a dual blood supply and are fed exclusively from the hepatic arterial branches that give off a vascular plexus around the bile ducts. Thus, ischemia of the intrahepatic bile ducts can easily occur after chemoembolization. The necrosis of the bile duct wall eventually leads to extravasation of bile; extravasated bile can track along the low-resistance connective tissue sheaths of the Glisson's capsule that surrounds the portal triads. According to one theory, the dilated bile ducts and the extravasated fluid in the Glisson's capsule can gradually compress and compromise the adjacent portal vein branches. CT findings of bile duct injury include linear or branching low-attenuating areas suggestive of bile duct dilatation with or without extravasation of bile along the portal tracts. Localized periportal tracking, that is, bilateral linear low-attenuating areas alongside the portal vein, due to gradual narrowing of the portal veins can also be revealed on CECT images.

Clinical History: 57-year-old man with history of longstanding alcohol abuse.

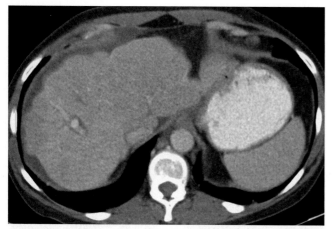

Figure 1.83   A

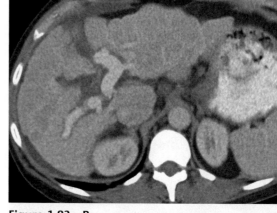

Figure 1.83   B

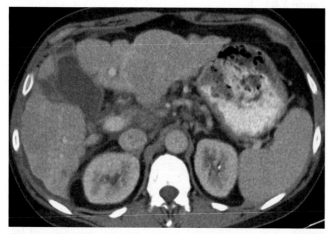

Figure 1.83   C

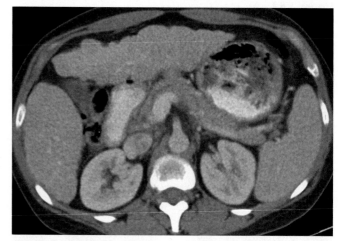

Figure 1.83   D

Findings: Axial CECT images show a nodular liver contour, hypertrophy of the left lateral segment and caudate lobe, and atrophy of the left medial segment and anterior segment of the right hepatic lobe.

Differential Diagnosis: Pseudocirrhosis, Budd-Chiari syndrome.

Diagnosis: Cirrhosis.

Discussion: Cirrhosis is a chronic disease of the liver that can be caused by a variety of etiologies, with alcohol being the most common in the United States. Other etiologies include hepatitis, inheritable diseases such as Wilsons disease, tyrosinemia, glycogen-storage disease, primary biliary cirrhosis, primary sclerosing cholangitis, and chronic right-sided heart failure. There are many CT findings in cirrhosis. This case demonstrates an enlarged caudate lobe. There are several theories for this finding. One suggests that the fibrosis and regeneration of the liver impairs the normal venous drainage, leading to atrophy. This process affects the caudate lobe less than the rest of the liver, because the caudate lobe has a separate drainage into the IVC. Therefore, blood is preferentially shunted to the caudate lobe, causing it to hypertrophy while the rest of the liver atrophies. Budd-Chiari syndrome can also cause caudate lobe hypertrophy by the same mechanism, but no other findings of Budd-Chiari are seen in this patient. Pseudocirrhosis causes the same morphologic changes as cirrhosis, but the patient is not known to have metastatic liver disease, especially from breast cancer.

CASE 1-84

Clinical History: 35-year-old woman who is taking oral contraceptives.

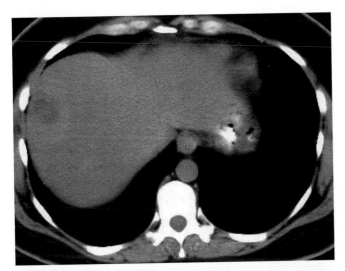

Figure 1.84   A

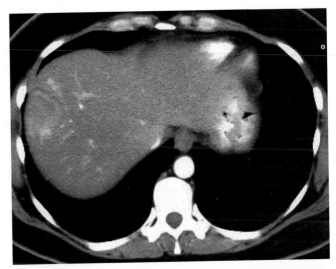

Figure 1.84   B

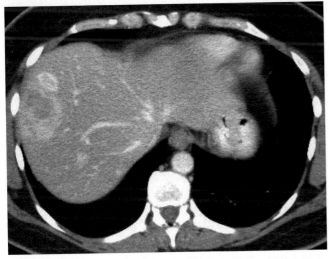

Figure 1.84   C

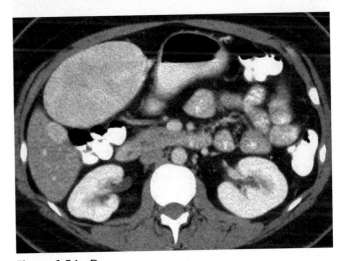

Figure 1.84   D

Findings: Axial NECT image (A) demonstrates a subcapsular lesion in the right lobe of the liver that has mixed high and low attenuation. Axial CECT images (B–D) show several heterogeneous hypervascular masses in the liver. The largest lesion is exophytically located in segment IV.

Differential Diagnosis: Focal nodular hyperplasia, hepatocellular carcinoma, metastases.

Diagnosis: Hepatocellular adenoma.

Discussion: Hepatocellular adenoma is a benign neoplasm of the liver composed of sheets of hepatocytes without veins or ducts. Typically, adenomas are solitary (80%). Oral contraceptive use is thought to lead to the development of adenomas as well as increase the risk for hemorrhage by the tumor. Although seen predominantly in females of childbearing age, males on anabolic steroids also have an increased risk. Glycogen storage disease is typically associated with multiple hepatocellular adenomas. Large adenomas are usually heterogeneous since they outgrow their blood supply and eventually hemorrhage or necrose. This case is somewhat unusual in that the large adenoma in segment IV still shows homogeneous enhancement. Areas of fat can also be found in adenomas. These hypervascular lesions could be focal nodular hyperplasia (FNH), although no central scar is seen, and FNH tend to enhance homogeneously. A hepatocellular carcinoma would be less likely because no cirrhosis or peritumoral halo is seen. The age and sex of the patient and the history of oral contraceptive use make hepatocellular adenoma the best choice. Further differentiation between adenoma and FNH could be done with a sulfur-colloid study or ferumoxides-enhanced MRI, since adenomas typically do not contain Kupffer cells.

Clinical History: 27-year-old man involved in a motor vehicle accident.

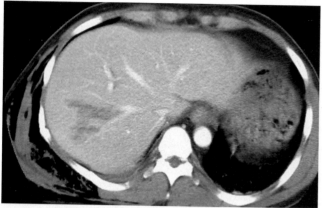

Figure 1.85   A

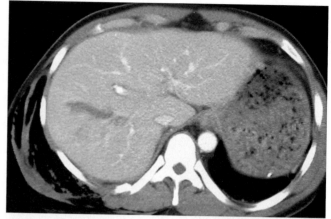

Figure 1.85   B

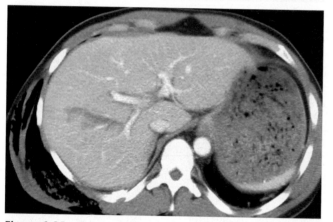

Figure 1.85   C

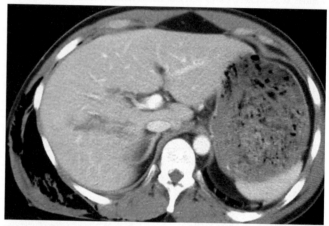

Figure 1.85   D

Findings: Axial CECT images demonstrate a linear low-attenuation area in the right hepatic lobe. Note right-sided rib fractures and subcutaneous emphysema.

Differential Diagnosis: None.

Diagnosis: Hepatic laceration.

Discussion: The liver is the most frequently injured abdominal organ in blunt trauma. Hepatic injuries occur in 3% to 10% of patients sustaining blunt abdominal trauma. CT is currently the diagnostic modality of choice for the evaluation of blunt liver trauma. Parenchymal liver injuries can be accurately detected on CECT scans. Hepatic parenchymal injuries can be categorized by CT as contusions, subcapsular and parenchymal hematomas, linear or stellate lacerations, and hepatic fractures. Hepatic lacerations are the most common type of parenchymal liver injury and appear as irregular linear or branching low-attenuation areas on CECT. Laceration of a major hepatic vein is a CT finding that indicates increased morbidity and the need for more aggressive management. Sonography has a limited role in initial diagnostic evaluation of hepatic trauma, but it may be useful in follow-up of patients who are treated conservatively. US and CT can also be used in diagnosing post-traumatic complications, such as hepatic or perihepatic abscesses or bilomas. The presence of rib fractures and subcutaneous emphysema are clues to the traumatic etiology of the liver abnormality.

CASE 1-86

Clinical History: 32-year-old woman referred to the hospital because of increasing right upper quadrant pain and back pain but no fever.

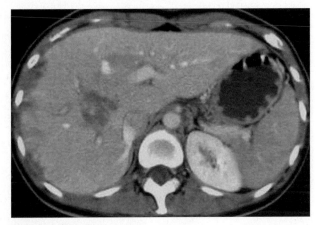

Figure 1.86   A

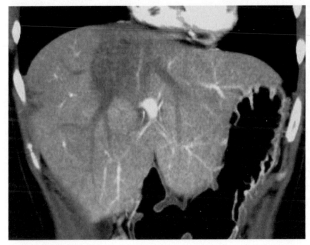

Figure 1.86   B

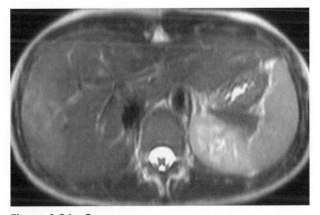

Figure 1.86   C

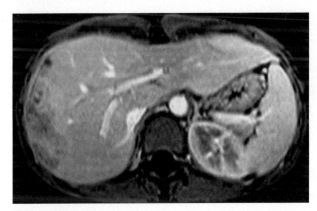

Figure 1.86   D

Findings: Axial (A) and coronal (B) CECT images show ill-defined low-attenuation areas in a subcapsular location. Note the linear appearance of some of the lesions. Axial T2-WI (C) shows the subcapsular lesions to be mildly hyperintense. Gadolinium-enhanced, fat-suppressed axial T1-WI (D) shows heterogeneous enhancement of the subcapsular area.

Differential Diagnosis: Metastases.

Diagnosis: Hepatic fascioliasis.

Discussion: Fascioliasis is a parasitic infection caused by *Fasciola hepatica*. The disease mainly involves the hepatobiliary system and manifests in two stages: the hepatic (acute, invasive) stage and the biliary (chronic, obstructive) stage. Cholestasis, obstructive jaundice, and recurrent cholangitis may be encountered in the biliary stage. Given the nonspecific nature of presenting signs and symptoms, such as abdominal pain, fever, and eosinophilia, fascioliasis can be confused with a wide spectrum of hepatobiliary diseases, and the diagnosis and treatment of human fascioliasis is, therefore, frequently delayed. Although serologic confirmation is mandatory for a final diagnosis, radiologic imaging plays a pivotal role in the detection and characterization of fascioliasis since some radiologic findings are quite specific. Reported CT imaging features include single or multiple hypodense nodular areas or tunnel-like branching or tortuous peripheral hypodensities that are the result of parasite migration though the liver; the presence of the latter are highly suggestive of the disease. In particular, the majority of migrating immature flukes become trapped in the immediate subcapsular tissues of the liver where they die, leaving a cavity filled with necrotic debris. As the parasite penetrates the Glisson's capsule, capsular hyperintensity on T2-WI or enhancement of the capsule in CT or MRI may be seen as an inflammatory response.

Case images courtesy of Dr. Manuel Fernandez, Clinica Las Condes, Santiago, Chile.

Clinical History: 68-year-old man with a history of malignant pleural mesothelioma and radiotherapy.

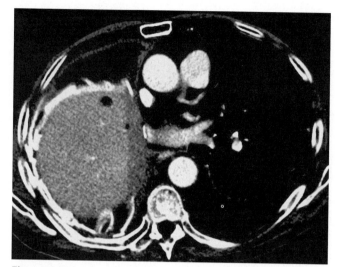

Figure 1.87   A

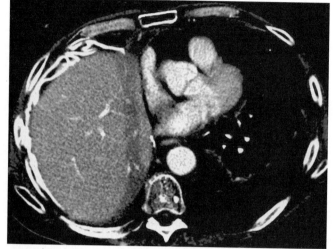

Figure 1.87   B

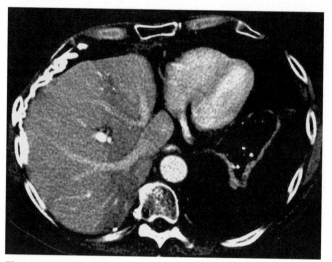

Figure 1.87   C

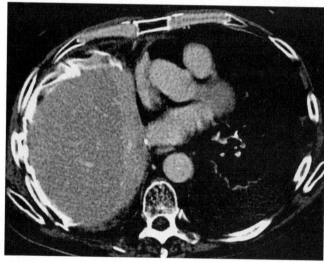

Figure 1.87   D

Findings: Axial early-phase CECT images (A–C) demonstrate a sharp linear area of low density within the medial portion of the liver. This area shows some degree of late enhancement (D). The well-circumscribed, round, low-density lesions are consistent with simple cysts. There is evidence of right extrapleural pneumonectomy with diaphragmatic reconstruction.

Differential Diagnosis: Metastatic disease.

Diagnosis: Radiation injury to liver.

Discussion: Radiation-induced liver disease, also known as radiation hepatitis, has been reported after a threshold dose of 30 to 35 Gy in adults. Histopathologically, two stages of radiation-induced liver disease have been defined: an acute phase, which occurs within 3 months after exposure and is characterized by sinusoidal congestion, hyperemia, and diffuse fatty change; and a later chronic phase in which fibrosis of the portal tract and disorganization of the lobular architecture occur. In acute radiation-induced liver injury, CT often demonstrates a nonspherical area of low attenuation with well-defined, linear borders. However, if the underlying liver tissue shows fatty change, the irradiated portion of the liver may appear hyperattenuating relative to the background fatty liver. The enhancement pattern after administration of intravenous contrast material is heterogeneous and variable. The irradiated portion of the liver may enhance during the arterial phase or during the delayed phase.

Clinical History: 50-year-old woman with recent history of liver biopsy.

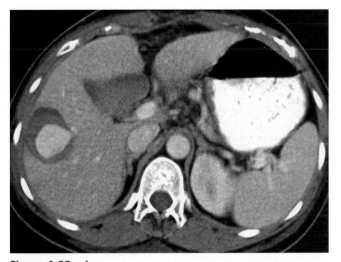

Figure 1.88   A

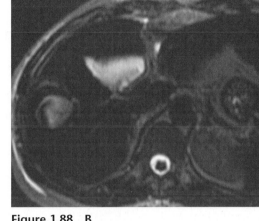

Figure 1.88   B

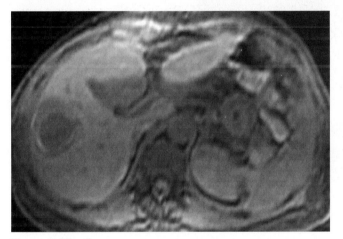

Figure 1.88   C

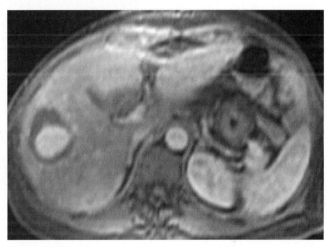

Figure 1.88   D

Findings: Axial CECT image (A) shows a lesion with focal central area of high attenuation and concentric outer rings of lower attenuation. The center of the lesion is hyperintense on the axial T2-WI (B) and hypointense on fat-suppressed axial T1-WI (C) and enhances strongly on the gadolinium-enhanced, fat-suppressed axial T1-WI (D).

Differential Diagnosis: None.

Diagnosis: Right hepatic artery pseudoaneurysm after liver biopsy.

Discussion: Hepatic artery pseudoaneurysms can be classified, according to their location, as intrahepatic or extrahepatic. Intrahepatic pseudoaneurysms are mostly related to previous procedures, such as liver biopsy and percutaneous

transhepatic biliary drainage. The most important risk factor for extrahepatic pseudoaneurysms is local sepsis, which is frequently associated with the formation of a Roux-en-Y hepaticojejunostomy. The latter creates the potential for colonization of the subhepatic space by enteric organisms. Clinical symptoms include right upper quadrant pain, hemobilia, gastrointestinal bleeding, intermittent jaundice, and bleeding from surgical drains. An abdominal mass with bruit may be detected on physical examination. The diagnosis can be made via CECT, US, MRI, or arteriography. Early enhancement of a round lesion that communicates with blood vessels on a CECT or MRI study is diagnostic in the proper clinical setting.

Clinical History: 35-year-old woman referred to CT because of an abnormal abdominal sonogram.

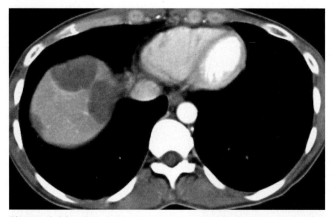

Figure 1.89   A

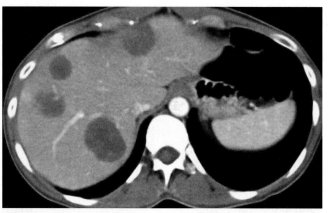

Figure 1.89   B

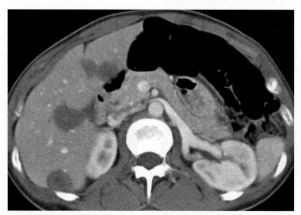

Figure 1.89   C

Findings: Axial CECT images demonstrate multiple hypodense lesions peripherally located in the liver. The lesions have a target appearance and cause capsular retraction.

Differential Diagnosis: Multiple abscesses, lymphoma, multiple metastases.

Diagnosis: Epithelial hemangioendothelioma.

Discussion: Epithelial hemangioendothelioma (EHE) is a rare malignant hepatic neoplasm of vascular origin. It develops in adults and should not be confused with infantile hemangioendothelioma, which occurs in young children. Some authors consider EHE an intermediate between hemangioma and angiosarcoma. Like hemangioma, EHE occurs more frequently in women than men. EHE is usually diagnosed incidentally; however, symptoms such as jaundice and liver failure may be present. EHEs appear as multiple nodules that grow, coalesce, and eventually form large confluent masses. Capsular retraction has been reported in 25% to 69% of cases. On NECT images, EHE is of low attenuation, corresponding to the presence of myxoid stroma. Portions of these large, low-attenuation masses may become isodense to the liver parenchyma after administration of contrast material, and therefore, it is often easier to identify the extent of the disease on unenhanced scans. A target sign of concentric zones may be seen on CT or MRI and is due to the presence of a central area of hemorrhage, coagulation necrosis, and calcifications and a peripheral region of cellular proliferation and edema.

Clinical History: 88-year-old man presenting with weight loss and right upper quadrant pain.

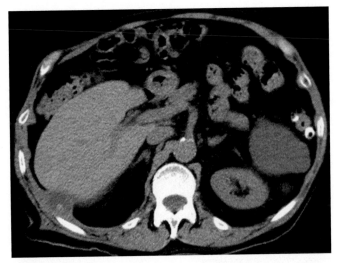

Figure 1.90   A

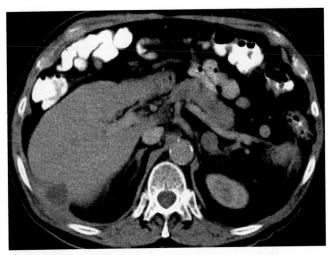

Figure 1.90   B

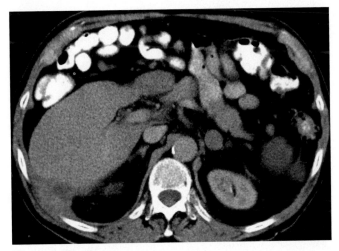

Figure 1.90   C

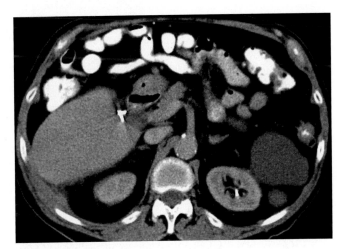

Figure 1.90   D

Findings: Axial NECT (A) and CECT (B–D) images show a lesion with a hypodense center abutting the posterior aspect of the liver and the right chest wall, with surrounding soft tissue thickening. There is a small hyperdense structure within the collection (A).

Differential Diagnosis: None.

Diagnosis: Dropped gallstone with abscess formation.

Discussion: Laparoscopy has become the procedure of choice for routine cholecystectomy. Despite the fact that the overall complication rate of the procedure is less than that observed with open cholecystectomy, there are two complications occurring more frequently at laparoscopy. One of them is bile duct injury or bile leakage, and the other is late infection due to dropped gallstones. If a spilled stone is retained in the abdominal cavity, recurrent intra-abdominal abscess may occur as a delayed complication. The diagnosis of dropped gallstone after laparoscopic cholecystectomy is important because simple abscess drainage or antibiotics therapy is typically not enough to treat such cases. In fact, surgical or percutaneous stone removal is essential for complete cure. In a patient with a recurrent intra-abdominal abscess, a history of laparoscopic cholecystectomy, and a hyperdense structure within a perihepatic collection on CT, the diagnosis of dropped gallstones should be rendered.

Clinical History: 50-year-old woman presenting right upper quadrant pain, nausea, and vomiting.

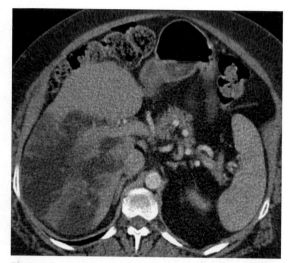

Figure 1.91   A

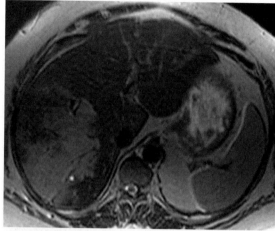

Figure 1.91   B

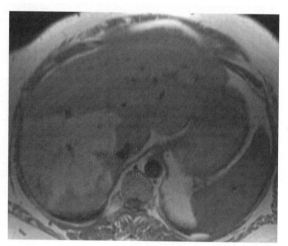

Figure 1.91   C

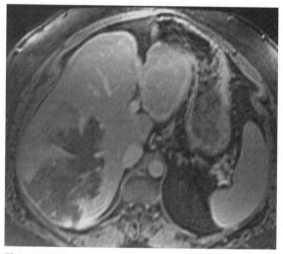

Figure 1.91   D

Findings: Axial CECT image (A) shows a large hypodense lesion in the right hepatic lobe. On the T2-WI (B) and T1-WI (C), the lesion appears hyperintense relatively to the normal liver parenchyma and has blood vessels coursing through it. The gadolinium-enhanced, fat-suppressed axial T1-WI (D) demonstrates signal drop in the lesion.

Differential Diagnosis: Alcoholic steatohepatitis, hepatocellular carcinoma.

Diagnosis: Nonalcoholic steatohepatitis.

Discussion: Nonalcoholic fatty liver disease (NAFLD) is a condition characterized by significant lipid deposition in the hepatocytes of a patient without a history of excessive alcohol ingestion. Histopathologic findings of NAFLD vary from steatosis alone to steatosis with inflammation, necrosis, and fibrosis. At the most severe end of the NAFLD continuum resides nonalcoholic steatohepatitis (NASH), with or without cirrhosis. Histopathologic findings of NASH include steatosis (predominately macrovesicular), mixed lobular inflammation, and hepatocellular ballooning. Unlike steatosis alone, NASH may progress to cirrhosis. NASH lowers liver parenchyma attenuation on NECT and can be diagnosed when hepatic attenuation is 10 HU or more lower than splenic attenuation. On MRI, the steatotic liver segments appear hyperintense on both T1-WI and T2-WI. Out-of-phase images demonstrate the typical signal decrease. In cases of mild involvement of the liver by NASH, diffuse fatty change is the only detectable imaging feature. Differentiation between NASH and a hepatic neoplasm is possible by the nonspherical shape of NASH and the absence of vascular invasion or distortion.

Clinical History: 53-year-old woman with an incidental liver finding on US performed for investigation of lower abdominal pain.

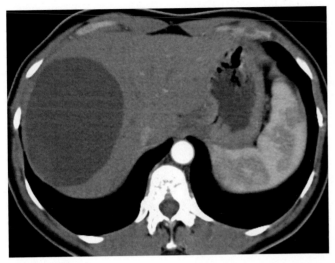

Figure 1.92   A

Figure 1.92   B

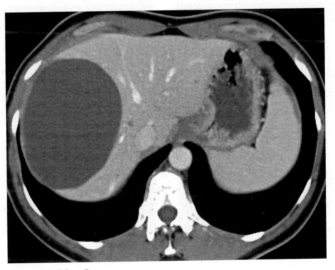

Figure 1.92   C

Findings: Axial CECT images obtained during the arterial (A), portal venous (B), and delayed (C) phases after contrast administration show a homogeneous cystic mass of water density in the right hepatic lobe. The mass does not show any enhancement.

Differential Diagnosis: Biliary cystadenoma, abscess.

Diagnosis: Bile duct cyst.

Discussion: Simple cysts are among the most common liver lesions; they are presumed to be present in 2.5% of the population. Simple cysts are thought to be benign developmental lesions that do not communicate with the biliary tree. Histopathologically, hepatic cysts contain serous fluid and are lined by a nearly imperceptible wall consisting of cuboidal epithelium. The presence of thick walls or enhancing internal components suggests the diagnosis of hepatic abscess or biliary cystadenoma rather than a simple cyst. A hepatic cyst appears as a homogeneous and hypoattenuating lesion on NECT images, with no enhancement of its wall or content after intravenous administration of contrast material. It is typically round or ovoid in shape and well defined.

CASE 1-93

Clinical History: 49-year-old woman with colon cancer (presenting with fever) after radiofrequency ablation and segmental right lobe resection of liver metastasis.

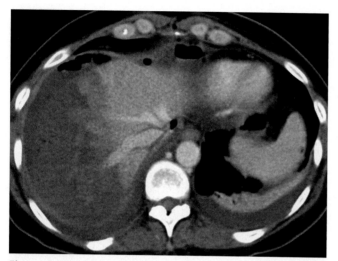

Figure 1.93   A

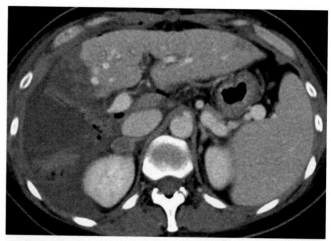

Figure 1.93   B

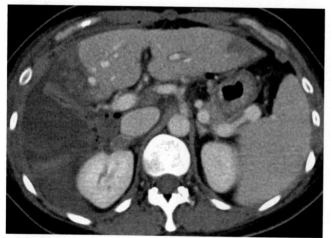

Figure 1.93   C

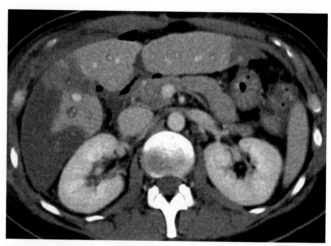

Figure 1.93   D

Findings: Axial CECT images demonstrate a diffuse area of low attenuation within segments V to VIII of the right lobe of the liver. Note lack of enhancement of the right portal vein and right hepatic artery. In addition, there is capsular disruption with an air-fluid level in the peritoneal space, a right-sided pleural effusion, gas bubbles in the right hepatic lobe, and low-density lesions in the left hepatic lobe.

Differential Diagnosis: Diffuse metastatic disease, diffuse hepatocellular carcinoma.

Diagnosis: Hepatic infarction due to right portal vein and right hepatic artery thrombosis.

Discussion: Hepatic infarction is thought to be a rare process because of the dual blood supply to the liver from the portal vein and hepatic artery. Although this is true, infarctions can be seen when either a portal branch or hepatic arterial branch is occluded, especially with coexistent hepatic outflow obstruction. Moreover, when both the hepatic arterial and portal venous supply to a segment of the liver is absent, the liver is likely to infarct, as seen in this case. The areas of infarction are usually hypodense and do not demonstrate enhancement with contrast. They appear either well circumscribed and wedge shaped, as is seen in this example, or ill defined and diffuse. Causes of hepatic infarction include emboli (usually from the heart), occlusion of the hepatic artery or portal vein from an infiltrating neoplasm, thrombosis of the hepatic artery, atherosclerosis, vasculitis, or iatrogenic causes.

Clinical History: 34-year-old man with acute myelogenous leukemia (AML) presenting with abnormal liver function tests and diarrhea 32 days after bone marrow transplantation.

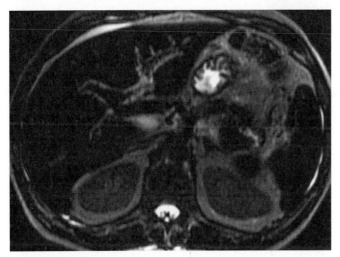

Figure 1.94 A

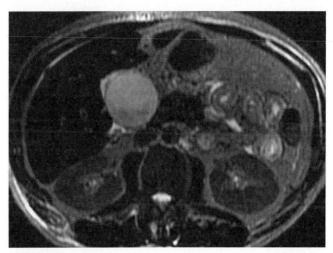

Figure 1.94 B

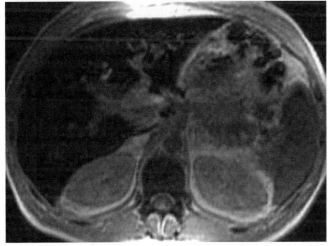

Figure 1.94 C

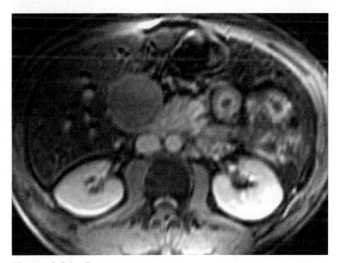

Figure 1.94 D

Findings: On T2-WI (A and B) and T1-WI (C), the liver and spleen show diffusely low T1 and T2 signal intensity consistent with diffuse iron deposition. The liver is enlarged, and there is evidence of mild periportal edema. The gallbladder is diffusely distended, and its wall is mildly thickened; there is some sludge within the gallbladder. There is a small amount of fluid accumulating in the gallbladder bed. Note wall thickening (B) and, on the gadolinium-enhanced, fat-suppressed T1-WI (D), mucosal hyperenhancement of the adjacent small bowel loops.

Differential Diagnosis: Hepatic veno-occlusive disease.

Diagnosis: Acute graft-versus-host disease.

Discussion: Acute graft-versus-host disease develops within 1 to 10 weeks of hematopoietic stem-cell transplantation.

In fact, it remains the primary cause of morbidity and mortality in patients with allogeneic bone marrow transplantation. The skin, gastrointestinal tract, and liver are the most commonly affected organ systems. Involvement of the gastrointestinal tract in cases of acute graft-versus-host disease is often severe and characterized by diarrhea, abdominal pain, nausea, vomiting, and fever. Intestinal involvement manifests itself as small bowel wall thickening, as seen in this case. Concomitant hepatic involvement is frequent. Extraintestinal imaging findings are nonspecific and include ascites, splenomegaly, periportal edema, pericholecystic fluid, biliary sludge, and gallbladder wall enhancement and thickening.

Clinical History: 58-year-old man presenting with weight loss and malaise.

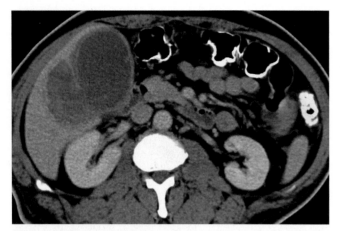

Figure 1.95   A

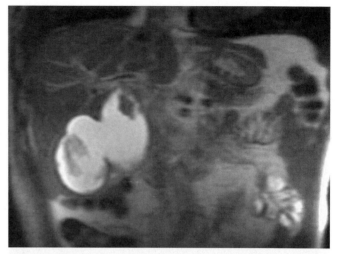

Figure 1.95   B

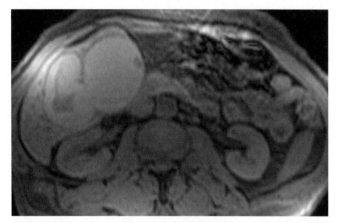

Figure 1.95   C

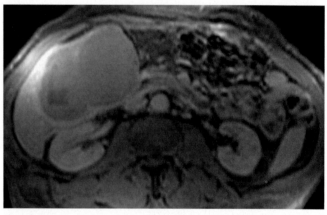

Figure 1.95   D

Findings: Axial CECT image (A) shows an ill-defined fluid collection with heterogeneous content adjacent to the gallbladder. The wall of the gallbladder is thickened. On the T2-WI (B), some hypointense structures are evident within the hyperintense collection and gallbladder, which appear to communicate. On the fat-suppressed T1-WI (C), both the collection and gallbladder content are hyperintense, suggesting high protein content. On the gadolinium-enhanced, fat-suppressed axial T1-WI (D), the collection shows rimlike enhancement.

Differential Diagnosis: Gallbladder carcinoma.

Diagnosis: Gallbladder perforation.

Discussion: Although gallbladder perforation is most often a complication of severe acute cholecystitis, it can occur in the setting of gallbladder carcinoma as well. Other causes include chronic cholecystitis, cholelithiasis, trauma, steroids, and vascular compromise. Gallbladder perforation is classified into three types: acute free perforation into the peritoneal cavity, subacute perforation with pericholecystic abscess, and chronic perforation with cholecystoenteric fistula. Imaging findings, such as distention of the gallbladder, thickening of the gallbladder wall, pericholecystic fluid, bulging of the gallbladder wall, and wall defect, are well defined on both CT and MRI. Due to its excellent soft tissue resolution and multiplanar capability, MRI can depict all the radiologic findings previously listed and others, such as inflammation of the adjacent pericholecystic and omental fat or associated abscesses. Evidence of irregular mural enhancement or frank tumor invasion is suggestive of perforated gallbladder carcinoma rather than perforated acute cholecystitis.

SUGGESTED READINGS

HEPATIC NEOPLASMS

- Albrecht T, Hohmann J, Oldenburg A, et al. Detection and characterisation of liver metastases. *Eur Radiol.* 2004;8:P25–P33.

- Baker ME, Pelly R. Hepatic metastases: basic principles and implications for radiologists. *Radiology* 1995;197:329–337.

- Boechat MI, Kangarloo H, Ortega J, et al. Primary liver tumors in children: comparison of CT and MR imaging. *Radiology* 1988; 169:727–732.

- Bogner B, Hegedus G. Ciliated hepatic foregut cyst. *Pathol Oncol Res.* 2002;8:278–279.

- Brancatelli G, Federle MP, Grazioli L, et al. Focal nodular hyperplasia: CT findings with emphasis on multiphasic helical CT in 78 patients. *Radiology* 2001;219:61–68.

- Brancatelli G, Federle MP, Vilgrain V, et al. Fibropolycystic liver disease: CT and MR imaging findings. *Radiographics* 2005;25:659–670.

- Choi BI, Lee JM, Han JK. Imaging of intrahepatic and hilar cholangiocarcinoma. *Abdom Imaging.* 2004;29:548–557.

- Choi H, Loyer EM, DuBrow RA, et al. Radio-frequency ablation of liver tumors: assessment of therapeutic response and complications. *Radiographics* 2001;21:S41–S54.

- Coumbaras M, Wendum D, Monnier-Cholley L, et al. CT and MR imaging features of pathologically proven atypical giant hemangiomas of the liver. *Am J Roentgenol.* 2002;179:1457–1463.

- Dachman AH, Lichtenstein JE, Friedman AC, et al. Infantile hemangioendothelioma of the liver: a radiologic-pathologic-clinical correlation. *Am J Roentgenol.* 1983;140:1091–1096.

- Danet IM, Semelka RC, Braga L, et al. Giant hemangioma of the liver: MR imaging characteristics in 24 patients. *Magn Reson Imaging.* 2003;21:95–101.

- Diaz-Ruiz MJ, Falco J, Martin J, et al. Hepatocellular carcinoma presenting as portal thrombosis with intrabiliary growth: US and MR findings. *Abdom Imaging.* 2000;25:263–265.

- Fang SH, Dong DJ, Zhang SZ. Imaging features of ciliated hepatic foregut cyst. *World J Gastroenterol.* 2005;11:4287–4289.

- Fennessy FM, Mortele KJ, Kluckert T, et al. Hepatic capsular retraction in metastatic carcinoma of the breast occurring with increase or decrease in size of subjacent metastasis. *Am J Roentgenol.* 2004;182:651–655.

- Freeny PC, Baron RL, Teefey SA. Hepatocellular carcinoma: reduced frequency of typical findings with dynamic contrast enhanced CT in a non-Asian population. *Radiology* 1992;182:143–148.

- Furui S, Yuji I, Yamauchi T. Hepatic epithelioid hemangioendothelioma: report of five cases. *Radiology* 1989;171:63–68.

- Gallego C, Velasco M, Marcuello P, et al. Congenital and acquired anomalies of the portal venous system. *Radiographics* 2002;22:141–159.

- Gibbs JF, Litwin AM, Kahlenberg MS. Contemporary management of benign liver tumors. *Surg Clin North Am.* 2004;84:463–480.

- Hussain SM, Terkivatan T, Zondervan PE, et al. Focal nodular hyperplasia: findings at state-of-the-art MR imaging, US, CT, and pathologic analysis. *Radiographics* 2004;24:3–17.

- Itai Y, Shin O, Kuni O, et al. Regenerating nodules of liver cirrhosis: MR imaging. *Radiology* 1987;165:419–423.

- Ito K, Higuchi M, Kada T, et al. CT of acquired abnormalities of the portal venous system. *Radiographics* 1997;17:897–917.

- Kadoya M, Matsui O, Nakanuma Y, et al. Ciliated hepatic foregut cyst: radiologic features. *Radiology* 1990; 175:475–477.

- Kanematsu M, Kondo H, Goshima S, et al. Imaging liver metastases: review and update. *Eur J Radiol.* 2006;58:217–228.

- Kanematsu M, Semelka RC, Leonardou P, et al. Hepatocellular carcinoma of diffuse type: MR imaging findings and clinical manifestations. *J Magn Reson Imaging.* 2003;18:189–195.

- Khan SA, Thomas HC, Davidson BR, et al. Cholangiocarcinoma. *Lancet* 2005;366:1303–1314.

- Koyama T, Fletcher JG, Johnson CD, et al. Primary hepatic angiosarcoma: findings at CT and MR imaging. *Radiology.* 2002;222:667–673.

- Levy AD. Malignant liver tumors. *Clin Liver Dis.* 2002;6:147–164.

- Lewin M, Mourra N, Honigman I, Flejou JF, et al. Assessment of MRI and MRCP in diagnosis of biliary cystadenoma and cystadenocarcinoma. *Eur Radiol.* 2006;16:407–413.

- Limanond P, Zimmerman P, Raman SS, et al. Interpretation of CT and MRI after radiofrequency ablation of hepatic malignancies. *Am J Roentgenol.* 2003;181:1635–1640.

- Lu DS, Yu NC, Raman SS, et al. Radiofrequency ablation of hepatocellular carcinoma: treatment success as defined by histologic examination of the explanted liver. *Radiology* 2005;234:954–960.

- Lyburn ID, Torreggiani WC, Harris AC, et al. Hepatic epithelioid hemangioendothelioma: sonographic, CT, and MR imaging appearances. *Am J Roentgenol.* 2003;180:1359–1364.

- Maetani Y, Itoh K, Watanabe C, et al. MR imaging of intrahepatic cholangiocarcinoma with pathologic correlation. *Am J Roentgenol.* 2001; 176:1499–1507.

- Marti-Bonmati L, Lonjedo E, Mathieu D, et al. Tumoural portal vein thrombosis. Enhancement with MnDPDP. *Acta Radiol.* 1997;38:655–659.

- Martin J, Sentis M, Zidan A, et al. Fatty metamorphosis of hepatocellular carcinoma: detection with chemical shift gradient-echo MR imaging. *Radiology* 1995;195:125–130.

- Mathieu D, Grenier P, Larde D, et al. Portal vein involvement in hepatocellular carcinoma: dynamic CT features. *Radiology* 1984;152:127–132.

- Mathieu D, Vasile N, Grenier P. Portal thrombosis: dynamic CT features and course. *Radiology* 1985;154:737–741.

- Matsui O, Masumi K, Tomiaki K. Benign and malignant nodules in cirrhotic livers: distinction based on blood supply. *Radiology* 1991; 178:493–497.

- Matsushita M, Shimizu S, Nagasawa M, et al. Epithelioid hemangioendothelioma of the liver: imaging diagnosis of a rare hepatic tumor. *Dig Surg.* 2005;22: 416–418.

- Mermuys K, Vanhoenacker PK, Roskams T, et al. Epithelioid hemangioendothelioma of the liver: radiologic-pathologic correlation. *Abdom Imaging.* 2004;29:221–223.

- Miller WJ, Dodd GD 3rd, Federle MP, et al. Epithelioid hemangioendothelioma of the liver: imaging findings with pathologic correlation. *Am J Roentgenol.* 1992;159:53–57.

- Mortele B, Mortele KJ, Seynaeve P, et al. Hepatic bile duct hamartomas (von Meyenburg complexes): MR and MR cholangiography imaging Findings. *J Comput Assist Tomogr.* 2002;26:438–443.

- Mortele KJ, De Keukeleire K, Praet M, et al. Malignant focal hepatic lesions complicating underlying liver disease: dual-phase contrast-enhanced spiral CT sensitivity and specificity in OLT patients. *Eur Radiol.* 2001;1:1631–1638.

- Mortele KJ, Mergo PJ, Urrutia M, et al. Dynamic gadolinium-enhanced MRI findings in infantile hepatic hemangioendothelioma. *J Comput Assist Tomogr.* 1998;22:714–717.

- Mortele KJ, Praet M, Van Vlierberghe H, et al. Focal nodular hyperplasia of the liver: assessment with plain and dynamic-enhanced MRI. *Abdom Imaging.* 2002;27:700–707.

- Mortele KJ, Praet M, Van Vlierberghe H, et al. CT and MR imaging findings in focal nodular hyperplasia of the liver: radiologic-pathologic correlation. *Am J Roentgenol.* 175:687–692, 2000.

- Mortele KJ, Ros PR. Benign liver neoplasms. *Clin Liver Dis.* 2002;6: 119–145.

- Mortele KJ, Ros PR. Cystic focal liver lesions in the adult: differential CT and MR imaging features. *Radiographics* 2001;21:895–910.

- Mortele KJ, Stubbe J, Praet M, et al. Intratumoral steatosis in focal nodular hyperplasia coinciding with diffuse hepatic steatosis: CT and MRI findings with histologic correlation. *Abdom Imaging.* 2000;25:179–181.

- Mortele KJ, Vanzieleghem B, Mortele B, et al. Gadolinium-enhanced MR imaging of infantile hemangioendothelioma: atypical features. *Eur Radiol.* 2002;12:862–865.

- Murakami T, Chikazumi K, Taro M, et al. Regenerating nodules in hepatic cirrhosis: MR findings with pathologic correlation. *Am J Roentgenol.* 1990;155:1227–1231.

- Murphy BJ, Casillas J, Ros PR, et al. The CT appearance of cystic masses of the liver. *Radiographics* 1989;9:307–322.
- Nascimento AB, Mitchell DG, Rubin R, et al. Diffuse desmoplastic breast carcinoma metastases to the liver simulating cirrhosis at MR imaging: report of two cases. *Radiology* 2001;221:117–121.
- Okuda K, Noguchi T, Kubo Y, et al. A clinical and pathological study of diffuse type hepatocellular carcinoma. *Liver* 1981;1:280–289.
- Outwater E, Tomaszewski J, Daly J, et al. Hepatic colorectal metastases: correlation of MR imaging and pathologic appearance. *Radiology* 1991;180:327–332.
- Peterson MS, Baron RL, Rankin SC. Hepatic angiosarcoma: findings on multiphasic contrast-enhanced helical CT do not mimic hepatic hemangioma. *Am J Roentgenol.* 2000;175:165–170.
- Powers C, Ros PR, Stoupis C, et al. Primary liver neoplasms: MR imaging with pathologic correlation. *Radiographics* 1994;14:459–482.
- Prasad SR, Wang H, Rosas H, et al. Fat-containing lesions of the liver: radiologic-pathologic correlation. *Radiographics* 2005;25:321–331.
- Quinn SF, Benjamin GG. Hepatic cavernous hemangiomas: simple diagnostic sign with dynamic bolus CT. *Radiology* 1992;182:545–548.
- Radin DR, Craig JR, Colletti PM, et al. Hepatic epithelioid hemangioendothelioma. *Radiology* 1988;169:145–148.
- Ros PR, Buck JL, Goodman ZD, et al. Intrahepatic cholangiocarcinoma: radiologic-pathologic correlation. *Radiology* 1988;167:689–693.
- Ros PR, Zachary DG, Ishak KG, et al. Mesenchymal hamartoma of the liver: radiologic-pathologic correlation. *Radiology* 1986;158:619–624.
- Sanders LM, Botet JF, Straus DJ, et al. CT of primary lymphoma of the liver. *Am J Roentgenol.* 1989;152:973–976.
- Sans N, Fajadet P, Galy-Fourcade D, et al. Is capsular retraction a specific CT sign of malignant liver tumor? *Eur Radiol.* 1999;9:1543–1545.
- Shamsi K, Deckers F, De Schepper A. Unusual cystic liver lesions: a pictorial essay. *Eur J Radiol.* 1993;16:79–84.
- Soyer P, Bluemke DA, Vissuzaine C, et al. CT of hepatic tumors: prevalence and specificity of retraction of the adjacent liver capsule. *Am J Roentgenol.* 1994;162:1119–1122.
- Stanley P, Hall TR, Wolley MM, et al. Mesenchymal hamartomas of the liver in childhood: sonographic and CT findings. *Am J Roentgenol.* 1986;147:1035–1039.
- Stocker JT, Ishak KG. Undifferentiated (embryonal) sarcoma of the liver. *Cancer* 1978;42:336–348.
- Sugawara Y, Yamamoto J, Yamasaki S, et al. Cystic liver metastases from colorectal cancer. *J Surg Oncol.* 2000;74:148–152.
- Takayasu K, Hiroyoshi F, Wakao Y, et al. CT diagnosis of early hepatocellular carcinoma: sensitivity, findings, and CT-pathologic correlation. *Am J Roentgenol.* 1995;164:885–890.
- Valls C, Iannacconne R, Alba E, et al. Fat in the liver: diagnosis and characterization. *Eur Radiol.* 2006;14:1–17.
- Valls C, Rene M, Gil M, et al. Giant cavernous hemangioma of the liver: atypical CT and MR findings. *Eur Radiol.* 1996;6:448–450.
- Vilgrain V, Boulos L, Vullierme MP, et al. Imaging of atypical hemangiomas of the liver with pathologic correlation. *Radiographics* 2000;20:379–397.
- Vogt DP, Henderson JM, Chmielewski E. Cystadenoma and cystadenocarcinoma of the liver: a single center experience. *J Am Coll Surg.* 2005;200:727–733.
- Wong LK, Link DP, Frey CF, et al. Fibrolamellar hepatocarcinoma: radiology, management, and pathology. *Am J Roentgenol.* 1982;139:172–175.
- Wu T, Boitnott J. Dysplastic nodules: a new term for premalignant hepatic nodular lesions. *Radiology* 1996;201:21–22.
- Yoshikawa J, Matsui O, Takashima T, et al. Fatty metamorphosis in hepatocellular carcinoma: radiologic features in 10 cases. *Am J Roentgenol.* 1988;15:717–720.

DIFFUSE LIVER DISEASES

- Adler D, Glazer G, Silver T. Computed tomography of liver infarction. *Am J Roentgenol.* 1984;142:315–318.
- Akhan O, Akpinar E, Oto A, et al. Unusual imaging findings in Wilson's disease. *Eur Radiol.* 2002;12(suppl 3):S66–S69.
- Basaran C, Karcaaltincaba M, Akata D, et al. Fat-containing lesions of the liver: cross-sectional imaging findings with emphasis on MRI. *Am J Roentgenol.* 2005;184:1103–1110.
- Benya EC, Sivit CJ, Quinones RR. Abdominal complications after bone marrow transplantation in children: sonographic and CT findings. *Am J Roentgenol.* 1993;161:1023–1027.
- Coy DL, Ormazabal A, Godwin JD, et al. Imaging evaluation of pulmonary and abdominal complications following hematopoietic stem cell transplantation. *Radiographics* 2005;25:305–317.
- Elsayes KM, Narra VR, Yin Y, et al. Focal hepatic lesions: diagnostic value of enhancement pattern approach with contrast-enhanced 3D gradient-echo MR imaging. *Radiographics* 2005; 25:1299–1320.
- Farman J, Ramirez G, Brunetti J, et al. Abdominal manifestations of sarcoidosis. CT appearances. *Clin Imaging.* 1995;19:30–33.
- Fennessy FM, Mortele KJ, Kluckert T, et al. Hepatic capsular retraction in metastatic carcinoma of the breast occurring with increase or decrease in size of subjacent metastasis. *Am J Roentgenol.* 2004;182:651–655.
- Goldman IS, Winkler ML, Raper SE, et al. Increased hepatic density and phospholipidosis due to amiodarone. *Am J Roentgenol.* 1985;144:541–546.
- Harrison SA, Torgerson S, Hayashi PH. The natural history of nonalcoholic fatty liver disease: a clinical histopathological study. *Am J Gastroenterol.* 2003;98:2042–2047.
- Hommeyer SC, Teefey SA, Jacobson AF, et al. Veno-occlusive disease of the liver: prospective study of US evaluation. *Radiology* 1992;184:683–686.
- Hood MN, Ho VB, Smirniotopoulos JG, et al. Chemical shift: the artifact and clinical tool revisited. *Radiographics* 1999;19:357–371.
- Jung G, Brill N, Poll LW, et al. MRI of hepatic sarcoidosis: large confluent lesions mimicking malignancy. *Am J Roentgenol.* 2004;183:171–173.
- Kalantari BN, Mortele KJ, Cantisani V, et al. CT features with pathologic correlation of acute gastrointestinal graft-versus-host disease after bone marrow transplantation in adults. *Am J Roentgenol.* 2003;181:1621–1625.
- Kawamoto S, Soyer PA, Fishman EK, et al. Nonneoplastic liver disease: evaluation with CT and MR imaging. *Radiographics* 1998;18:827–848.
- Kemper J, Jung G, Poll LW, et al. CT and MRI findings of multifocal hepatic steatosis mimicking malignancy. *Abdom Imaging.* 2002; 27:708–710.
- Koslin DB, Stanley RJ, Shin MS, et al. Hepatic perivascular lymphedema: CT appearance. *Am J Roentgenol.* 1988;150:111–113.
- Koyama T, Ueda H, Togashi K, et al. Radiologic manifestations of sarcoidosis in various organs. *Radiographics* 2004;24:87–104.
- Larson RE, Semelka RC. Magnetic resonance imaging of the liver. *Top Magn Reson Imaging.* 1995;7:71–81.
- Martin DR. Magnetic resonance imaging of diffuse liver diseases. *Top Magn Reson Imaging.* 2002;13:151–163.
- Mathieu D, Vasile N, Menu Y, et al. Budd-Chiari syndrome: dynamic CT. *Radiology* 1987;165:409–413.
- Mortele KJ, Ros PR. Imaging of diffuse liver disease. *Semin Liver Dis.* 2001;21:195–212.
- Mortele KJ, Ros PR. MR imaging in chronic hepatitis and cirrhosis. *Semin Ultrasound CT MR.* 2002;23:79–100.
- Mortele KJ, Van Vlierberghe H, Wiesner W, et al. Hepatic veno-occlusive disease: MRI findings. *Abdom Imaging.* 2002;27:523–526.
- Neiderau C, Fischer R, Sonnenberg A, et al. Survival and causes of death in cirrhotic and in noncirrhotic patients with primary hemochromatosis. *N Engl J Med.* 1985;313:1256–1262.
- Ohtomo K, Baron RL, Dodd GD 3rd, et al. Confluent hepatic fibrosis in advanced cirrhosis: appearance at CT. *Radiology* 1993;188:31–35.
- Ohtomo K, Baron RL, Dodd GD 3rd, et al. Confluent hepatic fibrosis in advanced cirrhosis: evaluation with MR imaging. *Radiology* 1993; 189:871–874.
- Oliva MR, Mortele KJ, Segatto E, et al. Computed tomography features of nonalcoholic steatohepatitis with histopathologic correlation. *J Comput Assist Tomogr.* 2006;30:37–43.
- Patrick D, White FE, Adams PC. Long-term amiodarone therapy: a cause of increased hepatic attenuation on CT. *Br J Radiol.* 1984;57:573–576.
- Prasad SR, Wang H, Rosas H, et al. Fat-containing lesions of the liver: radiologic-pathologic correlation. *Radiographics* 2005;25:321–331.

- Saadeh S, Younossi ZM, Remer EM, et al. The utility of radiological imaging in nonalcoholic fatty liver disease. *Gastroenterology* 2002;123: 745–750.
- Siegelman E, Mitchell D, Rubin R, et al. Parenchymal versus reticuloendothelial iron overload in the liver: distinction with MR imaging. *Radiology* 1991;179:361–366.
- Siegelman ES. MR imaging of diffuse liver disease. Hepatic fat and iron. *Magn Reson Imaging Clin North Am.* 1997;5:347–365.
- Stark D, Hahn P, Trey C, et al. MRI of the Budd-Chiari syndrome. *Am J Roentgenol.* 1986;146:1141–1148.
- Tom WW, Yeh BM, Cheng JC, et al. Hepatic pseudotumor due to nodular fatty sparing: the diagnostic role of opposed-phase MRI. *Am J Roentgenol.* 2004;183:721–724.
- Valls C, Iannacconne R, Alba E, et al. Fat in the liver: diagnosis and characterization. *Eur Radiol.* 2006;14:1–17.
- Van den Bosch MA, Van Hoe L. MR imaging findings in two patients with hepatic veno-occlusive disease following bone marrow transplantation. *Eur Radiol.* 2000;10:1290–1293.
- Vitellas KM, Tzalonikou MT, Bennett WF, et al. Cirrhosis: spectrum of findings on unenhanced and dynamic gadolinium-enhanced MR imaging. *Abdom Imaging.* 2001;26:601–615.
- Vogelzang R, Anschuetz S, Gore R. Budd-Chiari syndrome: CT observations. *Radiology* 1987;163:329–333.
- Yang DM, Kim HS, Cho SW, et al. Pictorial review: various causes of hepatic capsular retraction: CT and MR findings. *Br J Radiol.* 2002;75:994–1002.

BILIARY DISEASE

- Atri M, Bonifacio A, Ryan M, et al. Dropped gallstones post laparoscopic cholecystectomy mimicking peritoneal seeding: CT and ultrasound features. *J Comput Assist Tomogr.* 2002;26:1000–1005.
- Bennett GL, Balthazar EJ. Ultrasound and CT evaluation of emergent gallbladder pathology. *Radiol Clin N Am.* 2003;41:1203–1216.
- Chan F, Man S, Leong LL, et al. Evaluation of recurrent pyogenic cholangitis with CT: analysis of 50 patients. *Radiology* 1989;170:165–169.
- Fidler J, Paulson EK, Layfield L. CT evaluation of acute cholecystitis: findings and usefulness in diagnosis. *Am J Roentgenol.* 1996;166:1085–1088.
- Gore RM, Yaghmai V, Newmark GM, et al. Imaging benign and malignant disease of the gallbladder. *Radiol Clin North Am.* 2002;40:1307–1323.
- Grand D, Horton KM, Fishman EK. CT of the gallbladder: spectrum of disease. *Am J Roentgenol.* 2004;183:163–170.
- Ishak KG, Willis GW, Cummins SD, et al. Biliary cystadenoma and cystadenocarcinoma. *Cancer* 1977;38:322–338.
- Ito K, Mitchell DG, Outwater EK, et al. Primary sclerosing cholangitis: MR imaging features. *Am J Roentgenol.* 1999;172:1527–1533.
- Kim YJ, Kim MJ, Kim KW, et al. Preoperative evaluation of common bile duct stones in patients with gallstone disease. *Am J Roentgenol.* 2005;184:1854–1859.
- Kondo S, Isayama H, Akahane M, et al. Detection of common bile duct stones: comparison between endoscopic ultrasonography, magnetic resonance cholangiography, and helical-computed-tomographic cholangiography. *Eur J Radiol.* 2005;54:271–275.
- Korobkin M, Stephens DH, Lee JKT, et al. Biliary cystadenoma and cystadenocarcinoma: CT and sonographic findings. *Am J Roentgenol.* 1989;153:507–511.
- Maldjian C, Stancato-Pasik A, Shapiro RS. Abscess formation as a late complication of dropped gallstones. *Abdom Imaging.* 1995;20:217–218.
- Mortele KJ, Wiesner W, Cantisani V, et al. Usual and unusual causes of extrahepatic cholestasis: assessment with magnetic resonance cholangiography and fast MRI. *Abdom Imaging.* 2004;29:87–99.
- Mortele KJ, Ji H, Ros PR. CT and magnetic resonance imaging in pancreatic and biliary tract malignancies. *Gastrointest Endosc* 2002; 56(suppl 6):S206–S212.
- Rubens DJ. Hepatobiliary imaging and its pitfalls. *Radiol Clin North Am.* 2004;42:257–278.
- Sakamoto I, Iwanaga S, Nagaoki K, et al. Intrahepatic biloma formation (bile duct necrosis) after transcatheter arterial chemoembolization. *Am J Roentgenol.* 2003;181:79–87.
- Shanmugam V, Beattie GC, Yule SR, et al. Is magnetic resonance cholangiopancreatography the new gold standard in biliary imaging? *Br J Radiol.* 2005;78:888–893.
- Sood B, Jain M, Khandelwal N, et al. MRI of perforated gallbladder. *Australas Radiol.* 2002;46:438–440.
- Stefanidis D, Sirinek KR, Bingener J. Gallbladder perforation: risk factors and outcome. *J Surg Res.* 2006;131:204–208.
- Tsai HM, Lin XZ, Chen CY, et al. MRI of gallstones with different compositions. AJR *Am J Roentgenol.* 2004;182:1513–1519.
- Tseng JH, Pan KT, Hung CF, et al. Choledochal cyst with malignancy: magnetic resonance imaging and magnetic resonance cholangiopancreatographic features in two cases. *Abdom Imaging.* 2003;28:838–841.
- Tumer AR, Yuksek YN, Yasti AC, et al. Dropped gallstones during laparoscopic cholecystectomy: the consequences. *World J Surg.* 2005; 29:437–440.
- Vitellas KM, Keogan MT, Freed KS, et al. Radiologic manifestations of sclerosing cholangitis with emphasis on MR cholangiopancreatography. *Radiographics* 2000;20:959–975.
- Weiner SN, Koenigsberg M, Morehouse H, et al. Sonography and computed tomography in the diagnosis of carcinoma of the gallbladder. *Am J Roentgenol.* 1984;142:735–739.
- Yeh H. Ultrasonography and computed tomography of carcinoma of the gallbladder. *Radiology* 1979;133:167–173.
- Yoshikane H, Hashimoto S, Hidano H, et al. Multiple early bile duct carcinoma associated with congenital choledochal cyst. *J Gastroenterol.* 1998;33:454–457.
- Yu JS, Kim KW, Park MS, et al. Bile duct injuries leading to portal vein obliteration after transcatheter arterial chemoembolization in the liver: CT findings and initial observations. *Radiology* 2001;221: 429–436.
- Zissin R, Osadchy A, Shapiro-Feinberg M, et al. CT of a thickened-wall gall bladder. *Br J Radiol.* 2003;76:137–143.

INFECTION

- Acunas B, Izzet R, Levent C, et al. Purely cystic hydatid disease of the liver: treatment with percutaneous aspiration and injection of hypertonic saline. *Radiology* 1992;182:541–543.
- Balci NC, Semelka RC, Noone TC, et al. Pyogenic hepatic abscesses: MRI findings on T1- and T2-weighted and serial gadolinium-enhanced gradient-echo images. *J Magn Reson Imaging.* 1999;9:285–290.
- Balci NC, Sirvanci M. MR imaging of infective liver lesions. *Magn Reson Imaging Clin N Am.* 2002;10:121–135.
- Beggs I. The radiology of hydatid disease. *Am J Roentgenol.* 1985;145:639–648.
- Choliz J, Olaverri FJ, Casas T, et al. Computed tomography in hepatic echinococcosis. *Am J Roentgenol.* 1982;139:699–702.
- Elizondo G, Weissleder R, Stark D, et al. Amebic liver abscess: diagnosis and treatment evaluation with MR imaging. *Radiology* 1987; 165:795–800.
- Francis I, Glazer G, Amendola A, et al. Hepatic abscesses in the immunocompromised patient role of CT in detection, diagnosis, management, and follow-up. *Gastrointest Radiol* 1986;11:257–262.
- Mathieu D, Vasile N, Pierre-Louis F, et al. Dynamic CT features of hepatic abscesses. *Radiology* 1985;154:749–752.
- Mendez R, Schiebler M, Outwater E, et al. Hepatic abscesses: MR imaging findings. *Radiology* 1994;190:431–436.
- Mortele KJ, Segatto E, Ros PR. The infected liver: radiologic-pathologic correlation. *Radiographics* 2004;24:937–955.
- Oto A, Akhan O, Ozmen M. Focal inflammatory diseases of the liver. *Eur J Radiol.* 1999;32:61–75.
- Ralls P, Barnes P, Johnson M, et al. Medical treatment of hepatic amebic abscess: rare need for percutaneous drainage. *Radiology* 1987;165: 805–807.
- Ralls P, Henley D, Colletti P, et al. Amebic liver abscess: MR imaging. *Radiology* 1987;165:801–804.
- Shirkhoda A. CT findings in hepatosplenic and renal candidiasis. *J Comput Assist Tomogr.* 1987;11:795–798.

MISCELLANEOUS

- Bluemke DA, Fishman EK, Kuhlman JE, et al. Complications of radiation therapy: CT evaluation. *Radiographics* 1991;11:581–600.
- Casillas VJ, Amendola MA, Gascue A, et al. Imaging of nontraumatic hemorrhagic hepatic lesions. *Radiographics* 2000;20:367–378.
- Finley DS, Hinojosa MW, Paya M, et al. Hepatic artery pseudoaneurysm: a report of seven cases and a review of the literature. *Surg Today.* 2005;35:543–547.
- Florio F, Nardella M, Balzano S, et al. Congenital intrahepatic portosystemic shunt. *Cardiovasc Intervent Radiol.* 1998;21:421–424.
- Gallego C, Velasco M, Marcuello P, et al. Congenital and acquired anomalies of the portal venous system. *Radiographics* 2002;22:141–159.
- Ito K, Higuchi M, Kada T, et al. CT of acquired abnormalities of the portal venous system. *Radiographics* 1997;17:897–917.
- Kawamoto S, Soyer PA, Fishman EK, et al. Nonneoplastic liver disease: evaluation with CT and MR imaging. *Radiographics* 1998;18:827–848.
- Kim HJ, Kim KW, Kim AY, et al. Hepatic artery pseudoaneurysms in adult living-donor liver transplantation: efficacy of CT and Doppler sonography. *Am J Roentgenol.* 2005;184:1549–1555.
- Lee KH, Han JK, Jeong JY, et al. Hepatic attenuation differences associated with obstruction of the portal or hepatic veins in patients with hepatic abscess. *Am J Roentgenol.* 2005;185:1015–1023.
- Lipson JA, Qayyum A, Avrin DE, et al. CT and MRI of hepatic contour abnormalities. *Am J Roentgenol.* 2005;184:75–81.
- Parvey HR, Raval B, Sandler CM. Portal vein thrombosis: imaging findings. *Am J Roentgenol.* 1994;162:77–81.
- Romano L, Giovine S, Guidi G, et al. Hepatic trauma: CT findings and considerations based on our experience in emergency diagnostic imaging. *Eur J Radiol.* 2004;50:59–66.
- Shanmuganathan K. Multi-detector row CT imaging of blunt abdominal trauma. *Semin Ultrasound CT MR.* 2004;25:180–204.
- Tublin ME, Dodd GD 3rd, Baron RL. Benign and malignant portal vein thrombosis: differentiation by CT characteristics. *Am J Roentgenol.* 1997;168:719–723.
- Yoon W, Jeong YY, Kim JK, et al. CT in blunt liver trauma. *Radiographics* 2005;25:87–104.

CHAPTER TWO
PANCREAS

KOENRAAD J. MORTELE,
VINCENT PELSSER,
AND PABLO R. ROS

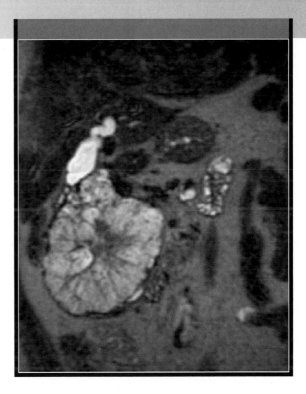

Clinical History: 57-year-old man presenting with symptoms of acute recurrent pancreatitis.

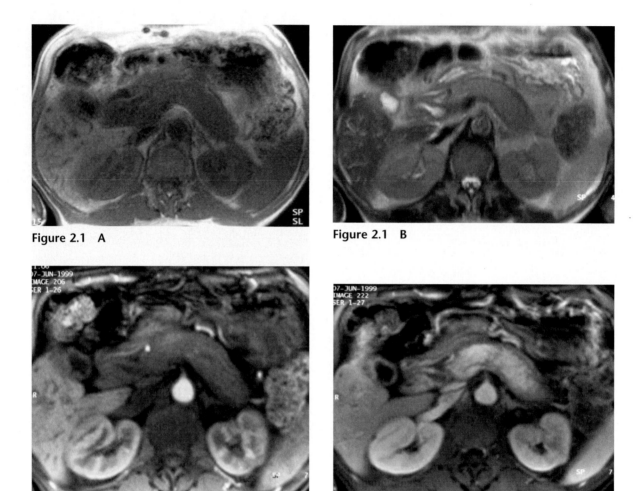

Figure 2.1 A

Figure 2.1 B

Figure 2.1 C

Figure 2.1 D

Findings: Axial T1-weighted image (WI) (A) and T2-WI (B) show a swollen pancreas and abnormal low signal of the pancreas on T1-WI and increased signal intensity on T2-WI. Also note peripheral hypointense rim surrounding the pancreas on T2-WI. After gadolinium administration, the pancreas shows a delayed enhancement on the pancreatic phase fat-saturated T1-WI (C) and shows lack of enhancement of the peripheral rim on the portal venous phase T1-WI (D). Also note abnormal rimlike enhancement of the common bile duct (CBD).

Differential Diagnosis: Diffuse pancreatic ductal adenocarcinoma, acute pancreatitis.

Diagnosis: Autoimmune pancreatitis.

Discussion: Autoimmune pancreatitis, also known as sclerosing or lymphoplasmacytic pancreatitis, is an increasingly recognized subtype of chronic pancreatitis. It is frequently associated with other autoimmune diseases, such as sclerosing cholangitis or retroperitoneal fibrosis. Immunoglobulin G4 levels are elevated in approximately 60% of cases. On

contrast-enhanced CT (CECT), the pancreas is typically swollen and appears sausagelike in shape. The normal pancreatic lobulations are absent. The biliary duct is typically dilated due to the periductal fibrosis in the pancreatic head. The enhancement of the gland is heterogeneous and delayed after iodinated contrast administration. On MRI, the pancreas is abnormally hypointense on T1-WI and normal or mildly hyperintense on T2-WI. A rim of fibrosis, hypointense on both T1-WI and T2-WI, is sometimes seen encircling the gland. After gadolinium administration, the enhancement of the gland is delayed, and lack of enhancement of the peripheral fibrotic rim is typically detected. Enhancing periductal fibrosis around the CBD may also be present. Magnetic resonance cholangiopancreatography (MRCP) is helpful in diagnosing associated strictures in the intra- or extrahepatic bile ducts. Despite the fact that autoimmune pancreatitis can be treated noninvasively by steroids, it is currently the most common benign condition for which Whipple procedures are performed.

CASE 2-2

Clinical History: 72-year-old man presenting with weight loss and hemoptysis.

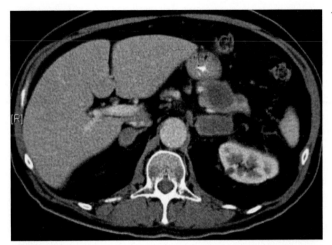

Figure 2.2 A

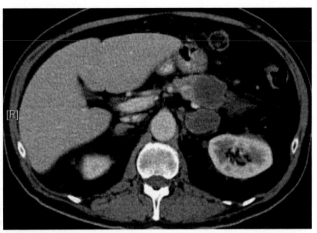

Figure 2.2 B

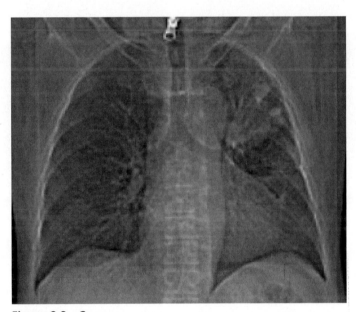

Figure 2.2 C

Findings: Consecutive axial CECT images (A and B) demonstrate bilateral adrenal masses and two low-attenuation lesions in the tail of the pancreas with mild rim enhancement. Anteroposterior chest x-ray (C) shows ill-defined mass in the left upper lung lobe.

Differential Diagnosis: Endocrine pancreatic tumor, lymphoma, metastases.

Diagnosis: Metastatic lung carcinoma.

Discussion: Metastasis to the pancreas is rare but does occur in tumors that spread hematogenously, such as lung cancer, renal cancer, breast cancer, sarcoma, and melanoma. Metastasis can also occur to the peripancreatic nodes from any source, which can subsequently invade the pancreas.

This is often difficult to distinguish from a primary pancreatic neoplasm. The finding of multiple pancreatic lesions is a limited differential. Besides metastases, primary endocrine tumors of the pancreas can also be multiple. Gastrinomas can be multiple in up to 50% of cases, especially if associated with multiple endocrine neoplasm type I (MEN I). Lymphoma of the pancreas can present as multiple solid masses or can diffusely involve the pancreas and simulate pancreatitis. The key to the diagnosis is that pancreatic metastases usually occur in advanced stages of the disease, in which a primary malignancy is already known. Pancreatic metastases can appear hypervascular (renal cell carcinoma, sarcoma, or melanoma) or hypovascular (lung carcinoma) depending on the primary tumor type.

Clinical History: 46-year-old man presenting with weight loss.

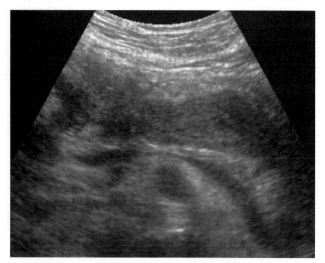

Figure 2.3   A

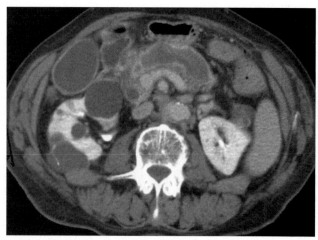

Figure 2.3   B

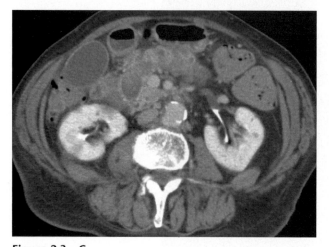

Figure 2.3   C

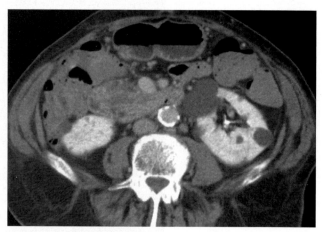

Figure 2.3   D

Findings: Sonographic axial image (A) through the pancreas shows markedly dilated pancreatic duct with presence of debris within the duct. Consecutive axial CECT images (B–D) demonstrate a dilated pancreatic duct extending to the papilla that is bulging within the duodenum. Note atrophy of the pancreatic parenchyma and enhancing soft tissue within the pancreatic duct. No obstructing pancreatic mass is identified. There is no history of pancreatitis or significant alcohol intake.

Differential Diagnosis: Chronic pancreatitis, ampullary carcinoma.

Diagnosis: Intraductal papillary mucinous neoplasm.

Discussion: Intraductal papillary mucinous neoplasm (IPMN) is a mucin-producing neoplasm that can involve the main duct, a side branch, or both. Side-branch IPMN is characterized by grapelike cystic dilatation of a side branch of the pancreatic duct predominantly affecting the uncinate process. An identifiable associated soft tissue mass is rarely seen by CT because side-branch IPMN tend to be benign. In patients with main duct IPMN, often the only finding is dilatation of the pancreatic duct and small cysts that communicate with the main duct. Presence of papillary projections, soft tissue masses, ductal dilatation more than 1 cm, bulging papilla, and calcifications have all been associated with an increased risk of malignancy. In this patient, without a history of alcohol ingestion and episodes of recurrent pancreatitis, chronic pancreatitis would be unlikely. Other findings of chronic pancreatitis, such as calcifications or a beaded pancreatic duct, are also absent. An ampullary carcinoma can cause dilatation of the pancreatic duct, but it is usually associated with dilatation of the CBD.

CASE 2-4

Clinical History: 55-year-old woman with a history of several years of intermittent epigastric pain and occasional fevers.

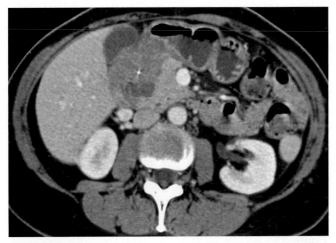

Figure 2.4   A

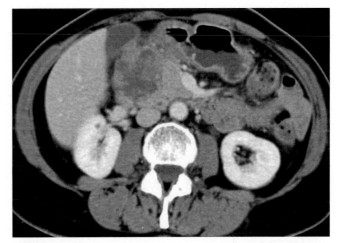

Figure 2.4   B

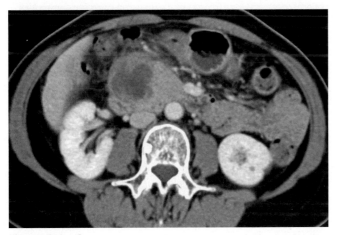

Figure 2.4   C

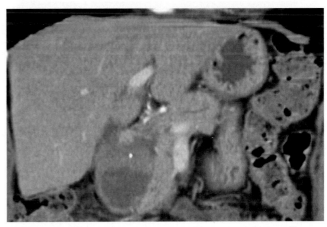

Figure 2.4   D

Findings: Axial CECT images (A–C) and coronal reformatted image (D) demonstrate a 5-cm mass in the head of the pancreas. The mass is well circumscribed and exophytic in location. There is central necrosis and presence of a punctate calcification. The CBD and pancreatic duct are not dilated.

Differential Diagnosis: Pancreatic ductal adenocarcinoma, endocrine pancreatic tumor, metastasis.

Diagnosis: Acinar cell carcinoma.

Discussion: Acinar cell carcinoma is a rare malignant neoplasm with poor prognosis due to the frequent presence of liver metastases at the time of diagnosis. Like pancreatic ductal adenocarcinomas, acinar cell carcinomas are seen in elderly patients with a mean age of 65 years old. Systemic lipase secretion by acinar cell neoplasms leads to distant fat necrosis in the skin, bone, and joints. The lipase hypersecretion also results in an erythematous rash, lytic bone lesions, and polyarthralgias in these patients. By CT, acinar cell carcinomas tend to be larger than the typical adenocarcinoma, measuring up to 15 cm, and are usually well circumscribed with little desmoplastic reaction. An exophytic location is typical. Because of their larger size, acinar cell neoplasms can have central necrosis, as is seen in this case. Also, calcifications may be present. A nonhyperfunctioning endocrine pancreatic tumor would be a good differential diagnosis for this case because those lesions tend to be large as well, may contain calcifications, and typically are heterogeneous when large.

Clinical History: 19-year-old woman presenting with left upper quadrant discomfort after minor trauma during an assault.

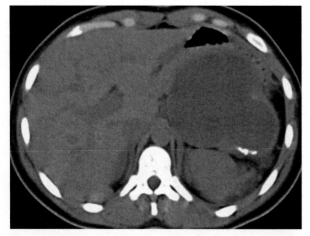

Figure 2.5 A

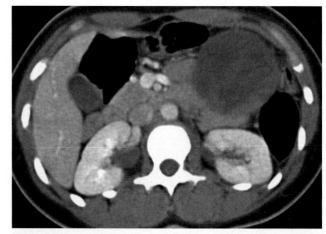

Figure 2.5 B

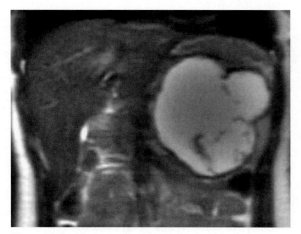

Figure 2.5 C

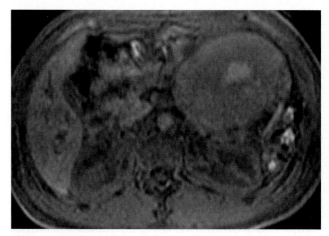

Figure 2.5 D

Findings: Nonenhanced CT (NECT) image (A) demonstrates a large 10-cm cystic mass arising from the body and tail of the pancreas. Note peripheral eggshell-like calcification. CECT image (B) demonstrates an enhancing soft tissue rind that surrounds the central cystic component. Coronal T2-WI (C) shows hyperintense aspect of the lesion because of its fluid content and presence of a hypointense capsule. Unenhanced fat-saturated T1-WI (D) shows hyperintense signal centrally due to the presence of methemoglobin (hemorrhage).

Differential Diagnosis: Mucinous cystic neoplasm, pseudocyst, nonhyperfunctioning endocrine pancreatic tumor.

Diagnosis: Solid and papillary epithelial neoplasm.

Discussion: Solid and papillary epithelial neoplasm of the pancreas is a rare low-grade malignancy seen most commonly in young women. The mean age of presentation is in the 20s, ranging between the second and sixth decades of life. There is no race predilection. Surgical resection is often curable. The lesion typically presents as a large, thick-walled, encapsulated cystic mass with hemorrhage and necrosis. The peripheral solid portions usually enhance with intravenous contrast and can have curvilinear calcifications as well. There is no location predilection. The differential diagnosis includes pseudocyst, mucinous cystic neoplasm, or a nonhyperfunctioning endocrine tumor that has undergone cystic degeneration. The lack of history for pancreatitis makes pseudocyst unlikely. Both mucinous cystic neoplasm and a nonhyperfunctioning endocrine tumor can have the same radiographic appearance as solid and papillary epithelial neoplasm; however, hemorrhage is uncommon in the former and the presence of a capsule excludes the latter. The treatment of all three lesions is nevertheless the same and consists of surgical resection.

CASE 2-6

Clinical History: 47-year-old man undergoing a follow-up scan 5 months after an attack of acute pancreatitis.

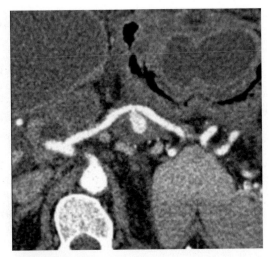

Figure 2.6 **A**

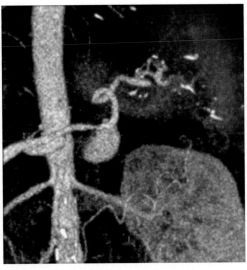

Figure 2.6 **B**

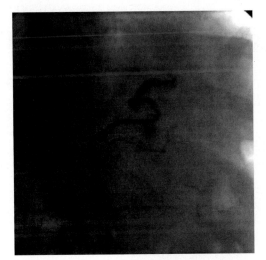

Figure 2.6 **C**

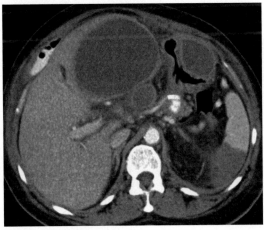

Figure 2.6 **D**

Findings: Curved reformatted CT image (A) along the splenic artery and three-dimensional volume-rendered image (B) of the splenic artery show the presence of a 2-cm enhancing nodule abutting the splenic artery. The nodule has the same density as the splenic artery. Digital subtraction angiography image (C) confirms the presence of an enhancing blush adjacent to the splenic artery. CECT image (D) obtained after attempted stenting of the splenic artery shows pseudocysts in the gastrohepatic and gastrosplenic ligaments, a splenic infarct, and the presence of a radiopaque stent in the splenic artery. Note that the nodule next to the splenic artery still enhances.

Differential Diagnosis: None.

Diagnosis: Pseudoaneurysm of the splenic artery from pancreatitis.

Discussion: Pseudoaneurysms can be seen as a late complication of pancreatitis secondary to the erosion of a peripancreatic artery by pancreatic enzymes. Commonly involved vessels include the splenic artery, gastroduodenal artery, and pancreaticoduodenal arcades. With contrast enhancement, the pseudoaneurysm can sometimes be demonstrated as an enhancing structure within or adjacent to a pseudocyst. Diagnosis can be confirmed by angiography. Rupture of a pseudoaneurysm has a high mortality rate of approximately 37%. Embolization of a pseudoaneurysm can be performed during the acute phase of pancreatitis until surgery can be performed at a later date. Unlike in this case, embolization by itself has been used therapeutically as well.

Clinical History: 44-year-old man with repeated bouts of pancreatitis.

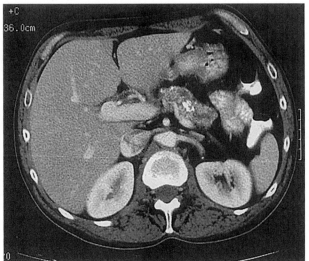

Figure 2.7   A

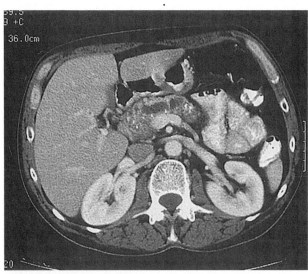

Figure 2.7   B

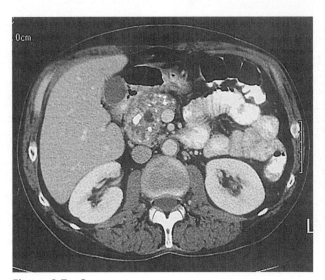

Figure 2.7   C

Findings: Axial consecutive CECT images demonstrate multiple pancreatic calcifications scattered throughout the gland with an irregularly dilated pancreatic duct.

Differential Diagnosis: None.

Diagnosis: Chronic pancreatitis.

Discussion: Chronic pancreatitis is most commonly secondary to underlying alcohol consumption in the United States. The alcohol alters the function of the acinar cells, resulting in concentration of proteins in the ducts. This leads to stone formation, ductal stenosis and dilatation, and acinar atrophy. The ductal dilatation in chronic pancreatitis is most commonly irregular in appearance (73%), followed by smooth (15%) and beaded (12%). Pancreatic ductal dilatation is seen

in 68% of patients with chronic pancreatitis, in 54% of patients with glandular atrophy, and in 50% of patients with calcifications. This case demonstrates the typical findings of chronic pancreatitis with calcifications and ductal dilatation. There is always a concern for an underlying pancreatic adenocarcinoma in a patient with chronic pancreatitis causing pancreatic ductal dilatation. The head of the pancreas, however, is diffusely calcified, with no focal low-attenuation mass present. Pancreatic adenocarcinomas rarely calcify. If there is continued concern for a malignancy, then endoscopic ultrasound (EUS), endoscopic retrograde cholangiopancreatography (ERCP), or biopsy is required. Correlation with serum CA 19-9 level is also helpful because it may be significantly elevated in pancreatic adenocarcinoma.

CASE 2-8

Clinical History: 59-year-old woman with increasing right upper quadrant pain.

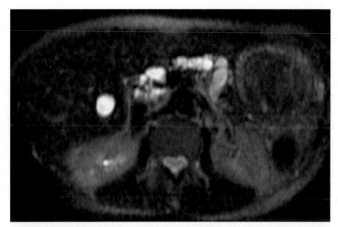

Figure 2.8 A

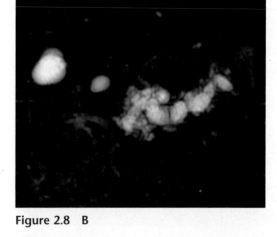

Figure 2.8 B

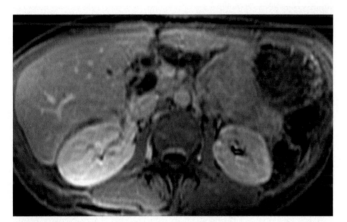

Figure 2.8 C

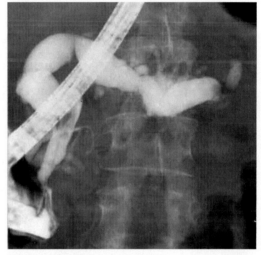

Figure 2.8 D

Findings: Axial heavily T2-WI (A) shows markedly dilated pancreatic duct. Projective coronal oblique thick-slab MRCP image (B) displays the dilated pancreatic duct in its entirety. Also note several dilated side branches. Gadolinium-enhanced, fat-suppressed axial T1-WI (C) shows no enhancing nodules (or papillary protrusions) within the duct. ERCP image (D) confirms the dilation of the pancreatic duct and its side branches and presence of mucin globs within the duct. No obstructing mass is seen.

Differential Diagnosis: Chronic pancreatitis, ampullary carcinoma.

Diagnosis: Intraductal papillary mucinous neoplasm, combined type.

Discussion: Intraductal papillary mucinous neoplasm (IPMN) is similar histologically to a mucinous cystic neoplasm but differs in that it doesn't contain ovarian stroma and it involves the main pancreatic duct or a side branch of the pancreatic duct or both. IPMN produces mucin that fills the pancreatic duct and causes it to dilate. By ERCP, there are multiple cystic cavities, usually in the uncinate process, which communicate with the main pancreatic duct. There is also a large amount of mucin coming from the ampulla as it is cannulated by the endoscopist. The papilla can be dilated, and this has been referred to as the "fishmouth" papilla. IPMN ranges histologically from benign adenoma to borderline lesions (dysplasia and carcinoma in situ) to frankly invasive neoplasms. Adenocarcinoma and colloid carcinoma are the two subtypes recognized among invasive IPMN. Spread of the cancer outside of the pancreas occurs late in the course of the disease, so this neoplasm has a fairly good prognosis after resection. Typically, main duct or combined involvement has a less favorable prognosis than side branch involvement only.

CASE 2-9

Clinical History: 17-year-old girl with daily abdominal pain starting 3 years ago.

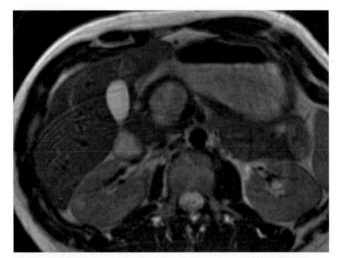

Figure 2.9 A

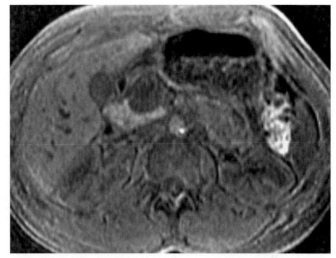

Figure 2.9 B

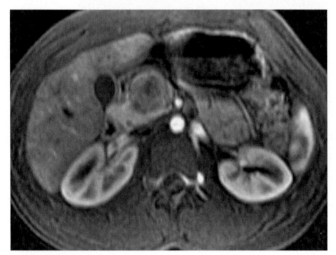

Figure 2.9 C

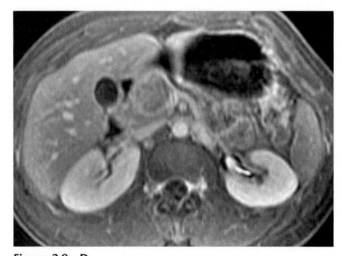

Figure 2.9 D

Findings: Axial T2-WI (A) shows an encapsulated cystic mass in the head of the pancreas. Axial fat-saturated T1-WI (B) shows the lesion to be hypointense and heterogeneous. Gadolinium-enhanced arterial phase (C) and delayed-phase (D) axial T1-WI demonstrate progressive enhancement of the capsule and lack of central enhancement.

Differential Diagnosis: Pseudocyst, mucinous cystic neoplasm, nonhyperfunctioning endocrine tumor.

Diagnosis: Solid and papillary epithelial neoplasm.

Discussion: Solid and papillary epithelial neoplasm (SPEN) is an uncommon tumor of the pancreas found most commonly in young females (daughter tumor). The lesion is typically large and well demarcated because it is encapsulated.

A thick rind of tissue is usually present with areas of necrosis centrally. Small nodules of soft tissue can often be seen protruding into the center of the lesion. SPEN is mildly hypervascular, and the thick wall demonstrates mild contrast enhancement. The differential diagnosis for a cystic mass in the pancreas in a young adult is limited. Excluding an abscess and hematoma, the differential diagnosis would include a pseudocyst, nonhyperfunctioning endocrine tumor with cystic degeneration, or a mucinous cystic tumor of the pancreas. The lack of history for pancreatitis would exclude pseudocyst, and the age would make a nonhyperfunctioning endocrine tumor and mucinous cystic neoplasm less likely. Prognosis for this patient is excellent with surgical excision because SPEN is benign or low-grade malignant.

Clinical History: 65-year-old woman who had a recent pneumonia and was found to have an incidental abdominal finding on CT scan of the thorax.

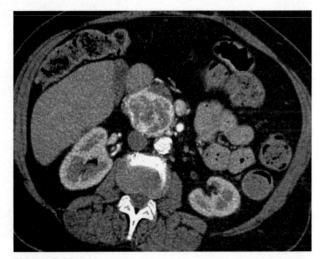

Figure 2.10   A

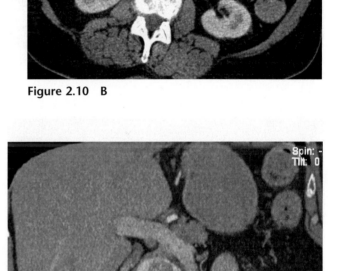

Figure 2.10   B

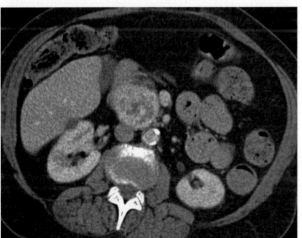

Figure 2.10   C

Figure 2.10   D

Findings: Consecutive axial arterial phase CECT images (A–C) demonstrate a 4-cm hypervascular mass in the head of the pancreas. The lesion is heterogeneous and well defined. Coronal reformatted arterial phase CECT image (D) demonstrates lack of vascular invasion.

Differential Diagnosis: Metastasis, acinar cell neoplasm, pancreatic ductal adenocarcinoma.

Diagnosis: Nonhyperfunctioning endocrine pancreatic tumor.

Discussion: Endocrine pancreatic neoplasms are typically classified in hyperfunctioning and nonhyperfunctioning tumors. Hyperfunctioning tumors overproduce a certain hormone and, based on the type of hormone (e.g., insulin, gastrin, somatostatin, glucagon, vasointestinal peptide), cause a specific syndrome. Nonhyperfunctioning tumors are more silent and, therefore, larger at diagnosis. They are most often located in the pancreatic tail due to a predominance of islet cells in the tail. Pancreatic endocrine tumors are hypervascular and demonstrate intense contrast enhancement on arterial or pancreatic phase CT images. The larger the lesions, the more likely the lesion will contain areas of necrosis. Endocrine tumors can be isodense or slightly hyperdense on the equilibrium phase of a CECT and can be difficult to detect. Pancreatic ductal adenocarcinomas are hypovascular and would not demonstrate intense enhancement, as is seen in this case, on the arterial phase of the CECT. Metastases are unlikely because the lesion is solitary and there is no known primary. Acinar cell carcinomas tend to be well defined but are generally hypovascular to the surrounding parenchyma.

Clinical History: 53-year-old woman with abdominal discomfort.

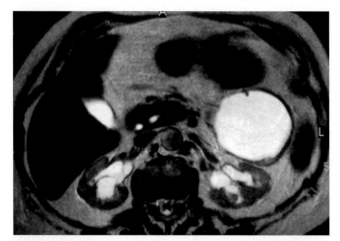

Figure 2.11   A

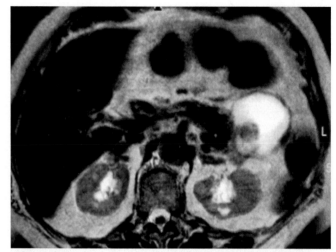

Figure 2.11   B

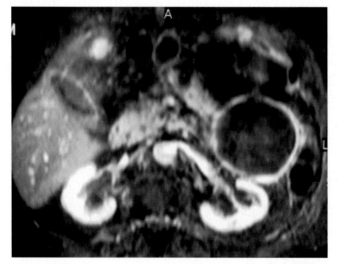

Figure 2.11   C

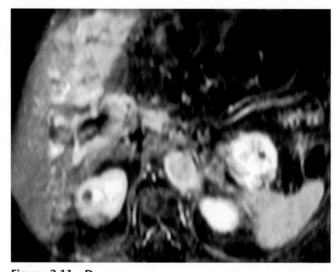

Figure 2.11   D

Findings: Axial consecutive heavily T2-WI (A and B) demonstrate the presence of a large encapsulated cystic pancreatic mass in the tail of the pancreas. A subtle mural nodule is shown in the inferior and posterior aspect of the lesion. Gadolinium-enhanced, fat-saturated axial T1-WI (C and D) show enhancement of the capsule of the lesion and the mural nodule.

Differential Diagnosis: Pancreatic pseudocyst, solid and papillary epithelial neoplasm.

Diagnosis: Mucinous cystadenocarcinoma.

Discussion: Mucinous cystadenocarcinoma is a primary cystic neoplasm of the pancreas. All mucinous cystic neoplasms are considered to have malignant potential, and

complete resection is recommended. Most of these lesions occur in patients between the ages of 40 and 60 years old ("mother tumor"), but the range is from 20 to 80 years of age. By CT imaging, these lesions are predominantly cystic, with the cysts being larger than 2 cm, hence the term macrocystic. They typically contain less than six individual cystic compartments. They can be septated and have eggshell-like peripheral calcifications. On MRI, the lesions vary in appearance depending on the cyst content. They are typically hypointense on the T1-WI and hyperintense on the T2-WI, as is seen in this case. If this lesion was encountered in a younger patient, one would favor a solid and papillary epithelial neoplasm or a pseudocyst from pancreatitis if that history was present.

Clinical History: 53-year-old woman with jaundice.

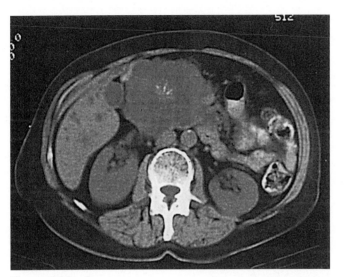

Figure 2.12   A

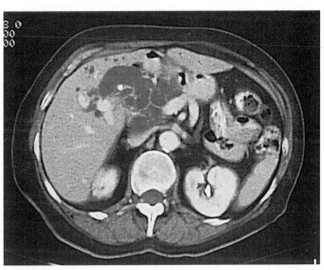

Figure 2.12   B

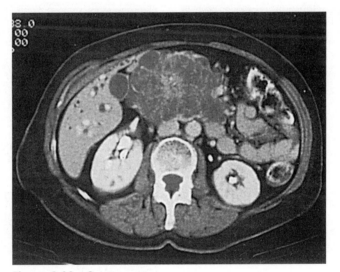

Figure 2.12   C

Findings: NECT image (A) demonstrates a low-attenuation lesion in the head of the pancreas with central punctate calcifications. CECT images (B and C) demonstrate the same lesion to have enhancing septations separating multiple small cysts. Note the dilated CBD and intrahepatic biliary ducts (B).

Differential Diagnosis: None.

Diagnosis: Microcystic serous pancreatic adenoma.

Discussion: Microcystic serous pancreatic adenoma is almost always a benign neoplasm of the pancreas arising from the duct cells. They typically occur in older women between the ages of 60 and 80 years ("grandmother tumor"). This lesion has been associated with von Hippel-Lindau disease. This lesion can occur anywhere within the pancreas, but there is a predilection for the pancreatic head. The cysts tend to be small, measuring less than 2 cm in size. Generally, there are more than six individual cystic components. The septations separating the cysts can enhance after intravenous contrast administration, and if the cysts are very small, the lesion can appear solid, especially on sonography and CT. Punctate calcifications within a central stellate fibrotic scar are characteristic of this lesion, as is seen in this example. Other cystic neoplasms of the pancreas include a mucinous cystic neoplasm, which tends to have larger cysts; a solid and papillary epithelial neoplasm, which is seen in younger patients; an intraductal papillary mucinous neoplasm, which connects to the pancreatic duct; and a necrotic islet cell tumor, which would not have innumerable small cysts.

Clinical History: 36-year-old woman with epigastric pain and bloating.

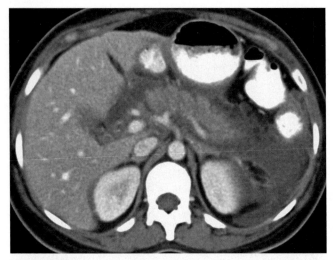

Figure 2.13   A

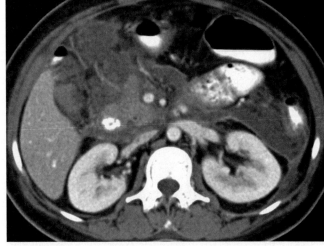

Figure 2.13   B

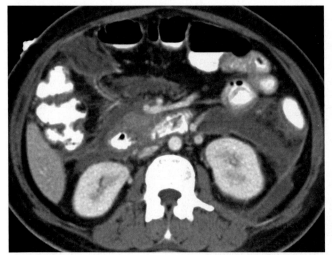

Figure 2.13   C

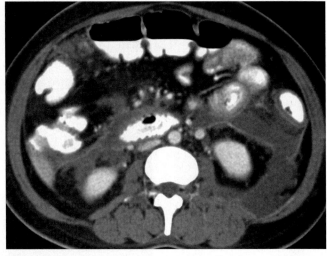

Figure 2.13   D

Findings: Consecutive axial CECT images demonstrate extensive peripancreatic inflammation within the anterior pararenal space. These fluid collections extend down into the transverse mesocolon on the right, the posterior pararenal space on the left, and the perirenal space on the right. Note that the pancreas appears edematous, but there are no areas of pancreatic necrosis.

Differential Diagnosis: None.

Diagnosis: Acute pancreatitis.

Discussion: This case demonstrates the spaces in the retroperitoneum. The pancreas is located within the anterior pararenal space just anterior to Gerota's fascia, which separates it from the kidney. Fluid and inflammation from pancreatitis will pool within the anterior pararenal space and frequently spare the kidney and the perirenal space, as is seen in this case. The fluid has also accumulated in the posterior pararenal space, which is not contiguous with the anterior pararenal space at this level. Fat and the lateroconal fascia separate them from each other. The three spaces, the anterior and posterior pararenal space and perirenal space, communicate in the infrarenal space. This anatomy is important to understand because it helps define the source of an abnormality in the retroperitoneum.

Clinical History: 66-year-old man presenting with a 4-week history of increasing nausea and vomiting, decreased appetite, and weight loss of about 9 kg.

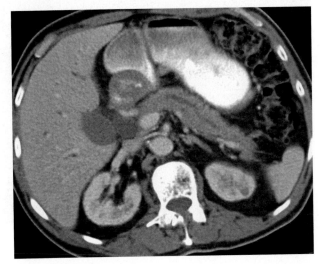

Figure 2.14   A

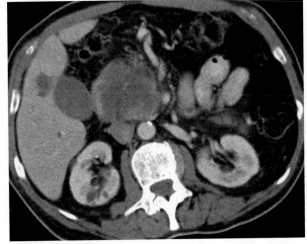

Figure 2.14   B

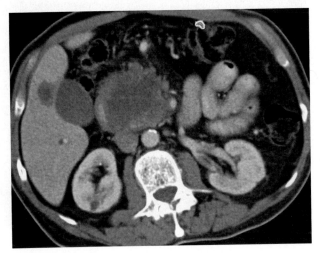

Figure 2.14   C

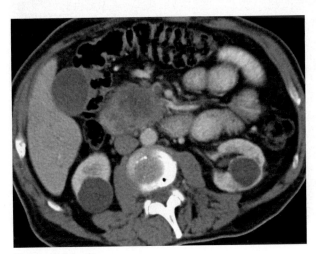

Figure 2.14   D

Findings: Consecutive axial CECT images demonstrate a low-attenuation, ill-defined lesion in the head of the pancreas. The lesion encases the superior mesenteric artery (SMA). There is thrombosis of the superior mesenteric vein (SMV). Note the collateral vessels anterior to the pancreas, the dilated pancreatic duct, and dilated intrahepatic ducts.

Differential Diagnosis: Pancreatitis.

Diagnosis: Pancreatic ductal adenocarcinoma with superior mesenteric vein thrombosis.

Discussion: Key roles for CT in the evaluation of pancreatic ductal adenocarcinoma are to confirm the diagnosis and to determine the resectability. One of the most reliable staging criteria for resectability is the presence of vascular invasion.

The fat plane between the pancreas and the SMV can be obliterated normally. This does not necessarily indicate vascular invasion by the malignancy. However, if the SMV is obstructed by the mass, then vascular invasion is likely present. In contradistinction, if the perivascular fat around the SMA is obliterated by the mass or there is thickening of the vessel, as seen in this case, then vascular invasion is suspected. Typically, encasement of more than 180 degrees of the circumference of the artery indicates vascular invasion. The presence of mesenteric, gastric, and omental collateral vessels should also suggest SMV or splenic vein thrombosis. These collaterals, typically the gastrocolic trunk entering the SMV, are seen well on CECT, as noted in this example.

Clinical History: 59-year-old woman with bilateral lower abdominal cramping.

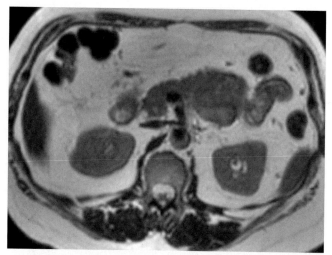

Figure 2.15   A

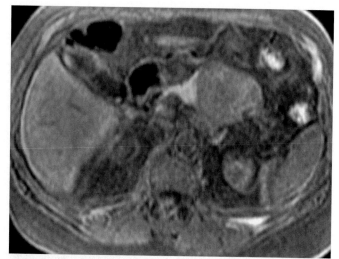

Figure 2.15   B

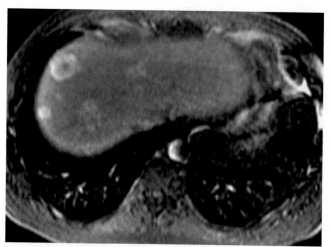

Figure 2.15   C

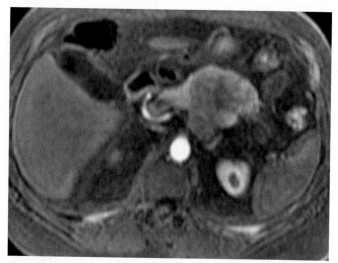

Figure 2.15   D

Findings: Axial T2-WI (A) and fat-saturated T1-WI (B) demonstrate a 4-cm lesion in the tail of the pancreas that is mildly hyperintense and hypointense, respectively. Gadolinium-enhanced, fat-saturated axial T1-WI show hypervascular lesions in the liver (C) and heterogeneous enhancement of the pancreatic mass (D).

Differential Diagnosis: Pancreatic adenocarcinoma, metastasis.

Diagnosis: Nonhyperfunctioning endocrine pancreatic tumor.

Discussion: Endocrine neoplasms of the pancreas secrete hormones, such as insulin, glucagon, and somatostatin. When the tumor is hyperfunctioning with excessive hormone secretion, these patients usually present early in the course of the disease when the lesion is still small. Except for insulinomas, the majority of these lesions are malignant but tend to be slow growing. Insulinoma is the most common pancreatic endocrine tumor and typically presents in the fourth through sixth decades of life. Insulinomas are small, with most being <1.5 cm and solitary (90%). Small calcifications (10%) can be present. Endocrine tumors are most often hypervascular, and their metastases, preferentially to the liver, also demonstrate hypervascularity, as shown in this case. Nonhyperfunctioning endocrine tumors tend to be larger at presentation, are more heterogeneous due to necrosis and hemorrhage, and tend to be malignant.

CASE 2-16

Clinical History: 18-year-old woman with abdominal pain and bloating.

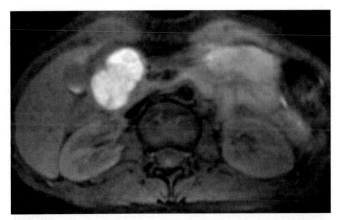

Figure 2.16 A

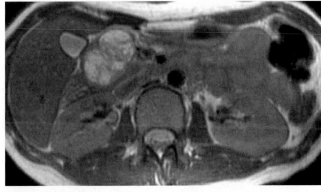

Figure 2.16 B

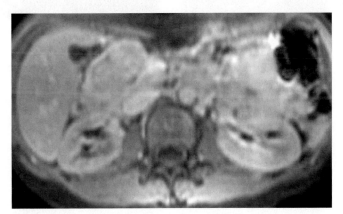

Figure 2.16 C

Findings: Axial fat-suppressed T1-WI (A) demonstrates a 3-cm hyperintense lesion in the head of the pancreas. Axial T2-WI (B) demonstrates the lesion to be encapsulated and hyperintense. Gadolinium-enhanced, fat-saturated axial T1-WI (C) shows capsular enhancement but lack of central enhancement.

Differential Diagnosis: Endocrine pancreatic tumor, hemorrhagic pseudocyst.

Diagnosis: Solid and papillary epithelial neoplasm.

Discussion: In an 18-year-old woman, there are not many diagnostic possibilities for a pancreatic mass. Of the pancreatic neoplasms, the most likely diagnosis is a solid and papillary epithelial neoplasm (SPEN). Because of its internal hemorrhage, a nonhyperfunctioning endocrine tumor is also a possibility. The patient is too young for an adenocarcinoma, microcystic adenoma, or a mucinous cystic neoplasm. Adolescents can get pancreatitis with pseudocyst formation from trauma, drugs, or postviral infections, but a history of pancreatitis is usually known. The lesion is completely hemorrhagic, which excludes a choledochal cyst or duplication cyst. On MRI, solid and papillary epithelial neoplasms typically present as large encapsulated masses with internal hemorrhage. Due to the paramagnetic effect of methemoglobin, hemorrhage is easily detected on fat-saturated T1-WI. The capsule in SPEN is hypointense on T1-WI and T2-WI and enhances after gadolinium administration.

Clinical History: 38-year-old man with history of peptic ulcer disease.

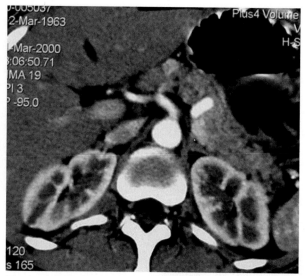

Figure 2.17   A

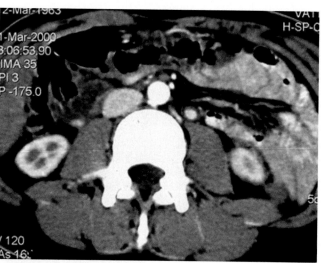

Figure 2.17   B

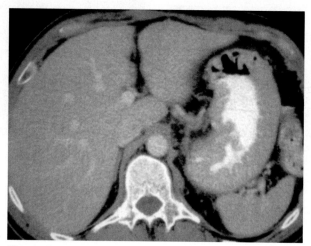

Figure 2.17   C

Findings: Consecutive axial CECT images (A and B) demonstrate two small hypervascular lesions in the body of the pancreas and the duodenal wall. Note the thickened stomach wall as well (C).

Differential Diagnosis: Metastases.

Diagnosis: Multiple gastrinomas in a patient with multiple endocrine neoplasia type I syndrome.

Discussion: Multiple endocrine neoplasia type I (MEN I) syndrome consists of a pituitary adenoma, parathyroid adenoma, and pancreatic endocrine tumor. The pancreatic endocrine tumors can be insulinomas, gastrinomas, or VIPomas. This patient had multiple gastrinomas resulting in Zollinger-Ellison syndrome, causing a thickened stomach wall. Few diseases will cause multiple lesions in the pancreas. These lesions did not appear cystic, excluding pseudocysts. Other lesions include metastases and lymphoma. Gastric cancer with metastases to the pancreas is a possibility, but no other metastases are present in the abdomen, and typically, gastric metastases are not hypervascular. Lymphoma can also involve the stomach and pancreas, but widespread lymphadenopathy is usually present; moreover, lymphoma is hypovascular. Gastrinomas can be multiple in up to 60% of cases and located outside the pancreas, especially if associated with MEN I. The thickened gastric wall is due to the excess acid produced by the stomach secondary to the elevated serum gastrin levels. A careful history of the patient's family revealed that other people in the family had similar problems as well.

CASE 2-18

Clinical History: 50-year-old woman with chronic epigastric pain radiating into the chest for 6 years requiring multiple hospitalizations.

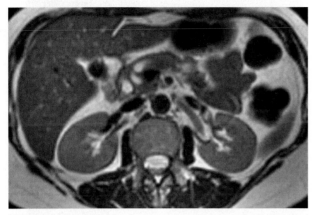

Figure 2.18 A

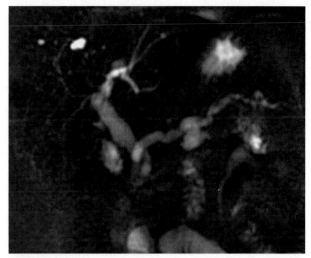

Figure 2.18 B

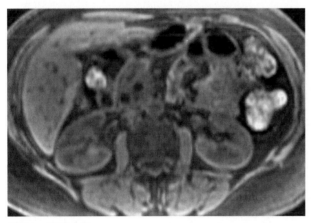

Figure 2.18 C

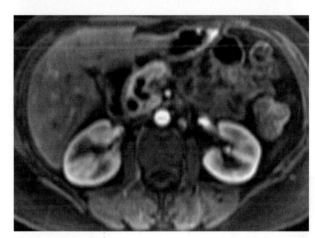

Figure 2.18 D

Findings: Axial T2-WI (A) at the level of the pancreatic head shows mildly atrophic pancreas with dilated duct of Wirsung. Projective oblique coronal thick-slab MRCP image (B) shows irregularly dilated pancreatic duct with several abnormal side branches. Unenhanced fat-suppressed axial T1-WI (C) shows abnormal low signal intensity of the pancreatic head. Gadolinium-enhanced, fat-saturated axial T1-WI (D) shows normal enhancement of the pancreatic head.

Differential Diagnosis: Intraductal papillary mucinous neoplasm, pancreatic ductal adenocarcinoma.

Diagnosis: Chronic pancreatitis.

Discussion: In the United States, the most common cause for chronic pancreatitis is oral intake of alcohol. Other causes have been implicated including hereditary pancreatitis, cystic fibrosis, hyperlipidemia, and hyperparathyroidism. Pathologically, there is progressive and irreversible fibrosis and destruction of the pancreas with atrophy of the acini. This leads to stone formation and loss of both endocrine and exocrine function. Radiologically, there are multiple calcifications throughout the pancreas, which are predominantly intraductal in location. There can be atrophy of the pancreas as well as pancreatic and biliary ductal dilatation, as seen in this case. The biliary dilatation is thought to be due to stenosis of the CBD as it passes through the fibrotic head of the pancreas. On MRI, chronic pancreatitis is characterized by abnormal low signal intensity of the parenchyma on fat-saturated T1-WI. Unlike pancreatic adenocarcinoma, chronic pancreatitis enhances after gadolinium administration. MRCP is helpful to evaluate the pancreatic duct and its side branches. Intraductal lithiasis and strictures are easily depicted. Secretin-enhanced MRCP is valuable to assess the exocrine pancreatic function in these patients.

Clinical History: 64-year-old woman undergoing CT colonography for an incomplete sigmoidoscopy.

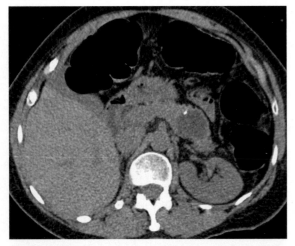

Figure 2.19 A

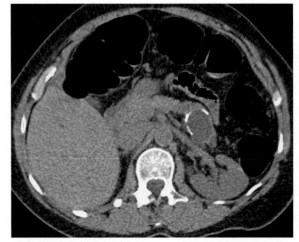

Figure 2.19 B

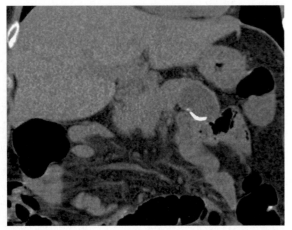

Figure 2.19 C

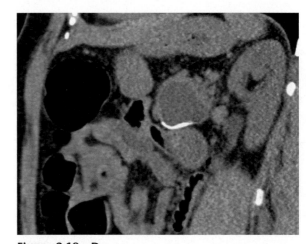

Figure 2.19 D

Findings: Consecutive axial unenhanced CT colonographic images (A–B) demonstrate a 4-cm cystic mass in the tail of the pancreas. Note the peripheral calcifications. Coronal (C) and sagittal (D) reformatted CT images illustrate the location of the cystic mass in the pancreas and its relationship to other abdominal organs and vessels.

Differential Diagnosis: Macrocystic variant serous pancreatic adenoma, pseudocyst.

Diagnosis: Mucinous cystic neoplasm.

Discussion: Approximately 85% to 90% of cysts in the pancreas are pseudocysts from pancreatitis. These lesions lack an inner epithelial lining. The other 10% to 15% of cysts are of duct cell origin. These consist of cysts (either congenital or associated with von Hippel-Lindau or autosomal dominant polycystic kidney disease) or cystic neoplasms (microcystic or macrocystic serous pancreatic adenomas, mucinous cystic neoplasms, IPMN, or SPEN). Mucinous cystic neoplasms tend to have cysts that are greater than 2 cm and few in number. There is often a thick wall present in the periphery of the tumor, which can calcify, as is seen in this case. The few septa that form these cysts enhance with contrast administration (gadolinium and iodinated contrast). Approximately 85% of these lesions are found in the tail of the pancreas, with a marked female preponderance (female-to-male ratio of 9:1). A microcystic serous pancreatic adenoma is unlikely because it tends to have tiny cysts with central calcifications rather than peripheral calcifications. Pseudocyst is a good differential diagnosis, and a thorough history is necessary to exclude it.

CASE 2-20

Clinical History: 82-year-old woman with chest pain found to have abnormal liver function tests.

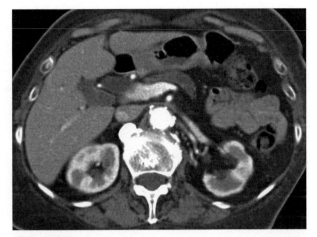

Figure 2.20   A

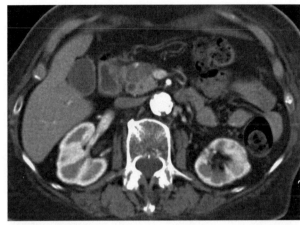

Figure 2.20   B

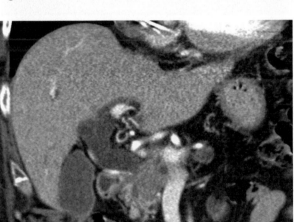

Figure 2.20   C

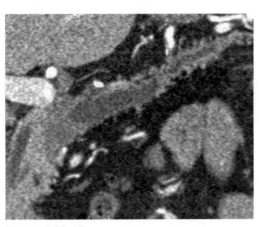

Figure 2.20   D

Findings: Consecutive axial CECT images (A and B) obtained during the pancreatic parenchymal phase demonstrate a 2-cm, low-attenuation lesion in the head of the pancreas. Note the dilated common bile and pancreatic ducts. Coronal (C) and curved (D) reformatted CT images show the relationship of the mass to the pancreatic duct and the obliteration of the fat plane between the mass and the superior mesenteric vein.

Differential Diagnosis: Focal chronic pancreatitis, autoimmune pancreatitis, metastasis.

Diagnosis: Pancreatic ductal adenocarcinoma.

Discussion: Risk factors for pancreatic adenocarcinomas include smoking, longstanding diabetes, and hereditary pancreatitis. Alcohol is a cause for pancreatitis but is not a risk factor for ductal adenocarcinoma. Elevated liver enzymes and laboratory findings of obstructive jaundice are commonly seen because most lesions occur in the head of the pancreas. The importance of CT for pancreatic adenocarcinoma is in both diagnosis and staging. CT findings that exclude resectability include retroperitoneal extension, vascular invasion, adjacent organ involvement (except the duodenum), lymphadenopathy, distant metastases, and ascites. In this case, there is no lymphadenopathy or ascites seen, but involvement of the superior mesenteric vein is questionable. Approximately 30% of patients who are thought to be resectable by CT are found to have local invasion or liver metastases at time of surgery.

Clinical History: 42-year-old man from Argentina presents with abdominal pain and fevers.

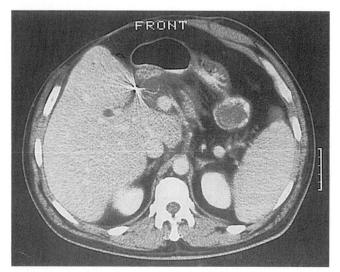

Figure 2.21   A

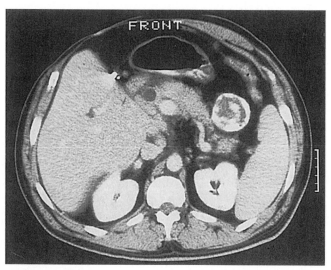

Figure 2.21   B

Findings: CECT images demonstrate a 4-cm peripherally calcified cystic lesion arising from the body of the pancreas.

Differential Diagnosis: Old hematoma, abscess, pseudocyst, mucinous cystic neoplasm.

Diagnosis: Hydatid cyst of the pancreas.

Discussion: The liver is the most common organ affected by the parasite *Echinococcus granulosus* (75–80% of cases), but other organs can also be involved, including the brain, lung, and kidney. Infection in humans is from the feces of the dog contaminated by the parasite. The eggs hatch in the gastrointestinal (GI) tract and enter the portal system where access to the rest of the body is obtained if not destroyed by the liver. The differential diagnosis for a calcified cystic lesion in the pancreas includes an old abscess, hematoma, or a pseudocyst. Cystic neoplasms can also have peripheral eggshell-like calcifications, such as a mucinous cystic neoplasm and solid and papillary epithelial neoplasm. This patient was found to have similar lesions in the liver that were confirmed as hydatid cysts.

CASE 2-22

Clinical History: 59-year-old woman with abdominal pain and steatorrhea.

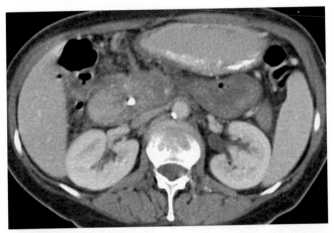

Figure 2.22   A

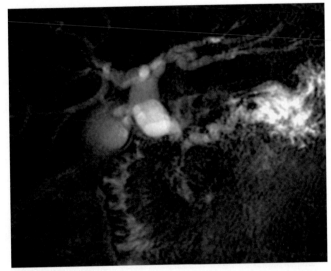

Figure 2.22   B

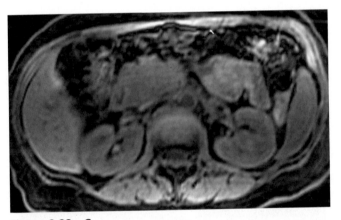

Figure 2.22   C

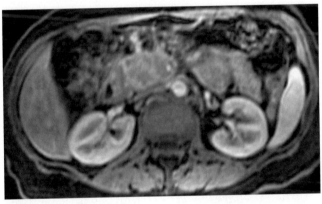

Figure 2.22   D

Findings: Axial CECT image (A) demonstrates a large, ill-defined, hypodense mass in the head of the pancreas with encasement of the SMA. The SMV is not identified. Note presence of a plastic stent in the CBD. Projective coronal oblique thick-slab MRCP image (B) shows the obstruction of pancreatic and CBD ("double duct sign"). Fat-suppressed axial T1-WI (C) demonstrates a low signal intensity mass in the head of the pancreas. Gadolinium-enhanced, fat-saturated axial T1-WI (D) shows hypovascular appearance of the pancreatic mass.

Differential Diagnosis: Pancreatitis, metastasis.

Diagnosis: Pancreatic ductal adenocarcinoma with SMV thrombosis.

Discussion: One of the critical factors in staging a patient with pancreatic adenocarcinoma is involvement of vascular structures, especially the SMV and SMA. Loss of the fat plane between the pancreas and the SMV can be seen normally. However, SMV thrombosis suggests vascular involvement by the tumor and would render the patient unresectable. On MRI, typically a flow void is seen in the vessels on T2-WI, with loss of the flow void and high signal intensity centrally indicative of a thrombosis of the vessel. Gradient-echo sequences can also be used to evaluate retroperitoneal vasculature. MRI can also be used to evaluate for peripancreatic extension, lymphadenopathy, liver metastases, and ductal dilatation.

Clinical History: 70-year-old man presenting with anemia.

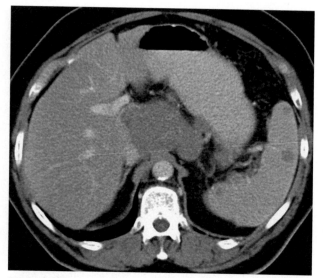

Figure 2.23 A

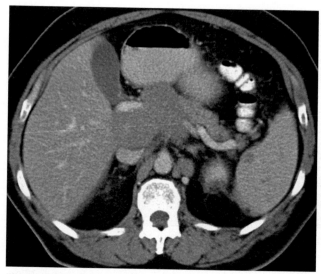

Figure 2.23 B

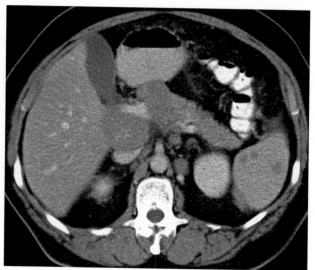

Figure 2.23 C

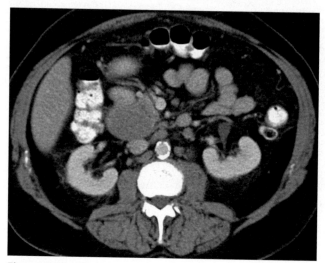

Figure 2.23 D

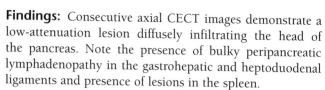

Findings: Consecutive axial CECT images demonstrate a low-attenuation lesion diffusely infiltrating the head of the pancreas. Note the presence of bulky peripancreatic lymphadenopathy in the gastrohepatic and heptoduodenal ligaments and presence of lesions in the spleen.

Differential Diagnosis: Pancreatic ductal adenocarcinoma, metastasis.

Diagnosis: Pancreatic lymphoma.

Discussion: Primary lymphoma of the pancreas is exceedingly rare, with peripancreatic lymphoma being much more common. Non-Hodgkin lymphoma is more common than Hodgkin lymphoma in the pancreas, with histiocytic and Burkitt lymphomas the most common subtypes. It is often difficult to distinguish between peripancreatic and pancreatic lymphoma because lymph nodes can often invade the pancreas due to its lack of serosa. Also confusing the picture is the presence of pancreatitis, which can sometimes accompany lymphoma due to obstruction of the pancreatic duct. Lymphoma of the pancreas can present either as a solitary mass or as multiple solid masses. Alternatively, the pancreas can be diffusely involved, simulating pancreatitis. Associated lymphadenopathy or splenic involvement, as seen in this case, can be present. The lack of a known primary tumor makes metastases unlikely.

Clinical History: 68-year-old woman with left lower quadrant pain and fever.

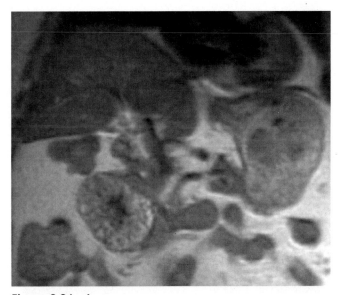

Figure 2.24   A

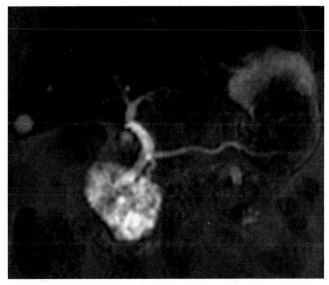

Figure 2.24   B

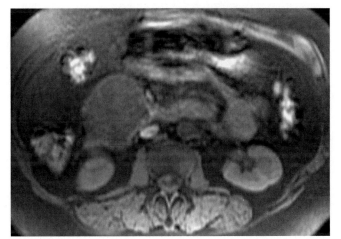

Figure 2.24   C

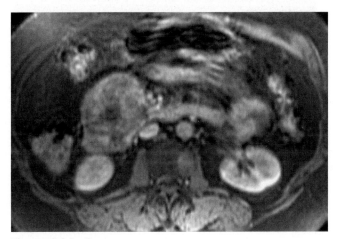

Figure 2.24   D

Findings: Coronal T2-WI (A) demonstrates a 6-cm hyperintense mass with multiple internal septations and a central scar in the head of the pancreas. Projective oblique coronal thick-slab MRCP image (B) confirms the cystic nature of the mass and shows normal pancreatic and common bile ducts. Pre- (C) and post- (D) gadolinium-enhanced, fat-saturated axial T1-WI show enhancement of the internal septations of the mass.

Differential Diagnosis: None.

Diagnosis: Microcystic serous pancreatic adenoma.

Discussion: Approximately 95% of the nonneoplastic cystic masses of the pancreas are pseudocysts. The remaining masses are true cysts either congenital in origin or associated with von Hippel-Lindau or polycystic kidney disease.

Cystic neoplasms include serous microcystic or macrocystic pancreatic adenoma, mucinous cystic neoplasm, SPEN, IPMN, lymphangioma, teratoma, and necrotic endocrine tumor. Except for the microcystic serous pancreatic adenoma, most of the other neoplasms tend to have one or a few large cysts (>2 cm) and resemble pseudocysts in appearance. The solid portion of cystic neoplasms varies depending on the cell type and aggressiveness of the lesion. Microcystic serous pancreatic adenoma, on the other hand, will have innumerable (>6) small (<2 cm) cysts, as is seen in this case. If the cysts are very small, the lesion can appear solid by CT; central calcifications are not uncommon. MRI and MRCP are very helpful to confirm the cystic nature of the lesion. The age, sex, and appearance of this lesion are characteristic for a microcystic serous pancreatic adenoma.

Clinical History: 46-year-old woman who recently started drinking alcohol presented with intermittent right-sided abdominal pain radiating to the back.

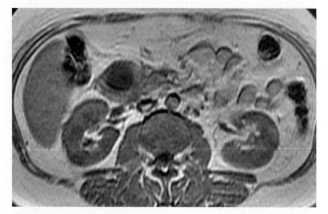

Figure 2.25   A

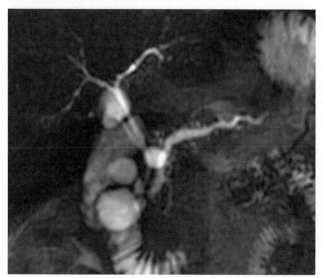

Figure 2.25   B

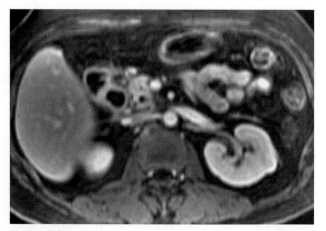

Figure 2.25   C

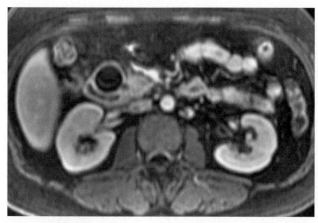

Figure 2.25   D

Findings: Axial T1-WI (A) shows a 3-cm homogenous low signal intensity lesion between the duodenum and the pancreatic head. Projective coronal oblique thick-slab MRCP image (B) shows irregular and beaded appearance of the pancreatic duct and three cystic masses overlying the duodenum. Gadolinium-enhanced, fat-saturated axial T1-WI (C and D) show lack of enhancement of the cystic structures in the duodenal wall and pancreatic head.

Differential Diagnosis: Pancreatic pseudocyst, mucinous cystic tumor.

Diagnosis: Groove pancreatitis.

Discussion: Groove pancreatitis is a subtype of chronic pancreatitis that is poorly understood. It has also been referred to as cystic dystrophy of the duodenal wall. Alcohol has been recognized as an important risk factor. The inflammation is typically restricted to the groove between the duodenal sweep and the pancreatic head. In the pure form, there is no involvement of the pancreatic duct or CBD. In the segmental form, there is displacement of the CBD medially and segmental involvement of the pancreatic parenchyma. Associated changes of chronic pancreatitis, as seen in this case, can be present in the pancreatic duct. Mucinous cystic tumor presents as a solitary lesion and doesn't have associated pancreatic ductal changes.

Clinical History: 49-year-old man with severe abdominal pain and weight loss over the past 6 months.

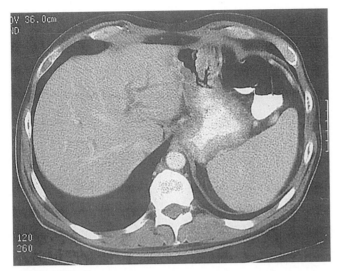

Figure 2.26   A

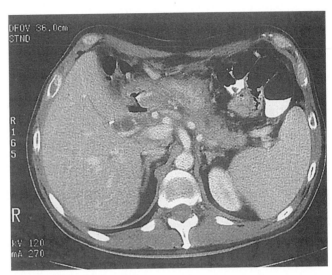

Figure 2.26   B

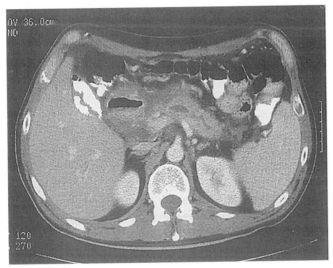

Figure 2.26   C

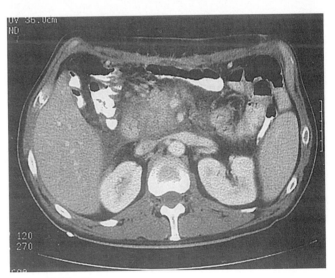

Figure 2.26   D

Findings: Consecutive axial CECT images demonstrate an edematous swollen pancreas with peripancreatic inflammation. Note the dilated intrahepatic and pancreatic ducts.

Differential Diagnosis: None.

Diagnosis: Acute pancreatitis secondary to a pancreatic ductal adenocarcinoma.

Discussion: Acute pancreatitis can be due to several causes, with alcohol and biliary stones accounting for the majority of cases. Other causes include iatrogenic (post-ERCP) trauma, postinfection, hereditary pancreatitis, and drugs. Pancreatic carcinoma is a rare cause of acute pancreatitis, making up less than 5% of the cases of pancreatitis.

It is often very difficult to diagnose pancreatic cancer in a patient with acute pancreatitis. The diagnosis should be suggested in a middle-aged or elderly patient with no identifiable cause for pancreatitis. Biliary dilatation and long-standing elevated bilirubin levels are less common in focal pancreatitis and would suggest the diagnosis of a ductal adenocarcinoma. Acute pancreatitis also tends to spread anteriorly in the retroperitoneum, whereas pancreatic cancer more commonly spreads in a retropancreatic direction. Obliteration of the fat surrounding vessels can be seen in both acute pancreatitis and cancer but is more typical in pancreatic cancer. Pancreatic cancer in this patient was suggested, and the diagnosis was confirmed by ERCP.

Clinical History: 54-year-old man with recurrent episodes of epigastric pain.

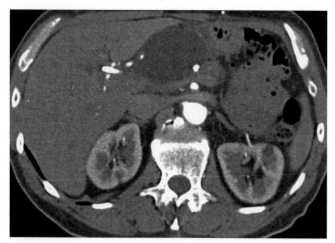

Figure 2.27 A

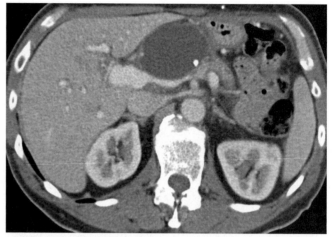

Figure 2.27 B

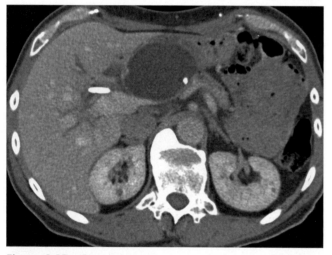

Figure 2.27 C

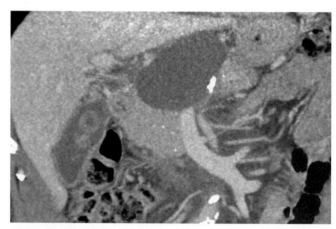

Figure 2.27 D

Findings: Axial consecutive CECT images (A and B) and portal venous phase (C) obtained during the pancreatic parenchymal phase demonstrate findings of chronic pancreatitis with a dilated pancreatic duct in an atrophic gland. A 7-cm, well-defined cystic lesion is seen in the region of the lesser sac with narrowing of the portal vein. Coronal reformatted CT image (D) shows the relationship of the homogeneous cyst to the pancreas. A plastic stent is seen in the bile ducts.

Differential Diagnosis: Mucinous cystic neoplasm, necrotic tumor (metastasis, nonhyperfunctioning endocrine tumor).

Diagnosis: Pancreatic pseudocyst.

Discussion: Pancreatic pseudocyst formation is one of the many complications of acute and chronic pancreatitis. The majority of peripancreatic fluid collections will resolve spontaneously without drainage. Approximately 10% of patients, however, will form a pseudocyst. These cysts differ from true congenital cysts in that they do not have an inner epithelial lining. A fluid collection is not usually considered a true pseudocyst until it is approximately 6 weeks old and has developed a mature fibrotic wall. At that time, it is unlikely to resolve on its own. Drainage of noninfected pseudocysts is usually reserved for those larger than 5 cm, those that are enlarging, or those that are symptomatic for the patient. The main differential diagnosis for a pseudocyst is a mucinous cystic neoplasm. Patients with mucinous cystic neoplasms do not usually have a history of pancreatitis or demonstrate signs of chronic pancreatitis, as is seen in this case. If no history of pancreatitis can be elicited, then a mucinous cystic neoplasm must be considered, especially if the patient is a middle-aged woman.

Clinical History: 9-year-old boy with epigastric pain and increasing abdominal girth.

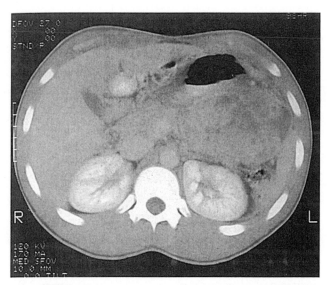

Figure 2.28   A

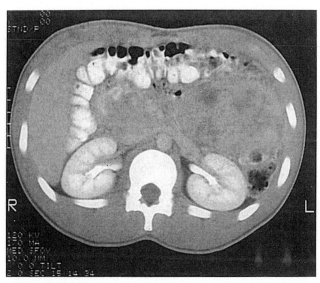

Figure 2.28   B

Findings: Axial CECT images demonstrate a large, 7-cm, heterogeneous enhancing mass arising from the tail of the pancreas.

Differential Diagnosis: Lymphoma, retroperitoneal sarcoma, hematoma, solid and papillary epithelial neoplasm.

Diagnosis: Pancreatoblastoma.

Discussion: Pancreatoblastoma is a rare neoplasm of the pancreas composed of epithelial cells sometimes intermixed with mesenchymal tissue. Pancreatoblastomas typically arise in children between the ages of 1 and 8 years old and are usually large at the time of presentation. Hemorrhage and necrosis are commonly present. Prognosis is fairly good if distant metastases have not occurred. The difficulty in diagnosing this lesion is discerning the organ of origin. If it arises from the pancreas, then, in this age group, the most likely diagnosis would be a pancreatoblastoma or, less likely, a solid and papillary epithelial neoplasm. Other large masses in the abdomen could be due to a retroperitoneal sarcoma or lymphoma. If there is a history of trauma, then a large hematoma could have this heterogeneous appearance as well. Pancreatoblastomas can present with an elevated alpha-fetoprotein serum level.

Clinical History: 63-year-old woman with back pain.

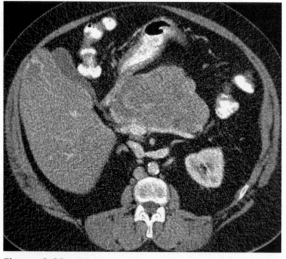

Figure 2.29   A

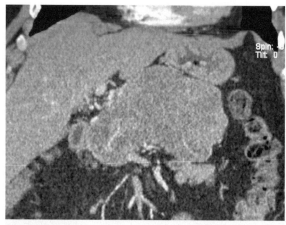

Figure 2.29   B

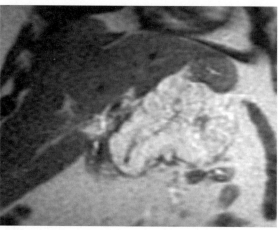

Figure 2.29   C

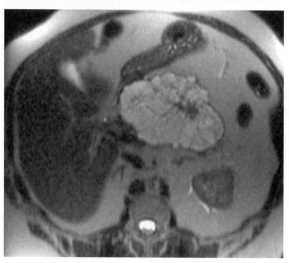

Figure 2.29   D

Findings: Axial and coronal reformatted CECT images (A and B) demonstrate a 9-cm, well-defined, low-attenuation lesion in the body of the pancreas with small cystic changes. Coronal (C) and axial (D) T2-WI demonstrate this lesion to be of high signal intensity. The signal characteristics follow that of water. Note the linear low signal intensity areas, which represent fibrous septations.

Differential Diagnosis: Mucinous cystic neoplasm, non-hyperfunctioning endocrine tumor.

Diagnosis: Microcystic serous pancreatic adenoma.

Discussion: Microcystic serous pancreatic adenoma is a benign cystic lesion of the pancreas that is often lobulated due to the presence of multiple small cysts. The cysts are filled with glycogen-rich fluid and range in size from 1 mm to 2 cm. On MRI, the cysts usually follow the signal characteristics of water depending on the amount of protein and glycogen within the fluid. Because they are hypervascular, the cysts can occasionally hemorrhage and be bright on T1-WI. The central scar and septa will typically be dark on both the T1-WI and T2-WI, as is seen in this case. MRI is very valuable in confirming the cystic nature of the lesion. Mucinous cystic neoplasms tend to have a few large cysts rather than multiple small cysts, as is seen in this case. They most often resemble a pseudocyst. Necrotic nonhyperfunctioning endocrine tumors can also have a cystic component but are usually much larger in size with more of a solid component than is seen here. Adenocarcinomas are typically solid and found in the head of the pancreas.

Clinical History: 67-year-old man known to have an abdominal aortic aneurysm presenting with back pain.

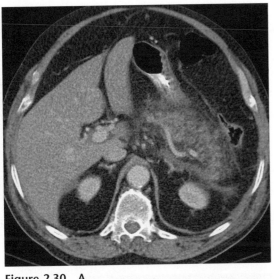

Figure 2.30   A

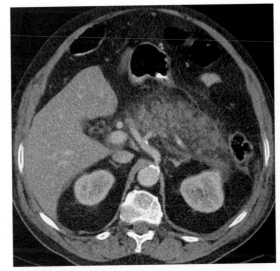

Figure 2.30   B

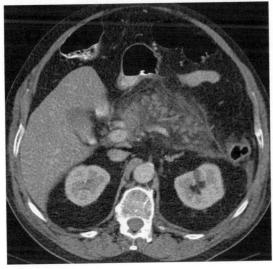

Figure 2.30   C

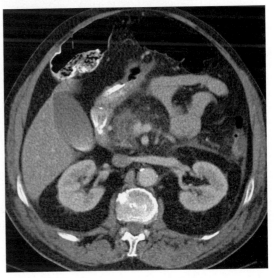

Figure 2.30   D

Findings: Consecutive axial CECT images demonstrate a swollen pancreas with peripancreatic inflammation. There are no peripancreatic fluid collections or necrotic areas in the pancreas.

Differential Diagnosis: None.

Diagnosis: Interstitial acute pancreatitis.

Discussion: Complications from pancreatitis can have devastating repercussions for the patient. A grading system for pancreatitis based on the amount of pancreatic and peripancreatic inflammation was devised by Balthazar et al. to help predict the outcome of these patients: grade A, normal pancreas radiographically; grade B, enlargement of the pancreas

with no peripancreatic disease; grade C, peripancreatic inflammation; grade D, single peripancreatic fluid collection or phlegmon; and grade E, two or more peripancreatic fluid collections or the presence of gas. Grades A and B carry a better prognosis with a shorter uncomplicated hospital stay than grades D and E. Later on, Balthazar refined his grading system by adding a score for the presence of pancreatic necrosis (<30%, 30–50%, or >50%); this CT severity index allows one to accurately differentiate patients with mild pancreatitis, who only need supportive therapy, from patients with severe pancreatitis, who typically are observed in the intensive care unit and are more likely to develop complications.

Clinical History: 36-year-old woman presenting with abdominal pain.

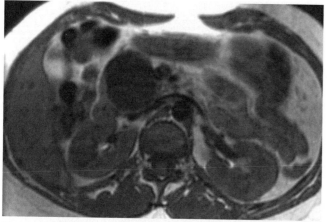

Figure 2.31   A

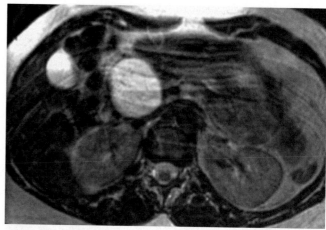

Figure 2.31   B

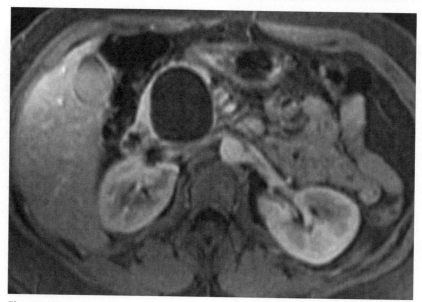

Figure 2.31   C

Findings: Axial T1-WI (A) and T2-WI (B) show well-defined unilocular cystic lesion in the pancreatic head. Gadolinium-enhanced, fat-saturated axial T1-WI (C) shows no enhancement of the lesion.

Differential Diagnosis: Pancreatic pseudocyst, mucinous cystic tumor.

Diagnosis: Macrocystic variant of the serous pancreatic adenoma.

Discussion: Serous cystic tumors are composed of epithelial cells that produce serous fluid and show evidence of ductal differentiation. Previously, these tumors were also known as "microcystic adenomas" because they were composed of a

large number (>6) of tiny cysts that were typically 2 cm or smaller. Recently, however, a variant of serous cystic tumors of the pancreas lined by epithelial cells indistinguishable from those in microcystic serous adenoma has been reported. This variant is termed "macrocystic serous adenoma of the pancreas" because the cysts are large and there are only a few cysts. Typically, this tumor is uni- or bilocular and contains no mural nodules, papillary projections, or calcifications. It is predominantly seen in women and typically located in the pancreatic head. The distinction between a mucinous cystic tumor and a macrocystic serous pancreatic adenoma cannot be made on the basis of radiologic features alone, and a fine-needle aspiration is typically needed.

Clinical History: 43-year-old woman with left lower quadrant pain, nausea, and vomiting for 3 weeks.

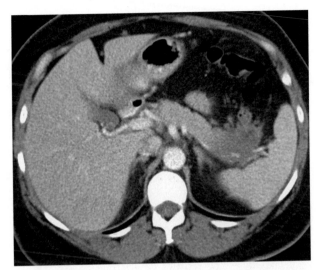

Figure 2.32   A

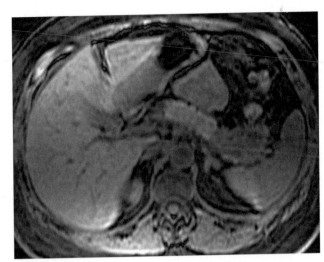

Figure 2.32   B

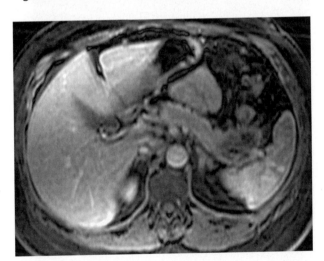

Figure 2.32   C

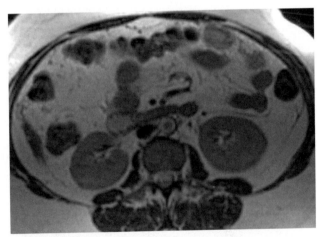

Figure 2.32   D

Findings: Axial CECT image (A) demonstrates a low-attenuation mass in the tail of the pancreas. No dilated ducts are present. Axial fat-suppressed T1-WI (B) shows the mass to be hypointense compared to normal pancreatic parenchyma. Gadolinium-enhanced, fat-suppressed axial T1-WI (C) shows hypovascular aspect of the lesion. Axial T2-WI (D) below the pancreas shows soft tissue masses in the greater omentum on the left.

Differential Diagnosis: Focal pancreatitis, metastases.

Diagnosis: Metastatic pancreatic ductal adenocarcinoma.

Discussion: Pancreatic ductal adenocarcinoma arises from the duct cells of the pancreas and accounts for approximately 80% to 95% of the nonendocrine malignancies of the pancreas. These tumors occur most commonly in the head of the pancreas and in patients between the ages of 50 and 70 years. It rarely occurs in patients younger than 40 years of age. Pancreatic ductal adenocarcinomas are hypovascular relative to the normal pancreas, and therefore, they have low attenuation on a CECT. Because they commonly occur in the head of the pancreas, they can present with symptoms of biliary obstruction even when the tumor is still small due to the desmoplastic reaction. Most lesions range in size between 2 and 5 cm. Other entities in the differential diagnosis of a hypovascular mass include segmental pancreatitis and metastases. Pancreatitis can usually be excluded by history. Metastases tend to be multiple, and a primary malignancy is typically known by the time a pancreatic metastasis is found.

Clinical History: 50-year-old woman who noted abdominal asymmetry, with the left side of her abdomen being more pronounced than the right.

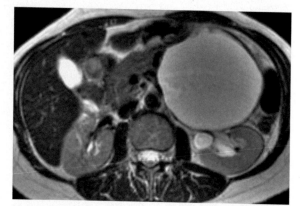

Figure 2.33　A

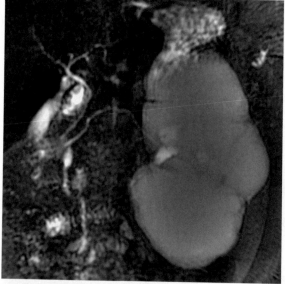

Figure 2.33　B

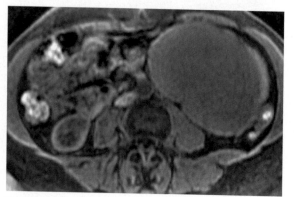

Figure 2.33　C

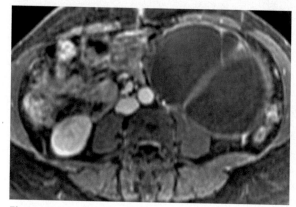

Figure 2.33　D

Findings: Axial T2-WI (A) and projective coronal oblique thick-slab MRCP image (B) demonstrate a 10 × 10 × 17 cm encapsulated cystic lesion with some septations arising from the tail of the pancreas. Pre- (C) and post- (D) gadolinium-enhanced, fat-suppressed axial T1-WI show subtle enhancement of the wall and septations.

Differential Diagnosis: Pseudocyst.

Diagnosis: Mucinous cystic neoplasm.

Discussion: Mucinous cystic neoplasm is lined by mucin-producing columnar cells and arises from the ductal epithelium. It is typically located in the pancreatic tail. There is a very strong female predominance (female-to-male ratio of 9:1), and women typically present with mucinous cystic tumors during their fifth or sixth decades of life. Pathologically, the tumor is characterized by the presence of ovarian stroma. Mucinous cystic tumor can be benign, borderline malignant, or frank malignant, and therefore, they are surgical lesions. Calcifications are present in approximately 30% of cases and are typically crescentlike in the wall or in the septations. Mural nodules and papillary projections can be seen in either benign or malignant lesions. However, the larger the solid portions of the lesion are, the worse the prognosis. A large cystic lesion in an older woman will most likely be a pseudocyst or mucinous cystic neoplasm. These two diagnoses are often difficult to distinguish if the history is equivocal. Both can become large and have thick walls and calcifications.

CASE 2-34

Clinical History: 66-year-old man presenting with bacteremia during the course of an acute pancreatitis attack.

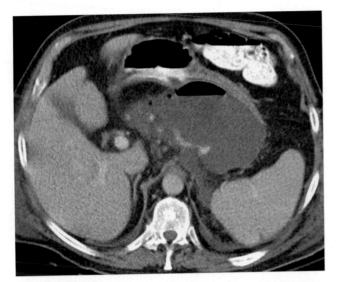

Figure 2.34   A

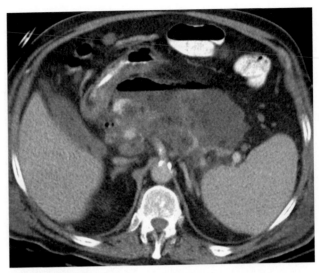

Figure 2.34   B

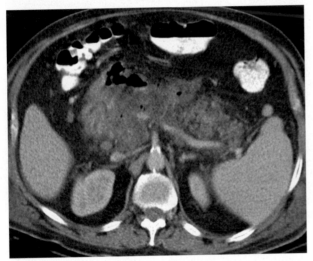
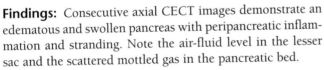

Figure 2.34   C

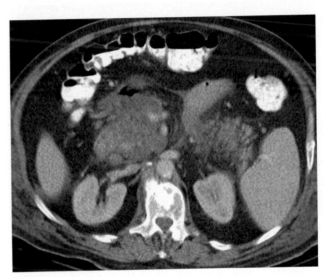

Figure 2.34   D

Findings: Consecutive axial CECT images demonstrate an edematous and swollen pancreas with peripancreatic inflammation and stranding. Note the air-fluid level in the lesser sac and the scattered mottled gas in the pancreatic bed.

Differential Diagnosis: None.

Diagnosis: Infected pancreatic necrosis.

Discussion: Many complications can occur in acute pancreatitis. Necrotizing pancreatitis is one of the most worrisome. In necrotizing pancreatitis, there is destruction of the pancreatic parenchyma due to the pancreatic enzymes. This can lead to infection of the pancreas by gram-negative bacteria, typically due to translocation of micro-organisms from the gut. Infected necrotizing pancreatitis carries a high mortality rate. CT findings include lack of enhancement of the normal pancreas after contrast administration and formation of a low-attenuation area in the pancreas region. The presence of gas bubbles within the pancreatic bed is highly suggestive of infected necrosis, but sterile necrosis cannot be excluded. Often percutaneous needle aspiration is needed to confirm the presence of infection. Treatment options for infected necrotizing pancreatitis include surgical debridement or aggressive percutaneous catheter drainage.

Clinical History: 64-year-old woman with a history of left nephrectomy 9 years ago.

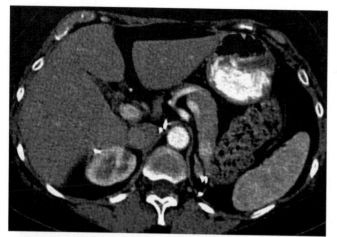

Figure 2.35   A

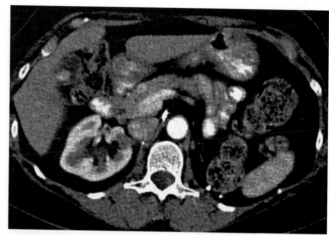

Figure 2.35   B

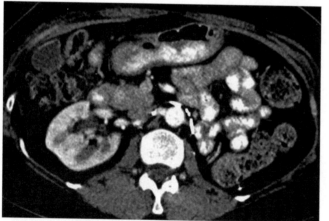

Figure 2.35   C

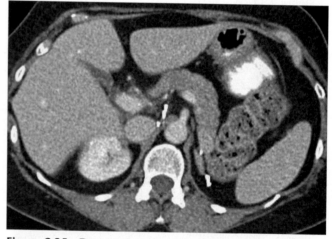

Figure 2.35   D

Findings: Consecutive axial CECT images (A–C) obtained during the pancreatic parenchymal phase demonstrate multiple small hypervascular lesions within the pancreas. Note that the patient is post left nephrectomy. Axial CECT image (D) obtained during the portal venous phase fails to demonstrate the pancreatic tail lesion.

Differential Diagnosis: Endocrine pancreatic tumors.

Diagnosis: Metastatic renal cell carcinoma.

Discussion: Metastatic disease to the pancreas is extremely rare and typically occurs during the advanced stages of a malignancy. Most metastases to the pancreas arise by direct extension from an adjacent organ. Other metastases are hematogenous in nature, such as renal cancer, lung cancer, breast cancer, and melanoma. Multiple masses in the pancreas are very rare but, when present, can be due to metastases, multiple endocrine pancreatic tumors (usually gastrinomas), or lymphoma. In this case, the history of prior nephrectomy and the absence of an endocrine syndrome are very suggestive of pancreatic metastases. Pancreatic lymphoma is typically hypovascular.

Clinical History: 53-year-old man with a previous history of pituitary and parathyroid tumor resection undergoing screening abdominal study.

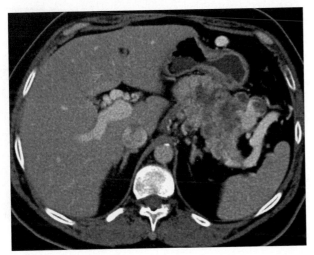

Figure 2.36   A

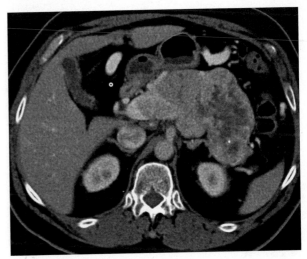

Figure 2.36   B

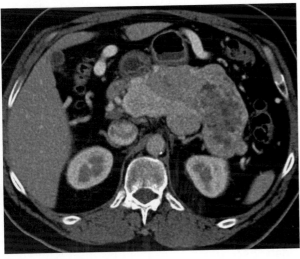

Figure 2.36   C

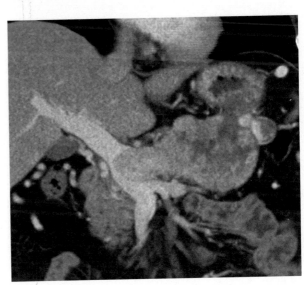

Figure 2.36   D

Findings: Consecutive axial CECT images (A–C) demonstrate a large, fairly well-defined, hypervascular and heterogeneous mass in the body and tail of the pancreas. Note the presence of numerous venous collaterals in the upper abdomen. Coronal reformatted CECT image (D) demonstrates invasion of the mass into the portal vein.

Differential Diagnosis: Metastasis, sarcoma, acinar cell tumor.

Diagnosis: Nonhyperfunctioning pancreatic endocrine tumor.

Discussion: Nonhyperfunctioning endocrine tumor of the pancreas accounts for approximately 15% to 30% of pancreatic endocrine tumors, and the vast majority have malignant biologic behavior. Nonhyperfunctioning endocrine tumors are similar to other endocrine tumors histologically, but they secrete only a small amount of hormones. Therefore, they are not easily detected clinically. These neoplasms are usually slow growing and will typically be large at the time of diagnosis. When discovered, liver and regional metastases are frequently present. Nonhyperfunctioning endocrine tumors have heterogeneous contrast enhancement on CECT with areas of hemorrhage and necrosis frequently seen due to their large size. Calcifications can be present as well. The differential diagnosis is limited for a large hypervascular lesion in the pancreas. Sarcoma and acinar cell tumor are frequently large lesions but are rare.

Clinical History: 26-year-old woman with lymphoma after lung transplantation.

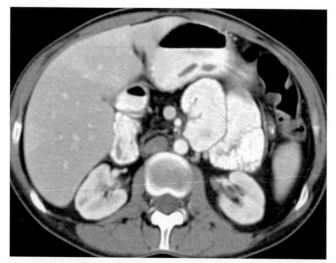

Figure 2.37   A

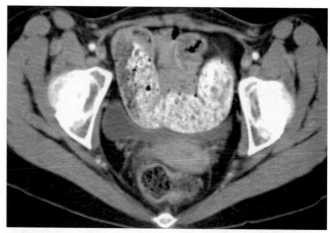

Figure 2.37   B

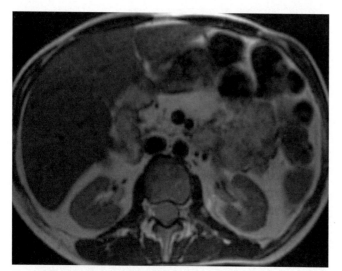

Figure 2.37   C

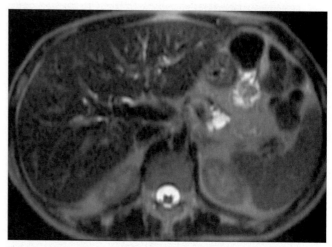

Figure 2.37   D

Findings: Axial CECT images of the abdomen (A) and pelvis (B) demonstrate complete fatty replacement of the pancreas and dilated fecaloid material containing small bowel loops. Axial T2-WI (C and D) show a hyperintense pancreas consistent with lipomatosis and the presence of a small cystic structure in the pancreatic body.

Differential Diagnosis: Severe malnutrition, Shwachman-Diamond syndrome, diabetes, Cushing syndrome.

Diagnosis: Cystic fibrosis with meconium ileus equivalent.

Discussion: Cystic fibrosis is characterized by the formation of thick secretions due to dysfunction of the exocrine glands, including the pancreas. There is also dysfunction of the mucociliary transport system, which results in recurrent pulmonary infections; slow transit of GI content is also characteristic. A typical finding in cystic fibrosis is complete fatty replacement of the pancreas. Other CT and MRI features include pancreatic fibrosis, seen as hypointense signal on T1-WI, and the presence of retention cysts, which are caused by obstruction of side branches and appear hyperintense on T2-WI. The diagnosis is confirmed in this case by the age of the patient and the coexisting meconium ileus equivalent. The fatty replacement seen in elderly patients, obese patients, and patients with Cushing syndrome tends to be marbled in appearance rather than diffuse replacement, as is seen in this case. Shwachman-Diamond syndrome is a rare disorder in the family of metaphyseal dysplasias that has coexisting fatty replacement of the pancreas.

Clinical History: 48-year-old man with severe intermittent abdominal pain, nausea, and vomiting.

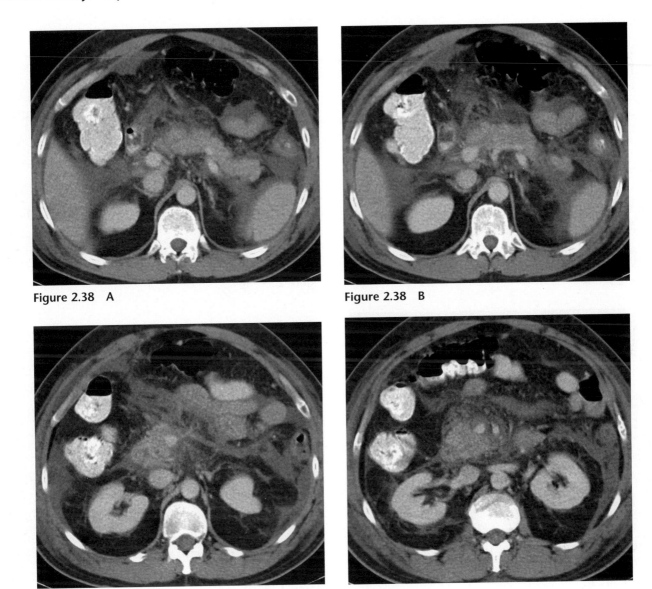

Figure 2.38 **A** Figure 2.38 **B**

Figure 2.38 **C** Figure 2.38 **D**

Findings: Consecutive axial CECT images demonstrate peripancreatic inflammation spreading anteriorly into the transverse mesocolon.

Differential Diagnosis: None.

Diagnosis: Acute pancreatitis.

Discussion: This case nicely demonstrates one of the many pathways of spread to and from the pancreas. Although the pancreas resides in the anterior pararenal space of the retroperitoneum, it has access to many parts of the abdomen. Pancreatitis or a pancreatic malignancy can spread by direct extension to other organs in the anterior pararenal space such as the duodenum and ascending and descending colon. A pancreatic process can also reach the transverse colon via the transverse mesocolon. As can be seen in this example, the inflammation from the acute pancreatitis tracks anteriorly through the transverse mesocolon to eventually reach the transverse colon. This can produce a thickened mucosa seen by barium enema or CT scan. Note that this process involves no loops of small bowel since the small bowel is attached to the retroperitoneum via the small bowel mesentery, which is not directly involved by the pancreatitis in this case. A pancreatic malignancy can also spread to the transverse colon in a similar manner.

Clinical History: 52-year-old woman with a history of Crohn disease.

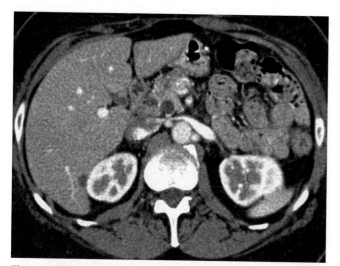

Figure 2.39   A

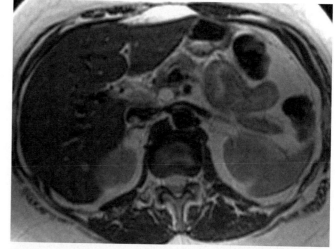

Figure 2.39   B

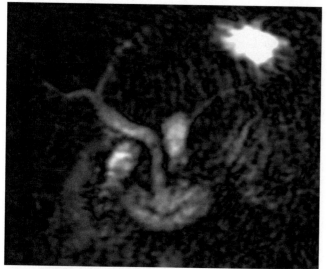

Figure 2.39   C

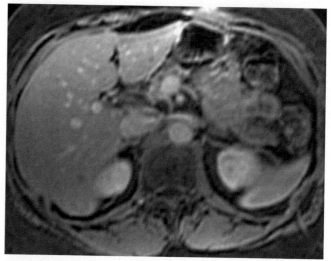

Figure 2.39   D

Findings: Axial CECT image (A) demonstrates a 1.5-cm well-defined cystic mass in the uncinate process. Heavily T2-WI (B) shows the lesion to be hyperintense. Projective coronal oblique thick-slab MRCP image (C) demonstrates a connection between the lesion and the pancreatic duct that is otherwise normal. Gadolinium-enhanced, fat-suppressed axial T1-WI (D) shows no enhancement of the lesion.

Differential Diagnosis: Pseudocyst, macrocystic serous pancreatic adenoma, mucinous cystic tumor.

Diagnosis: Intraductal papillary mucinous neoplasm.

Discussion: Intraductal papillary mucinous neoplasm (IPMN) is a relatively new and increasingly reported entity (synonyms include mucin-producing tumor, intraductal mucin-hypersecreting neoplasm, mucin-hypersecreting tumor, mucinous ductal ectasia, and ductectatic mucinous cystic tumor). This tumor is one of the mucin-producing tumors of the pancreas and is thought to originate in the pancreatic duct or its branches. It has papillary hyperplastic, atypical, or malignant epithelium. On CT and MRI, a dilated main pancreatic duct with a uni- or multilocular cystic lesion is typical. Communication between the main pancreatic duct and the cystic lesion may be depicted and excludes other cystic pancreatic neoplasms, such as serous or mucinous cystic tumors. Papillary projections or papillary neoplasm may be depicted in thin-section CT images. The bulging papilla and large caliber of the main pancreatic duct are more common in patients with malignant IPMNs. Side-branch IPMN is most often located in the uncinate process.

Clinical History: 42-year-old woman with left lower quadrant pain.

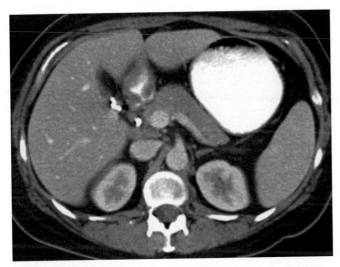

Figure 2.40   A

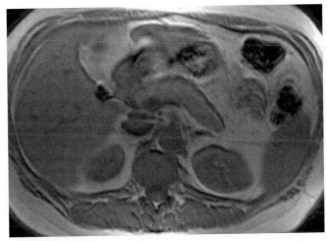

Figure 2.40   B

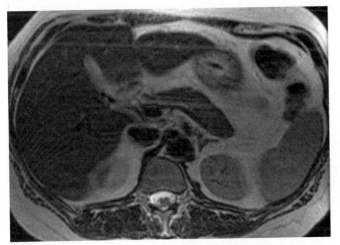

Figure 2.40   C

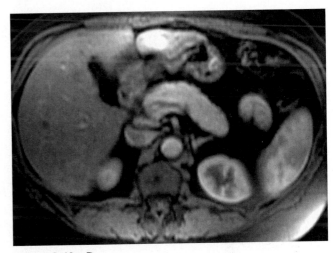

Figure 2.40   D

Findings: Axial CECT image (A) demonstrates absence of the pancreatic tail. Axial T1-WI (B), T2-WI (C), and gadolinium-enhanced, fat-suppressed axial T1-WI (D) show normal signal intensity and enhancement of the pancreas.

Differential Diagnosis: None.

Diagnosis: Truncated (hypoplastic) pancreas.

Discussion: Hypoplasia (partial agenesis) results from the absence of the ventral or dorsal anlage. The dorsal anlage absence, visualized as short or truncated pancreas, is more common and can be partial or complete. It may be seen as a solitary finding or in association with heterotaxia syndromes. Partial agenesis of the dorsal pancreas is relatively more common than agenesis of the ventral portion, but complete agenesis of the dorsal pancreas is extremely rare. Patients with agenesis of the dorsal pancreas often present with nonspecific abdominal pain, which may or may not be caused by pancreatitis. Many patients also have diabetes mellitus. When the diagnosis of agenesis of the dorsal pancreas is suspected, it is critical to rule out pancreatic carcinoma with upstream atrophy of the gland. On imaging, complete dorsal pancreatic hypoplasia is recognized as a short, rounded pancreatic head adjacent to the duodenum and absence of the pancreatic neck, body, and tail. In cases of partial agenesis or hypoplasia of the dorsal pancreas, the size of the body of the pancreas varies, there is a remnant of the duct of Santorini, and the minor duodenal papilla is present.

Clinical History: 45-year-old man imaged with MRI 9 months after acute pancreatitis.

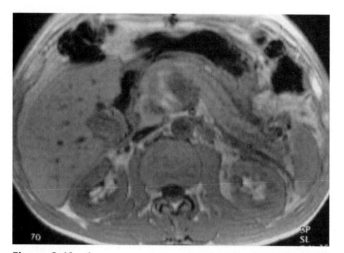

Figure 2.41 A

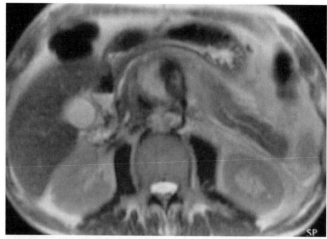

Figure 2.41 B

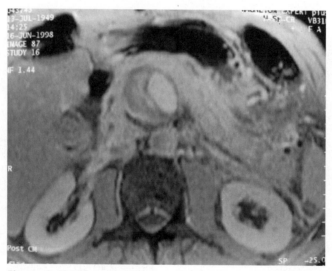

Figure 2.41 C

Findings: Axial T1-WI (A), T2-WI (B), and gadolinium-enhanced T1-WI (C) show a rounded vascular mass adjacent to the pancreatic head. Note nonenhancing hemorrhagic thrombus (hyperintense on T1-WI, hypointense on T2-WI) at the right side of the mass.

Differential Diagnosis: Nonhyperfunctioning endocrine tumor, solid and papillary epithelial neoplasm.

Diagnosis: Pseudoaneurysm of common hepatic artery.

Discussion: Acute pancreatitis is a common illness with a relatively unpredictable severity course. In most patients, fortunately, the acute pancreatic inflammatory disease is mild, only presenting with minimal abdominal pain that usually resolves within a few days. However, in 20% to 30% of cases, the pancreatitis can be severe and associated with potentially life-threatening complications, such as extensive pancreatic necrosis, pancreatic abscess formation, multiorgan failure, and development of peripancreatic vascular complications. Arterial hemorrhage in patients with pancreatitis results of autodigestion of arterial walls by pancreatic enzymes, especially elastase, and is considered the most severe manifestation of the spectrum of vascular complications. Acute hemorrhage may develop from direct vascular erosion or rupture of a pseudoaneurysm. The surgical and radiologic literature has stressed the importance of its early detection because severe peripancreatic hemorrhage can have catastrophic consequences, with an estimated mortality rate of 37%. Pseudoaneurysm formation typically manifests itself as a late complication of acute pancreatitis and does not usually develop within the first weeks or months after the initial pancreatitis event.

CASE 2-42

Clinical History: 50-year-old woman with multiple cerebral surgeries who presents with abdominal pain.

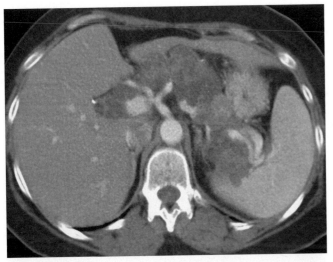

Figure 2.42   A

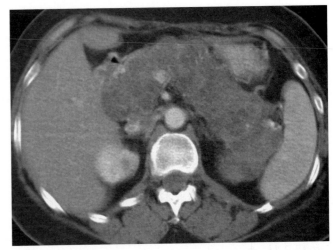

Figure 2.42   B

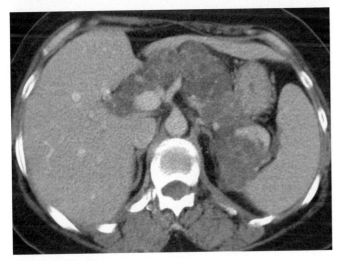

Figure 2.42   C

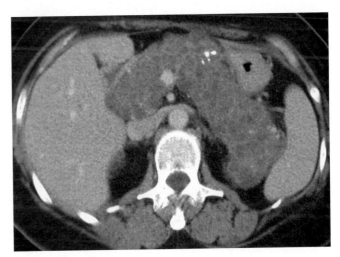

Figure 2.42   D

Findings: Axial consecutive CECT images obtained during the arterial phase (A and B) and portal venous phase (C and D) show complete replacement of the pancreatic gland by small cysts. Also note the presence of some punctate calcifications in the wall of some of the cysts.

Differential Diagnosis: Microcystic serous pancreatic adenoma, hepatorenal polycystic disease.

Diagnosis: Pancreatic cystosis in von Hippel-Lindau disease.

Discussion: Congenital pancreatic cysts are exceedingly rare. They have a female predominance and typically present as an asymptomatic palpable mass. Patients may also present with epigastric pain, jaundice, and vomiting related to compression of surrounding structures. These cysts can be single or multiple and are more commonly located in the tail and body of the pancreas. Multiple congenital cysts are associated with other anomalies, such as von Hippel-Lindau (VHL) disease and hepatorenal polycystic disease. VHL disease is an autosomal dominant disorder with variable penetrance that is characterized by retinal angiomas and central nervous system hemangioblastomas. Pancreatic cysts are relatively common in VHL, and involvement can range from a single cyst to cystic replacement of the gland. Peripheral calcifications can also be present. Pancreatic lesions may be the only manifestation of the disease by many years. Other pancreatic neoplasms not infrequently seen in VHL disease include microcystic serous pancreatic adenomas and endocrine pancreatic tumors.

Clinical History: 32-year-old woman with acute recurrent pancreatitis.

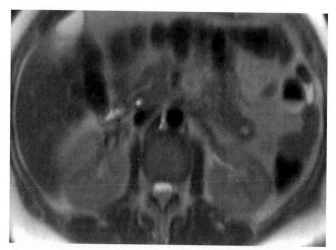

Figure 2.43   A

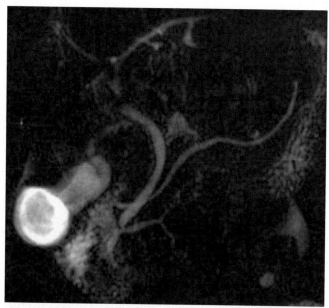

Figure 2.43   B

Findings: Axial T2-WI (A) at the level of the pancreatic head shows drainage of the pancreatic duct in the minor papilla and drainage of the CBD through the major papilla. Projective coronal oblique thick-slab MRCP image (B) shows lack of fusion between the main pancreatic duct and the duct of Wirsung (ventral duct). Note that the main pancreatic duct drains via the duct of Santorini into the minor papilla.

Differential Diagnosis: Dorsal dominant duct syndrome.

Diagnosis: Pancreas divisum.

Discussion: Pancreas divisum (PD) is the most common congenital anomaly of the pancreatic ductal system, being reported in 4% to 10% of the population. This anomaly results when the ventral and dorsal pancreatic ducts fail to fuse. The ventral duct (duct of Wirsung) drains only the ventral pancreatic anlage, while the majority of the gland empties into the minor papilla through the dorsal duct or duct of Santorini. Focal dilatation of the terminal portion of the dorsal duct, coined santorinicele, is described in association with PD and relative obstruction at the minor papilla. PD usually causes no symptoms, but it is found more frequently in patients with chronic abdominal pain and idiopathic pancreatitis than in the general population. The definitive diagnosis of PD is made with endoscopic retrograde pancreatography (ERP). MRCP has been shown to be highly sensitive and specific for depicting PD. MRCP with secretin stimulation helps in identifying PD and santorinicele. In dorsal dominant duct syndrome, the majority of the gland drains through the dorsal duct, but there is still a connection with the duct of Wirsung.

Clinical History: 28-year-old man imaged with CT for the evaluation of multiple stab wounds.

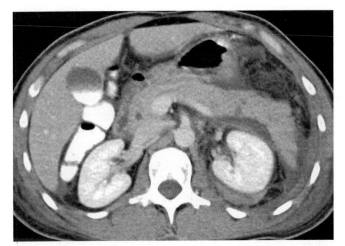

Figure 2.44 A

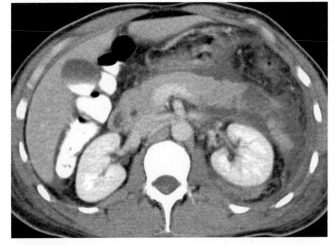

Figure 2.44 B

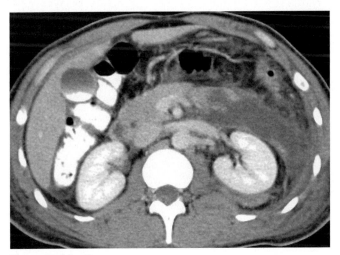

Figure 2.44 C

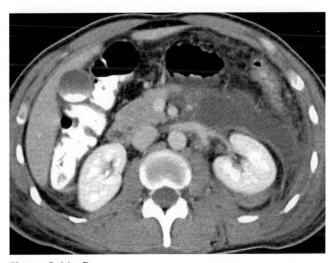

Figure 2.44 D

Findings: Consecutive axial CECT images through the upper abdomen show fluid in the anterior pararenal space and left perirenal space and a linear interruption in the pancreatic parenchyma.

Differential Diagnosis: Acute pancreatitis.

Diagnosis: Pancreatic laceration.

Discussion: Trauma to the pancreas can be iatrogenic because of surgery or biopsy, direct because of stab or gunshot injury, as seen in this case, or result from indirect trauma (e.g., a motor vehicle accident). The gland is typically swollen, and peripancreatic hemorrhage is present in the retroperitoneum. An unenhanced CT study may be valuable to demonstrate fresh high-density blood in the retroperitoneum. In cases of indirect trauma, it is important to look for associated injury to the gastrointestinal tract, especially the duodenum. An associated pancreatic ductal injury will lead to acute pancreatitis and fluid accumulation in the retroperitoneum.

Clinical History: 28-year-old man imaged with MRI 3 weeks after an episode of acute pancreatitis.

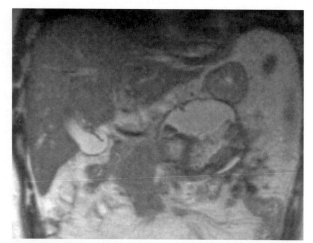

Figure 2.45   A

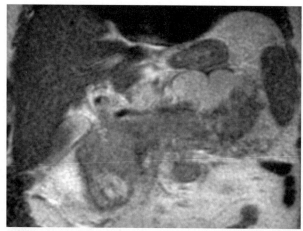

Figure 2.45   B

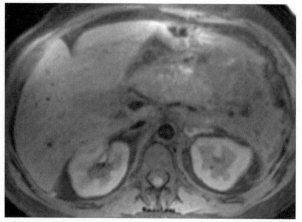

Figure 2.45   C

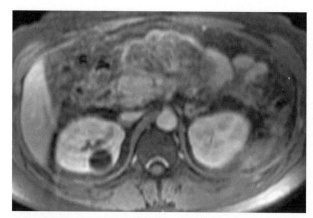

Figure 2.45   D

Findings: Coronal T2-WI (A and B) show the presence of a complex fluid collection in the lesser sac and a swollen appearance of the pancreatic gland. Note abnormal increased signal intensity of the pancreas when compared to the liver and the presence of peripancreatic fat stranding. Axial fat-suppressed T1-WI (C) shows small area of high signal intensity representing hemorrhage in the pancreatic bed. The pancreas has abnormal low signal intensity. Gadolinium-enhanced, fat-suppressed axial T1-WI (D) shows lack of enhancement of the majority of the pancreatic gland.

Differential Diagnosis: None.

Diagnosis: Organized pancreatic necrosis post acute necrotizing pancreatitis.

Discussion: In assessment of acute pancreatitis, MRI, as well as CT, can depict the presence and extent of necrosis and peripancreatic fluid collections. Several authors recommend intravenous gadolinium administration in imaging severe acute pancreatitis, particularly for the assessment of pancreatic parenchymal perfusion and presence of necrosis. Gadolinium has a good renal tolerance and is better tolerated than the iodinated contrast agents used in CT. The enlargement of the gland is well demonstrated on any sequence. Parenchymal edema is better shown on unenhanced T1-WI. Pancreatic enhancement is maximal within 20 to 40 seconds after gadolinium administration, and the extent of parenchymal necrosis is well demonstrated on sequential, multislice acquisition obtained during the first 1 to 2 minutes after injection. T2-WI sequences are the most sensitive in demonstrating fluid collections. Despite these results, CT retains several advantages; CT is widely accessible and less costly than MRI and is more sensitive in detecting small gas bubbles and calcifications. However, MRI combined with MRCP has become important in the evaluation of patients with suspected biliary pancreatitis.

Clinical History: 21-year-old woman with chronic left upper abdominal pain.

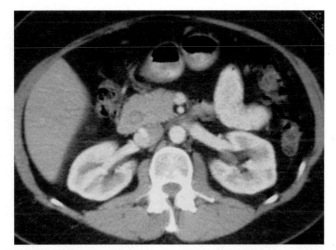

Figure 2.46   A

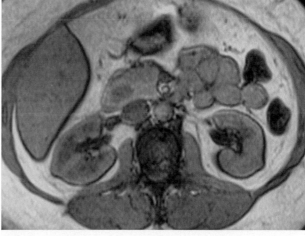

Figure 2.46   B

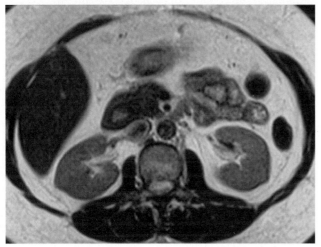

Figure 2.46   C

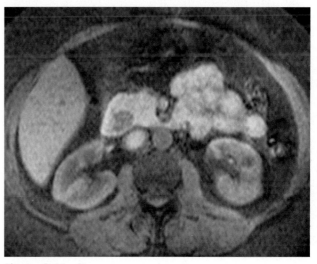

Figure 2.46   D

Findings: Axial CECT image (A) shows a round low-density lesion within the pancreatic head. The duodenum is not visualized. Axial T1-WI (B), T2-WI (C), and fat-saturated T1-WI shows that the tissue surrounding the cystic lesion follows the signal intensity of normal pancreatic parenchyma.

Differential Diagnosis: Cystic pancreatic neoplasm, pseudocyst.

Diagnosis: Annular pancreas.

Discussion: Annular pancreas is a rare congenital anomaly in which incomplete rotation of the ventral anlage leads to a segment of the pancreas encircling the second part of the duodenum. The incidence of annular pancreas is 1 in 2000, occurring as either an isolated finding or in association with other congenital abnormalities. In approximately half of symptomatic cases, annular pancreas will present in the neonate with gastrointestinal obstruction or bile duct obstruction possibly associated with pancreatitis. In the adult, it may manifest with symptoms of peptic ulcer disease, duodenal obstruction, or pancreatitis. In general, annular pancreas obstructs the duodenum in 10% of cases. There are two types of annular pancreas: the extramural and the intramural types. In the extramural type, the ventral pancreatic duct runs around the duodenum to join the main pancreatic duct. In the intramural type, the pancreatic tissue is intermingled with muscle fibers in the duodenal wall, and small ducts drain directly into the duodenum. Annular pancreas can be diagnosed on the basis of CT and MR findings that reveal pancreatic tissue and an annular duct encircling the descending duodenum.

Clinical History: 29-year-old woman found to have abnormal liver function tests before treatment for positive purified protein derivative (PPD).

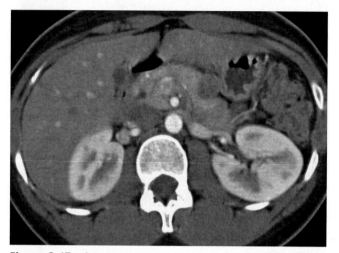

Figure 2.47   A

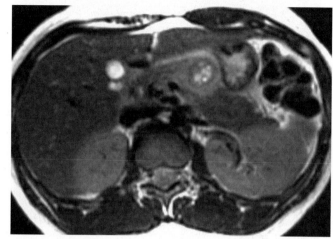

Figure 2.47   B

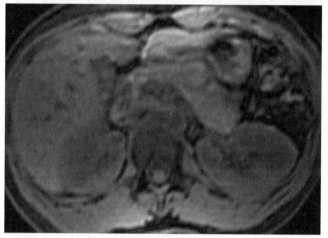

Figure 2.47   C

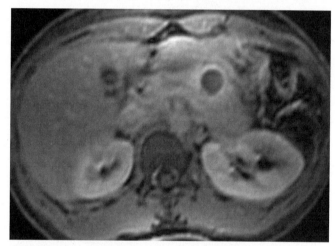

Figure 2.47   D

Findings: Axial CECT image (A) shows round cystic and multiloculated lesion within the pancreatic body. Axial T2-WI (B), fat-saturated T1-WI (C), and gadolinium-enhanced, fat-suppressed T1-WI (D) shows spontaneous hyperintense signal within the center of the lesion and peripheral rimlike enhancement.

Differential Diagnosis: Solid and papillary epithelial neoplasm, endocrine pancreatic tumor.

Diagnosis: Pancreatoblastoma.

Discussion: Pancreatoblastoma is a rare primary tumor of the pancreas most commonly seen in patients 1 to 8 years of age; however, rare cases in neonates and the elderly have been reported. Although the majority of cases are sporadic, a congenital form is associated with Beckwith-Wiedemann syndrome. There is a slight male predominance, and two thirds of cases in the medical literature have occurred in patients of Asian descent. There is no apparent predilection for the pancreatic head, body, or tail. Tumors are often large at presentation, with 85% measuring >8.0 cm. Elevated alpha-fetoprotein is the most common abnormal serologic marker and is seen in up to one third of pediatric cases. The majority of pancreatoblastomas are large, well-defined, at least partially circumscribed, and heterogeneous masses with low to intermediate signal intensity on T1-WI and high signal intensity on T2-WI. Enhancement is a common feature on CECT and MRI. This case is atypical because of the age of the patient and the small size of the mass.

Clinical History: 26-year-old woman presenting with hypoglycemia.

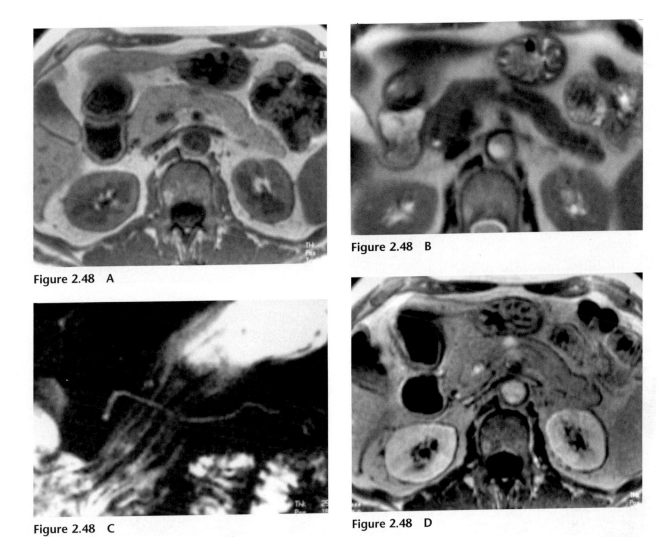

Figure 2.48   A

Figure 2.48   B

Figure 2.48   C

Figure 2.48   D

Findings: Axial T1-WI (A) and T2-WI (B) demonstrate a small lesion in the pancreatic body that is hypointense and markedly hyperintense, respectively. Projective coronal oblique thick-slab MRCP image (C) shows the lesion as hyperintense, and no obvious connection with the pancreatic duct is identified. Axial gadolinium-enhanced T1-WI (D) shows marked homogeneous enhancement of the lesion.

Differential Diagnosis: Solid and papillary epithelial tumor.

Diagnosis: Insulinoma.

Discussion: Insulinoma is the most common endocrine tumor of the pancreas (~60%), but only 5% to 10% are malignant. The Whipple triad (starvation attack, hypoglycemia after a fasting period, and relief by intravenous dextrose) is typically associated with the clinical onset of an insulinoma.

At the time of diagnosis, 50% of the tumors are smaller than 1.5 cm. Malignant insulinomas present with a larger diameter (mean diameter, 6.2 cm). In only 5% to 10% of cases, multiple insulinomas are found, and there is a slightly higher incidence for the body and tail. On multiphasic CECT, insulinomas present as hypervascularized lesions that are best seen in the early phases of pancreatic enhancement. The most striking evidence for malignancy is evidence of metastatic disease to the liver or local lymph nodes. On MRI, insulinomas appear as lesions with low signal intensity on T1-WI and as lesions with high signal intensity on T2-WI. Fat-suppression sequences are useful in emphasizing the signal intensity differences between tumor and normal pancreatic tissue. The use of intravenous gadolinium-chelates is helpful in the detection of endocrine tumors because these tumors are hypervascularized.

Clinical History: 57-year-old woman presenting with fever and jaundice.

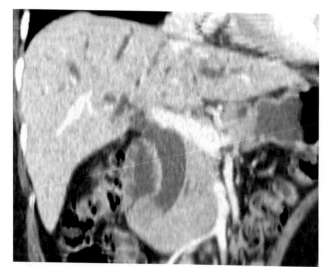

Figure 2.49 **A**

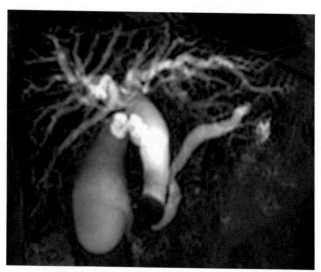

Figure 2.49 **B**

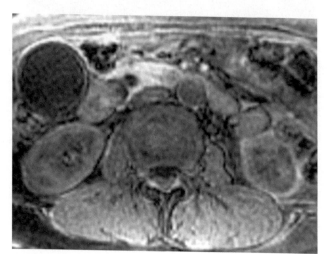

Figure 2.49 **C**

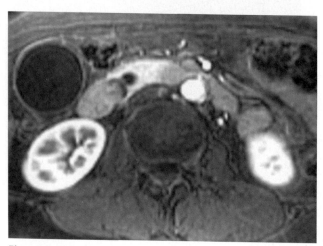

Figure 2.49 **D**

Findings: Coronal reformatted CECT image (A) shows dilated CBD and intrahepatic ducts caused by an obstructing mass at the level of the pancreatic head. Projective coronal oblique thick-slab MRCP image (B) demonstrates dilated pancreatic duct and CBD and acute amputation of the CBD. Axial fat-suppressed T1-WI (C) and gadolinium-enhanced, fat-suppressed T1-WI (D) show enhancement of the mass obstructing the CBD.

Differential Diagnosis: Pancreatic ductal adenocarcinoma, distal cholangiocarcinoma.

Diagnosis: Ampullary carcinoma.

Discussion: Ampullary malignant tumor, usually a polypoid adenocarcinoma protruding from the papilla, is less common than pancreatic carcinoma and is best identified at endoscopy. Tumors are usually small (50% are <3 cm) at

presentation because the lumen of the common bile duct does not permit much encroachment before it becomes obstructed. Cancer of the ampulla generally obstructs both the distal CBD and the pancreatic duct. Shouldering of the obstructed CBD is frequently seen, as demonstrated in this case. Pancreatic duct dilatation is mostly absent when the duct of Santorini and minor papilla are patent. On MRCP, ampullary lesions display a true double duct sign with obstruction of the distal CBD and pancreatic duct. In patients with pancreatic ductal adenocarcinoma, MRCP shows the so-called four-segment sign (i.e., an obstructed pancreatic duct and CBD with a short normal intrasphincteric segment of pancreatic duct and CBD).

Case images courtesy of Dr. Giovanni Artho, McGill University Health Center, Montreal, Canada.

CASE 2-50

Clinical History: 28-year-old woman presenting with epigastric pain.

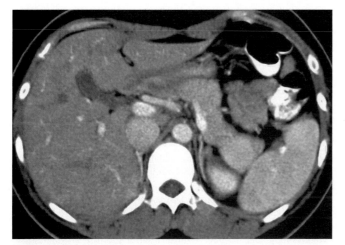

Figure 2.50   A

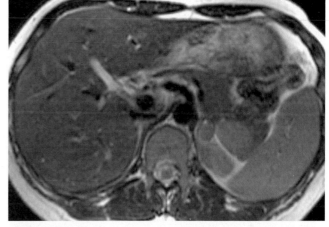

Figure 2.50   B

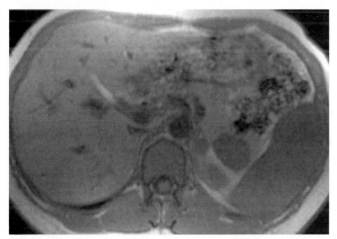

Figure 2.50   C

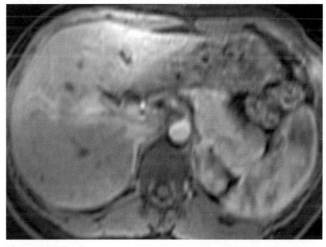

Figure 2.50   D

Findings: Axial CECT image (A) demonstrates a well-defined hypervascular mass in the pancreatic tail. Axial T2-WI (B), T1-WI (C), and gadolinium-enhanced T1-WI (D) show the lesion as hyperintense, hypointense, and hypervascular, respectively.

Differential Diagnosis: Endocrine pancreatic neoplasm, solid and papillary epithelial neoplasm.

Diagnosis: Intrapancreatic accessory spleen.

Discussion: Supernumerary spleens or splenunculi result from failure of the splenic anlagen to fuse and are present in approximately 15% of the population. They can be located anywhere within the retroperitoneum, but intrapancreatic locations are rare. An accurate CT or MRI diagnosis can be made by recognizing a similar density, intensity, or enhancement pattern of the accessory spleen when compared to the main spleen. Tagged RBC scan or ferumoxides-enhanced MRI is valuable to confirm the diagnosis in doubtful cases.

SUGGESTED READINGS

INFLAMMATION

- Amano Y, Oishi T, Takahashi M. Nonenhanced magnetic resonance imaging of mild acute pancreatitis. *Abdom Imaging.* 2001;26:59–63.

- Balthazar E, Ranson BM, Naidich D, et al. Acute pancreatitis: prognostic value of CT. *Radiology* 1985;156:767–772.

- Balthazar E, Robinson D, Megibow A, et al. Acute pancreatitis: value of CT in establishing prognosis. *Radiology* 1990;174:331–336.

- Balthazar EJ. CT diagnosis and staging of acute pancreatitis. *Radiol Clin North Am.* 1989;27:19–37.

- De Backer AI, Mortele KJ, Ros PR, et al. Chronic pancreatitis: diagnostic role of computed tomography and magnetic resonance imaging. *JBR-BTR.* 2002;85:304–310.

- Elmas N. The role of diagnostic radiology in pancreatitis. *Eur J Radiol.* 2001;38:120–132.

- Freeny PC. Classification of pancreatitis. *Radiol Clin North Am.* 1989;27:1–3.

- Johnson PT, Outwater EK. Pancreatic carcinoma versus chronic pancreatitis: dynamic MR imaging. *Radiology* 1999;212:213–218.

- Lecesne R, Laurent F, Drouillard J, et al. Chronic pancreatitis. In: Baert AL, Delorme G, Van Hoe L, eds. *Radiology of the pancreas.* 2nd ed. Heidelberg, Germany: Springer-Verlag; 1999:145–180.

- Lecesne R, Taourel P, Bret PM, et al. Acute pancreatitis: interobserver agreement and correlation of CT and MR cholangiopancreatography with outcome. *Radiology* 1999;211:727–735.

- Matos C, Metens T, Deviere J, et al. Pancreatic duct: Morphologic and functional evaluation with dynamic MR pancreatography after secretin stimulation. *Radiology* 1997;203:435–441.

- Mortele KJ, Banks PA, Silverman SG. State-of-the-art imaging of acute pancreatitis. *JBR-BTR.* 2003;86:193–208.

- Mortele KJ, Mergo PJ, Taylor HM, et al. Peripancreatic vascular abnormalities complicating acute pancreatitis: Contrast-enhanced helical CT findings. *Eur J Radiol.* 2004;52:67–72.

- Mortele KJ, Mergo PJ, Taylor HM, et al. Renal and perirenal space involvement in acute pancreatitis: state-of-the-art spiral CT findings. *Abdom Imaging.* 2000;25:272–278.

- Mortele KJ, Wiesner W, Cantisani V, et al. Usual and unusual causes of extrahepatic cholestasis: assessment with magnetic resonance cholangiography and fast MRI. *Abdom Imaging.* 2004;29:87–99.

- Mortele KJ, Wiesner W, Intriere L, et al. A modified CT severity index for evaluating acute pancreatitis: improved correlation with patient outcome. *Am J Roentgenol.* 2004;183:1261–1265.

- Robinson PJA, Sheridan MB. Pancreatitis: computed tomography and magnetic resonance imaging. *Eur Radiol.* 2000;10:401–408.

- Sahani DV, Kalva SP, Farrell J, et al. Auto-immune pancreatitis: imaging features. *Radiology* 2004:233:345–352.

- Sica GT, Braver J, Cooney MJ, et al. Comparison of endoscopic retrograde cholangiopancreatography with MR cholangiopancreatography in patients with pancreatitis. *Radiology* 1999;210:605–610.

- Ward J, Chalmers AG, Guthrie AJ, et al. T2-weighted and dynamic enhanced MRI in acute pancreatitis: comparison with contrast-enhanced CT. *Clin Radiol.* 1997;52:109–114.

NEOPLASMS

- Baek SY, Sheafor DH, Keogan MT, et al. Two-dimensional multiplanar and three-dimensional volume-rendered vascular CT in pancreatic carcinoma: interobserver agreement and comparison with standard helical techniques. *Am J Roentgenol.* 2001;176:1467–1473.

- Boland GW, O'Malley ME, Saez M, et al. Pancreatic-phase versus portal vein-phase helical CT of the pancreas: optimal temporal window for evaluation of pancreatic adenocarcinoma. *Am J Roentgenol.* 1999;172:605–608.

- Buetow PC, Parrino TV, Buck JL, et al. Islet cell tumors of the pancreas: pathologic-imaging correlation among size, necrosis and cysts, calcification, malignant behavior and functional status. *Am J Roentgenol.* 1995;165:1175–1179.

- Cantisani V, Mortele KJ, Levy A, et al. MR imaging features of solid-pseudopapillary tumor of the pancreas in adult and pediatric patients. *Am J Roentgenol.* 2003;181:395–401.

- Choi BI, Chung MJ, Han JK et al. Detection of pancreatic adenocarcinoma: Relative value of arterial and late phases of spiral CT. *Abdom Imaging.* 1997;22:199–203.

- Choi BI, Kim KW, Han MC, et al. Solid and papillary epithelial neoplasms of the pancreas: CT findings. *Radiology* 1988;166:413–416.

- Chung MJ, Choi BI, Han JK, et al. Functioning islet cell tumor of the pancreas: localization with dynamic spiral CT. *Acta Radiol.* 1997;38:135–138.

- Compagno J, Oertel JE. Mucinous cystic neoplasms of the pancreas with overt and latent malignancy (cystadenocarcinoma and cystadenoma). *Am Soc Clin Pathol.* 1978;69:573–580.

- Diehl SJ, Lehmann KJ, Sadick M, et al. Pancreatic cancer: value of dual-phase helical CT in assessing resectability. *Radiology* 1998;206:373–378.

- Ellsmere J, Mortele KJ, Sahani D, et al. Does multidetector-row CT eliminate the role of diagnostic laparoscopy in assessing the resectability of pancreatic head adenocarcinoma? *Surg Endosc.* 2005;19:369–373.

- Erturk SM, Mortele KJ, Oliva MR, et al. State-of-the-art computed tomographic and magnetic resonance imaging of the gastrointestinal system. *Gastrointest Endosc Clin N Am.* 2005;15:581–614.

- Fishman EK, Horton KM, Urban BA. Multidetector CT angiography in the evaluation of pancreatic carcinoma: preliminary observation. *J Comput Assist Tomogr.* 2000;24:849–853.

- Freeny PC, Mark, WM, Ryan JA, et al. Pancreatic ductal adenocarcinoma: diagnosis and staging with dynamic CT. *Radiology* 1988;166:125–133.

- Friedman AC, Lichtenstein JE, Dachman AH. Cystic neoplasms of the pancreas. *Radiology* 1983;149:45–50.

- Friesen SR. Tumors of the endocrine pancreas. *N Engl J Med.* 1982;306:580–590.

- Frucht H, Doppman JL, Norton JA, et al. Gastrinomas: comparison of MR imaging with CT, angiography, and US. *Radiology* 1989;171:713–717.

- Gabata T, Matsui O, Kadoya M, et al. Small pancreatic adenocarcinoma: efficacy of MR imaging with fat-suppression and gadolinium enhancement. *Radiology* 1994;193:683–688.

- Graf O, Boland GW, Warshaw AL, et al. Arterial versus portal venous helical CT for revealing pancreatic adenocarcinoma: conspicuity of tumor and critical vascular anatomy. *Am J Roentgenol.* 169:119–123.

- Ichikawa T, Haradome H, Hachiya J, et al. Pancreatic ductal adenocarcinoma: Preoperative assessment with helical CT versus dynamic MR imaging. *Radiology* 1997;202:655–662.

- Itai Y, Ohhashi K, Furui S, et al. Microcystic adenoma of the pancreas: spectrum of computed tomographic findings. *J Comput Assist Tomogr.* 1988;12:797–803.

- Johnson CD, Stephens DH, Charboneau JW, et al. Cystic pancreatic tumors: CT and sonographic assessment. *Am J Roentgenol.* 1988;151:1133–1138.

- Kanematsu M, Shiratori Y, Hoshi H, et al. Pancreas and peripancreatic vessels: effect of imaging delay on gadolinium enhancement at dynamic gradient-recalled-echo MR imaging. *Radiology* 2000;215:95–102.

- Keogan MT, McDermott VG, Paulson EK, et al. Pancreatic malignancy: effect of dual-phase helical CT in tumor detection and vascular opacification. *Radiology* 1997;205:513–518.

- Khurana B, Mortele KJ, Glickman JN, et al. Macrocystic serous adenoma of the pancreas: radiologic-pathologic correlation. *Am J Roentgenol.* 2003;181:119–123.

- Kim T, Murakami T, Takamura M, et al. Pancreatic mass due to chronic pancreatitis: Correlation of CT and MR imaging features with pathologic findings. *Am J Roentgenol.* 2001;177:367–371.

- Kraus BB, Ros PR. Insulinoma: diagnosis with suppressed MR imaging. *Am J Roentgenol.* 1994;162:69–70.

- McNulty N, Francis IR, Platt JF, et al. Multi-detector row helical CT of the pancreas: effect of contrast-enhanced multiphasic imaging on enhancement of the pancreas, peripancreatic vasculature, and pancreatic adenocarcinoma. *Radiology* 2001;220:97–102.

- Mortele KJ, Ji H, Ros PR. CT and magnetic resonance imaging in pancreatic and biliary tract malignancies. *Gastrointest Endosc.* 2002; 56(suppl 6):S206–S212.

- Mortele KJ, Mortele B, Silverman SG. CT features of the accessory (supernumerary) spleen. *Am J Roentgenol.* 2004;183:1653–1657.

- Mortele KJ, Wiesner W, Cantisani V, et al. Usual and unusual causes of extrahepatic cholestasis: assessment with magnetic resonance cholangiography and fast MRI. *Abdom Imaging.* 2004;29:87–99.

- Nishiharu T, Yamashota Y, Abe Y, et al. Local extension of pancreatic carcinoma: Assessment with thin-section helical CT versus breath-hold fast MR imaging: ROC analysis. *Radiology* 1999;212:445–452.

- Peters HE, Vitellas KM. Magnetic resonance cholangiopancreatography (MRCP) of intraductal papillary-mucinous neoplasm (IPMN) of the pancreas: case report. *Magn Reson Imaging.* 2001;19:1139–1143.

- Procacci C, Carbognin G, Accordini S, et al. Nonfunctioning endocrine tumors of the pancreas: possibilities of spiral CT characterization. *Eur Radiol.* 2001;11:1626–1630.

- Radin DR, Colletti PM, Forrester DM. Pancreatic acinar cell carcinoma with subcutaneous and intraosseous fat necrosis. *Radiology* 1986;158: 67–68.

- Raptopoulos V, Steer ML, Sheiman RG, et al. The use of helical CT and CT angiography to predict vascular involvement from pancreatic cancer: correlation with findings at surgery. *Am J Roentgenol.* 1997;168:971–977.

- Ros PR, Hamrick-Turner JE, Chiechi MV, et al. Cystic masses of the pancreas. *Radiographics* 1992;12:673–686.

- Rosebrook JL, Glickman JN, Mortele KJ. Pancreatoblastoma in an adult woman: sonography, CT, and dynamic gadolinium-enhanced MRI features. *Am J Roentgenol.* 2005;184:S78–S81.

- Scott J, Martin I, Redhead D, et al. Mucinous cystic neoplasms of the pancreas: Imaging features and diagnostic difficulties. *Clin Radiol* 2000;55:187–192.

- Semelka RC, Kroeker MA, Shoenut JP, et al. Pancreatic disease: prospective comparison of CT, ERCP and 1.5 Tesla MR imaging with dynamic gadolinium enhancement and fat suppression. *Radiology* 1991;181:785–791.

- Sugiyama M, Atomi Y, Hachiya J. Intraductal papillary tumors of the pancreas: Evaluation with magnetic resonance cholangiopancreatography. *Am J Gastroenterol.* 1998;93:156–159.

- Tabuchi T, Itoh K, Ohshio G, et al. Tumor staging of pancreatic adenocarcinoma using early and late-phase helical CT. *Am J Roentgenol.* 1999;173:375–380.

- Taouli B, Vilgrain V, Vullierme MP, et al. Intraductal papillary mucinous tumors of the pancreas: Helical CT with histopathologic correlation. *Radiology* 2000;217:757–764.

- Tatli S, Mortele KJ, Levy AD, et al. CT and MR imaging features of pure acinar cell carcinoma of the pancreas in adults. *Am J Roentgenol.* 2005; 184:511–519.

- Teefey SA, Stephens DH, Sheedy PF, et al. CT appearance of primary pancreatic lymphoma. *Gastrointest Radiol.* 1986;11:41–43.

DEVELOPMENTAL ANOMALIES

- Agha FP, Williams KD. Pancreas divisum: incidence, detection and clinical significance. *Am J Gastroenterol.* 1987;82:315–320.

- Bret PM, Reinhold C, Taourel P, et al. Pancreas divisum: evaluation with MR cholangiopancreatography. *Radiology* 1996;199:99–103.

- Guclu M, Serin E, Ulucan S. Agenesis of the dorsal pancreas in a patient with recurrent acute pancreatitis: case report and review. *Gastrointest Endosc.* 2004;60:472–475.

- Hough DM, Stephens DH, Johnson CD, et al. Pancreatic lesions in von Hippel-Lindau disease: prevalence, clinical significance, and CT findings. *Am J Roentgenol.* 1994;162:1091–1094.

- Inoue Y, Nakamura H. Aplasia or hypoplasia of the pancreatic uncinate process: comparison in patients with and patients without intestinal nonrotation. *Radiology* 1997;205:531–533.

- Jimenez JC, Emil S, Podnos Y, et al. Annular pancreas in children: a recent decade's experience. *J Ped Surg.* 2004;39:1654–1657.

- Kamisawa T, Yuyang T, Egawa N, et al. A new embryologic hypothesis of annular pancreas. *Hepatogastroenterology* 2001;48:277–278.

- Klein SD, Affronti JP. Pancreas divisum, an evidence-based review: part I, pathophysiology. *Gastrointest Endosc.* 2004;60:419–425.

- Leyendecker JR, Elsayes KM, Gratz BI, et al. MR cholangiopancreatography: spectrum of pancreatic duct abnormalities. *Am J Roentgenol.* 2002;179:1465–1471.

- Manfredi R, Costamagna G, Brizi MG, et al. Pancreas divisum and "santorinicele": diagnosis with dynamic MR cholangiopancreatography with secretin stimulation. *Radiology* 2000;217:403–408.

- Mortele KJ, Wiesner W, Silverman SG, et al. Asymptomatic non-specific serum hyperamylasemia and hyperlipasemia: spectrum of MRCP findings and clinical implications. *Abdom Imaging.* 2004;29:109–114.

- Nijs E, Callahan MJ, Taylor GA. Disorders of the pediatric pancreas: imaging features. *Pediatr Radiol.* 2005;35:358–373.

- Schulte SJ. Embryology, normal variation, and congenital anomalies of the pancreas. In: *Margulis' and Burhenne's alimentary tract radiology.* 5th ed. St Louis: Mosby; 1994;1039–1051.

- Soto JA, Lucey BC, Stuhlfaut JW. Pancreas divisum: depiction with multi-detector row CT. *Radiology* 2005;235:503–508.

CHAPTER THREE

GASTROINTESTINAL TRACT

KOENRAAD J. MORTELE,
VINCENT PELSSER,
AND PABLO R. ROS

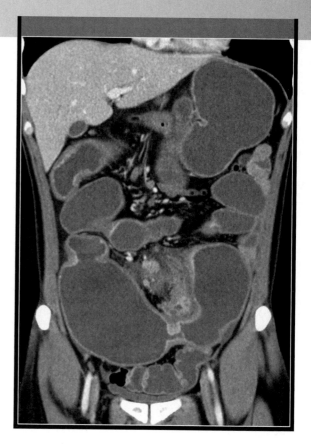

CASE 3-1

Clinical History: 49-year-old woman presenting with longstanding history of abdominal pain and diarrhea.

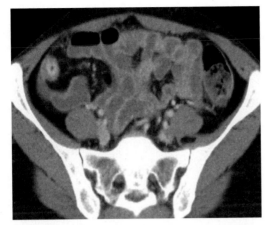

Figure 3.1   A

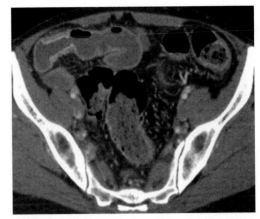

Figure 3.1   B

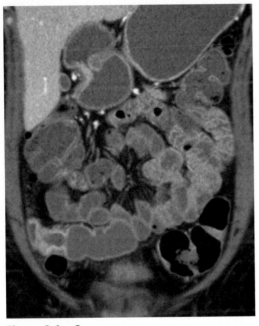

Figure 3.1   C

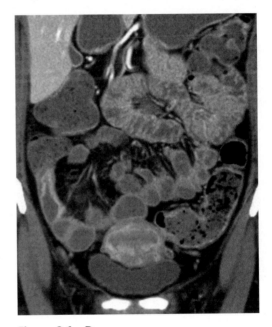

Figure 3.1   D

Findings: Axial (A and B) and coronal reformatted (C and D) contrast-enhanced CT (CECT) images of the pelvis (after oral administration of neutral contrast agent) demonstrate mild thickening of the terminal ileum with mucosal hyperenhancement. A second abnormal segment with similar features is identified in the mid ileum (B).

Differential Diagnosis: Infectious enteritis (tuberculosis, *Yersinia*), ischemia, lymphoma.

Diagnosis: Crohn disease of the ileum.

Discussion: Crohn disease is a chronic disease of the gastrointestinal (GI) tract, which is characterized by transmural inflammatory reaction, granulomas, skip lesions, fistula formation, and mesenteric abnormalities. Within the mesentery, there will be inflammatory changes including stranding, phlegmon, and abscess formation. The use of neutral oral contrast agents allows easy depiction of mucosal hyperenhancement, an established CT feature of active Crohn disease. Almost any segment of the GI tract can be involved by Crohn disease, although the terminal ileum and ascending colon are the most commonly involved areas. Ischemia would most likely involve more loops of small and large bowel rather than just the terminal ileum. Infectious enteritis and lymphoma could both appear similar on CT and would have to be considered. In this case, however, the bowel wall thickening of the terminal ileum as well as the discontinuous mucosal hyperenhancement (skip areas) makes Crohn disease the best diagnosis.

CASE 3-2

Clinical History: 30-year-old man with acute lymphocytic leukemia presenting with fever after bone marrow transplantation.

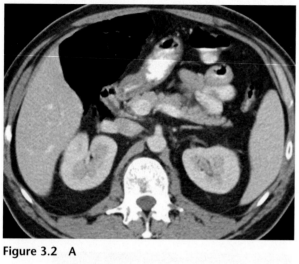
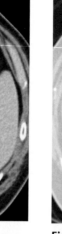

Figure 3.2   A

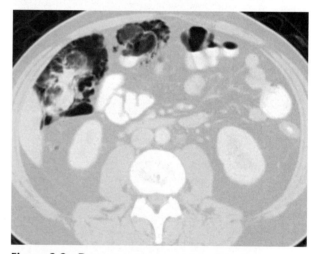

Figure 3.2   B

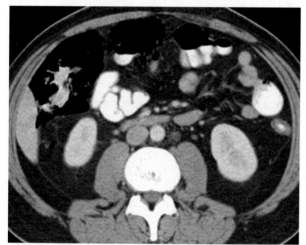

Figure 3.2   C

Figure 3.2   D

Findings: Axial CECT images displayed in soft tissue (A and C) and lung (B and D) windows demonstrate extensive accumulation of air in the colonic wall at the level of the hepatic flexure.

Differential Diagnosis: Pneumatosis intestinalis due to ischemia, pneumatosis cystoides.

Diagnosis: Benign colonic pneumatosis due to mucosal denudation (chemotherapy effect).

Discussion: It is generally accepted that bowel ischemia and bowel infarction are the most common causes of pneumatosis and that this constellation is associated with a bad prognosis and a high mortality rate. However, pneumatosis may occur in certain nonischemic conditions as well, where

it is not automatically associated with an unfavorable outcome. The pathogenesis of pneumatosis following intestinal mucosal injury is obvious since mucosal and submucosal bowel wall damage may allow some intraluminal air to enter the damaged or dissected bowel wall; therefore, it is not surprising that pneumatosis may be associated with bone marrow transplantation, where it may be related, at least partially, to GI mucosal damage caused by the chemotherapeutic agents themselves. Pneumatosis has also been reported to occur secondary to diverticulitis, graft-versus-host disease, ulcerative colitis, Crohn disease, and gastric and colon cancers. Pneumatosis cystoides intestinalis, also known as primary pneumatosis, is characterized by bubblelike gas collections along the bowel wall and only involves the colon.

CASE 3-3

Clinical History: 67-year-old woman with hysterectomy and radiation for uterine sarcoma presenting with weight loss and chronic abdominal pain.

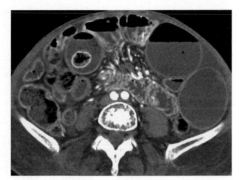

Figure 3.3   A

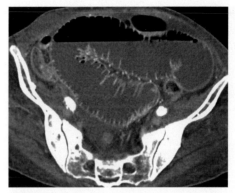

Figure 3.3   B

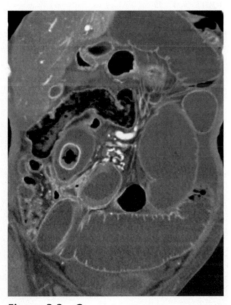

Figure 3.3   C

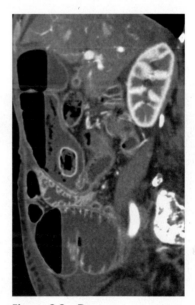

Figure 3.3   D

Findings: Axial (A and B) and coronal reformatted (C and D) CECT images demonstrate multiple dilated loops of small bowel (up to 6 cm), with an acute transition point at the level of the proximal ileum. Note the presence of an enterolith (3 cm) located proximally to the point of obstruction and a small amount of ascites.

Differential Diagnosis: Radiation enteritis.

Diagnosis: Small bowel obstruction secondary to an adhesion.

Discussion: CT has traditionally been used to reveal the site, level, and cause of obstruction and to display the signs of threatened bowel viability. Oral contrast agents may not be necessary because the fluid and gas in the dilated bowel provide sufficient contrast. Intravenous (IV) administration of contrast material is preferred for the evaluation of ischemia. The criterion of small bowel dilatation is defined as 2.5 cm calculated from outer wall to outer wall. The transition point is determined by identifying a caliber change between dilated proximal and collapsed distal small bowel loops. Multiplanar reformations may aid in determining the site and level of obstruction. Complete versus partial obstruction of the small bowel is determined by the degree of distal collapse, proximal bowel dilatation, and transit of ingested contrast material. Adhesions are responsible for more than half of all small bowel obstructions, followed by hernias and extrinsic compression due to neoplastic growths. Radiation enteritis frequently involves loops of small bowel located within the radiation therapy port. The normal loops of small bowel in the pelvis make radiation enteritis unlikely.

Clinical History: 56-year-old woman with a history of lymphoma presenting with diarrhea.

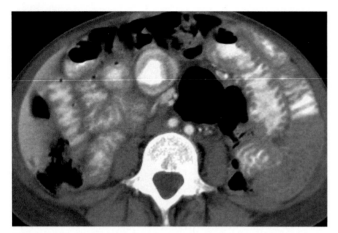

Figure 3.4　A

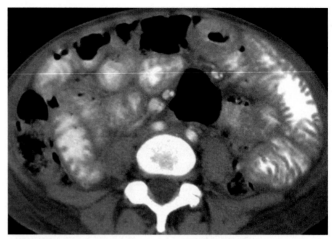

Figure 3.4　B

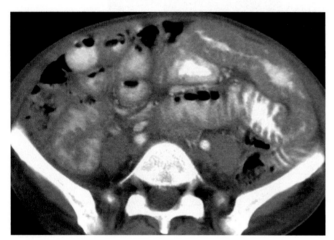

Figure 3.4　C

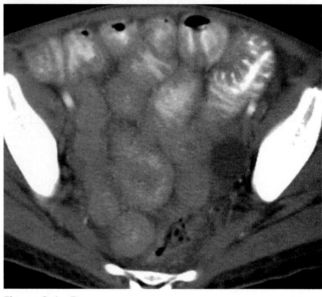

Figure 3.4　D

Findings: Axial CECT images demonstrate nodular thickening and dilatation of the small bowel loops. The colon appears normal.

Differential Diagnosis: Ischemia, infectious enteritis, Crohn disease, lymphoma.

Diagnosis: Amyloidosis of the small bowel.

Discussion: Amyloidosis is a heterogeneous group of disorders that results in deposition of proteins in various tissues of the body. This leads to tissue hypoxia, mucosal edema, and ulceration. Amyloidosis can be primary or secondary. Primary amyloidosis is probably an inherited disorder of plasma cell function, whereas secondary amyloidosis is a reactive disease to a chronic inflammatory process or illness. CT findings of amyloidosis in the GI tract include loss of haustrations or valvulae conniventes with thickening and nodularity of the mucosa and muscular wall. The bowel can be dilated or narrowed by this process. This appearance is often nonspecific. Amyloidosis can involve both the small and large bowel. Simultaneous diffuse thickening of the small bowel and colon can also be seen in low-flow ischemia, infectious enterocolitis (e.g., *Candida*), Crohn disease, and lymphoma.

CASE 3-5

Clinical History: 68-year-old man with positive occult blood stool test. Colonoscopy revealed a rectal mass.

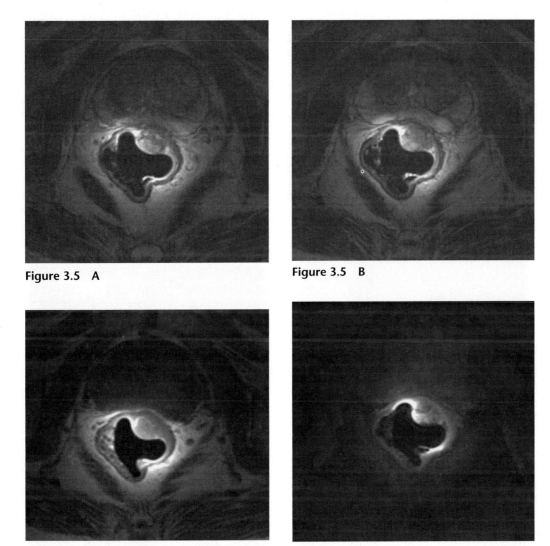

Figure 3.5   A

Figure 3.5   B

Figure 3.5   C

Figure 3.5   D

Findings: Axial T2-weighted image (WI) (A and B), axial T1-WI (C), and gadolinium-enhanced, fat-suppressed axial T1-WI (D) obtained after endorectal coil placement demonstrate the presence of a rectal solid mass in the anterolateral wall. The mass is hyperintense on T2-WI, hypointense on T1-WI, and enhances following contrast administration. Note invasion of the muscularis propria of the rectum (hypointense outer layer) by the mass. No enlarged lymph nodes are present in the mesorectal fat.

Differential Diagnosis: GI stromal tumor, carcinoid.

Diagnosis: Rectal adenocarcinoma (T2N0Mx).

Discussion: Endorectal MRI is performed by placing an endorectal coil into the rectum. This allows superb detail of structures adjacent to the rectum, such as the uterus, cervix, prostate, and particularly the rectal wall. MRI is advantageous over CT because multiple planes can be performed. This case demonstrates a typical adenocarcinoma of the rectum. On MRI, rectal adenocarcinomas are isointense to muscle on the T1-WI. Because the surrounding fat is of high signal intensity, perirectal extension, if present, is well seen. In this example, the outer margin is well defined, and the tumor is confined to the rectal wall. On the T2-WI, the tumor is hyperintense relative to muscle, making it possible to see the margins of the lesion in relation to the muscularis propria of the rectum. The ability to see the lesion in multiple planes is important to delineate crucial anatomy, such as the distance between the cancer and the anal sphincter or mesorectal fascia. All these findings are important in the preoperative staging to determine the best approach.

Clinical History: 56-year-old woman with history of breast cancer and hysterectomy.

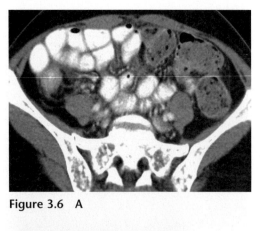

Figure 3.6   A

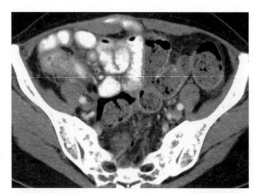

Figure 3.6   B

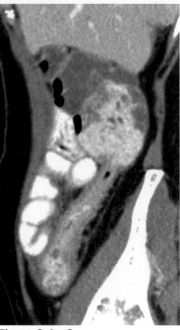

Figure 3.6   C

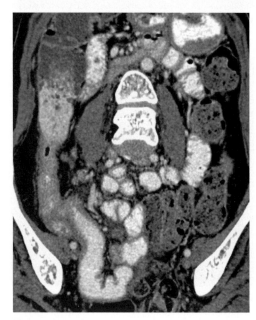

Figure 3.6   D

Findings: Axial (A and B), sagittal (C), and curved reformatted (D) CECT images demonstrate circumferential wall thickening of the terminal ileum, cecum, and ascending colon.

Differential Diagnosis: Crohn disease, ischemia, adenocarcinoma, lymphoma.

Diagnosis: Breast cancer metastases to proximal colon and distal small bowel.

Discussion: Metastases to the colon are fairly common but often are asymptomatic and are found incidentally by autopsy. Malignancies can spread to the colon by way of direct extension, as is seen in prostate, ovarian, uterine, and cervical carcinomas. Intraperitoneal seeding and hematogenous spread can also occur. The most common malignancies to spread hematogenously include melanoma, breast, and lung cancer. Breast metastases can present as an eccentric mass or as an irregular circumferential stricture (linitis plastica), as seen in this case. The stricture appearance can simulate Crohn disease of the colon. An eccentric mass is most often going to be confused with an adenocarcinoma of the colon. A metastasis, however, will appear as an extrinsic mass invading into the lumen, whereas a colon cancer will be a mass growing out from the colonic mucosa. Lymphoma tends to involve the cecum and often is large. Lymphoma, however, will not cause obstruction but aneurysmal dilatation of the involved bowel segment.

Clinical History: 69-year-old woman presenting with abdominal pain, nausea, and vomiting.

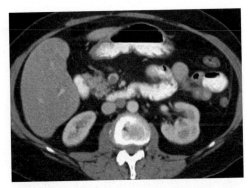

Figure 3.7 A

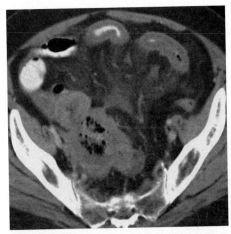

Figure 3.7 B

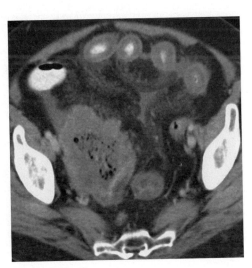

Figure 3.7 C

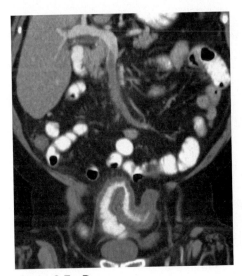

Figure 3.7 D

Findings: Axial (A–C) CECT images demonstrate extensive bowel wall thickening of the distal small bowel with associated stranding in the small bowel mesentery and some interloop fluid accumulation. A filling defect is seen in the superior mesenteric vein (SMV), as better shown on the curved reformatted CECT image (D). The associated 8.3 × 6.2 cm right lower quadrant lesion is an excavated cecal cancer.

Differential Diagnosis: Infectious enteritis, Crohn disease.

Diagnosis: Small bowel ischemia due to SMV thrombosis.

Discussion: Acute mesenteric arterial ischemia is commonly seen in the elderly due to cardiac problems (arrhythmias, congestive heart failure, and myocardial infarction) and atherosclerotic disease. In other age groups, mesenteric ischemia can be due to sepsis, hypotension, and hypovolemia. This leads to decreased blood flow in the superior mesenteric artery (SMA), which causes ischemia of the ileum and proximal colon. Thrombosis of the SMV due to iatrogenic, infectious, neoplastic, or paraneoplastic causes may also lead to bowel ischemia due to venous congestion. CT findings include bowel wall thickening of the small bowel and the "double halo" sign. The double halo sign represents enhancement of the mucosa and muscularis propria, with edema of the submucosa. Pneumatosis, portal venous air, or air in the mesenteric veins all signify bowel ischemia and are easily seen on CT. Atherosclerotic disease or a clot in the SMA or SMV can sometimes be depicted with CT as well, as shown in this case. Crohn disease does not usually involve a large amount of small bowel. The presence of an SMV clot, double halo sign, and extensive small bowel involvement makes ischemic bowel the best diagnosis in this case.

Clinical History: 62-year-old woman with intermittent abdominal discomfort.

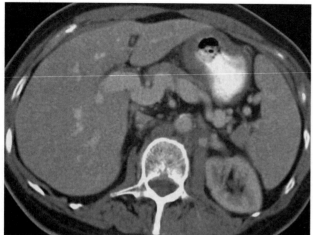

Figure 3.8   A

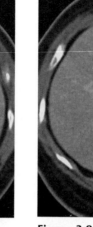

Figure 3.8   B

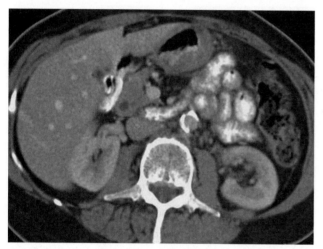

Figure 3.8   C

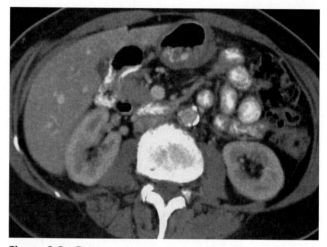

Figure 3.8   D

Findings: Axial CECT images demonstrate circumferential wall thickening of the stomach antrum up to 1.6 cm.

Differential Diagnosis: Adenocarcinoma, metastasis, gastritis.

Diagnosis: Non-Hodgkin lymphoma of the stomach.

Discussion: Lymphoma of the stomach accounts for approximately 3% to 5% of gastric neoplasms, with non-Hodgkin lymphoma (B-cell origin) making up the majority of these cases. The stomach is nevertheless the most frequently involved part of the GI tract in patients with lymphoma. More than 50% of cases represent primary involvement of the stomach. Radiographically, lymphoma can present as a solitary submucosal mass or as a necrotic, ulcerating exophytic mass in the gastric wall. Lymphoma can also be an infiltrating process, presenting as thickened gastric folds that are difficult to distinguish from gastritis. Hodgkin disease rarely involves the stomach but, when present, may mimic linitis plastica. For any mass arising from the gastric wall, the differential diagnosis includes gastric adenocarcinoma, GI stromal tumor (GIST), lymphoma and metastasis. In most cases, biopsy is necessary to confirm the diagnosis. Gastric adenocarcinoma arises from the mucosa and is typically associated with perigastric lymphadenopathy. GIST are typically hypervascular and don't present as linitis plastica. Most patients with gastric metastases (most commonly from breast cancer or melanoma) have a known underlying cancer at diagnosis.

Clinical History: 67-year-old woman taking a nonsteroidal anti-inflammatory drug presents with vomiting and abdominal pain of 2 days in duration.

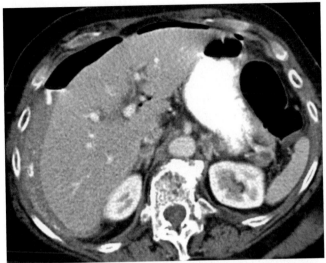

Figure 3.9   A

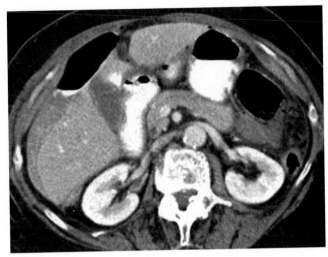

Figure 3.9   B

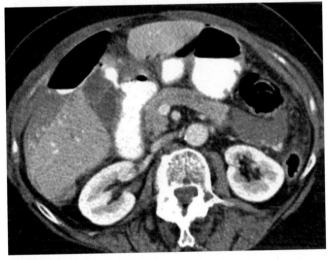

Figure 3.9   C

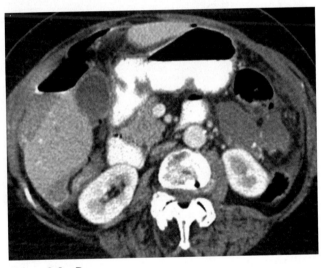

Figure 3.9   D

Findings: Axial CECT images demonstrate extraluminal air and oral contrast material in the peritoneal space. Extravasation of contrast is identified from the first portion of the duodenum.

Differential Diagnosis: None.

Diagnosis: Perforated duodenal bulb ulcer with pneumoperitoneum.

Discussion: Peptic ulcers can occur in the stomach or the duodenum. Duodenal ulcers are 2 to 3 times more common than gastric ulcers. Patients typically present with symptoms of epigastric pain often precipitated by food. Almost all duodenal ulcers are benign, whereas a percentage of gastric ulcers can be malignant (ulcerated gastric adenocarcinomas).

The majority of duodenal ulcers are located on the anterior wall of the duodenal bulb, which has an intraperitoneal location. Complications of peptic ulcer disease include GI hemorrhage, perforation, obstruction, and fistula formation. Because of the mixed peritoneal-retroperitoneal location of the duodenum, perforations may manifest as spillage of intraluminal content and air in the peritoneum in cases of perforation of the duodenal bulb, as seen in this case, or in the retroperitoneum if the perforation arises from the second or third portion of the duodenum. The differential diagnosis of pneumoperitoneum includes bowel perforation secondary to blunt or penetrating trauma, perforated ulcer, diverticulitis, neoplasm, iatrogenic bowel injury, and surgery.

Clinical History: 62-year-old man with increasing nausea, vomiting, and diarrhea following an episode of acute diverticulitis.

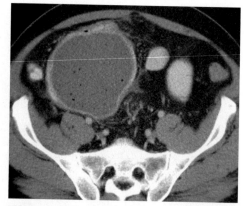

Figure 3.10 A

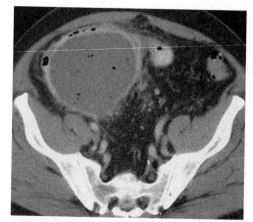

Figure 3.10 B

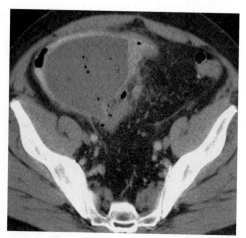

Figure 3.10 C

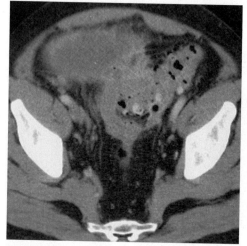

Figure 3.10 D

Findings: Axial CECT images demonstrate an 11-cm inflammatory mass that contains air anterior to the sigmoid colon. Note extensive wall thickening of the sigmoid colon, presence of diverticular disease, and displacement of small bowel loops.

Differential Diagnosis: Crohn colitis, traumatic perforation, perforated neoplasm.

Diagnosis: Diverticular abscess.

Discussion: Diverticulitis most commonly occurs in the elderly patient population in whom diverticulosis is more prevalent. It is characterized by perforation of colonic diverticula, which are acquired herniations of the mucosa and submucosa through the muscularis propria of the bowel wall. In debilitated elderly patients, the diagnosis of diverticulitis is often delayed because many of the symptoms are less pronounced and masked by underlying medical problems, such as diabetes, renal failure, and medications. When diverticulitis occurs in the younger patient (<40 years of age), it is often more severe and may require emergent surgery. CT findings of diverticulitis include bowel wall thickening, fat stranding in the mesocolon, free peritoneal fluid, and intramural or pelvic abscess formation. In this case, there is extraluminal air from the adjacent sigmoid colon that is segmentally inflamed. Although this can be due to fistula or abscess formation from Crohn colitis, no findings suggestive of Crohn disease are present. Prior trauma or a perforated neoplasm can also have this appearance, and therefore, an underlying neoplasm must be excluded by colonoscopic evaluation after the symptoms resolve.

Clinical History: 56-year-old man presenting with purplish rash on the legs and abdominal discomfort.

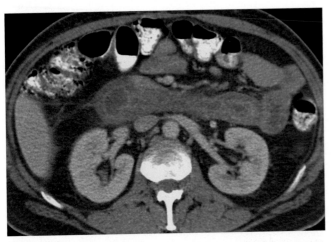

Figure 3.11 A

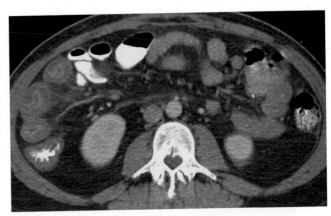

Figure 3.11 B

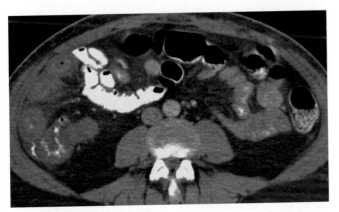

Figure 3.11 C

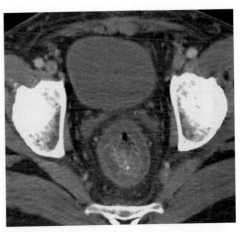

Figure 3.11 D

Findings: Axial CECT images show segmental mural thickening and stratification of the duodenum (A), ileum (B), ascending colon (C), and rectum (D). Mild mesenteric and mesocolonic fat stranding is present.

Differential Diagnosis: Mesenteric ischemia, Crohn disease.

Diagnosis: Henoch-Schönlein purpura.

Discussion: Henoch-Schönlein purpura (HSP) is an immunoglobulin A–mediated, autoimmune, hypersensitivity, small-vessel vasculitis that results in a triad of symptoms, including a purpuric rash occurring on the lower extremities, abdominal pain or renal involvement, and arthritis (especially ankles and knees). However, any of the triad may be absent, which often leads to confusion in diagnosis. Although the etiology is unknown, HSP is frequently associated with infectious agents, such as group A streptococci and *Mycoplasma*. It has also been associated with food reactions, exposure to cold, insect bites, and drug allergies. It has an incidence of 14 cases per 100,000 people, is more likely to occur in children, and occurs most frequently in the spring and fall. It is twice as common in males than in females. The second most frequent symptom of HSP, after the skin rash, is abdominal pain, which occurs in up to 65% of cases. The most common complaint is colicky abdominal pain, which may be severe and associated with vomiting. Stools may show gross or occult blood; hematemesis may also occur. Severe cases may proceed to intussusception, hemorrhage, and shock. Younger children are less likely to exhibit GI symptoms. Endoscopic evaluation often shows mucosal erosions and swelling. Radiologic findings are nonspecific. Mural thickening, thickened folds, ulceration, and spasm are seen radiographically. The CT appearance of segmental mural thickening and luminal narrowing correlates well with the abnormalities seen on upper endoscopy.

Clinical History: 78-year-old man presenting with epigastric discomfort.

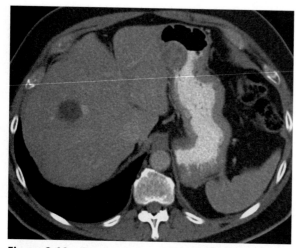

Figure 3.12   A

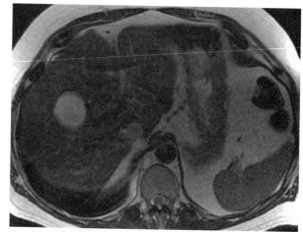

Figure 3.12   B

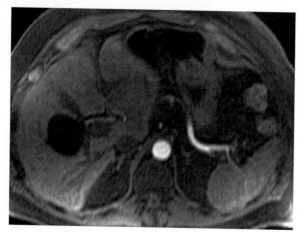

Figure 3.12   C

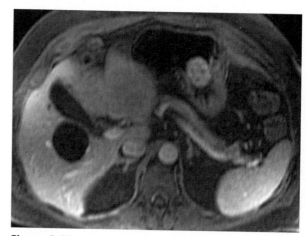

Figure 3.12   D

Findings: Axial CECT image (A) shows a 2-cm, well-defined heterogeneous mass arising from the lesser curvature of the stomach. Axial T2-WI (B) and early (C) and late (D) gadolinium-enhanced, fat-suppressed axial T1-WI demonstrate the hyperintense and hypervascular characteristics of the mass, respectively.

Differential Diagnosis: Adenocarcinoma, metastasis, lymphoma.

Diagnosis: GI stromal tumor of the stomach.

Discussion: GI stromal tumor (GIST) is the most common extramucosal tumor of the stomach and usually presents as an encapsulated intramural mass. GIST is characterized by immunoreactivity for the receptor c-KIT. At diagnosis, the majority of lesions are benign. Although GIST may arise anywhere in the GI tract, 70% of all GISTs occur in the stomach. Exophytic tumor growth is occasionally observed, resulting in a subserosal exogastric lesion. These lesions may grow to be among the largest tumors of the stomach because of their inclination to remain silent. They also have a limited tendency to cause GI bleeding, which is, in contrast, a common complication of gastric adenocarcinoma. Conventional barium examinations or endoscopy are often nonconclusive in patients with subserosal exogastric GIST because these lesions pass unrecognized due to the normal appearing overlying gastric mucosa. Other intramural gastric lesions include leiomyoma, leiomyoblastoma, lipoma, hemangioma, lymphangioma, schwannoma, and neurofibroma. Because they are composed of smooth muscle cells, GISTs typically show a hypervascular appearance on contrast-enhanced CT and MRI scans.

Clinical History: 61-year-old man presenting with rectal bleeding.

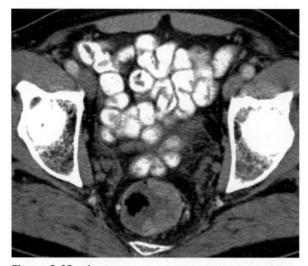

Figure 3.13   A

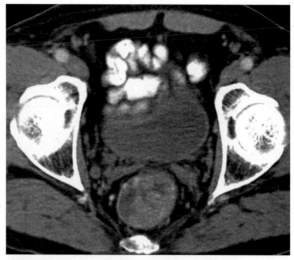

Figure 3.13   B

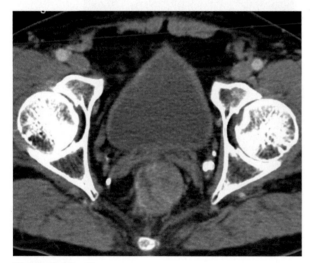

Figure 3.13   C

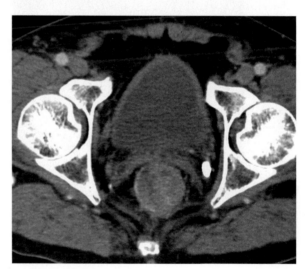

Figure 3.13   D

Findings: Axial CECT images demonstrate a large circumferential mass in the rectum. The rectal lumen, which contains fluid, is almost completely obliterated by the mass. Also note minimal extension of the mass within the mesorectal fat.

Differential Diagnosis: Lymphoma, metastasis, ulcerative colitis.

Diagnosis: Adenocarcinoma of the rectum.

Discussion: Colon cancer is the most common malignancy of the GI tract. More than 50% of the cases occur in the rectosigmoid. Metastases to the liver via the portal venous system occur in lesions located in the proximal two thirds of the rectum. The lesions in the distal one third of the rectum metastasize to the lung via the hemorrhoidal plexus. Rectosigmoid lesions demonstrate spread to lymph nodes in the mesorectum, inferior mesenteric chains, external iliac chain, and para-aortic chain. CT is good at detecting gross extension of the tumor outside the colonic wall, but microscopic invasion is often missed. The polypoid lesion in this example is typical for an adenocarcinoma. The size of the lesion (>1 cm) and extension outside the wall into the mesorectal fat suggest malignancy. These lesions can present as annular constricting, polypoid, or infiltrating. The most common lesion is the annular constricting lesion. The lumen is almost obliterated by the tumor. Both lymphoma and metastases could have this appearance, although they much less commonly involve the rectum. Ulcerative colitis does not produce localized bowel wall thickening with mesorectal extension, as seen in this case.

Clinical History: 92-year-old man presenting with diarrhea after antibiotic therapy.

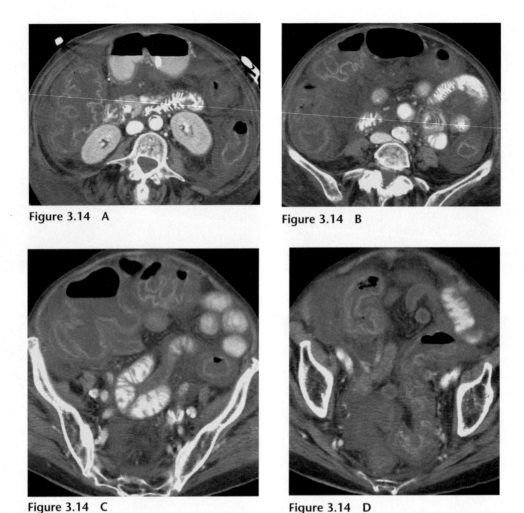

Figure 3.14   A

Figure 3.14   B

Figure 3.14   C

Figure 3.14   D

Findings: Axial CECT images demonstrate marked thickening of the ascending, transverse, and descending colon. Fluid is also seen in the paracolic gutters and mesocolon. An image in the pelvis (D) demonstrates thickening of the sigmoid colon and rectum. Free fluid is again noted.

Differential Diagnosis: Ulcerative colitis, infectious colitis, ischemic colitis.

Diagnosis: Pseudomembranous colitis.

Discussion: Pseudomembranous colitis (PMC) is a toxin-mediated disease with no evidence of microbial invasion into the bowel wall mucosa. Isolating the toxin in the stool of the affected patient makes the diagnosis. PMC forms characteristic yellow or creamy white plaques related to the overgrowth of *Clostridium difficile*. This occurs after the use of almost any antibiotic but is most closely associated with clindamycin and lincomycin. The patients typically have watery diarrhea, crampy abdominal pain, and occasionally fever. The characteristic CT features include diffuse pancolitis with marked mural thickening and with minimal pericolonic inflammatory changes. The thickening is homogeneously low in attenuation and is thought to be due to edema in the bowel wall. The pericolonic stranding that is present is out of proportion to the degree of bowel wall thickening. Ascites is seen in up to 77% of patients with PMC and suggests the acute nature of this disease. Crohn colitis would typically involve the terminal ileum, which was spared in this case. Ulcerative colitis usually has only mild to moderate bowel wall thickening. Involvement of the entire colon without small bowel involvement is unusual for ischemia. Infectious colitis can present in this manner, but the history of antibiotic therapy makes PMC the best diagnosis in this case.

Clinical History: 63-year-old woman with hysterectomy and radiotherapy for cervical cancer presenting with weight loss.

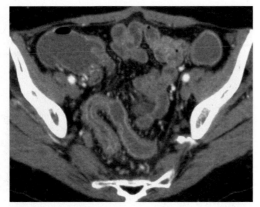

Figure 3.15   A

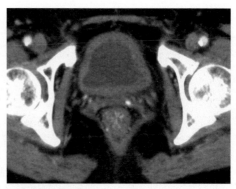

Figure 3.15   B

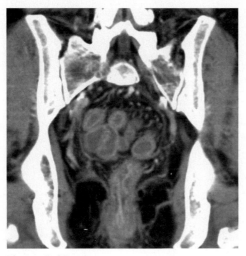

Figure 3.15   C

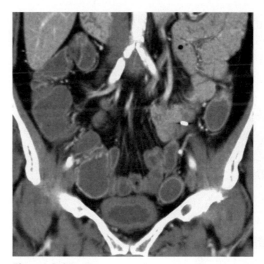

Figure 3.15   D

Findings: Axial (A and B) and coronal reformatted (C and D) CECT images demonstrate thickening of small bowel wall, rectosigmoid wall, and bladder wall in the pelvis. There is extensive mucosal hyperenhancement of the affected bowel segments and hyperemia of the mesenteric vessels.

Differential Diagnosis: Ischemia, Crohn disease, lymphoma.

Diagnosis: Radiation enterocolitis.

Discussion: Radiation changes in the GI tract are commonly seen in the rectum, sigmoid, and small bowel with the use of external-beam radiation therapy for many pelvic malignancies. A good clinical history will suggest the diagnosis and often eliminate the need for a lengthy workup. Radiation enteritis and colitis can occur several years after radiation therapy. Most commonly, it is seen in women with cervical cancer who present with crampy abdominal pain and diarrhea. CT findings suggestive of radiation enteritis include bowel wall thickening of loops of bowel within the radiation port. Because of the mesenteric edema, the loops of bowel are often separated in the pelvis. Mucosal hyperenhancement, as seen in this case, is suggestive of active inflammation. It is unusual to have involvement of both the sigmoid colon and small bowel at the same time by the same disease process. This can occur in Crohn disease with skip lesions and ischemia with involvement of multiple branch vessels from vasculitis or emboli. Lymphoma, which is considered a systemic disease, can also affect various loops of bowel. Other CT findings in radiation disease include increased attenuation of the mesenteric fat and hyperemia of the mesenteric vessels supplying the involved bowel segments.

Clinical History: 46-year-old woman with history of diarrhea and abdominal pain.

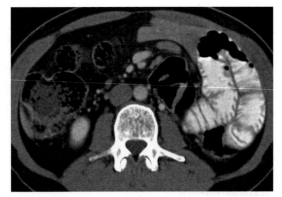

Figure 3.16 A

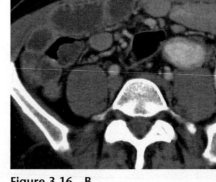

Figure 3.16 B

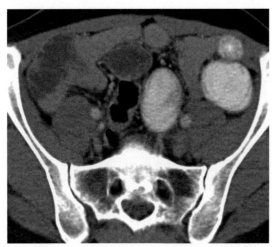

Figure 3.16 C

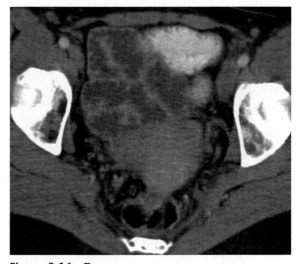

Figure 3.16 D

Findings: Axial CECT images demonstrate mildly dilated contrast-filled loops of small bowel. The involved loops of ileum in the pelvis show the presence of a jejunal fold pattern.

Differential Diagnosis: Scleroderma, small bowel obstruction, ileus.

Diagnosis: Nontropical sprue (celiac disease).

Discussion: Celiac disease or sprue is related to intake of dietary gluten, which causes an immunologic reaction with resultant atrophy of the small bowel villi leading to malabsorption. Genetic factors have been identified in this disease, and there is an increased risk for development of jejunal T-cell lymphoma and carcinoma of the jejunum. The malabsorption results in diarrhea, steatorrhea, and abdominal pain possibly related to intermittent intussusception. Diagnosis of sprue is usually made by mucosal biopsy by endoscopy. The CT findings of sprue are similar to those seen on a small bowel series. There is small bowel dilatation usually involving the duodenum and jejunum with loss of the normal valvulae conniventes. The folds present are thickened probably from the associated hypoalbuminemia. Jejunization of the ileum is a key CT feature and is characterized by the presence of jejunal-like folds in the ileum. Other entities to consider in patients with dilated small bowel include scleroderma, small bowel obstruction, and ileus. The small bowel folds in scleroderma and obstruction tend to be normal. Scleroderma does not tend to have excess fluid, as is seen in sprue and obstruction. The dilated small bowel with jejunization of the ileum in this case makes sprue the best diagnosis.

Clinical History: 77-year-old man with a history of stage IV lung cancer on chemotherapy and morphine presenting with constipation.

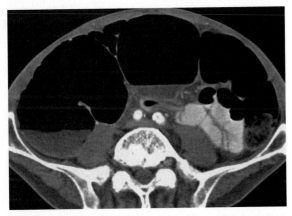

Figure 3.17   A

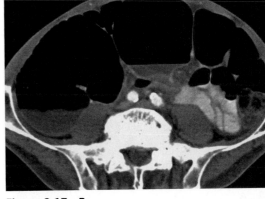

Figure 3.17   B

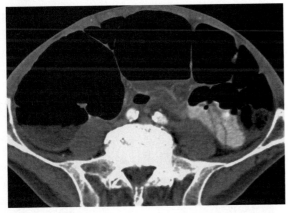

Figure 3.17   C

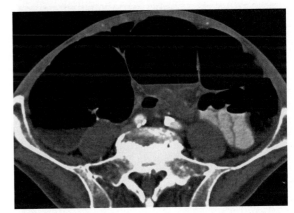

Figure 3.17   D

Findings: Axial CECT images demonstrate a markedly dilated transverse colon. A loop of bowel is seen in the right lower quadrant, which tapers to a point with vessels coursing into it.

Differential Diagnosis: Obstructed sigmoid colon from other etiologies (e.g., neoplasm, adhesions, hernia), ileus.

Diagnosis: Sigmoid volvulus.

Discussion: Any loop of bowel can volvulate at its mesenteric attachment. The majority of colonic volvulus occurs in the sigmoid colon. In the United States, the typical patient is from a nursing home or mental institution. These patients usually have chronic constipation and paralytic ileus due to a combination of medications, immobility, and handicapped mental status, leading to dilated loops of colon that volvulate. Radiographically on plain films, there is a dilated loop of sigmoid colon that is bean shaped, with its long axis pointing toward the right upper quadrant. The same finding can be seen on a CT scan as well. The dilated colon can be followed to the point of obstruction in the pelvis ("beak sign"), with a swirling of vessels ("whirl sign") to the point of volvulus. Sigmoid volvulus is the third most common cause of colonic obstruction, and CT is extremely helpful in excluding other causes of a colonic obstruction, such as a neoplasm or hernia. An ileus is unlikely because the distal rectum is decompressed. In this case, the volvulus was reduced by sigmoidoscopy.

Clinical History: 57-year-old man with crampy abdominal pain.

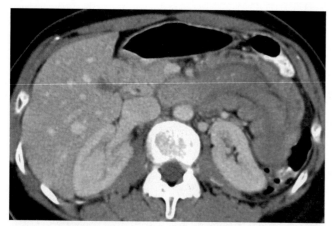

Figure 3.18   A

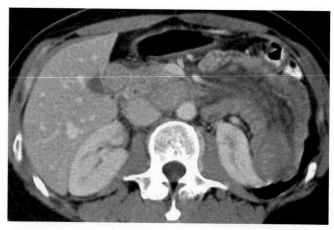

Figure 3.18   B

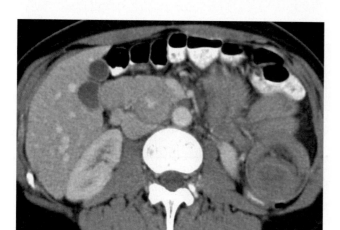

Figure 3.18   C

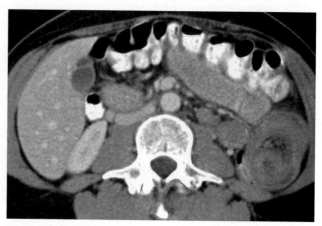

Figure 3.18   D

Findings: Axial CECT images demonstrate a circular mass in the proximal jejunum. This mass appears to be intraluminal and contains a crescent of fat at its periphery. Note the lack of obstruction of the proximal small bowel.

Differential Diagnosis: Lymphoma, adenocarcinoma.

Diagnosis: Jejuno-jejunal intussusception.

Discussion: Intussusception represents invagination of a proximal segment of bowel (intussusceptum) into the lumen of a distal segment of bowel (intussuscipiens). It is typically seen in children (95%) and may be transient or persistent. Intussusceptions are easily identified on CT because there typically is a round soft tissue mass with concentric rings ("target" sign) made up of the walls of the small bowel. The peripheral fat attenuation layer represents herniated mesenteric fat, which has traveled with the loop of jejunum. Diagnosis is crucial because ischemia can occur if the intussusception should persist. Intussusception is classified into two types in adults: the more common short-segment intussusception, which typically is not obstructing and not caused by a lead mass; and long-segment intussusception, which is caused by a lead mass and is obstructing the proximal bowel. Most intussusceptions occur in the ileum; in the small bowel, benign tumors are more common causes than malignant neoplasms.

CASE 3-19

Clinical History: 44-year-old woman with history of multiple endocrine neoplasm type I (MEN I) syndrome.

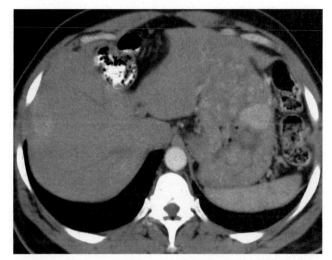

Figure 3.19 A

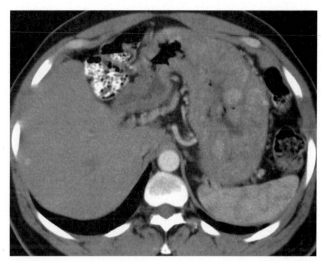

Figure 3.19 B

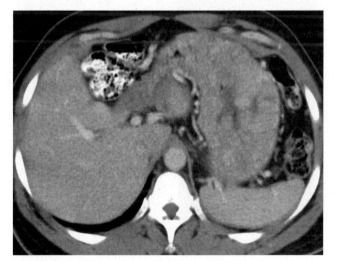

Figure 3.19 C

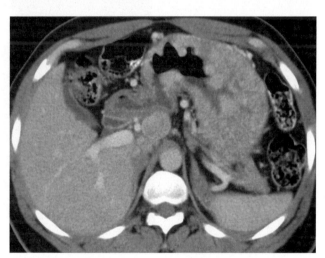

Figure 3.19 D

Findings: Axial CECT images obtained in the arterial (A and B) and portal venous phase (C and D) show marked thickening of the gastric folds and presence of hypervascular lesions in the stomach wall and liver.

Differential Diagnosis: Gastritis, gastric carcinoma, Ménétrier disease, lymphoma, metastases.

Diagnosis: Zollinger-Ellison syndrome.

Discussion: Zollinger-Ellison syndrome is characterized by peptic ulcer disease as a result of marked increase in gastric acid due to a gastrin-producing endocrine tumor (gastrinoma). Most gastrinomas (75%) are located in the pancreas or duodenum. CT features of Zollinger-Ellison syndrome include the presence of hypervascular (primary and secondary) masses in the pancreas, liver, and GI tract and inflammatory changes in the stomach, duodenum, and proximal small bowel. Thickening of the folds throughout the stomach, luminal narrowing, and even signs of ulcer perforation may be present. MEN I is a syndrome that includes tumors of the pituitary, parathyroid, adrenal cortex, and pancreas, especially gastrinomas. The history of MEN I syndrome in this patient and the presence of hypervascular lesions in the stomach (gastrinoma) and liver (metastasis) make Zollinger-Ellison the best diagnosis in this case.

Clinical History: 65-year-old woman with epigastric pain and weight loss.

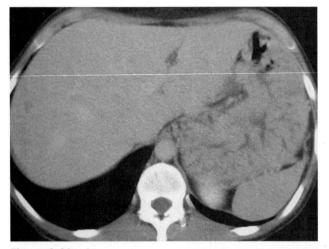

Figure 3.20   A

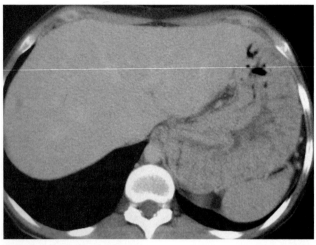

Figure 3.20   B

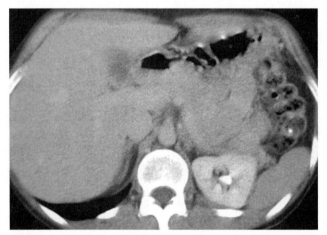

Figure 3.20   C

Findings: Axial CECT images demonstrate marked thickening of gastric folds with sparing of the antrum.

Differential Diagnosis: Lymphoma, adenocarcinoma, peptic ulcer disease, eosinophilic gastritis, Zollinger-Ellison syndrome.

Diagnosis: Ménétrier disease.

Discussion: Ménétrier disease is characterized by hyperplasia of the gastric mucous glands, causing increased secretions of mucus and protein. Patients also have decreased acid production, resulting in thickened gastric folds, hypochlorhydria, and hypoproteinemia. There is a slight male predominance. Patients typically present with abdominal pain, weight loss, diarrhea, and peripheral edema from protein loss.

Radiographically, there is marked thickening of the gastric folds with sparing of the antrum in the majority of the cases. Frequently, there is abrupt change from abnormal to normal gastric mucosa, as seen in this case. The greatest degree of thickening of the gastric mucosa is commonly seen along the greater curvature. Often the folds become so enlarged that they can appear as a polypoid mass on both CT and upper GI studies. The main differential diagnoses are lymphoma and adenocarcinoma of the stomach. Biopsy is necessary to exclude a malignancy. Peptic ulcer disease and gastritis do not usually cause gastric thickening to this extent. Other entities such as Crohn disease, eosinophilic gastritis, and tuberculosis are rare but could be considered as well.

Clinical History: 44-year-old man with a history of pneumonia that did not respond to typical antibiotics now presents with abdominal pain and diarrhea.

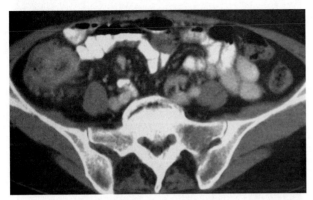

Figure 3.21 A

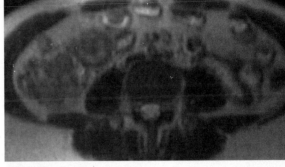

Figure 3.21 B

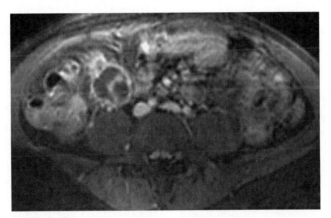

Figure 3.21 C

Findings: Axial CECT image (A) shows asymmetrical thickening of the cecal wall and pericolonic lymphadenopathy. Axial T2-WI (B) shows the intermediate signal of the wall thickening and a large sentinel lymph node. Gadolinium-enhanced, fat-suppressed axial T1-WI (C) shows enhancement of the cecal wall and necrosis of the sentinel lymph node.

Differential Diagnosis: Crohn colitis, lymphoma, amebiasis, *Yersinia* infection, ischemic colitis.

Diagnosis: Tuberculosis of the cecum.

Discussion: Intestinal tuberculosis is thought to be due to hematogenous spread, swallowing of infected sputum, or infected cow's milk. Typically, GI tract tuberculosis is associated with pulmonary tuberculosis, and an abnormal radiograph or positive sputum stain and cultures can suggest diagnosis. However, positive chest film findings are present in only 50% of cases of GI tract tuberculosis. The findings of tuberculosis are similar to those seen in Crohn disease, and tuberculosis should be considered when Crohn disease is a potential diagnosis. Early in the disease, there is thickening and nodularity of the mucosa, which involves the cecum more than the terminal ileum. Ulcers form that heal and form strictures. The cecum can become rigid from the inflammation and scarring and appear cone shaped. This can simulate a carcinoma. Several pathologic processes involve both the terminal ileum and the cecum. Crohn colitis is the most common, but other entities, such as *Yersinia* colitis, amebiasis, and ischemia, can have this appearance as well. The segmental involvement of the cecum and the coexistence of a necrotic lymph node in a patient with antibiotic-resistant pneumonia make tuberculosis the best diagnosis in this case.

Case images courtesy of Dr. Adelard De Backer, St-Lucas Ziekenhuis, Ghent, Belgium.

Clinical History: 67-year-old woman with a history of alcohol abuse presenting with melena and abdominal pain.

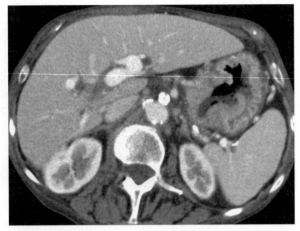

Figure 3.22   A

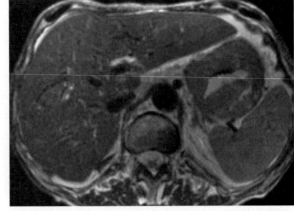

Figure 3.22   B

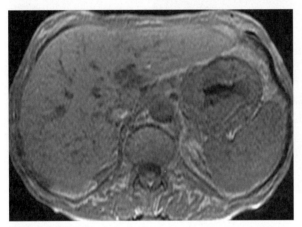

Figure 3.22   C

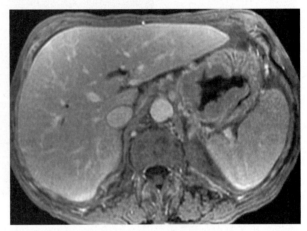

Figure 3.22   D

Findings: Axial CECT image (A) shows thickening of the medial aspect of the gastric wall (lesser curvature). Axial T2-WI (B), T1-WI (C), and gadolinium-enhanced, fat-suppressed axial T1-WI (D) show the mass is isointense, hypointense, and hypovascular, respectively, compared to the rest of the stomach.

Differential Diagnosis: Lymphoma, metastasis, GI stromal tumor.

Diagnosis: Gastric adenocarcinoma.

Discussion: Worldwide, gastric adenocarcinoma is the second most common cancer (second to lung cancer). The global incidence of gastric cancer differs by 10-fold. The lowest incidence (<3.7 cases per 100,000 people) is in North America, Western Europe, Australia, and New Zealand. Gastric carcinoma is typically diagnosed in middle-aged to elderly people; there is a male predominance (male-to-female ratio of 1.5–2.5:1). Gastric carcinoma is also 1.5 to 2.5 times more common in African American, Hispanic, and American Indian individuals than in whites. Some associated risk factors include *Helicobacter pylori* infection, pernicious anemia, partial gastrectomy, and smoking. The imaging appearance of gastric adenocarcinoma is variable, and the tumor may appear polypoid, ulcerative, or infiltrative (scirrhous). Associated perigastric metastatic lymph nodes and liver metastases are often present at diagnosis. Krukenberg tumors represent metastatic deposits to the ovaries. Ninety-five percent of gastric cancers are adenocarcinoma, and in the United States, they represent the third most common GI malignancy after colorectal and pancreatic carcinoma. To differentiate gastric adenocarcinoma from lymphoma, a deep-tissue biopsy is usually required. Gastric adenocarcinoma primarily involves the mucosa, while GI stromal tumor is an intramural lesion, frequently exophytic and exogastric in location. Gastric metastases are uncommon, and typically, the primary tumor is known at the time of diagnosis.

Clinical History: 61-year-old woman presenting with intermittent abdominal pain.

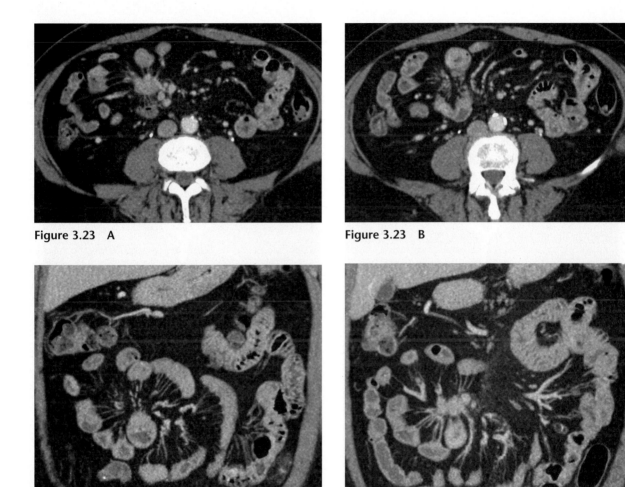

Figure 3.23   A

Figure 3.23   B

Figure 3.23   C

Figure 3.23   D

Findings: Axial (A and B) and coronal reformatted (C and D) CECT images demonstrate a dilated loop of ileum with the presence of an enhancing submucosal mass. Note the large amount of soft tissue stranding and nodularity within the mesentery adjacent to the mass.

Differential Diagnosis: Adenocarcinoma, lymphoma, Crohn disease, tuberculosis, metastases.

Diagnosis: Carcinoid of the terminal ileum.

Discussion: Carcinoid is a slow-growing tumor with malignant potential that arises from the enterochromaffin cells of the bowel. The most common location for a carcinoid tumor in the GI tract is the appendix, followed by the distal small bowel and rectum. Within the small bowel, the majority of carcinoids are found in the ileum, followed by the jejunum and duodenum. When the lesions are small

(<1 cm), they will present as a submucosal lesion. As the tumor grows, it can penetrate the mucosa and cause ulceration and obstruction. Hormonally active substances are secreted by this tumor, such as serotonin, histamine, and bradykinin. The serotonin causes an intense desmoplastic reaction, which can lead to kinking of the bowel and obstruction. In this example, there is a relatively small submucosal mass, but extensive stranding and nodularity is seen in the mesentery adjacent to the mass. This represents the desmoplastic reaction and metastatic spread of the tumor. Adenocarcinoma, lymphoma, and hemorrhage will not invoke as much desmoplastic reaction as is seen in this case. Crohn disease can have inflammatory changes around the involved bowel but will typically present as segmental thickening or stricture of the bowel and not as a focal mass.

Clinical History: 36-year-old man presenting with left lower quadrant pain.

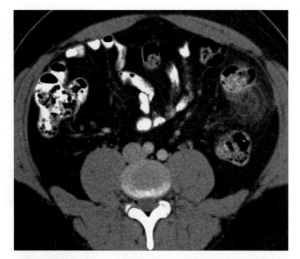

Figure 3.24   A

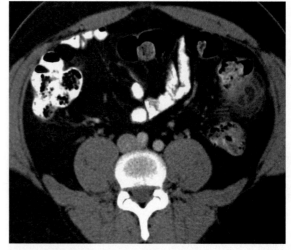

Figure 3.24   B

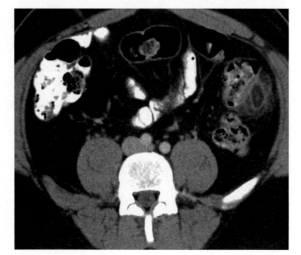

Figure 3.24   C

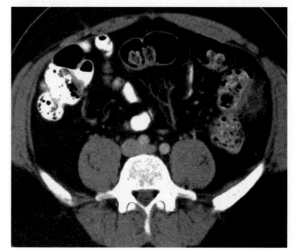

Figure 3.24   D

Findings: Axial CECT images demonstrate a small fatty mass with a central punctate hyperdensity surrounded by a dense rim (C) and fat stranding adjacent to the descending colon. The latter shows focal wall thickening laterally (B and D).

Differential Diagnosis: Acute diverticulitis, omental infarct.

Diagnosis: Epiploic appendagitis.

Discussion: An epiploic appendage is a peritoneal pouch arising from the serosal surface of the colon that is composed of fat and vascular structures. Acute inflammation of an appendage, called epiploic appendagitis, results from presumed torsion and secondary vascular compromise of the appendage. Affected patients are usually obese men in their fourth or fifth decades of life and present with acute onset of abdominal pain, mostly in the left lower quadrant. Sigmoid appendages are most commonly the culprits, followed by descending and right colon appendages. CT features of epiploic appendagitis include the presence of an oval fat-containing mass abutting the colon, less than 5 cm in size, with a hyperattenuating peripheral rim and surrounding fat stranding. A hyperattenuating central dot representing the thrombosed appendiceal vein may be present, as seen in this case. The adjacent colonic wall is typically of normal thickness but may become secondarily thickened. If accurately diagnosed, treatment is conservative, with anti-inflammatory medication and no need for antibiotics. The absence of colonic diverticula makes acute diverticulitis unlikely. Omental infarcts occur almost exclusively on the right side of the abdomen and are typically larger in size.

Clinical History: 24-year-old man presenting with suprapubic abdominal pain, nausea, and vomiting.

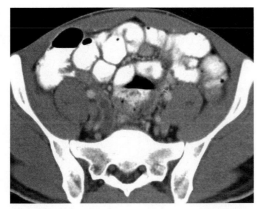

Figure 3.25   A

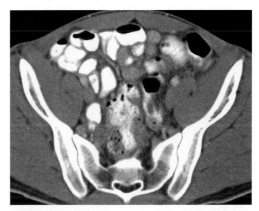

Figure 3.25   B

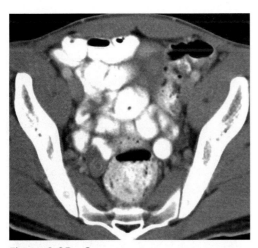

Figure 3.25   C

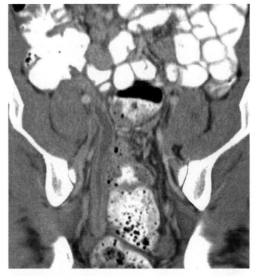

Figure 3.25   D

Findings: Axial CECT images (A–C) demonstrate an enlarged, edematous appendix measuring up to 12 mm in width. Curved reformatted CECT image (D) shows the appendix tracking along the iliac vessels posteriorly into the lower pelvis, with its tip just superior to the seminal vesicles. There is associated fat stranding in the surrounding mesentery.

Differential Diagnosis: Mesenteric adenitis, Crohn disease, cecal diverticulitis.

Diagnosis: Acute appendicitis.

Discussion: Appendicitis is typically a clinical diagnosis based on laboratory findings and physical exam. Like diverticulitis, the prevalence is higher in Western countries due to the low-fiber diet, resulting in impaction of the appendiceal content. Appendicitis is more commonly seen in children and adolescents but can be seen in the elderly as well. In the elderly, the diagnosis can be difficult due to the milder symptoms. The CT findings of appendicitis include a dilated (>6 mm) and inflamed appendix, cecal ("cecal bar" sign) and pericecal inflammation, an appendicolith, and pericecal fluid collections. CT is excellent for depicting acute appendicitis (accuracy = 95%) and differentiating between mild inflammation versus abscess or extensive phlegmon formation. If there is a periappendiceal abscess present, CT can also be used to guide percutaneous drainage. In mesenteric adenitis, the appendix is normal, and the CT findings include enlarged lymph nodes in the ileocolic mesentery. Both Crohn disease and cecal diverticulitis may secondarily involve the appendix, but presence of associated features of both diseases may be helpful to obtain an accurate presumptive diagnosis.

Clinical History: 73-year-old woman presenting with weight loss.

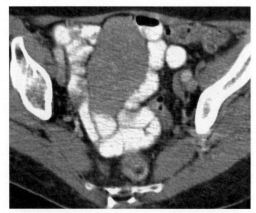

Figure 3.26 A

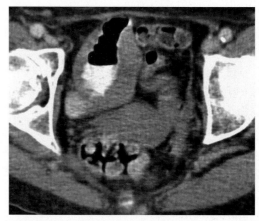

Figure 3.26 B

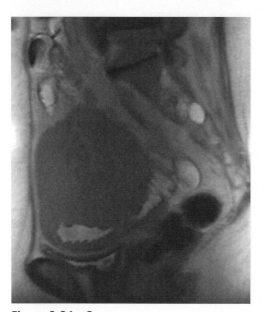

Figure 3.26 C

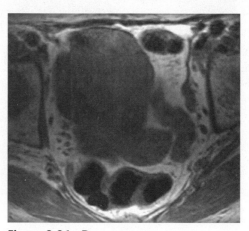

Figure 3.26 D

Findings: Axial CECT images (A and B) through the pelvis show circumferential wall thickening of an ileal loop with mild aneurysmal dilatation of the involved bowel segment. Sagittal T2-WI (C) and axial T1-WI (D) show the homogeneous appearance of the mass and the asymmetric involvement of the bowel wall.

Differential Diagnosis: Adenocarcinoma, abscess, hemorrhage.

Diagnosis: Lymphoma of the ileum.

Discussion: Lymphoma accounts for approximately 50% of all primary malignant small bowel tumors, and the small bowel is the second most common site of involvement, after the stomach, in the GI tract. The majority constitutes non-Hodgkin lymphomas from B-cell origin. The terminal ileum is the most common location of small bowel lymphoma. Small bowel lymphoma can present as a large exophytic mass or as an infiltrating mass (most common) causing an annular stricture. Typically, only a short segment of bowel is involved, and the mass at presentation is large (measuring up to 12 cm in size), as seen in this case. These large lesions can necrose, ulcerate, and fistulize to adjacent structures. Associated lymphadenopathy in the mesentery is common. In this example, the large circumferential bulky mass should suggest a malignancy, such as adenocarcinoma or lymphoma. Hemorrhage and an abscess could also present as a bulky mass, but low-attenuation fluid is normally present in or around the mass. Enteritis, ischemia, and inflammatory bowel disease usually involve a longer segment of bowel with diffuse bowel wall thickening rather than a large bulky mass.

Clinical History: 61-year-old woman presenting with acute abdominal pain and elevated white blood cell count.

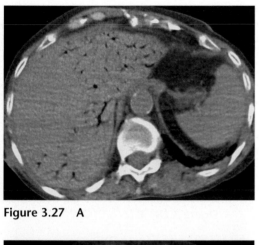

Figure 3.27   A

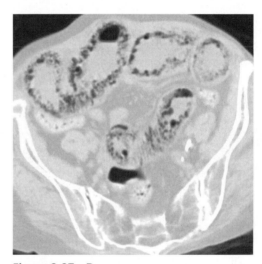

Figure 3.27   B

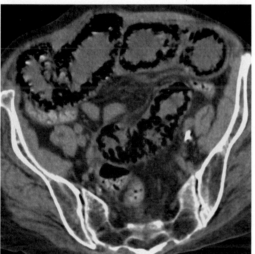

Figure 3.27   C

Figure 3.27   D

Findings: Axial nonenhanced CT (NECT) images (A–C) demonstrate air in the peripheral portal venules in the liver (A) and dilated loops of small bowel that contain air in their wall (B and C). This is better seen when the same image is displayed in lung windows (D).

Differential Diagnosis: None.

Diagnosis: Mesenteric ischemia with pneumatosis and portal venous air.

Discussion: The primary causes of insufficient blood flow to the small intestine are various and include thromboembolism (50% of cases), nonocclusive causes, bowel obstruction, neoplasms, vasculitis, abdominal inflammatory conditions, trauma, chemotherapy, radiation, and corrosive injury. CT can demonstrate changes due to ischemic bowel accurately, may be helpful in determining the primary cause of ischemia, and can demonstrate important coexistent complications. However, CT findings in acute small bowel ischemia are not specific, and therefore, it is often a combination of clinical, laboratory, and radiologic signs that lead to a correct diagnosis. The CT findings include thickened bowel within a vascular territory or watershed zone, stranding and inflammation around the affected bowel, and pneumatosis. Although pneumatosis can be due to benign causes, with the appropriate history, ischemic bowel must be ruled out first. In addition to pneumatosis, venous air in the mesenteric and portal veins can also be present in an ischemic bowel. This is often difficult to see on standard soft tissue windows and is often better seen in either lung or bone windows, as demonstrated in this example.

Clinical History: 46-year-old man with history of ileum and proximal colon resection presenting with diarrhea and abdominal pain.

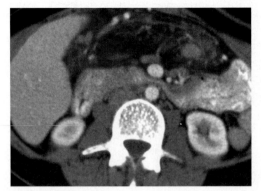

Figure 3.28 A

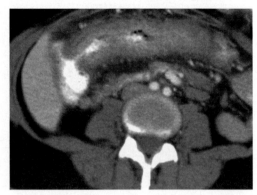

Figure 3.28 B

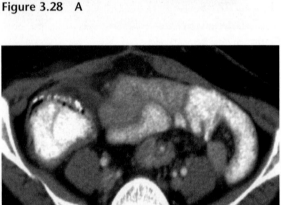

Figure 3.28 C

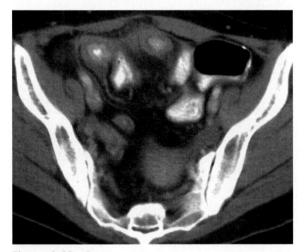

Figure 3.28 D

Findings: Axial CECT images show fat proliferation and lymphadenopathy in the transverse mesocolon (A), segmental wall thickening of the transverse colon (B), suture material following prior ileocolic anastomosis (C), and segmental wall thickening of small bowel loops in the pelvis (D).

Differential Diagnosis: Ulcerative colitis, pseudomembranous colitis.

Diagnosis: Crohn colitis.

Discussion: Crohn disease is of unknown etiology and characterized by transmural inflammation in a discontinuous fashion (skip lesions) usually involving the terminal ileum. Involvement of the colon and terminal ileum is seen in approximately 40% to 45% of patients, and colonic involvement alone is seen in 30% of patients. Complications include fistula and abscess formation and adenocarcinoma. Changes of Crohn colitis include aphthous ulcers, thickening of the bowel wall, deep ulcers, rigidity of the bowel wall, and a "cobblestone" appearance of the mucosa. The cobblestone appearance is due to linear ulcers separated by areas of edematous mucosa. Finally, there is stricture formation of the bowel. "Creeping fat" represents fibrofatty proliferation typically seen in patients with Crohn disease, as demonstrated in this case. It is thought to occur as a response to repeated episodes of inflammation resulting in separation of loops of bowel; it is most frequently seen in the small bowel mesentery but can occur in the colon as well. Pseudomembranous colitis typically involves the entire colon, and there is a greater degree of bowel wall thickening. Ulcerative colitis begins in the rectum, progresses proximally without skip lesions, and does not involve the terminal ileum.

CASE 3-29

Clinical History: 51-year-old woman with prior surgery for gastric cancer presenting with painless jaundice.

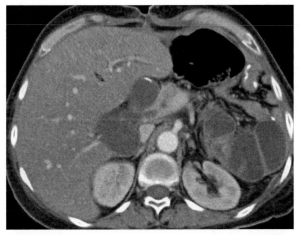

Figure 3.29   A

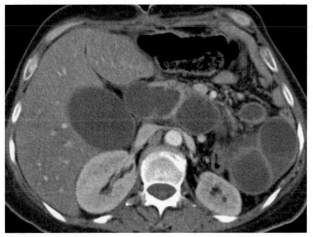

Figure 3.29   B

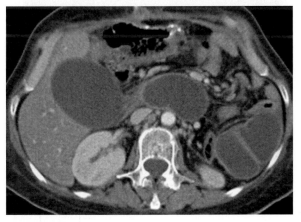

Figure 3.29   C

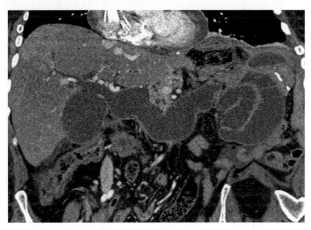

Figure 3.29   D

Findings: Axial (A–C) and coronal curved reformatted images (D) show marked dilation of the afferent loop following Bilroth II procedure. The efferent loop is unremarkable. Note the associated mild biliary dilatation, minimal ascites, and soft tissue stranding along the peritoneum (D).

Differential Diagnosis: Paralytic ileus, postoperative anastomotic stricture.

Diagnosis: Afferent loop syndrome due to peritoneal metastases.

Discussion: Afferent loop syndrome (ALS) is a purely mechanical complication that infrequently (<1%) occurs following construction of a gastrojejunostomy. Creation of an anastomosis between the stomach and jejunum leaves a segment of small bowel, most commonly consisting of duodenum and proximal jejunum, lying upstream from the gastrojejunostomy. This limb of intestine conducts bile, pancreatic juices, and other proximal intestinal secretions toward the gastrojejunostomy and is thus termed the afferent loop. Patients with ALS may present with acute, complete obstruction or with chronic, partial obstruction. The syndrome can manifest at any time from the first postoperative day to many years after surgery; the acute form usually occurs in the early postoperative period (1–2 weeks). On CT, the afferent limb appears as a dilated (average, 5 cm), fluid-filled, tubular mass. Valvulae conniventes and intraluminal air is observed in nearly all cases. The dilated loop is confined to the subhepatic area in 60% of cases, but it can cross the midline, as seen in this case. Biliary dilation is typically present in all patients. Notably, orally administered contrast usually fails to opacify the afferent limb.

Clinical History: 58-year-old woman with history of abdominal pain presenting with vomiting.

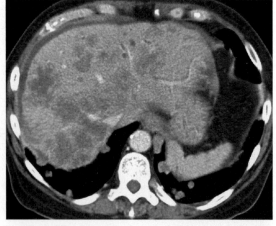

Figure 3.30   A

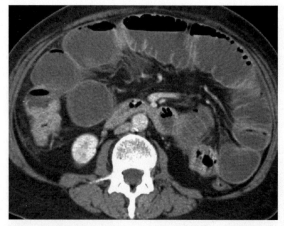

Figure 3.30   B

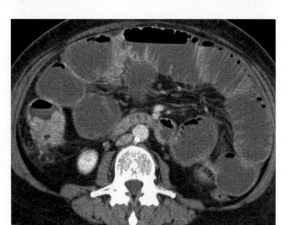

Figure 3.30   C

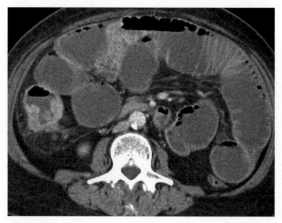

Figure 3.30   D

Findings: Axial CECT image (A) of the upper abdomen demonstrates numerous pulmonary nodules and low-attenuation masses in the liver. Axial CECT images of mid abdomen (B–D) reveal a constricting lesion of the ascending colon. Note the lymphadenopathy in the mesocolon and associated bowel obstruction.

Differential Diagnosis: Lymphoma, metastasis.

Diagnosis: Metastatic colon cancer.

Discussion: Colon cancer is the second most common cancer in men and ranks third in frequency in women living in Western countries. The incidence of colon cancer varies in different parts of the world. In the United States, the incidence is approximately 36 cases per 100,000 people. In many developing countries, the incidence is less than 10 per 100,000 people. Colon carcinoma typically presents on CT as a short segment of luminal irregular wall thickening.

Fifty-five percent of colon cancers arise in the rectosigmoid colon; only 15% arise in the ascending colon. Colon cancers arising in the right colon tend to be larger at presentation due to lack of symptoms. A constricting lesion in the ascending colon and cecum can be due to a variety of etiologies. Tuberculosis (tuberculoma) and amebiasis (ameboma) can have this appearance, and both are more common in the right colon. A stricture from ischemia is also a possibility, although no other signs of ischemia in the remaining bowel are seen, and associated lymphadenopathy, as seen in this case, would be unusual. Although possible, Crohn colitis without terminal ileum involvement is rare. The presence of numerous solid liver lesions, adenopathy in the mesocolon, and an "apple-core" lesion suggest a malignancy. Both lymphoma and adenocarcinoma would be good possibilities in this case.

Clinical History: 44-year-old woman presenting with acute right lower quadrant pain and fever.

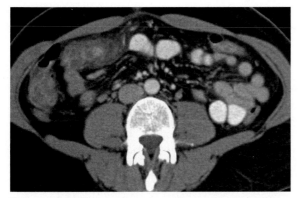

Figure 3.31   A

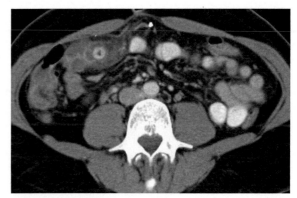

Figure 3.31   B

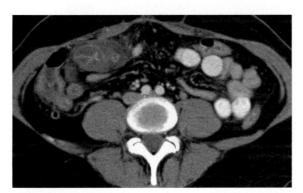

Figure 3.31   C

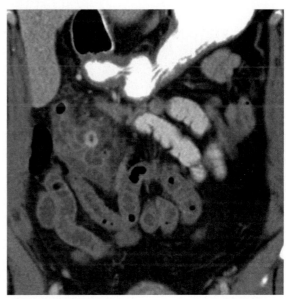

Figure 3.31   D

Findings: Axial (A–C) and coronal reformatted (D) CECT images demonstrate thickening of the wall of the transverse colon with stranding and inflammatory changes in the mesocolon surrounding a diverticulum. Note presence of other diverticula at the level of the hepatic flexure.

Differential Diagnosis: Epiploic appendagitis, inflammatory bowel disease.

Diagnosis: Diverticulitis.

Discussion: Diverticula of the colon are acquired herniations of mucosa and submucosa through the muscular layers of the bowel wall. They are found most commonly in the sigmoid colon and are thought to be related to the low-fiber diet found in Western countries. Diverticulitis occurs secondary to perforation of a diverticulum. This can lead to bowel wall inflammation and spasm, a localized ileus, and abscess formation. Because the perforation usually walls itself off quickly, there is rarely free air present on plain films. On CT, however, extraluminal air can be seen as well as an inflammatory mass, which represents a phlegmon or focal abscess. In the colon, the sigmoid has the smallest lumen requiring the highest pressures. The colonic wall is weakest where the blood vessels penetrate the wall to reach the submucosa, around the taenia mesocolica, and on the mesenteric side of the taenia libera and taenia omentalis, where diverticula are found. This case demonstrates a subtle case of diverticulitis. There is inflammation seen in and around the wall of the transverse colon with extension into the pericolonic fat. This finding, in conjunction with the presence of multiple diverticula, makes diverticulitis the most likely diagnosis. Epiploic appendagitis also most likely involves the sigmoid colon, is not associated with diverticula, and rarely would cause such marked colonic wall thickening.

Clinical History: 71-year-old man on warfarin (Coumadin) with a history of atrial fibrillation presents with an international normalized ratio (INR) of 8.4 and vague abdominal discomfort.

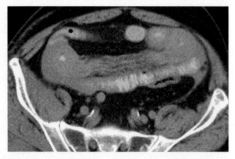

Figure 3.32 A

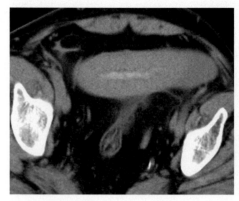

Figure 3.32 B

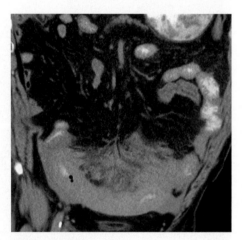

Figure 3.32 C

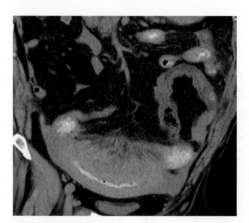

Figure 3.32 D

Findings: Axial (A and B) and coronal reformatted (C and D) NECT images show hyperdense thickened appearance of mid ileal small bowel loops and associated high-density stranding in the small bowel mesentery.

Differential Diagnosis: Lymphoma, adenocarcinoma, Crohn disease, shock bowel.

Diagnosis: Small bowel hematoma.

Discussion: Nontraumatic spontaneous intramural small bowel hematoma, once considered a rare complication of oral anticoagulation therapy, is being reported with increasing frequency. Overanticoagulation by warfarin is the most common cause of spontaneous intramural small bowel hematoma. Other risk factors include hemophilia, idiopathic thrombocytopenic purpura, leukemia, lymphoma, myeloma, chemotherapy, vasculitis, pancreatitis, and pancreatic cancer. The presentation of patients who have spontaneous intramural small bowel hematoma can vary from mild and vague abdominal pain to intestinal tract obstruction and an acute abdomen. The hemorrhage is usually located in the submucosal layer of the bowel and originates from a small vessel that produces slow bleeding. In addition to intramural bleeding, intraluminal, intramesenteric, and retroperitoneal hemorrhage can occur, especially when the duodenum is involved. Hemorrhagic ascites can be present and is related to leakage of blood from an engorged, thickened, and inflamed bowel wall, with submucosal bleeding extending into all layers. CT findings of small bowel wall hematoma include circumferential small bowel wall thickening and obstruction. Although mural hyperdensity is a rather uncommon finding, it is pathognomonic of spontaneous intramural small bowel hematoma when the mural hyperdensity occurs in patients who are overanticoagulated with warfarin. The involved bowel appears longer in spontaneous hematomas than in traumatic hematomas. Spontaneous small bowel wall hematomas most often are single lesions and most commonly involve the jejunum, followed by the ileum and the duodenum. These findings are different from those seen in traumatic small bowel hematomas, which most commonly affect the duodenum.

Clinical History: 24-year-old woman presenting with a 1-week history of abdominal pain.

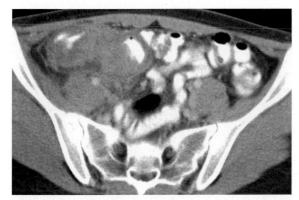

Figure 3.33 A

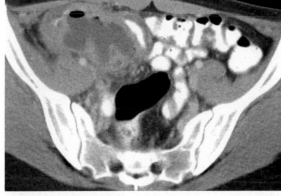

Figure 3.33 B

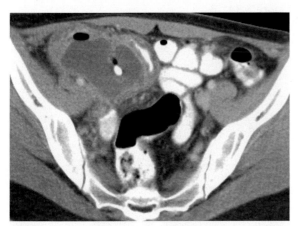

Figure 3.33 C

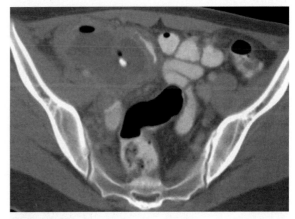

Figure 3.33 D

Findings: Axial CECT images (A–C) demonstrate marked thickening of the wall of the cecum and terminal ileum. A thick-walled fluid collection containing air and high-density material is displacing the cecum and terminal ileum. Axial CECT image displayed in bone windows (D) shows that the high-density material in the collection represents a stone.

Differential Diagnosis: Crohn colitis, typhlitis, tubo-ovarian abscess.

Diagnosis: Perforated appendix with periappendiceal abscess.

Discussion: Appendicitis is the most common abdominal surgical emergency in the United States. It occurs most commonly in the late teens and twenties but has been seen in the elderly as well. Obstruction of the appendix leading to appendicitis can be due to an appendicolith, foreign body, adhesion, neoplasm, or Crohn colitis. CT findings of appendicitis include appendiceal dilatation (>6 mm), the presence of an appendicolith, wall thickening of the appendix (>3 mm), mucosal hyperenhancement of the appendix, periappendiceal/pericecal stranding, abscess or phlegmon formation, and cecal and ascending colon wall thickening. In patients with perforated appendicitis, it is often difficult to identify an abnormal appendix. More commonly, a periappendiceal abscess/phlegmon is seen, which is similar in appearance to a perforated neoplasm or diverticulitis. In this patient's age group and especially because of the presence of an appendicolith, perforated appendicitis is the most likely diagnosis. Alternative diagnoses include Crohn colitis with an abscess, typhlitis if the patient had neutropenia and tubo-ovarian abscess if the patient had a history of pelvic inflammatory disease.

Clinical History: 59-year-old woman with peritoneal carcinomatosis from pancreatic cancer presenting with abdominal pain and vomiting.

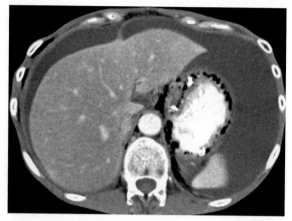

Figure 3.34 A

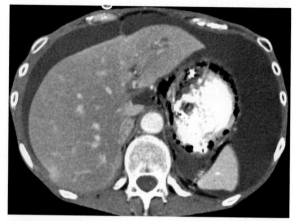

Figure 3.34 B

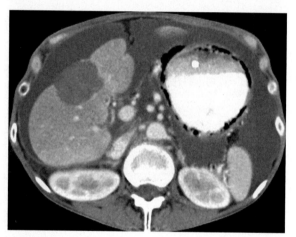

Figure 3.34 C

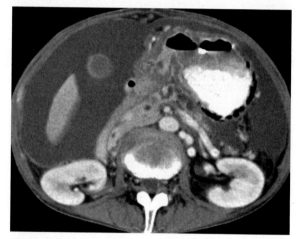

Figure 3.34 D

Findings: Axial CECT images show gastric dilatation, air bubbles in the gastric wall, and soft tissue masses in the liver. Note presence of a nasogastric tube in the stomach.

Differential Diagnosis: Interstitial gastritis.

Diagnosis: Emphysematous gastritis.

Discussion: Emphysematous gastritis is a condition involving gastric wall inflammation, radiologic evidence of intramural gas, and systemic toxicity. It is caused by mucosal disruption characterized by gas in the stomach wall. The most common cause of emphysematous gastritis is corrosive ingestion; however, other causes include trauma or gastric infarction. Organisms most commonly involved are

Escherichia coli, Streptococcus species, *Enterobacter* species, and *Pseudomonas aeruginosa*. The main differential diagnosis for intramural gas is emphysematous gastritis and interstitial gastritis. In patients with interstitial gastritis, the appearance of intramural gas tends to be sharply defined and linear. Some patients may have recently undergone a gastric procedure. Emphysematous gastritis is an almost uniformly fatal disease. Surgical intervention after development of emphysematous gastritis has been unsuccessful. A protocol of early treatment with a broad-spectrum antibiotic and surgical revascularization performed immediately after diagnostic angiography has been reported to successfully reverse gastric ischemia.

CASE 3-35

Clinical History: 73-year-old woman post allograft bone marrow transplantation for chronic myelogenous leukemia presenting with intractable nausea, vomiting, and diarrhea.

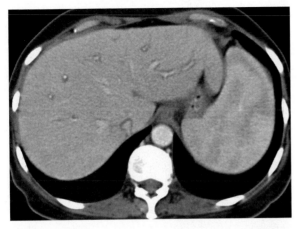

Figure 3.35   A

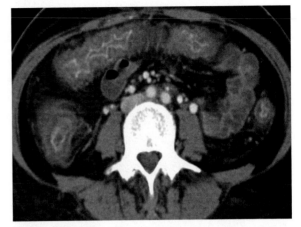

Figure 3.35   B

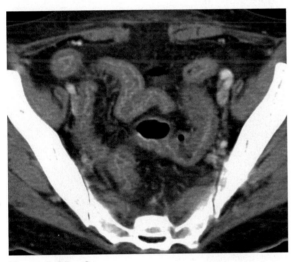

Figure 3.35   C

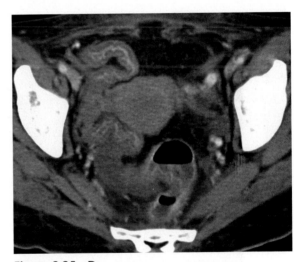

Figure 3.35   D

Findings: Axial CECT image (A) of the liver shows periportal edema. Axial CECT images (B–D) of the pelvis demonstrate marked thickening and mucosal hyperenhancement of multiple loops of small and large bowel with mesenteric edema and inflammation. A small amount of free fluid is seen in the pelvis.

Differential Diagnosis: Viral enteritis, mesenteric ischemia, radiation enteritis.

Diagnosis: Graft-versus-host disease.

Discussion: Graft-versus-host disease (GVHD) is due to the presence of immunocompetent cells in the donor marrow that are reacting with cells in the recipient. Acute GVHD can occur up to 100 days after transplantation. It commonly affects the skin, liver, and GI tract. In the GI tract, the small bowel is most commonly involved, but the stomach, duodenum, and colon can also demonstrate changes as well. There is prolonged coating of the small bowel, which can appear as circular collections of barium in cross section or parallel tracks in longitudinal sections. Bowel wall thickening with mural stratification due to mucosal hyperenhancement, mesenteric edema, mesenteric hyperemia, and adenopathy can also be seen. The affected bowel may be normal in caliber or less commonly dilated. This appearance can be indistinguishable from viral enteritis, which can also be a complication of bone marrow transplantation. Mesenteric ischemia would typically involve the proximal portion of the colon. Radiation enteritis would be within the confines of the radiation field. Diagnosis of GVHD is typically made by rectal biopsy.

Clinical History: 79-year-old woman with lower GI bleed who failed optic colonoscopy.

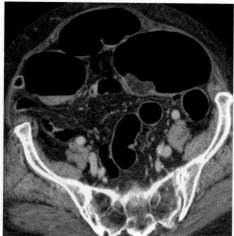

Figure 3.36 A

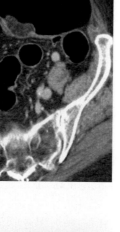

Figure 3.36 B

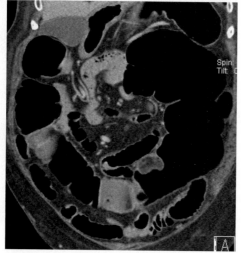

Figure 3.36 C

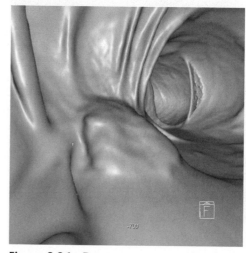

Figure 3.36 D

Findings: Axial CECT image (A) demonstrates a 3-cm mass of homogeneous fat density in the transverse colon. Coronal reformatted CECT images displayed in lung window (B) and soft tissue window (C) show a polypoid lesion in the transverse colon. Note the oblong shape of the lesion. A three-dimensional, volume-rendered image (D) shows the polypoid appearance of the mass.

Differential Diagnosis: Colonic polyp, colon cancer.

Diagnosis: Colonic lipoma.

Discussion: Intestinal lipomas are slow-growing, usually incidentally discovered tumors that may occur anywhere along the bowel. The colon, specifically the cecum and the right colon, is the most common location, accounting for 65% to 75% of the cases, followed by the distal small bowel and the stomach. Intestinal lipomas are submucosal lesions but may project completely endoluminally, as seen in this case. Most lipomas are asymptomatic, but they may be the cause of intussusception, and when they reach over 2 cm in size, they may ulcerate and cause anemia due to chronic GI bleeding. On CT scan, they appear as well-delineated homogeneous lesions of fat density (between −80 and −120 Hounsfield units). Soft tissue strands within the mass due to ulceration may be seen. Because lipomas are soft tumors, their shape may change from one examination to another and with peristalsis or compression. The shape and density of this lesion is pathognomonic for a colonic lipoma. On three-dimensional virtual colonography images, however, lipomas will present as polypoid masses. Therefore, careful review of the two-dimensional images in soft tissue windows is crucial to avoid misdiagnosis.

Clinical History: 33-year-old man with diarrhea and rectal bleeding.

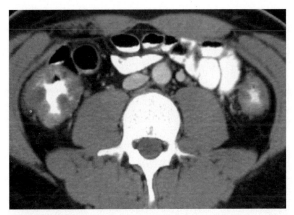

Figure 3.37   A

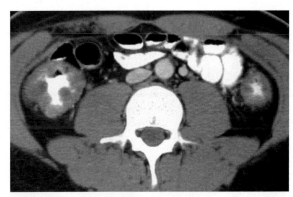

Figure 3.37   B

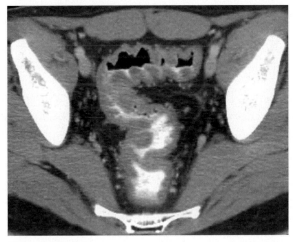

Figure 3.37   C

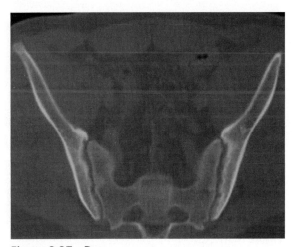

Figure 3.37   D

Findings: Axial CECT images (A–C) demonstrate smooth thickening of the wall of the ascending, transverse, descending, and rectosigmoid colon without mesocolonic changes. Axial CECT image (D) displayed in bone window shows bilateral sacroiliitis.

Differential Diagnosis: Crohn disease, cathartic abuse, radiation colitis, pseudomembranous colitis.

Diagnosis: Ulcerative colitis.

Discussion: Ulcerative colitis is predominantly a mucosal disease that begins in the rectum and progresses proximally to involve the entire colon. Early in the course of the disease, the mucosa is edematous and hyperemic with areas of ulceration. Thumbprinting can often be seen during this stage as well. Eventually the mucosa becomes friable and denuded with islands of edematous mucosa-forming "pseudopolyps." With further episodes of inflammation and healing, there is distortion of the haustral pattern with eventual loss of haustration and shortening of the colon, leading to a "lead pipe" colon in the chronic phases of ulcerative colitis. Other entities can also cause loss of haustration including cathartic abuse, which predominantly involves the left side of the colon. In ulcerative colitis, the terminal ileum can be involved with backwash ileitis, but in contrast to Crohn disease, the lumen is usually enlarged rather than strictured. Also, Crohn colitis spares the rectum. The age of onset is typically in the twenties, but ulcerative colitis can be seen at almost any age. On CT, the bowel wall thickening is less pronounced than with other colitides, with an average thickening of approximately 8 mm. Ischemia would be unlikely because this would involve both the SMA and inferior mesenteric artery (IMA) vascular distributions. Pseudomembranous colitis typically has a much thicker wall, and typically there is a history of antibiotic use.

Clinical History: 34-year-old man presenting with periumbilical pain.

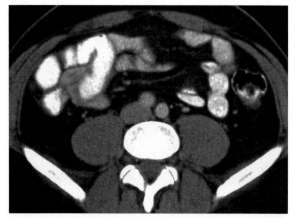

Figure 3.38   A

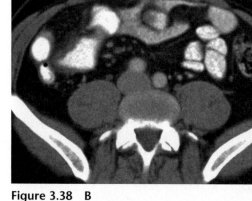

Figure 3.38   B

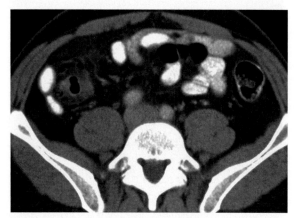

Figure 3.38   C

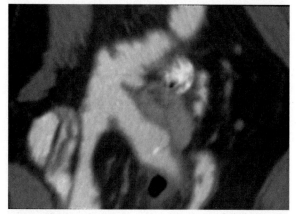

Figure 3.38   D

Findings: Axial CECT images (A–C) and curved reformatted CECT image (D) demonstrate a 5-cm long and 2.8-cm wide, blind-ended structure that arises from the side of the mid ileum. It fills with oral contrast proximally, but near its tip, it demonstrates focal wall thickening and adjacent fat stranding. A small focus of extraluminal gas is identified.

Differential Diagnosis: Appendicitis.

Diagnosis: Perforated Meckel diverticulitis.

Discussion: Meckel diverticulum is the most common form of congenital abnormality of the small intestine, resulting from an incomplete obliteration of the vitelline duct (omphalomesenteric duct, yolk stalk). Most patients are asymptomatic; Meckel diverticulum is usually an incidental finding when a barium study, CT, or laparotomy is performed for other abdominal conditions. On CT, the diverticulum has been reported to appear as a rounded or tubular collection of air and fluid located in the abdomen or pelvis and communicating with the adjacent small bowel. Like other diverticula in the body, the Meckel diverticulum can become inflamed. Diverticulitis is seen usually in older patients. Meckel diverticulum is less prone to inflammation than the appendix because most diverticula have a wide mouth, have very little lymphoid tissue, and are self-emptying. If an inflammatory process is visualized on CT in the lower abdomen or pelvis, particularly at midline, one should carefully search for the presence of an inflamed Meckel diverticulum. If a normal appendix is identified, the likelihood of this diagnosis increases. Luminal opacification of the small bowel with oral contrast material facilitates the identification of the diverticulum.

CASE 3-39

Clinical History: 43-year-old woman presenting with rectal bleeding and anemia.

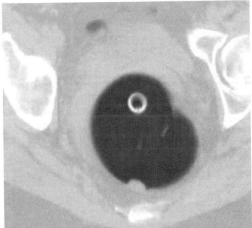

Figure 3.39 A

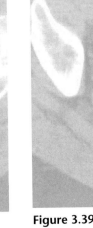

Figure 3.39 B

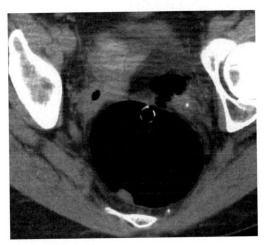

Figure 3.39 C

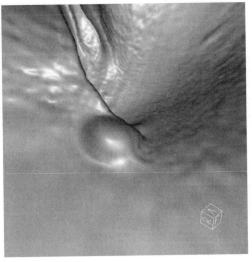

Figure 3.39 D

Findings: Axial NECT images obtained with the patient in supine position (A) and prone position (B) and displayed in lung windows show a 1.6-cm polypoid lesion arising from the posterior rectal wall. Axial NECT image displayed in soft tissue windows (C) shows the mass is homogeneous. A three-dimensional volume rendered endoluminal image (D) confirms its polypoid appearance.

Differential Diagnosis: Adherent stool, colon cancer.

Diagnosis: Colonic adenomatous polyp.

Discussion: On CT-colonography, colorectal polyps appear as round, oval, or lobulated intraluminal projections and are homogeneous in attenuation and enhance after contrast administration. Villous tumors often appear heterogeneous and can mimic stool. The majority of colonic adenomas that will develop into cancer are polypoid or villous in shape. A small proportion of adenomas are "flat" or depressed and have been

shown to be difficult to identify on CT-colonography. Positive predictive characteristics of adenoma with increased propensity to develop into cancer are its size and the total number of adenomas. Polyps greater than 10 mm in diameter and more than three polyps, regardless of size, have been reported as risk factors for transformation into colorectal cancer through the "adenoma-carcinoma sequence." Retained stool often has a heterogeneous aspect due to incorporated air or high-density food particles. Lack of wall attachment, enhancement, and changing location on prone/supine images favors fecal origin. An entity to keep in mind when observing mobile filling defects is pedunculated polyps with a long stalk. The morphology of the polyp with head and stalk is helpful in differentiating these lesions from mobile fecal material. Fecal material can be round, oval, or lobulated but often presents angled borders and irregular geometric morphology. Fecal tagging also helps to differentiate immobile retained stool from real lesions.

Clinical History: 37-year-old woman with abdominal pain, diarrhea, and new onset of asthma. Biochemical analysis revealed eosinophilia.

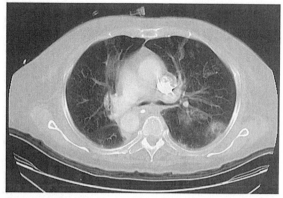

Figure 3.40   A

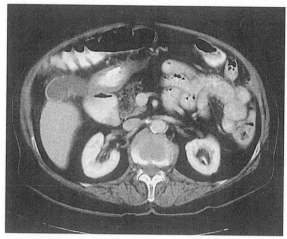

Figure 3.40   B

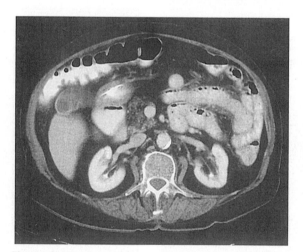

Figure 3.40   C

Findings: Axial CECT image (A) of the chest demonstrates bilateral consolidations. Axial CECT images of the abdomen (B and C) demonstrate thickening and distension of the proximal duodenum.

Differential Diagnosis: Peptic ulcer disease, eosinophilic gastroenteritis, tuberculosis, Crohn disease, lymphoma.

Diagnosis: Strongyloidiasis.

Discussion: *Strongyloides stercoralis* is a parasite endemic in Africa, Asia, and South America. Cases in the United States are usually present in patients who have migrated from these areas or in the acquired immunodeficiency syndrome (AIDS) population, in which *S. stercoralis* presents as an opportunistic infection. The larvae of the parasite enter the skin and subsequently reach the lungs via the venous system. Patients frequently present with new-onset reactive airway disease due to the pneumonitis from the parasite. As with other parasitic infections, peripheral eosinophilia is commonly seen. From the lung, the larvae then migrate to the proximal small bowel, predominantly the proximal duodenum. Radiographically, there are edematous folds, ulcerations, and spasm of the proximal duodenum. As the process progresses, there can be narrowing of the third and fourth portions of the duodenum, resulting in proximal dilatation. Thickening of the wall of the proximal duodenum is nonspecific, but with coexistent pulmonary infiltrates, the differential diagnosis is limited to *Strongyloides* and tuberculosis. With new onset of asthma and peripheral eosinophilia, the diagnosis of *Strongyloides* is most likely.

CASE 3-41

Clinical History: 74-year-old woman with a history of melanoma.

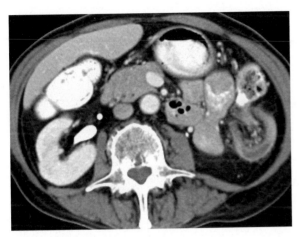

Figure 3.41 A

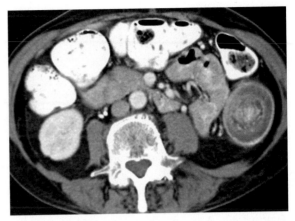

Figure 3.41 B

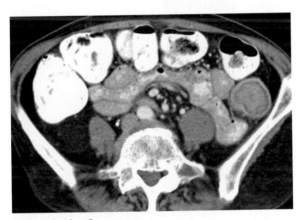

Figure 3.41 C

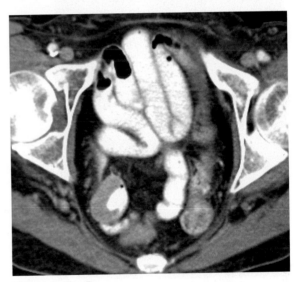

Figure 3.41 D

Findings: Axial CECT images demonstrate a round soft tissue mass in the left abdomen composed of concentric rings; the middle ring measures fat density. In addition, soft tissue masses are identified in the wall of the proximal jejunum and distal ileum.

Differential Diagnosis: None.

Diagnosis: Colocolic intussusception due to large bowel metastasis from melanoma.

Discussion: This case demonstrates the classic CT appearance of an intussusception. An intussusception represents the invagination of one loop of bowel (intussusceptum) into another loop of bowel (intussuscipiens) by peristalsis. The mass in the left abdomen corresponds to the intussusception scanned in the short axis. In this mass, invaginated mesenteric fat can be seen. Three distinct layers of bowel wall can be distinguished. The outermost layer represents the edematous wall of the intussuscipiens. The next two layers are the herniated intussusceptum with its associated mesenteric fat; the latter separates both bowel walls. Chronic intussusception can lead to bowel ischemia. This example represents a fairly early stage of intussusception since three distinct layers of bowel wall can still be identified. As the intussusception progresses, there will be loss of the layers secondary to edema in the bowel wall eventually leading to bowel wall ischemia and necrosis. In adults, intussusceptions can be caused by a mass in the bowel wall that serves as a lead point; due to intestinal peristalsis, the mass invaginates into distal bowel. Primary malignant bowel neoplasms are the most common causes of large bowel intussusceptions. However, in patients with a known primary, especially when additional small bowel masses are identified, intussusception due to metastatic disease is the most likely diagnosis.

Clinical History: 27-year-old woman presenting with acute abdominal pain following head and neck surgery.

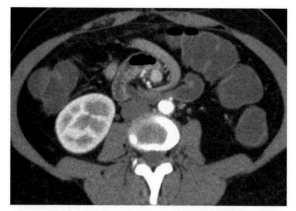

Figure 3.42 A

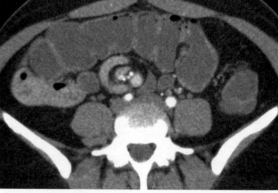

Figure 3.42 B

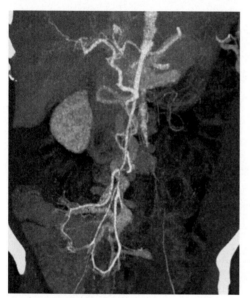

Figure 3.42 C

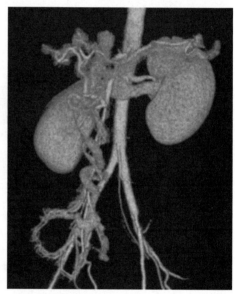

Figure 3.42 D

Findings: Axial CECT images (A and B) obtained after oral administration of a neutral contrast agent demonstrate a swirling appearance of the mesenteric vessels and an abnormal location of the ileum lateral to the cecum. Coronal maximum-intensity projection (MIP) CECT image (C) and three-dimensional, volume-rendered image (D) show a twisted appearance of the SMA and SMV.

Differential Diagnosis: Malrotation.

Diagnosis: Midgut volvulus.

Discussion: Malrotation of the intestine results when the normal embryologic sequence of bowel development is interrupted. In the normal embryo, herniation of the gut through the umbilicus at 6 weeks is accompanied by a 270-degree counterclockwise rotation of the developing intestine around the SMA. Malrotation is caused by incomplete rotation (<270 degrees) occurring between weeks 5 and 12. The disease is estimated to occur in 1 in 500 live births. Malrotation is associated with a narrow stalk of mesentery about which the gut may twist, resulting in midgut volvulus. Accompanying superior mesenteric vascular compromise (first venous, followed by arterial) can lead to life-threatening ischemia of the small bowel and gangrenous necrosis. The mortality rate for midgut volvulus is approximately 15%. In malrotation with midgut volvulus, findings may include a dilated, fluid-filled duodenum, proximal small bowel obstruction, a "corkscrew" pattern (proximal jejunum spiraling downward in right or mid upper abdomen), mural edema, and the "whirlpool sign" on color Doppler and CT indicating flow within the SMV wrapping around the SMA (in a clockwise direction).

CASE 3-43

Clinical History: 38-year-old woman presenting with constipation and sensation of incomplete stool evacuation.

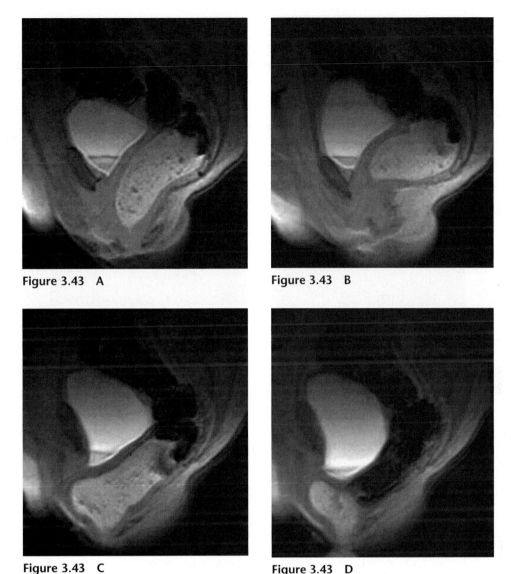

Figure 3.43 A

Figure 3.43 B

Figure 3.43 C

Figure 3.43 D

Findings: Sagittal T1-WI (A) obtained during relaxation shows a normal position of the bladder, vagina, and anorectal junction in relation to the pubococcygeal line. Sagittal T1-WI (B) obtained during contraction of the sphincter shows motion of all three compartments suggestive of competence of the pelvic floor muscles; there is normal sharpening of the anorectal angle. Sagittal T1-WI (C) obtained during straining shows descent of the anorectal junction with widening of the anorectal angle. Sagittal T1-WI (D) obtained during defecation shows that the anterior wall of the rectum projects approximately 3 cm more anteriorly than expected. Also note incomplete evacuation of the contrast retained in the anterior rectal outpouching. The base of the bladder projects 4 cm below the pubococcygeal line.

Differential Diagnosis: None.

Diagnosis: Anterior rectocele.

Discussion: Pelvic organ prolapse is very common, and it is the indication for more than 300,000 surgeries in the United States annually. Rectocele is defined as herniation or bulging of the posterior vaginal wall, with the anterior wall of the rectum in direct apposition to the vaginal epithelium. Etiologically, most cases are the result of vaginal childbirth and chronic increases in intra-abdominal pressure. In some patients, rectocele is thought to develop as a result of congenital or inherited weaknesses within the pelvic support system. Rectocele is a defect of the rectovaginal septum, not the rectum. Rectoceles are commonly found on proctograms, and small bulges of the anterior rectal wall detected upon evacuation proctography might be normal findings. Rectoceles should be considered abnormal if contrast trapping (the rectocele does not completely empty upon evacuation) is noted.

Clinical History: 59-year-old woman presenting with rectal incontinence.

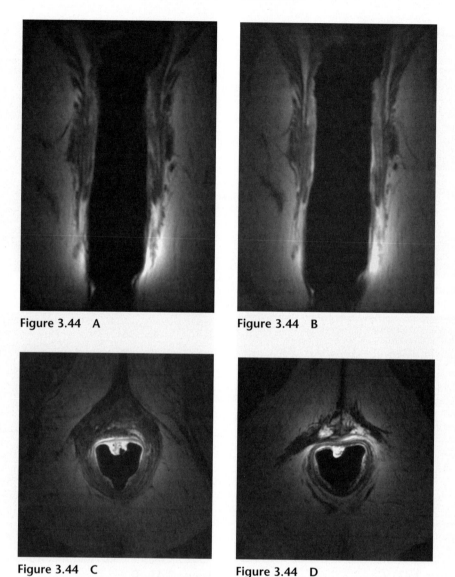

Figure 3.44 A

Figure 3.44 B

Figure 3.44 C

Figure 3.44 D

Findings: Coronal T2-WI (A and B) and axial T2-WI (C and D) show thinning of the inferior part of the external anal sphincter. Also note the abnormally increased signal intensity of the external sphincter (puborectal muscle). The internal sphincter is circular and normal in thickness and signal intensity.

Differential Diagnosis: Anal sphincter tear, anal sphincter scarring.

Diagnosis: External anal sphincter atrophy.

Discussion: Fecal incontinence is the inability to voluntarily control defecation. The prevalence of fecal incontinence ranges from 3 to 10 per 1,000 people but may actually be much higher. Women are affected more often than men; the condition is often a consequence of childbirth. Because of the fine demonstration of muscle layers, endoanal MRI allows detection of local thinning and atrophy of the sphincter, usually a result of denervation injury. Atrophy of the external sphincter, defined as an extreme generalized thinning, has been proven to be a predictive factor for a negative outcome of sphincteric surgery. On coronal images, the thickness of all anal muscles may be compared; such comparison makes external sphincteric atrophy easy to detect. Several studies have demonstrated a good correlation between atrophy as seen at endoanal MRI and the findings at surgery and histopathologic investigation of the biopsy specimens. Therefore, endoanal MRI is of major importance in the preoperative assessment of fecal incontinence. A sphincteric defect is defined as a discontinuity of the muscle ring. Scarring is defined as a hypointense deformation of the normal pattern of the muscle layer due to replacement of muscle cells by fibrous tissue.

CASE 3-45

Clinical History: 57-year-old man with intermittent crampy abdominal pain.

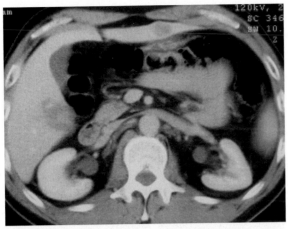

Figure 3.45   A

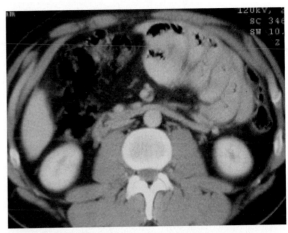

Figure 3.45   B

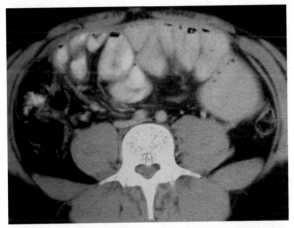

Figure 3.45   C

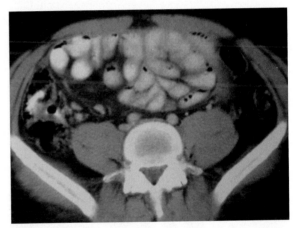

Figure 3.45   D

Findings: Axial CECT images demonstrate mildly dilated small bowel loops grouped together in the mid abdomen. A thickened layer of peritoneum that separates them from other small bowel and large bowel segments surrounds the dilated loops. Minimal mesenteric stranding is seen within the enclosed area.

Differential Diagnosis: Small bowel obstruction due to adhesions.

Diagnosis: Internal small bowel hernia.

Discussion: Internal hernias are defined by the protrusion of a viscus through a normal or abnormal peritoneal or mesenteric aperture within the confines of the peritoneal cavity. The orifice can be either acquired, such as a postsurgical, traumatic, or postinflammatory defect, or congenital, including both normal apertures, such as the foramen of Winslow, and abnormal apertures arising from anomalies

of internal rotation and peritoneal attachment. Internal hernias, including paraduodenal (traditionally the most common), pericecal, foramen of Winslow, and intersigmoid hernias, account for approximately 0.5% to 5.8% of all cases of intestinal obstruction and are associated with a high mortality rate, exceeding 50% in some series. Also, the incidence of internal hernias is increasing because of a number of relatively new surgical procedures now being performed. General CT features include apparent encapsulation of distended bowel loops with an abnormal location, arrangement or crowding of small bowel loops within the hernial sac, and evidence of obstruction with segmental dilatation and stasis, with additional features of apparent fixation. Additional findings include mesenteric vessel abnormalities, with engorgement, crowding, twisting, and stretching of these vessels commonly found.

Clinical History: 63-year-old man presenting with anemia, weight loss, and hematochezia.

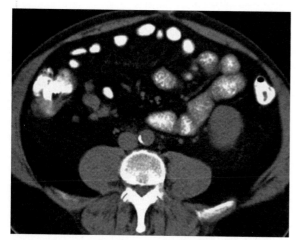

Figure 3.46   A

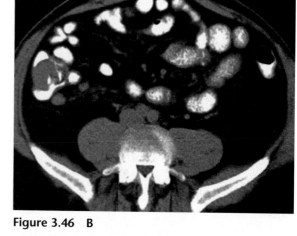

Figure 3.46   B

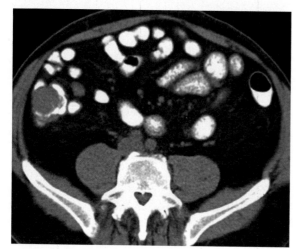

Figure 3.46   C

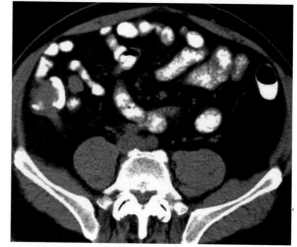

Figure 3.46   D

Findings: Axial CECT images (A–D) demonstrate a rounded cecal mass causing a filling defect. No mesocolonic stranding is visible, but there is extensive ileocolic lymphadenopathy (A–C), and the mass extends to the appendix (D).

Differential Diagnosis: Adenocarcinoma, GI stromal tumor, metastasis.

Diagnosis: Colonic lymphoma.

Discussion: When evaluating a soft tissue mass in the cecum, it is important to determine if the mass is inflammatory or neoplastic. If characteristics suggest an inflammatory process, the differential diagnosis should include diverticulitis, appendicitis, or typhlitis. The most common neoplastic possibilities include adenocarcinoma, lymphoma, GI stromal tumor, carcinoid, and metastases. Colonic lymphoma is less common than lymphoma involving the stomach or small bowel. In fact, lymphoma represents less than 1% of all colonic neoplasms, although it is found with increased frequency in patients with AIDS, Crohn disease, and ulcerative colitis. It is also more common in men than in women and typically occurs in patients between the ages of 50 and 70 years. When present in the colon, lymphoma most commonly involves the cecum and the rectum and is usually of the non-Hodgkin type. Types of presentation include nodules that can ulcerate and cause perforation; discrete masses, usually without obstruction; focal or diffuse infiltration of the colonic wall causing fold thickening; and aneurysmal dilatation by destruction of the bowel wall innervation. The prognosis of colonic lymphoma depends on tumor bulk as defined by staging.

Clinical History: 55-year-old woman presenting with severe epigastric pain.

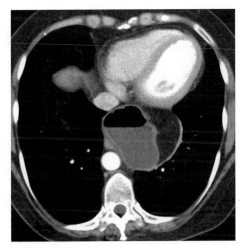

Figure 3.47 A

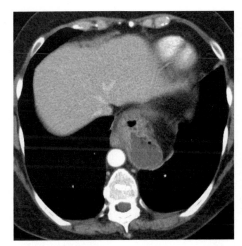

Figure 3.47 B

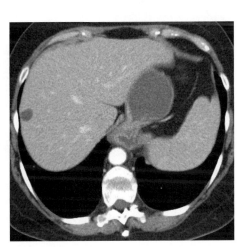

Figure 3.47 C

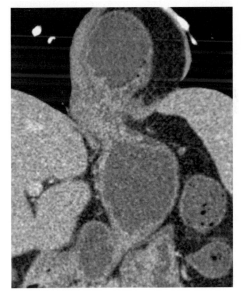

Figure 3.47 D

Findings: Axial (A–C) and curved reformatted (D) CECT images demonstrate intrathoracic location of part of the stomach. Note normal caliber esophagus running along the intrathoracic stomach and position of the gastroesophageal junction just above the diaphragm.

Differential Diagnosis: Sliding hernia, paraesophageal hernia.

Diagnosis: Mixed hiatal hernia.

Discussion: There are three main types of hiatal hernia: sliding, paraesophageal, and mixed. In a paraesophageal hernia, the stomach bulges up through the opening in the diaphragm (hiatus) alongside the esophagus (upside down stomach). The lower esophageal sphincter (LES) remains in its normal location inside the opening of the diaphragm. This type of hernia most commonly occurs when there is a large opening in the diaphragm next to the esophagus. In a sliding hiatal hernia, part of the stomach moves through the diaphragm so that it is positioned outside of the abdomen and in the chest. The LES often moves up above its normal location in the opening of the diaphragm. In a mixed hiatal hernia, the LES is above the diaphragm, as in a sliding hiatal hernia, and the stomach is alongside the esophagus, as in a paraesophageal hiatal hernia. Paraesophageal and mixed hiatal hernias often have no symptoms or only minimal symptoms. Symptoms may include vague, nonspecific abdominal complaints, such as feeling full after a meal and indigestion. If not treated, the hernia can grow. This can result in twisting (volvulus) of the stomach (possibly leading to gangrene), which requires emergency surgical treatment. Because of the risk involved in emergency treatment, it generally is recommended that all people with these types of hernias undergo surgery regardless of the symptoms.

Clinical History: 30-year-old man who made a recent trip to India presenting with fever and diarrhea.

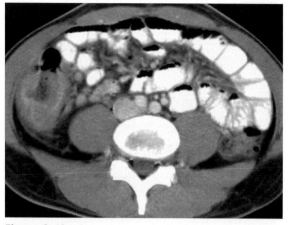

Figure 3.48 A

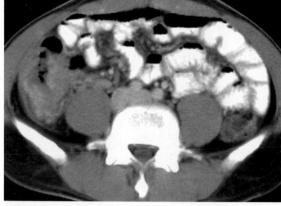

Figure 3.48 B

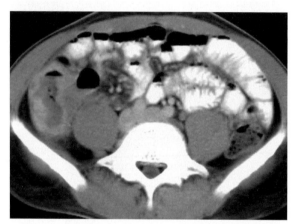

Figure 3.48 C

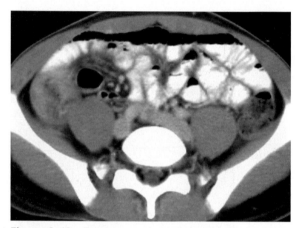

Figure 3.48 D

Findings: Axial CECT images show asymmetrical thickening of the cecal wall and ascending colon with associated ileocolic lymphadenopathy. Note that the terminal ileum is mildly dilated, but its wall is unremarkable.

Differential Diagnosis: Tuberculosis, Crohn colitis, lymphoma, *Yersinia* infection, ischemic colitis.

Diagnosis: Colonic amebiasis.

Discussion: *Entamoeba histolytica* is a protozoan that is endemic in various parts of the world, including some areas of the United States. Infection is acquired by the fecal-oral route, either by person-to-person contact or indirectly by eating or drinking fecally contaminated food or water. The incubation period is commonly 2 to 4 weeks but ranges from a few days to years. The clinical spectrum of intestinal amebiasis ranges from asymptomatic infection to fulminant colitis and peritonitis. The parasite initially infects the colon, but it occasionally may spread to other organs, most commonly the liver (amebic liver abscess). It may live in the large bowel in its cyst form without harming the host (commensalism), or for as yet poorly understood reasons, it may invade the tissues as a trophozoite-producing invasive amebiasis of the colon. In a review of over 3,000 cases of invasive amebiasis, the clinicopathologic forms of the disease were: ulcerative rectocolitis (95%), typhloappendicitis (3%), ameboma (1.5%), and fulminating colitis and toxic megacolon (0.5%). Typhloappendicitis is localized to the cecum and appendix, as shown in this example. The appendix is usually secondarily involved from disease in the cecum. An ameboma is a segmental lesion characterized by marked thickening of the bowel wall producing an excrescent mass that narrows the intestinal lumen.

Case images courtesy of Dr. Giovanni Artho, McGill University Health Center, Montreal, Canada.

Clinical History: 48-year-old woman presenting with severe acute abdominal pain and vomiting.

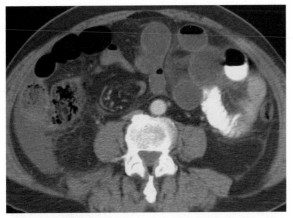

Figure 3.49 A

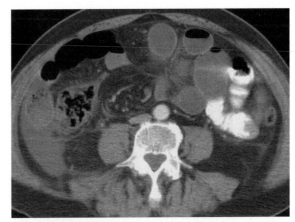

Figure 3.49 B

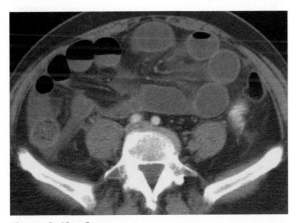

Figure 3.49 C

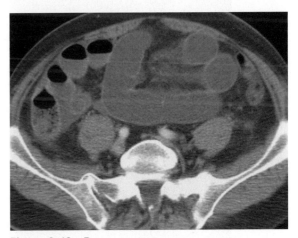

Figure 3.49 D

Findings: Axial CECT images show dilation of small bowel loops in the mid abdomen. The loops are arranged in an O-shaped fashion, and several points of transition are identified. Note presence of interloop fluid and stranding.

Differential Diagnosis: Paralytic ileus, uncomplicated mechanical small bowel obstruction.

Diagnosis: Closed-loop obstruction.

Discussion: The obstruction of a segment of bowel at two points results in a closed-loop obstruction. Progression to strangulation is not an invariable component of this entity when surgical intervention is delayed. CT findings in closed-loop obstruction depend on the length, degree of distention, and orientation of the closed loop in the abdomen. When a closed small bowel loop is horizontally oriented, it has a U- or C-shaped configuration at cross-sectional imaging. A radial configuration with stretched mesenteric vessels converging toward the site of torsion may be detected depending on the orientation of different small bowel loops within the incarcerated bowel segment. At the site of obstruction, the collapsed loops are round, oval, or triangular. The "beak sign" seen at the site of torsion appears as a fusiform tapering at longitudinal bowel imaging. A tightly twisted mesentery is occasionally seen in patients with volvulus and has been described as the "whirl sign." Ascites may be present in patients with closed-loop obstruction without ischemia or with simple bowel obstruction, but it is more commonly seen in patients with strangulation, and, therefore, should be considered a suspicious finding.

Clinical History: 61-year-old man with a history of Crohn disease presenting with perineal discharge.

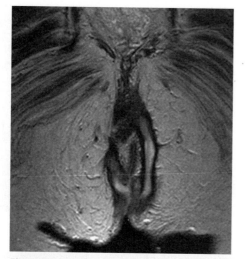

Figure 3.50   A

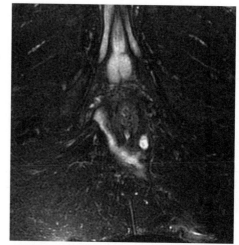

Figure 3.50   B

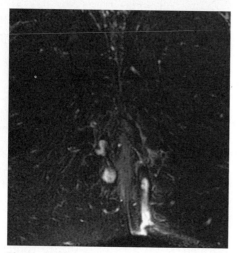

Figure 3.50   C

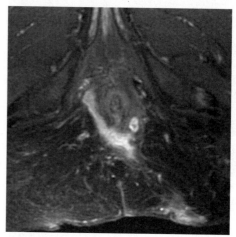

Figure 3.50   D

Findings: Coronal T2-WI (A), fat-suppressed axial T2-WI (B and C), and gadolinium-enhanced, fat-suppressed axial T1-WI (D) show the presence of bilateral fluid-filled tracts bridging the anal canal to the skin. Hyperenhancement of the tract wall and a posterior defect in the internal anal sphincter (D) are seen.

Differential Diagnosis: None.

Diagnosis: Anal fistula.

Discussion: Fistula-in-ano is a common condition defined by an abnormal perianal track that connects two epithelialized surfaces, usually the anal canal to the perianal skin. Perianal fistulas occur in about 10 out every 10,000 individuals; however, in referred tertiary centers, the disease is a common problem. Fistulous disease in the perirectal-perianal region may be due to a complication of chronic local inflammation, Crohn disease, infiltrating malignancy, radiation therapy, surgical treatment, or a traumatic delivery. For many years, examination under anesthesia (EUA) by an experienced colorectal surgeon was considered the reference standard for the detection of fistulas, but it is now accepted that preoperative MRI has a sensitivity surpassing EUA. The Parks classification system defines four types of fistula-in-ano that result from cryptoglandular infections: intersphincteric, transsphincteric, suprasphincteric, and extrasphincteric. Fat-suppressed T2-WI show the fluid fistulas the best and allow differentiating between active tracts (hyperintense) versus chronic scarring (hypointense). Active tracts also show enhancement following gadolinium administration.

CASE 3-51

Clinical History: 69-year-old woman with history of swallowing difficulty and hand contracture.

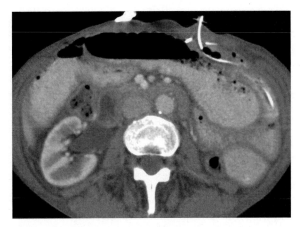

Figure 3.51   A

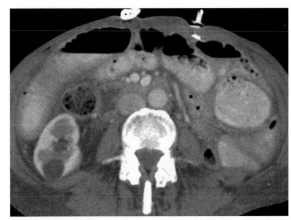

Figure 3.51   B

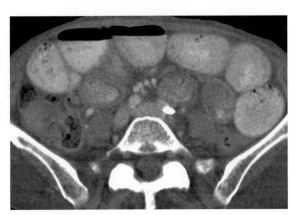

Figure 3.51   C

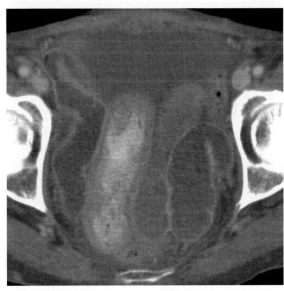

Figure 3.51   D

Findings: Axial CECT images show dilation of fluid-filled small bowel loops. Several loops of small bowel demonstrate bowel wall thickening. Particulate material is identified in distal small bowel loops. Note presence of jejunostomy tube.

Differential Diagnosis: Mechanical bowel obstruction, celiac sprue.

Diagnosis: Scleroderma.

Discussion: Scleroderma is a systemic disease that affects many organ systems. It is most obvious in the skin; however, the GI tract, the respiratory, renal, cardiovascular, genitourinary systems, and numerous vascular structures are frequently involved. The symptoms result from inflammation and progressive tissue fibrosis and occlusion of the microvasculature by excessive production and deposition of types I and III collagen. In scleroderma, the small bowel becomes dilated and often very atonic. The small bowel when dilated loses its propulsive function. Bacteria, which do not normally grow in the small bowel, now begin to grow. Sometimes, there is a markedly dilated small bowel, resulting in a condition called intestinal pseudo-obstruction. In pseudo-obstruction, the small bowel may require venting. Venting means to put a small jejunostomy into the jejunum to aspirate out the air, which keeps the patient from becoming severely distended. Another variance of scleroderma is dilated small bowel with spiculations causing a hide-bound appearance. It is due to fibrosis and atrophy in the small bowel usually in patients with severe malabsorption and weight loss.

Clinical History: 35-year-old woman presenting with abdominal pain.

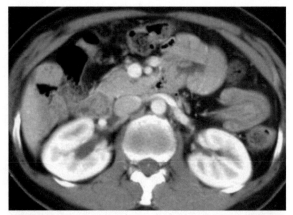

Figure 3.52 A

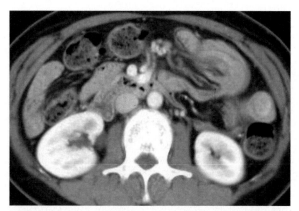

Figure 3.52 B

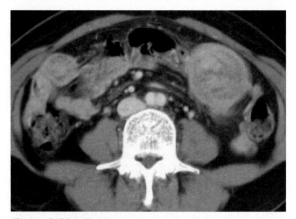

Figure 3.52 C

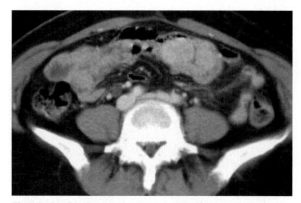

Figure 3.52 D

Findings: Axial CECT images demonstrate several large enhancing lesions within the lumen of the small bowel, causing intussusceptions.

Differential Diagnosis: Cronkhite-Canada syndrome, Gardner variant of familial adenomatous polyposis, juvenile polyposis syndrome.

Diagnosis: Peutz-Jeghers syndrome.

Discussion: Peutz-Jeghers syndrome (PJS) is an autosomal dominant inherited disorder characterized by intestinal hamartomatous polyps in association with mucocutaneous melanocytic macules of the lips and other parts of the face, hands, and feet. PJS has been described in all races; the occurrence in males and females is about equal, and the average age at diagnosis is approximately 25 years. A 15-fold elevated relative risk of developing cancer exists in PJS over that of the general population; cancer primarily is of the GI tract and of the female and male reproductive tracts. The hamartomas in the small intestine have a low risk of becoming cancerous; however, polyps in the stomach and colon are more likely to do so and should be monitored endoscopically. The principal causes of morbidity in PJS stem from the intestinal location of the polyps (i.e., small intestine, colon, stomach). Morbidity includes small intestinal obstruction and intussusception (43%), abdominal pain (23%), hematochezia (14%), and prolapse of a colonic polyp (7%). The polyposis syndromes may be classified as familial inherited (autosomal dominant) or nonfamilial. The inherited polyposis syndromes can be further subdivided into two groups depending on whether the polyps are adenomas or hamartomas. The adenomatous polyposis syndromes include the classic familial adenomatous polyposis (FAP), Gardner syndrome, and Turcot syndrome. Hamartomatous familial polyposis syndromes include PJS, juvenile polyposis syndrome, Cowden disease, and Ruvalcaba-Myhre-Smith syndrome. The noninherited polyposis syndromes include Cronkhite-Canada syndrome and a variety of miscellaneous nonfamilial polyposes.

Clinical History: 47-year-old woman presenting with abdominal pain, nausea, and vomiting.

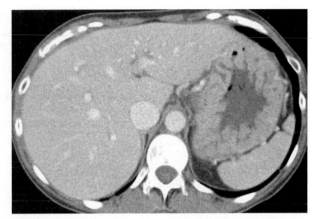

Figure 3.53   A

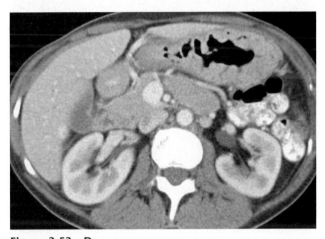

Figure 3.53   B

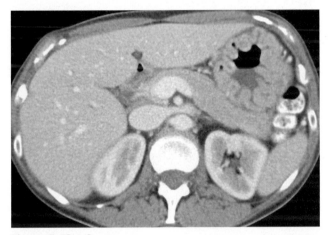

Figure 3.53   C

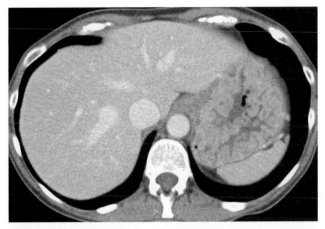

Figure 3.53   D

Findings: Axial CECT images show diffuse marked thickening of the gastric folds with mucosal hyperenhancement.

Differential Diagnosis: Gastric lymphoma, gastric cancer.

Diagnosis: Hypertrophic gastropathy.

Discussion: Hypertrophic gastropathies are characterized by hyperrugosity or enlarged folds, usually in the body and fundus of stomach. Hypertrophic gastropathies encompass a collection of disorders, including hypertrophic hypersecretory gastropathy, hypertrophic hypersecretory gastropathy with protein loss, Zollinger-Ellison syndrome, and Ménétrier disease. The latter is also known as giant hypertrophic gastritis, a premalignant disorder of the stomach characterized by overgrowth of the stomach mucosa and hypoalbuminemia due to loss of albumin by the stomach. The abnormalities of the stomach are highly characteristic with giant folds,

excess mucus secretion, and hypochlorhydria. The cause of the disease is not known, although infections with cytomegalovirus and *Helicobacter pylori* have been suspected to play a role. In some families, siblings have the disease, due possibly to autosomal recessive inheritance. The most classic CT finding in patients with hypertrophic gastritis is thickening of the gastric folds and wall. In severe cases, the gastric wall will demonstrate low attenuation compatible with submucosal edema and inflammation. At the same time, the mucosa may enhance due to hyperemia. This enhancement may give the wall a layered appearance, which is most pronounced at arterial phase imaging. This layering or "halo" will help distinguish gastritis from other conditions that cause gastric wall thickening (e.g., neoplasms). Neoplasms will not penetrate the layers of the GI tract wall and, therefore, will not create this striated or halo appearance.

Clinical History: 53-year-old man presenting with hematemesis.

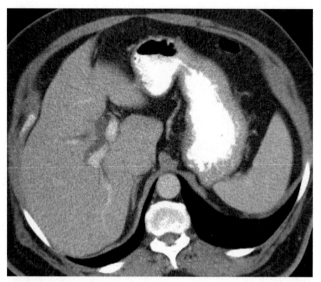

Figure 3.54 A

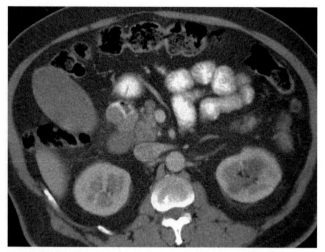

Figure 3.54 B

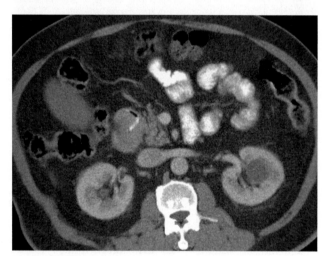

Figure 3.54 C

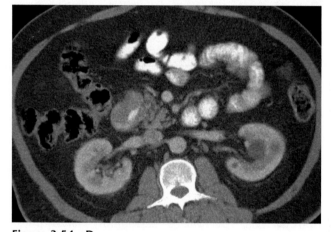

Figure 3.54 D

Findings: Axial CECT images show a soft tissue mass within the second portion of the duodenum. Note associated intrahepatic ductal dilatation.

Differential Diagnosis: Duodenal lymphoma, GI stromal tumor, metastasis.

Diagnosis: Duodenal adenocarcinoma.

Discussion: Duodenal carcinoma occurs in both sexes worldwide with no predisposing factors in the majority of cases. There is an increased risk in patients with familial adenomatous polyposis and adenomas of the duodenum. Duodenal carcinoma occurs about 22 years from the diagnosis of familial adenomatous polyposis in about 2% of patients; they constitute over 50% of upper GI cancers occurring in these patients. Carcinomatous changes occur in 30% to 60% of duodenal villous adenomas and much less in tubulovillous

and tubular adenomas. These categories of patients should be screened and adequately followed up. The general 5-year survival rate is 17% to 33%, but some centers have achieved 5-year survival rates of 40% to 60% with aggressive management. Small bowel adenocarcinomas frequently appear as solitary proximal small bowel masses and are rarely greater than 8 cm in diameter. Ulceration is seen in a third of adenocarinomas; lymphadenopathy is seen in a half of the tumors. Lymphomas, by contrast, appear as large, annular, aneurysmally ulcerated masses, with big lymphadenopathy. Carcinoid tumors are seen as mesenteric masses associated with desmoplastic changes and possibly hepatic metastases and lymphadenopathy. GI stromal tumors are large, locally spreading, bulky, heterogeneous tumors on CT, occasionally with calcifications. Lipomas are well-circumscribed, homogeneous, fat-density masses.

Clinical History: 66-year-old man with a history of longstanding Crohn disease presenting with abdominal pain.

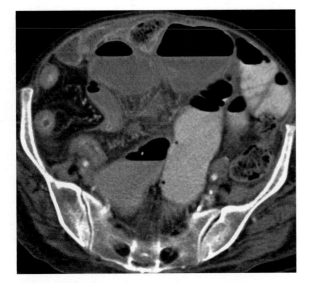

Figure 3.55   A

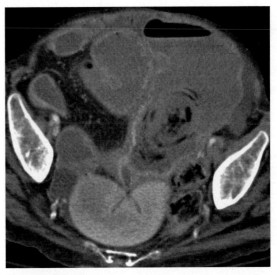

Figure 3.55   B

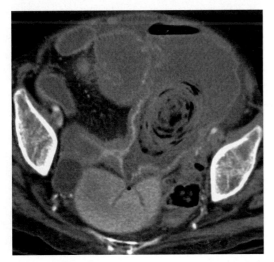

Figure 3.55   C

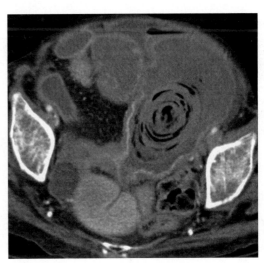

Figure 3.55   D

Findings: Axial CECT images obtained after oral administration of a neutral contrast agent shows an alternating pattern of dilated and strictured small bowel segments. Sharply delineated areas of mucosal hyperenhancement are present. Also note the intraluminal mass in the mid abdomen; the mass consists of concentric rings, of which some contain air. A small amount of ascites is seen.

Differential Diagnosis: Radiation enteritis.

Diagnosis: Small bowel Crohn disease (acute on chronic) with bezoar formation.

Discussion: Crohn disease is an inflammatory condition of the bowel that affects approximately half a million patients in North America. Symptomatic patients with Crohn disease may be affected by active inflammatory disease or inactive chronic disease (e.g., fibrous stricture). CT findings of mural stratification, mucosal and mural hyperenhancement, edema in the perienteric mesenteric fat, and engorged ileal vasa recta correlate with active inflammation. Submucosal fat deposition and mural thickening without enhancement or mural stratification typically correlate with fibrotic or quiescent disease. The sensitivity of CT for Crohn disease is estimated to be 71%, with lower detection of early mucosal disease. A bezoar is a ball of swallowed foreign material (usually hair or fiber) that collects in the intestines, especially the stomach. When a bezoar is composed of hair, it is referred to as a hairball or trichobezoar. When a bezoar is composed of vegetable materials, it is referred to as a phytobezoar or food ball. When a bezoar is composed of hair and food, it is referred to as a trichophytobezoar or hairy food ball.

Clinical History: 65-year-old woman presenting with sudden abdominal pain and diarrhea.

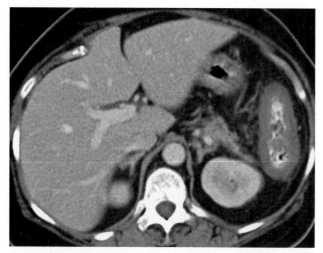

Figure 3.56   A

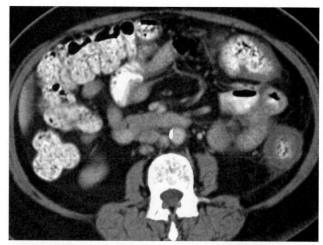

Figure 3.56   B

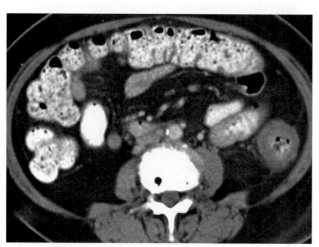

Figure 3.56   C

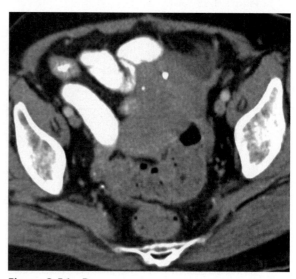

Figure 3.56   D

Findings: Axial CECT images show homogeneous hypodense thickening of the wall of the descending colon. The ascending and transverse and sigmoid colon are unremarkable. Note acute transition between normal and abnormal colon at the level of the splenic flexure.

Differential Diagnosis: Crohn colitis, infectious colitis, pseudomembranous colitis, ulcerative colitis.

Diagnosis: Ischemic colitis.

Discussion: Ischemic colitis is a common cause of abdominal pain in the elderly. Most patients are over 70 years of age, and many have a history of cardiac disease. Ischemic colitis results when blood flow to the colon is compromised, usually as a result of hypoperfusion and vasospasm of the splanchnic arteries. Clinical situations associated with nonocclusive ischemic colitis include heart failure with low cardiac output, hemorrhagic or septic shock, and the use of vasopressor drugs. Colonic ischemia can also result from occlusion of the mesenteric vasculature by a thrombus, embolus, or invasive tumor. Both arterial and venous occlusion can result in colonic ischemia. The extent and severity of the ischemia vary with its cause (hypoperfusion vs. thrombus) and the vessels involved (superior or inferior mesenteric artery). Therefore, ischemic colitis can be diffuse or segmental. Watershed areas of the colon (the splenic flexure and rectosigmoid) are particularly susceptible to ischemia due to hypovolemia. These regions represent areas of relatively poor perfusion at the border of major vascular territories. Left-sided involvement, as seen in this case, is typical in elderly patients with hypoperfusion.

Clinical History: 79-year-old man presenting with proctalgia.

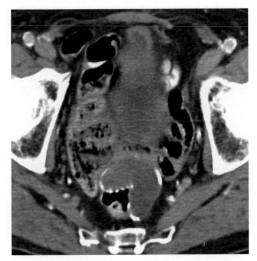

Figure 3.57   A

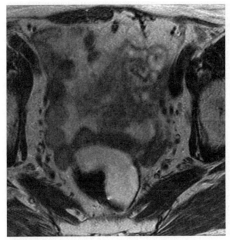

Figure 3.57   B

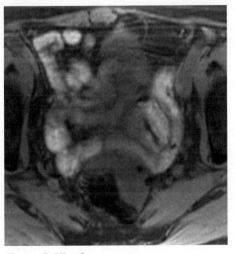

Figure 3.57   C

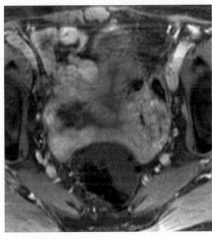

Figure 3.57   D

Findings: Axial CECT image (A) demonstrates a 7-cm, L-shaped cystic structure in front of the rectum. Peripherally, calcifications are present. Note that the cystic mass abuts the deep-lying cecum. Axial T2-WI (B) and fat-suppressed T1-WI (C) show the mass to be hyperintense and mildly hypointense, respectively. The calcifications are seen as areas of signal void. No enhancement of the mass is seen on the gadolinium-enhanced, fat-suppressed axial T1-WI (D).

Differential Diagnosis: Meckel diverticulum, abscess, rectal duplication cyst.

Diagnosis: Mucocele of the appendix.

Discussion: Mucocele of the appendix is a descriptive term for mucinous distension of the appendiceal lumen, regardless of the underlying pathology. The incidence of mucocele in appendectomy specimens is about 0.25%. The male-to-female ratio is 1:4, with a mean age of 55 years at diagnosis. The most common symptom is right lower abdominal pain mimicking appendicitis, although mucocele can also be asymptomatic. Most mucoceles are probably neoplastic in nature and thought to be the result of a pathologic spectrum consisting of hyperplasia, mucinous cystadenoma, and mucinous cystadenocarcinoma. Wall thickness of the mucocele has not been proven to be a reliable differential point between neoplastic and nonneoplastic causes; thus the presence of relatively thin wall in our case cannot exclude malignancy. Curvilinear nodular or punctuate wall calcifications, as in this case, have been reported in both malignant and benign mucoceles. Rupture of mucocele might result in pseudomyxoma peritonei and possibly a fatal outcome.

Clinical History: 37-year-old woman presenting with rectal pressure sensation.

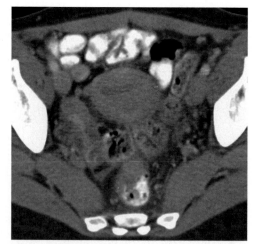

Figure 3.58 A

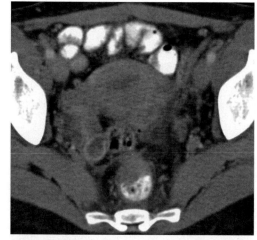

Figure 3.58 B

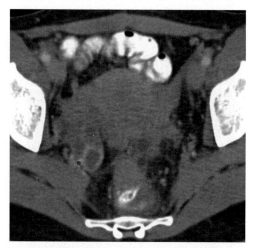

Figure 3.58 C

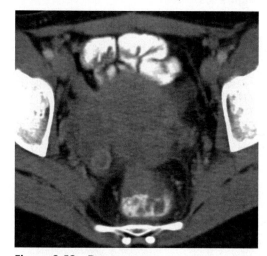

Figure 3.58 D

Findings: Axial CECT images demonstrate a 3-cm soft tissue mass arising from the anterior aspect of the rectal wall. The rectal lumen is slightly narrowed. The right ovary appears to contain a rim-enhancing corpus luteum cyst.

Differential Diagnosis: Rectal adenocarcinoma, drop metastasis, GI stromal tumor, carcinoid.

Diagnosis: Rectal endometriosis.

Discussion: Endometriosis is defined as the presence of endometrial tissue outside the endometrium and the myometrium. The most common locations of endometriosis are the ovaries and the pelvic peritoneum, followed in order of decreasing frequency by deep lesions of the pelvic subperitoneal space, the intestinal system, and the urinary system. Although peritoneal endometriosis can be asymptomatic, deep pelvic endometriosis is a cause of pelvic pain, dysmenorrhea, dyspareunia, dyschezia, and urinary symptoms and is associated with infertility. The histologic

findings of deep pelvic endometriosis are mainly characterized by fibromuscular hyperplasia that surrounds foci of endometriosis, and the foci sometimes contain small cavities. Between 7% and 35% of all women with endometriosis have been reported to have bowel involvement. Endometriosis of the rectum and/or rectosigmoid may be serosal or adventitial, in the muscle (muscularis), or full thickness involving both the muscularis and the lamina propria of the mucosa; the mucosal surface is rarely broken. The lesions are anterior or lateral. Posterior wall endometriosis is rare but can form a "napkin ring" deformity. Fibrotic endometriosis nodules infiltrating the anterior rectal wall are most common and may be focal (cicatrixal) or linear (a transverse bar often with associated stricture where the rectum is fused to the posterior vagina). When endometriosis is juxtaposed to the rectal wall, as seen in this case, invasion of the muscle wall can be difficult to diagnose with CT or MRI.

Clinical History: 83-year-old woman with a history of colon cancer presenting with abdominal pain and vomiting.

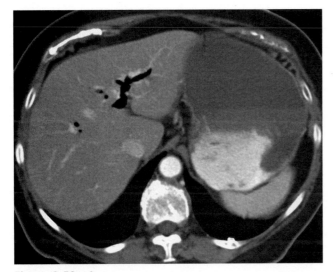

Figure 3.59   A

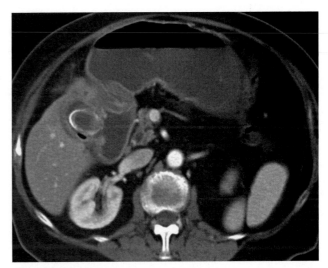

Figure 3.59   B

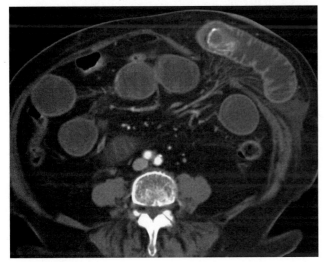
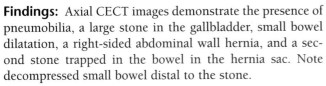

Figure 3.59   C

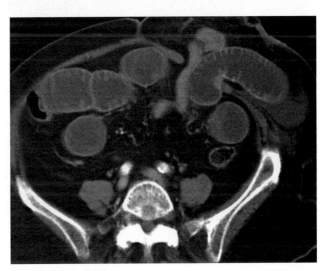

Figure 3.59   D

Findings: Axial CECT images demonstrate the presence of pneumobilia, a large stone in the gallbladder, small bowel dilatation, a right-sided abdominal wall hernia, and a second stone trapped in the bowel in the hernia sac. Note decompressed small bowel distal to the stone.

Differential Diagnosis: None.

Diagnosis: Gallstone ileus.

Discussion: Gallstone ileus is a mechanical obstruction caused by impaction of gallstone(s) in any part of the GI tract. Gallstone ileus is responsible for up to 2% of cases of small bowel obstruction. It is more prevalent in elderly patients, and the majority of cases occur in females. Mortality rates have been reported as high as 27% often due to coexisting medical conditions in this age group. The gallstone enters the GI tract through a fistula between a gangrenous gallbladder and duodenum or other parts of the GI tract. Occasionally, a stone may come into the intestine through a fistulous communication between the bile duct and the GI tract. Intestinal obstruction is usually caused when the gallstones are greater than 2.5 cm in diameter. The most common site of impaction of gallstones is in the distal ileum, followed by the jejunum and stomach. Presenting features may be nonspecific, but radiologic findings comprising Rigler's classic triad of small bowel obstruction, pneumobilia, and ectopic gallstones may occasionally be detected by plain radiograph, ultrasound, or CT. In addition, CT may demonstrate a fistulous communication between the gallbladder and duodenum, as seen in this case.

Clinical History: 62-year-old woman with a history of aortic surgery presenting with hematemesis.

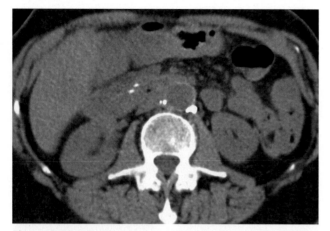

Figure 3.60   A

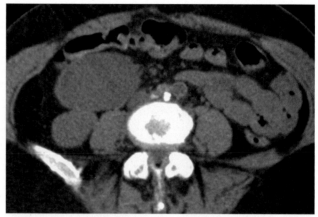

Figure 3.60   B

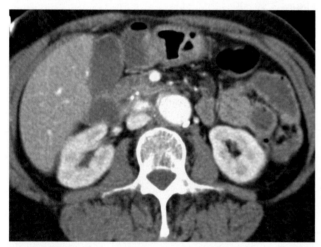

Figure 3.60   C

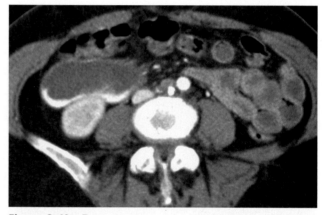

Figure 3.60   D

Findings: Axial NECT images (A and B) show a status post aortic aneurysm repair, a dilated third portion of the duodenum, and soft tissue density stranding between the duodenum and aorta. Following intravenous administration of iodinated contrast, axial CECT images (C and D) show extravasation of contrast into the duodenum.

Differential Diagnosis: None.

Diagnosis: Aortoduodenal fistula.

Discussion: The aorta lies in proximity with the GI tract for much of its thoracic and abdominal course. Aortoenteric fistulas, therefore, can potentially involve the gut anywhere from the esophagus to the colon. The majority of cases occur in the presence of aortic aneurysm disease, either as a primary event or a secondary complication following surgical repair. The duodenum participates in the majority of aortoenteric fistulas, owing to the proximity between its third portion and the abdominal aorta. Primary aortoduodenal fistula is a rare life-threatening cause of GI bleeding that results most commonly from an atherosclerotic aortic aneurysm. Unusual causes of a primary fistula include aortitis, radiation therapy, malignancy, and peptic ulcer disease. Most patients have GI bleeding, but the classic triad of abdominal pain, GI bleeding, and pulsatile mass is present in fewer than 25% of cases. A "herald bleed" frequently precedes lethal exsanguination, and patient survival hinges on prompt diagnosis and emergent therapeutic laparotomy. Unfortunately, a correct preoperative diagnosis is determined in only a minority of cases, underscoring the importance of heightened clinical suspicion. CT provides rapid and effective evaluation in hemodynamically stable patients suspected of having an aortoenteric fistula. CT findings, such as perianeurysmal hematoma, pseudoaneurysm, contrast agent extravasation, periaortic or intraluminal gas, and focal duodenal wall thickening, are highly suggestive of a fistula in the appropriate clinical setting.

SUGGESTED READINGS

NEOPLASM

- Balthazar EJ, Megibow AJ, Hulnick D, et al. Carcinoma of the colon: detection and preoperative staging by CT. *Am J Roentgenol.* 1988;150: 301–306.
- Bleday R, Telford JJ, Mortele KJ. Evaluation and staging of rectal cancer. *Sem Colon Rectal Surg.* 2002;13:139–143.
- Buck JL, Sobin LH. Carcinoids of the gastrointestinal tract. *Radiographics* 1990;10:1081–1095.
- de Lange EE, Fechner RE, Edge SB, et al. Preoperative staging of rectal carcinoma with MR imaging: surgical and histopathologic correlation. *Radiology* 1990;176:623–628.
- Fiscback W, Kestel W, Kirchner T, et al. Malignant lymphomas of the upper gastrointestinal tract. *Cancer* 1992;70:1075–1080.
- Freeny PC, Marks, WM, Ryan JA, et al. Colorectal carcinoma evaluation with CT: preoperative staging and detection of postoperative recurrence. *Radiology* 1986;158:347–353.
- Gould M, Johnson RJ. Computed tomography of abdominal carcinoid tumor. *Br J Radiol.* 1986;59:881–885.
- Hong X, Choi H, Loyer EM, et al. Gastrointestinal stromal tumor: role of CT in diagnosis and in response evaluation and surveillance after treatment with imatinib. *Radiographics* 2006;26:481–495.
- Megibow AJ, Balthazar EJ, Naidich DP, et al. Computed tomography of gastrointestinal lymphoma. *Am J Roentgenol.* 1983;141:541–547.
- Picus D, Glazer HS, Levitt RG, et al. Computed tomography of abdominal carcinoid tumors. *Am J Roentgenol.* 1984;143:581–584.
- Tatli S, Mortele KJ, Breen EL, et al. Local staging of rectal cancer using pelvic phased-array and endorectal coil. *J Magn Reson Imaging.* 2006;23:535–540.
- Weingrad DN, Decosse JJ, Sherlock P, et al. Primary gastrointestinal lymphoma: a 30-year review. *Cancer* 1982;49:1258–1265.
- Williams SM, Berk RN, Harned RK. Radiologic features of multinodular lymphoma of the colon. *Am J Roentgenol.* 1984;143:87–91.

INFLAMMATION

- Balthazar EJ, Megibow AJ, Hulnick D, et al. CT of appendicitis. *Am J Roentgenol.* 1986;147:705–710.
- Balthazar EJ, Megibow AJ, Schinella RA, et al. Limitations in the CT diagnosis of acute diverticulitis: comparison of CT, contrast enema, and pathologic findings of 16 patients. *Am J Roentgenol.* 1990;154:281–285.
- Balthazar EJ, Yen BC, Gordon RB. Ischemic colitis: CT evaluation of 54 cases. *Radiology* 1999;211:381–388.
- Bartlett JG. *Clostridium difficile*: clinical considerations. *Rev Infect Dis.* 1990;12:S243–S251.
- Bartram CI. Radiology in the current assessment of ulcerative colitis. *Gastrointest Radiol.* 1997;1:383–392.
- Berkmen YM, Rabinowitz J. Gastrointestinal manifestations of the strongyloidiasis. *Am J Roentgenol Radium Ther Nucl Med.* 1972;115: 306–311.
- Cardoso JM, Kimura K, Stoopen M, et al. Radiology of invasive amebiasis of the colon. *Am J Roentgenol.* 1977;128:935–941.
- Del Frate C, Mortele KJ, Tuncali K, et al. Myometrial abscess caused by diverticulitis. *J Women's Imaging.* 2003;5:187–191.
- Fishman EK, Kavuru BS, Jones B, et al. Pseudomembranous colitis: CT evaluation of 26 cases. *Radiology* 1991;180:57–60.
- Fultz PJ, Skucas J, Weiss SL. CT in upper gastrointestinal tract perforations secondary to peptic ulcer disease. *Gastrointest Radiol.* 1992; 17:5–8.
- Gore RM, Marn CS, Kirby DF, et al. CT findings in ulcerative, granulomatous, and indeterminate colitis. *Am J Roentgenol.* 1984;143:279–284.
- Horton KM, Corl FM, Fishman EK. CT evaluation of the colon: Inflammatory disease. *Radiographics* 2000;20:399–418.
- Hulnick DH, Megibow AJ, Balthazar EJ, et al. Computed tomography in the evaluation of diverticulitis. *Radiology* 1984;152:491–495.
- Jang HJ, Lim HK, Park CK, et al. Segmental wall thickening in the colonic loop distal to colonic carcinoma at CT: importance and histopathological correlation. *Radiology* 2000;216:712–717.
- Liberman JM, Haaga JR. Computed tomography of diverticulitis. *J Comput Assist Tomogr.* 1983;7:431–433.
- Louisy CL, Barton CJ. The radiological diagnosis of *Strongyloides stercoralis* enteritis. *Radiology* 1971;98:535–541.
- Merine D, Fishman EK, Jones B. Pseudomembranous colitis: CT evaluation. *J Comput Assist Tomogr.* 1987;6:1017–1020.
- Philpotts LE, Heiken JP, Westcott MA, et al. Colitis: use of CT findings in differential diagnosis. *Radiology* 1994;190:445–449.
- Ros PR, Buetow PC, Pantograg-Brown L. Pseudomembranous colitis. *Radiology* 1996;198:1–9.
- Segatto E, Mortele KJ, Hoon J, et al. Acute small bowel ischemia: CT imaging findings. *Semin Ultrasound, CT, MRI.* 2003;24:364–376.
- Trinh T, Jones B, Fishman EK. Amyloidosis of the colon presenting as ischemic colitis: a case report and review of the literature. *Gastrointest Radiol.* 1991;16:133–136.
- Wiesner W, Mortele KJ, Glickman JN, et al. Cecal gangrene: a rare cause of right-sided inferior abdominal quadrant pain, fever, and leukocytosis. *Emergency Radiol.* 2002;9:292–295.
- Wiesner W, Mortele KJ, Barthi K, et al. CT findings in isolated ischemic proctosigmoiditis. *Eur Radiol.* 2002;12:1762–1767.
- Wiesner W, Mortele KJ, Glickman JN, et al. Normal colonic wall thickness and its relation to colonic distension: how thick may a normal colonic wall appear at CT? *J Comput Assist Tomogr.* 2002;26:102–106.
- Wiesner W, Mortele KJ, Glickman JN, et al. Pneumatosis intestinalis and portomesenteric venous gas in intestinal ischemia: correlation of CT findings with severity of ischemia and clinical outcome. *Am J Roentgenol.* 2001;177:1319–1323.
- Wiesner W, Mortele KJ, Glickman JN, et al. Portal venous gas unrelated to bowel ischemia. *Eur Radiol.* 2002;12:1432–1437.
- Wold PB, Fletcher JG, Johnson CD, et al. Assessment of small bowel Crohn disease: noninvasive perioral CT enterography compared with other imaging methods and endoscopy—feasibility study. *Radiology* 2003;229:275–281.
- Wolfe MM, Jenson RT. Zollinger-Ellison syndrome. *N Engl J Med.* 1987;317:1200–1209.

MISCELLANEOUS

- Ballantyne GH, Brandner MD, Beart RW, et al. Volvulus of the colon. *Ann Surg.* 1985;202:83–92.
- Boudiaf M, Soyer P, Terem C, et al. CT evaluation of small bowel obstruction. *Radiographics* 2001;21:613–624.
- Bova JC, Friedman AC, Weser E, et al. Adaptation of the ileum in nontropical sprue: reversal of the jejunoileal fold pattern. *Am J Roentgenol.* 1985;144:299–302.
- Cantisani V, Mortele KJ, Viscomi SG, et al. Rectal inflammation as first manifestation of graft-versus-host disease: radiologic-pathologic findings. *Eur Radiol.* 2003;13:75–78.
- Cundiff GW, Fenner D. Evalaution and treatment of women with rectocele: focus on associated defecatory and sexual dysfunction. *Obstet Gynecol.* 2004;104:1403–1421.
- De Backer AI, Van Overbeke LN, Mortele KJ, et al. Inflammatory pseudopolyposis in a patient with toxic megacolon due to pseudomembranous colitis. *JBR-BTR.* 2001;84:201.
- Doubleday LC, Bernardino ME. CT findings in the perirectal area following radiation therapy. *J Comp Assist Tomogr.* 1980;4:634–638.
- Fishman EK, Zinreich ES, Jones B, et al. Computed tomographic diagnosis of radiation ileitis. *Gastrointest Radiol.* 1984;9:149–152.
- Fisk JD, Shulman HM, Greening RR, et al. Gastrointestinal radiographic features of human graft-vs-host disease. *Am J Roentgenol.* 1981;136: 329–336.

- Gardner EJ, Burt RW, Freston JW. Gastrointestinal polyposis: syndromes and genetic mechanisms. *West J Med.* 1980;132:488–499.
- Gayer G, Barsuk D, Hertz M, et al. CT diagnosis of afferent loop syndrome. *Clin Radiol.* 2002;57:835–839.
- Hill LD. Incarcerated paraesophageal hernia. *Am J Surg.* 1973;126: 286–291.
- Hillyard RW, El-Mandi M, Schellhammer PF. Intestinal strictures complicating preoperative radiation therapy followed by radical cystectomy. *J Urol.* 1986;136:98–101.
- Horton KM, Fishman EK. Current role of CT in imaging the stomach. *Radiographics* 2003;23:75–87.
- Iko BO, Teal JS, Siram SM, et al. Computed tomography of adult colonic intussusception: clinical and experimental studies. *Am J Roentgenol.* 1984;143:769–772.
- Jones B, Kramer SS, Saral R, et al. Gastrointestinal inflammation after bone marrow transplantation: graft-versus-host disease or opportunistic infection? *Am J Roentgenol.* 1988;150:277–281.
- Kalantari BN, Mortele KJ, Cantisani V, et al. CT features with pathologic correlation of acute gastrointestinal graft-versus-host disease after bone marrow transplantation in adults. *Am J Roentgenol.* 2003;181:1621–1625.
- Long FR, Kramer SS, Markowitz RI. Intestinal malrotation in children: tutorial on radiographic diagnosis in difficult cases. *Radiology* 1996; 198:775–780.
- Loren I, Lasson A, Anders A, et al. Gallstone ileus demonstrated by CT. *J Comp Assist Tomogr.* 1994;18:262–265.
- Martin LC, Merkle EM, Thompson WM. Review of internal hernias: radiographic and clinical findings *Am J Roentgenol.* 2006;186:703–717.
- Mori H, Hayashi K, Futagawa S. Vascular compromise in chronic volvulus with midgut malrotation. *Pediatr Radiol.* 1987;17:277–281.
- Mortele KJ, Govaere F, Vogelaerts D, et al. Giant Meckel diverticulum containing enteroliths: CT imaging findings. *Eur Radiol.* 2002;2:82–84.
- Odulate AS, Mortele KJ. The eligable patient: indications and contraindications. In: Lefere P, Gryspeerdt S, eds. *Virtual colonoscopy.* Berlin: Springer-Verlag; 2006:13–22.
- Olmsted WW, Cooper PH, Madewell JE. Involvement of the gastric antrum in Menetrier's disease. *Am J Roentgenol.* 1976;126:524–529.
- Patak MA, Mortele KJ, Ros PR. Multidetector row CT of the small bowel. *Radiol Clin North Am.* 2005;43:1063–1077.
- Pickhardt PJ, Bhalia S, Balfe DM. Acquired gastrointestinal fistulas: classification, etiologies, and imaging evaluation. *Radiology* 2002;224: 9–23.
- Reese DF, Hodgson JR, Dockerty MB. Giant hypertrophy of the gastric mucosa (Menetrier's disease): a correlation of the roentgenographic pathologic, and clinical findings. *Am J Roentgenol.* 1962;88: 619–626.
- Rociu E, Stoker J, Zwamborn AW, et al. Endoanal MR imaging of the anal sphincter in fecal incontinence. *Radiographics* 1999;19:171–177.
- Rosen A, Korobkin M, Silverman PM, et al. Mesenteric vein thrombosis: CT identification. *Am J Roentgenol.* 1984;143:83–86.
- Rosenberg HK, Seola FT, Koch P, et al. Radiographic features of gastrointestinal graft-vs-host disease. *Radiology* 1981;138:371–374.
- Searcy RM, Malagelada JR. Menetrier's disease and idiopathic hypertrophic gastropathy. *Ann Intern Med.* 1984;100:555–570.
- Siskind BN, Burrell MI, Pun H, et al. CT demonstration of gastrointestinal involvement in Henoch-Schonlein syndrome. *Abdom Imaging.* 1985;10:352–354.
- Skaane P, Schindler G. Computed tomography of adult ileocolic intussusception. *Gastrointest Radiol.* 1985;10:355–357.
- Styles RA, Larsen CR. CT appearance of adult intussusception. *J Comp Assist Tomogr.* 1983;7:331–333.
- Swift SE, Spencer JA. Gallstone ileus: CT findings. *Clin Radiol.* 1998; 53:451–456.
- Trier JS. Celiac sprue. *N Engl J Med.* 1991;325:1709–1719.
- Vandaele P, Oliva MR, Barish MA, et al. CT colonography: the essentials. *Appl Radiol.* 2006;35:8–17.
- Zerin JM, DiPietro MA. Mesenteric vascular anatomy at CT: normal and abnormal appearances. *Radiology* 1991;179:739–742.

CHAPTER FOUR
SPLEEN

Koenraad J. Mortele,
Vincent Pelsser,
and Pablo R. Ros

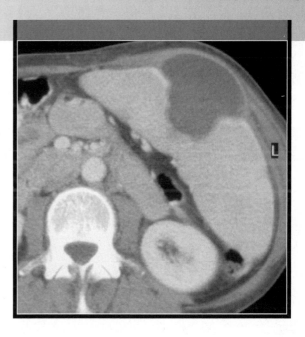

Clinical History: 47-year-old woman who noticed a lump in her right breast, staged with CT scan.

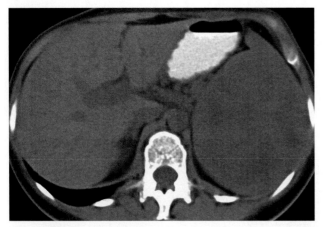

Figure 4.1   A

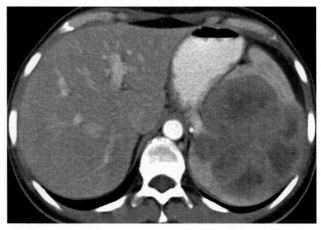

Figure 4.1   B

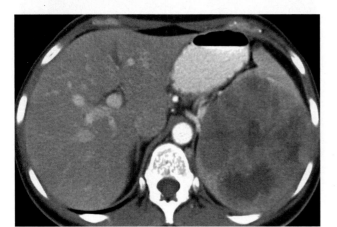

Figure 4.1   C

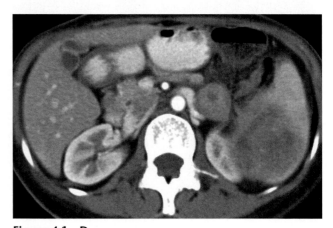

Figure 4.1   D

Findings: Axial nonenhanced CT (NECT) (A) and contrast-enhanced CT (CECT) (B–D) images demonstrate a heterogeneously enhancing splenic mass that measures 14.8 × 11.2 cm. No lesions are seen in the liver.

Differential Diagnosis: Abscess, lymphoma.

Diagnosis: Breast metastasis.

Discussion: Metastatic disease to the spleen is uncommon and typically occurs in patients with widespread metastatic disease (i.e., metastasis to three or more organs). Most metastases spread hematogenously via the splenic artery. Less common pathways include the splenic vein in patients with portal hypertension, lymphatics, and intraperitoneal seeding, such as in ovarian cancer. The most common primaries to metastasize to the spleen include melanoma (50%), breast (21%), lung (18%), ovary, prostate, colon, and stomach. One third of splenic metastases are microscopic aggregates and are not visible on imaging. Enhancement is seen in the periphery of these lesions with central areas of necrosis. This excludes predominantly other splenic cystic lesions, such as hydatid cysts and pancreatic pseudocysts. The large size makes a hemangioma less likely. This case is unusual because liver metastases are typically present when splenic metastases of this size occur. Both abscess and lymphoma can present with large, hypodense lesions in the spleen without hepatic involvement. They would be excellent diagnostic considerations.

Clinical History: 37-year-old woman found to have an enlarged spleen on physical examination.

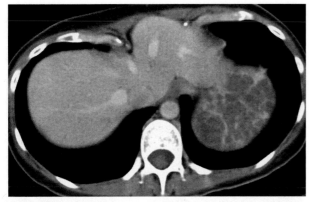

Figure 4.2 A

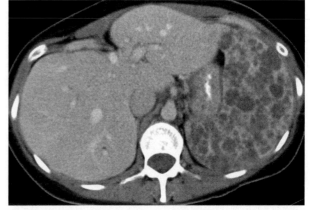

Figure 4.2 B

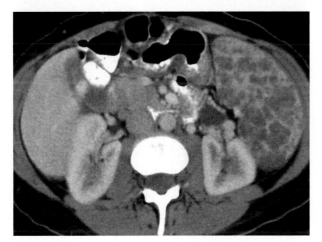

Figure 4.2 C

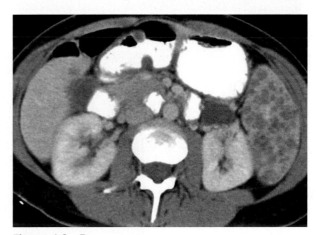

Figure 4.2 D

Findings: Axial CECT images show that the spleen is markedly enlarged, measuring 11.8 cm anteroposteriorly and 18 cm craniocaudally. The spleen is heterogeneous with presence of multiple, small (5 mm to 1 cm), hypodense lesions involving the entire spleen.

Differential Diagnosis: Lymphangioma, lymphoma, microabscesses, metastases.

Diagnosis: Splenic hemangiomatosis.

Discussion: Splenic hemangiomas may be single or multiple (as part of a generalized angiomatosis, such as Klippel-Trenaunay-Weber syndrome), sometimes replacing the entire spleen (hemangiomatosis), and may range from a few millimeters to many centimeters in size. Individual hemangiomas are characterized by an unencapsulated proliferation of vascular channels of variable size that are lined with a single layer of endothelium and filled with red blood cells. These vascular channels vary in size from capillary to cavernous. Most lesions are under 2 cm in diameter; when larger, they may rupture, causing hemorrhage in about 25% of cases. CT shows low-attenuation lesions resembling cysts with delayed enhancement of the solid portions following iodinated contrast administration.

Clinical History: 55-year-old woman presenting with fatigue and anemia.

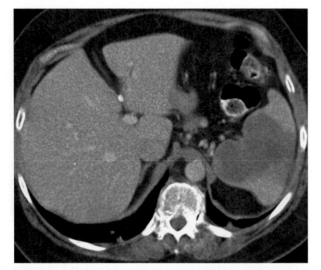

Figure 4.3   A

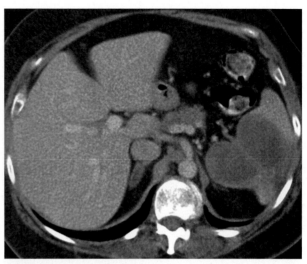

Figure 4.3   B

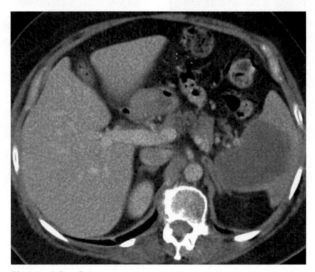

Figure 4.3   C

Findings: Axial CECT images demonstrate a 6.0 × 3.0 × 9.1 cm, low-attenuation, solid lesion in the spleen.

Differential Diagnosis: Abscess, infarct, metastasis, hemangioma, lymphangioma.

Diagnosis: Splenic lymphoma.

Discussion: Lymphoma constitutes the most common primary malignant splenic neoplasm. Laparotomy with splenectomy reveals clinically unsuspected splenic involvement in 23% to 34% of patients with Hodgkin lymphoma and 30% to 40% of patients with non-Hodgkin lymphoma. A single large mass in the spleen from lymphoma is unusual and is more commonly seen in high-grade lymphoma in its advanced stages. Splenic lymphoma can become large and extend through the splenic capsule and involve adjacent organs, such as the stomach or pancreas. Lymphoma enhances poorly on CECT, but cystic necrosis is rare. The large mass seen in this example may be difficult to distinguish from an abscess or infarct. The accuracy of detecting splenic lymphoma with CT ranges from 50% to 65%. The presence of splenomegaly is nonspecific, and one third of patients with lymphoma and splenomegaly do not have splenic lymphoma. Diffuse lymphomatous involvement of the spleen (<5 mm) is also difficult to detect by CT. The presence of abdominal lymphadenopathy with splenomegaly or focal splenic lesions is highly suggestive of splenic lymphoma and may obviate the need for biopsy or splenectomy.

Clinical History: 19-year-old woman involved in a motor vehicle accident.

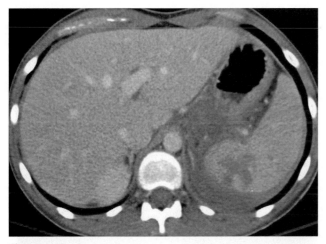

Figure 4.4 A

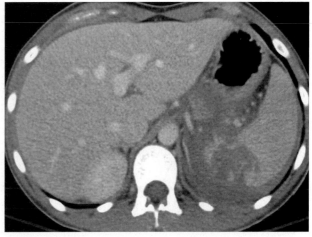

Figure 4.4 B

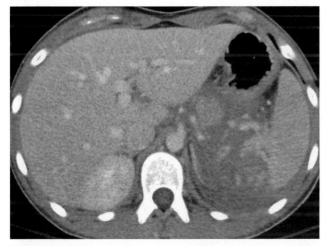

Figure 4.4 C

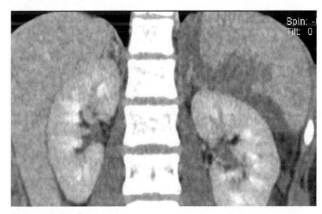

Figure 4.4 D

Findings: Axial (A–C) and coronal reformatted (D) CECT images demonstrate a stellate area of low attenuation in the medial aspect of the spleen with extension to the splenic hilum. Note perisplenic high-density fluid (blood).

Differential Diagnosis: None.

Diagnosis: Splenic fracture.

Discussion: The reported sensitivity of CT scans in the detection of splenic injury varies from 96% to nearly 100%. Injury to the spleen can be demonstrated with CT scan in several ways. There can be an intrasplenic or subcapsular hematoma that typically appears as focal areas of low attenuation on CECT. Areas of high attenuation representing acute to subacute hemorrhage, best appreciated on NECT, can also be present. A laceration can occur, and it will appear as a linear area of low attenuation that does not extend completely across the spleen. This is in contradiction to a fracture that will extend across the spleen, commonly to the splenic hilum. A "shattered" spleen involves multiple areas of fracture and hematoma, which results in a "fragmented" spleen. This case demonstrates a fracture of the spleen that extends completely across the spleen to involve the splenic hilum. In addition, larger focal areas of low attenuation are present, representing intrasplenic hematomas. Luckily for this patient, the hilar vessels were not injured and the hematocrit remained stable, thus requiring only conservative management.

Clinical History: 32-year-old man with a longstanding history of anemia.

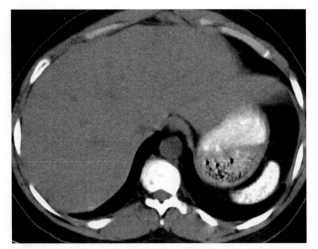

Figure 4.5   A

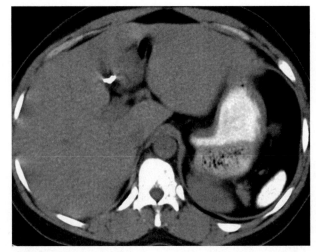

Figure 4.5   B

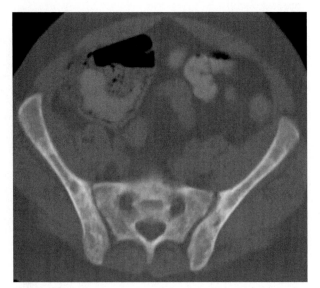

Figure 4.5   C

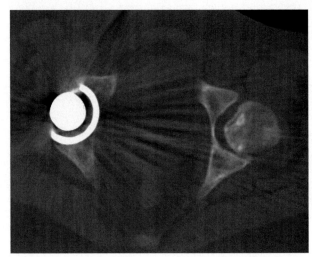

Figure 4.5   D

Findings: Axial NECT images (A and B) of the upper abdomen demonstrate a densely calcified small spleen. Axial NECT images (C and D) of the pelvis (displayed in bone window) show diffuse patchy increased bone density and right hip prosthesis.

Differential Diagnosis: Hemosiderosis, Thorotrast accumulation.

Diagnosis: Autosplenectomy from sickle cell disease.

Discussion: Sickle cell disease is a common hereditary disorder caused by a hemoglobinopathy. Autosplenectomy or end-stage spleen is typically seen in patients who have homozygous sickle cell disease. During the first year of life, microinfarctions of the spleen occur secondary to the veno-occlusive disease. This leads to perivascular fibrosis with subsequent decrease in

function and size of the spleen. In addition, there is hemosiderin and calcium deposition. Occasionally, the splenic calcifications can be seen on plain film, but they are much better detected on CT. The typical CT finding in sickle cell's autosplenectomy is a small calcified nonfunctioning spleen. Other causes for a dense spleen include hemosiderosis and Thorotrast administration. In these processes, however, the liver is also frequently involved and will demonstrate increased attenuation on a NECT. Also, the small size of the spleen due to the microinfarcts and fibrosis is more commonly seen in sickle cell disease rather than hemosiderosis. The spleen in Thorotrast administration is also small, but Thorotrast accumulation is also seen in the liver and abdominal lymph nodes. The age of the patient would also make it unlikely because Thorotrast use was discontinued in the 1950s.

Clinical History: 62-year-old man with a history of renal cell carcinoma.

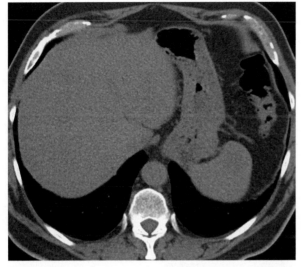

Figure 4.6 A

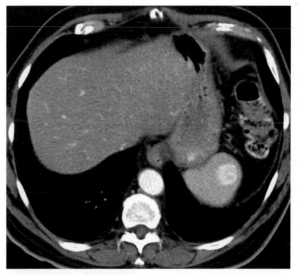

Figure 4.6 B

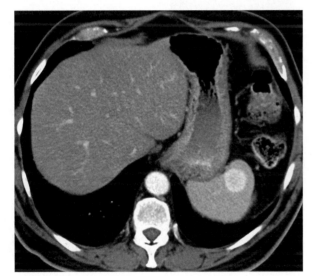

Figure 4.6 C

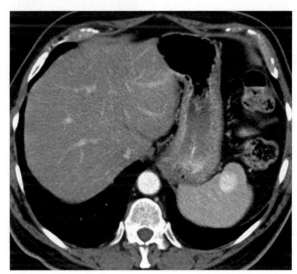

Figure 4.6 D

Findings: Axial NECT image (A) shows a normal-sized spleen without focal lesions. Axial CECT images (B–D) demonstrate a 2.0-cm hypervascular lesion in the lateral portion of the spleen.

Differential Diagnosis: Angiosarcoma, metastasis.

Diagnosis: Splenic hemangioma.

Discussion: Hemangioma is the most common benign primary tumor of the spleen. They can appear solid or cystic (30%) with central or peripheral calcifications. Coarse thick calcifications can occur in the solid portions. These calcifications appear in areas of fibrosis corresponding to previously thrombosed zones. Typically, hemangiomas are asymptomatic but can rupture in up to 20% of cases when they become large. A hyperdense lesion in the spleen on a CECT is typical of a hemangioma. Most other lesions in the spleen are hypodense with variable contrast enhancement. Angiosarcomas can be hyperdense by CECT but are extremely rare and are secondary to Thorotrast (thorium dioxide) administration. No other evidence of Thorotrast use is present, such as a hyperdense liver and spleen. Excluding lymphoma, metastases to the spleen are uncommon, occurring in approximately 7% of patients with widespread malignancy. The most common metastases to the spleen are from melanoma followed by breast, lung, ovary, and gastrointestinal (GI) tract malignancies. The majority of metastases from these primaries are multiple, but they can be solitary or diffusely infiltrating as well.

Clinical History: 29-year-old man who underwent CT scanning after an assault.

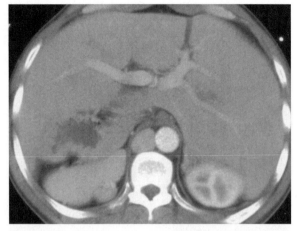

Figure 4.7 A

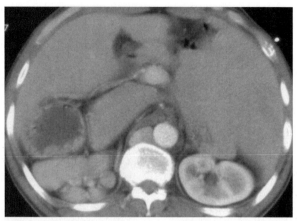

Figure 4.7 B

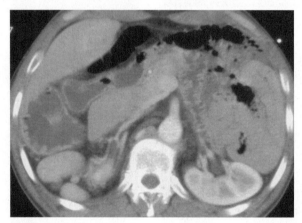

Figure 4.7 C

Findings: Axial CECT images demonstrate a large midline liver and multiple soft tissue masses in the right upper quadrant. Azygos continuation of the inferior vena cava is present.

Differential Diagnosis: None.

Diagnosis: Polysplenia.

Discussion: Polysplenia syndrome is a congenital abnormality involving multiple organ systems characterized by bilateral left sidedness. It occurs predominantly in males. These patients have bilateral morphologic left lungs (66%), multiple spleens (2–16 nodules), azygos or hemiazygos continuation of the inferior vena cava (50–85%), truncated pancreas, and abdominal situs ambiguous. Other congenital abnormalities include cardiac anomalies (dextrocardia, ventricular septal defects, and transposition of the great vessels) and gastrointestinal anomalies (esophageal atresia and biliary atresia). The key findings in this case to make the diagnosis of polysplenia are the presence of a midline liver and azygos continuation of the inferior vena cava. With these findings and the multiple soft tissue masses in the right upper quadrant, the diagnosis of polysplenia is made. A nuclear medicine scan could be performed to confirm that the upper quadrant masses are multiple spleens.

Case images courtesy of Dr. Angela D. Levy, Armed Forces Institute of Pathology, Washington, DC.

Clinical History: 45-year-old woman presenting with right upper quadrant pain.

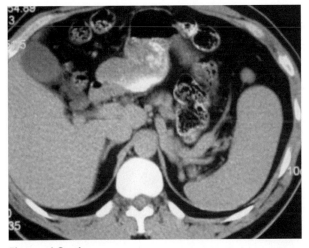

Figure 4.8 A

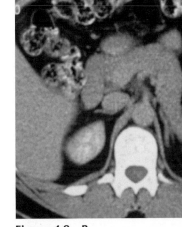

Figure 4.8 B

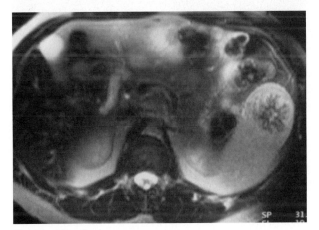

Figure 4.8 C

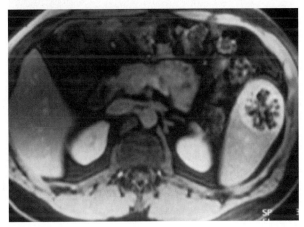

Figure 4.8 D

Findings: Axial NECT (A) and delayed-phase CECT (B) images demonstrate contour deformity of the anterior aspect of the spleen and minimal delayed enhancement of a mass in the anterior aspect of the spleen. Note nonenhancing central scar. Axial T2-weighted image (WI) (C) and portal venous phase, gadolinium-enhanced, fat-suppressed axial T1-WI (D) image show heterogeneous hyperintense appearance of the mass (with central scar) and marked peripheral enhancement, respectively.

Differential Diagnosis: Hemangioma, angiosarcoma.

Diagnosis: Splenic hamartoma.

Discussion: Splenic hamartoma, also known as nodular hyperplasia of the spleen, is a rare, benign tumor composed of anomalous mixtures of normal elements of splenic tissue, with red pulp predominance. Hamartomas are usually solitary. They are usually discovered incidentally or because of mass-related symptomatology. On NECT, hamartomas are usually isodense, causing only an abnormality of the contour of the spleen. Because of the red pulp predominance, they show marked and prolonged heterogeneous enhancement after contrast administration. MRI shows a well-defined mass that is isointense on T1-WI and moderately hyperintense on T2-WI. If the presence of fibrous tissue is substantial, hamartomas may have central areas of low signal intensity on T2-WI. After gadolinium administration, hamartomas show intense, diffuse, heterogeneous enhancement. This enhancement pattern allows distinction from splenic hemangiomas.

Clinical History: 32-year-old man with a history of Hodgkin disease presenting with generalized malaise and fever.

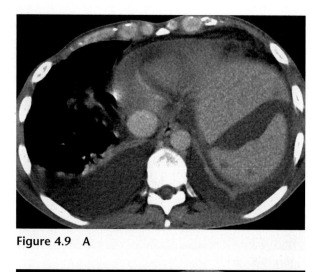

Figure 4.9   A

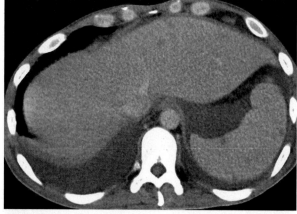

Figure 4.9   B

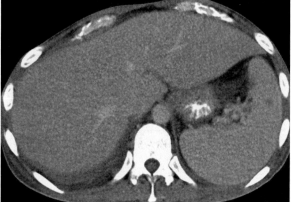

Figure 4.9   C

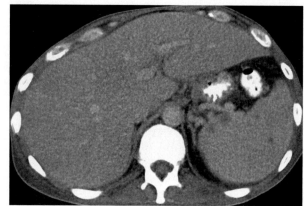

Figure 4.9   D

Findings: Axial CECT images demonstrate multiple small low-attenuation lesions in the spleen and liver. Note presence of ascites and bilateral pleural effusions.

Differential Diagnosis: Metastases, leukemia, lymphoma.

Diagnosis: Splenic candidiasis.

Discussion: Splenic fungal infections occur in patients who are immunocompromised from chemotherapy, leukemia, lymphoproliferative disorders, and human immunodeficiency virus (HIV). The most common fungal organism is *Candida* followed by *Aspergillus* and *Cryptococcus*. Splenomegaly is common, and the liver and kidneys are often involved. Persistent fever, malaise, and weight loss are some of the clinical findings. Infection of the spleen is thought to be due to colonization of the gastrointestinal tract with widespread dissemination once the patient becomes neutropenic. Diagnosis is often difficult because blood cultures are negative in up to 50% of cases, and the symptoms are nonspecific. The CT appearance of fungal microabscesses is nonspecific, with metastases and lymphoma having similar imaging findings. The most common CT pattern consists of multiple, scattered, rounded areas of decreased attenuation. The second type is the bull's-eye pattern and is only demonstrated occasionally. Numerous areas of punctate hyperdensity are seen later in the course of the disease and are compatible on pathology with areas of calcification. CT is helpful in guiding biopsies and assessing response to treatment.

CASE 4-10

Clinical History: 41-year-old woman with weight loss and night sweats.

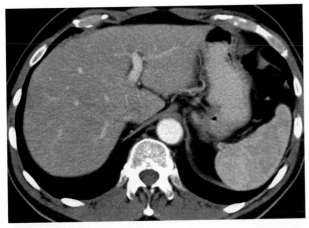

Figure 4.10 A

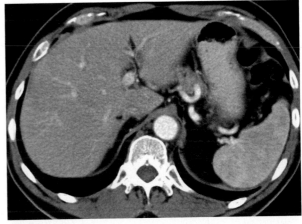

Figure 4.10 B

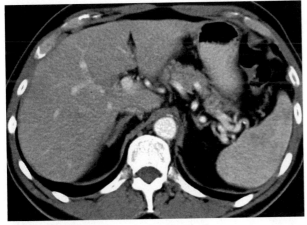

Figure 4.10 C

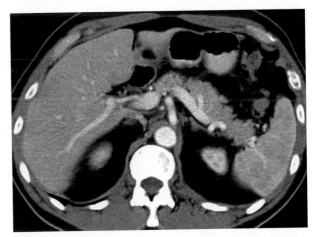

Figure 4.10 D

Findings: Axial CECT images of the upper abdomen demonstrate a mildly enlarged spleen that is heterogeneously enhancing.

Differential Diagnosis: Artifact (red and white pulp mixing).

Diagnosis: Diffuse splenic lymphoma.

Discussion: Lymphomatous involvement of the spleen associated with nodal disease and systemic involvement is much more common than primary splenic lymphoma without nodal disease. Involvement of the spleen can be seen in both Hodgkin and non-Hodgkin lymphoma and occurs more commonly in an older population (older than 50 years of age). Patients typically have nonspecific symptoms of fever, night sweats, and left upper quadrant pain. These symptoms can mimic an abscess. CECT is accurate in detecting splenic lymphoma in its late stages but is less accurate in early stages where the lesions are small or diffusely infiltrating the spleen. In these cases, splenectomy is often necessary to confirm the diagnosis. Splenic lymphoma can present by CT imaging as diffuse splenic enlargement, multiple small masses (<2 cm), and one or multiple large masses. The presence of multiple hypodense lesions in the spleen is nonspecific and can be seen in metastases and abscesses.

Clinical History: 75-year-old woman with a history of metastatic colon cancer and remote history of motor vehicle accident 20 years ago.

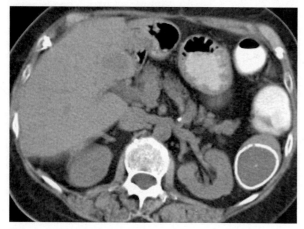

Figure 4.11   A

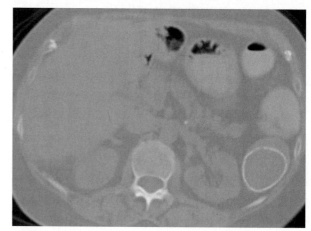

Figure 4.11   B

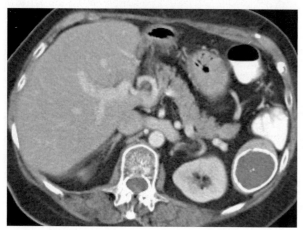

Figure 4.11   C

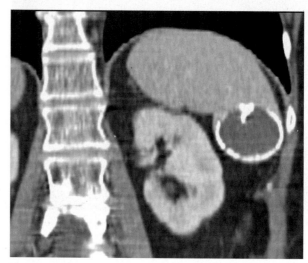

Figure 4.11   D

Findings: Axial NECT images in soft tissue (A) and bone window (B) show a rim-calcified cystic splenic lesion in the lower pole measuring 4.3 × 3.7 cm. Axial (C) and coronal (D) CECT images confirm lack of enhancement of the lesion and location within the spleen.

Differential Diagnosis: Epidermoid cyst, postinfectious cyst, hydatid cyst, infarct, pancreatic pseudocyst.

Diagnosis: Posttraumatic cyst.

Discussion: Cysts in the spleen can be divided into true cysts (primary or epidermoid) and false cysts (secondary or posttraumatic). Posttraumatic cysts account for 80% of all splenic cysts. True cysts possess an epithelial lining, are usually unilocular, and are detected most often in childhood and adolescents. Secondary cysts do not possess an epithelial lining but have a fibrous capsule. They are a result of prior infections, infarctions, or hematoma within the spleen. False cysts are usually smaller than true cysts and may contain internal debris. False cysts tend to be subcapsular in location and can calcify in the periphery in up to 50% of the cases. Other lesions that can present with eggshell calcifications include epidermoid cysts, hydatid cysts, and pancreatic pseudocysts. Clinical history is helpful in these situations to help narrow the differential diagnosis. The remote history of trauma and lack of clinical symptoms are suggestive of the diagnosis of posttraumatic (false) cyst.

Clinical History: 24-year-old man with Sturge-Weber syndrome presenting with left-sided abdominal pain.

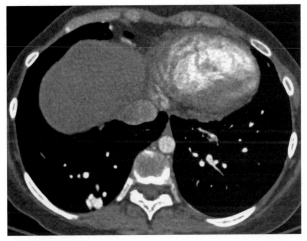

Figure 4.12   A

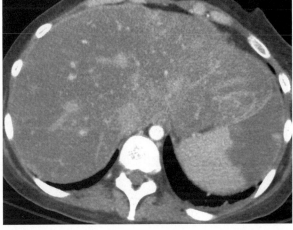

Figure 4.12   B

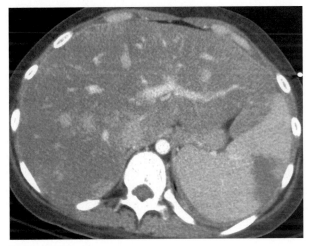

Figure 4.12   C

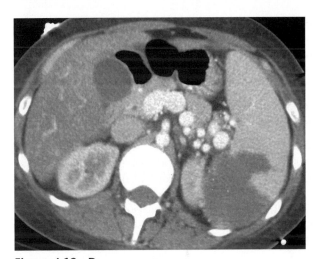

Figure 4.12   D

Findings: Axial CECT image (A) through the lower chest shows a right-sided arteriovenous fistula. Axial CECT images (B–D) through the upper abdomen demonstrate splenomegaly and multiple peripheral wedge-shaped, low-density defects in the spleen. Also note the diffuse fatty change of the liver.

Differential Diagnosis: Subcapsular hematoma, metastases.

Diagnosis: Splenic infarcts due to pulmonary arteriovenous fistula (Sturge-Weber syndrome).

Discussion: The classic appearance of splenic infarcts on CT is multiple peripheral wedge-shaped, low-attenuation defects in the spleen. This classical appearance, however, is present in less than half of all acute splenic infarcts. Other reported CT patterns include a multinodular appearance with ill-defined margins and a globally low-attenuation spleen. Thus, splenic infarcts frequently have an appearance indistinguishable from that of other lesions, including hematomas, neoplasms, and abscesses. A subcapsular hematoma typically causes compression of the splenic parenchyma in a crescentic manner with scalloping of the surface. Hematogenous metastases can present with multiple peripheral defects, but they typically involve the spleen diffusely. Serosal metastases such as from ovarian cancer, however, will typically scallop the surface of the spleen but will often demonstrate mass effect and bulge out beyond the expected contour of the spleen. Infarcts tend to preserve the splenic contour unless there is an associated subcapsular bleed. The finding of pulmonary arteriovenous fistula and splenic lesions is very suggestive of splenic infarcts.

Clinical History: 35-year-old asymptomatic woman noted to have splenomegaly by physical examination.

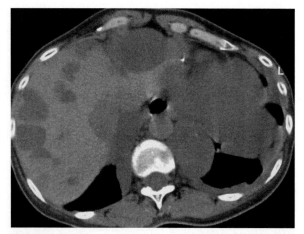

Figure 4.13 A

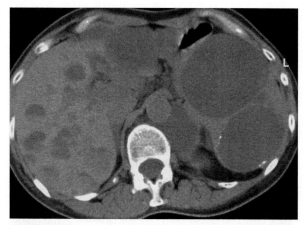

Figure 4.13 B

Findings: Axial NECT images demonstrate numerous low-density lesions in the spleen, liver, retrocrural area, and retroperitoneum. Note thin peripheral calcifications along the wall of some lesions and fluid-fluid level in some of the hepatic lesions.

Differential Diagnosis: Hemangiomatosis, metastases, abscesses, hydatid cysts.

Diagnosis: Lymphangiomatosis.

Discussion: Lymphangiomas are benign vascular lesions containing cystic spaces typically filled with proteinaceous and fatty material (lymph) rather than blood. These vascular spaces are lined by endothelium and can be single or multiple (lymphangiomatosis). Although most commonly encountered in the neck and axillary region, lymphangiomas, albeit rarely, also occur in the abdominal viscera. Most lymphangiomas occur at a young age but can present later in life secondary to pain from hemorrhage into the vascular spaces, as seen in some hepatic lesions in this case. The CT and MRI characteristics of these lesions are similar to those of other cystic lesions. They will be hypodense on CT, hypointense on the T1-WI, and hyperintense on the T2-WI. Because they contain proteinaceous/fatty material and can hemorrhage, these cystic spaces can have areas of high density on CT and high signal intensity on the T1-WI. Small, linear, peripheral calcifications may be present, as seen in this case. Lymphangiomas can be indistinguishable from metastases, abscesses, and hydatid cysts. Clinical history is often helpful in narrowing the differential diagnoses.

CASE 4-14

Clinical History: 51-year-old man from Argentina presents with fever.

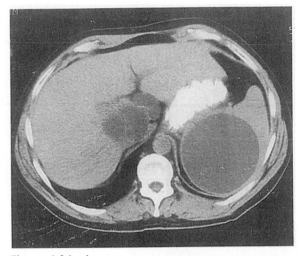

Figure 4.14   A

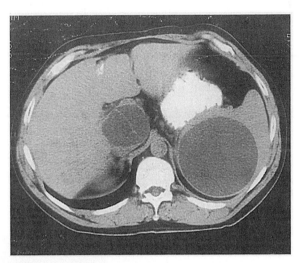

Figure 4.14   B

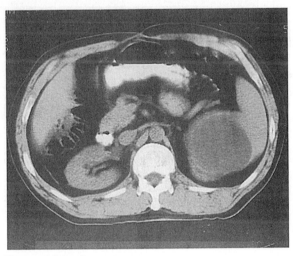

Figure 4.14   C

Findings: Axial NECT images demonstrate an 8.0-cm cyst in the posterior portion of the spleen. There is also a septated cystic lesion in the caudate lobe of the liver.

Differential Diagnosis: Epidermoid cyst, posttraumatic cyst, pancreatic pseudocyst, pyogenic abscess, infarct, neoplasm (hemangioma, lymphoma, lymphangioma, metastases).

Diagnosis: Splenic echinococcal (hydatid) cyst.

Discussion: Cystic splenic lesions can be congenital (epidermoid cyst), inflammatory (abscess, hydatid cyst), vascular (infarct, peliosis), posttraumatic (hematoma, false cyst), or neoplastic (hemangioma, lymphangioma, lymphoma, metastases). The finding of a second cystic lesion in the liver narrows the differential diagnosis considerably and can be seen in metastases, abscesses, and hydatid cysts.

Echinococcus granulosus is the organism that causes hydatid disease and typically involves the liver, lung, bone, and brain. Endemic areas for *Echinococcus granulosus* include Argentina, Greece, Spain, Middle East countries, and Australia. Often, the clinical findings are nonspecific including splenomegaly, fever, and abdominal pain. Available immunologic studies are specific for hydatid disease and can be used to confirm the diagnosis. CT findings of hydatid cysts include a well-defined wall of splenic parenchyma called the pericyst or ectocyst. This can contain peripheral eggshell calcifications. Low-attenuation internal septa can be seen representing the walls of the daughter cysts, which are budding from the inner germinal layer (endocyst). The high-attenuation contents of the cyst represent the hydatid sand, which is composed of scolices and debris.

Case images courtesy of Dr. Luis Ros, Zaragoza, Spain.

Clinical History: 44-year-old man presenting with right upper quadrant pain.

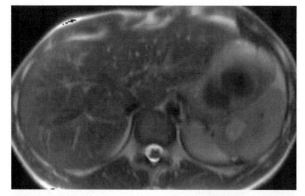

Figure 4.15 A

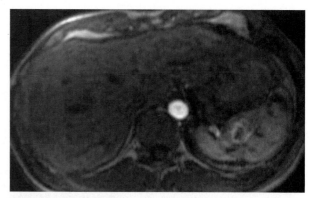

Figure 4.15 B

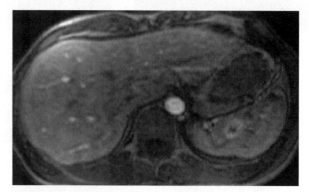

Figure 4.15 C

Findings: Axial T2-WI (A) demonstrates a 2.0-cm, well-defined hyperintense lesion in the spleen. Multiphasic gadolinium-enhanced, fat-suppressed axial T1-WI (B and C) show early peripheral rimlike enhancement of the lesion with progressive fill-in.

Differential Diagnosis: Lymphoma, metastasis, hamartoma, angiosarcoma.

Diagnosis: Splenic hemangioma.

Discussion: Hemangioma is the most common benign primary tumor of the spleen. It is most frequently seen in adults in their fourth through sixth decades of life. Hemangiomas are typically less than 2 cm in size and are frequently found incidentally on CT scans. Patients are usually asymptomatic unless the lesion is very large. Large hemangiomas can lead to anemia, thrombocytopenia, and coagulopathy. Hemangioma can be divided histologically into three types: capillary, cavernous, and mixed. Cavernous hemangiomas typically have a combination of both solid and cystic components. The solid components enhance with intravenous contrast, giving the lesion a heterogeneous appearance. Cavernous hemangiomas can have the centripetal enhancement as seen in hepatic hemangiomas. Capillary hemangiomas have early homogeneous enhancement. Most other primary lesions of the spleen, such as a hamartoma, angiosarcoma, and lymphoma will not have such a homogeneous bright signal on T2-WI. Metastases will typically be multiple. Both abscesses and infarcts will not have enhancement of the central areas, as is seen in this example.

Clinical History: 57-year-old woman presenting with progressive abdominal distension.

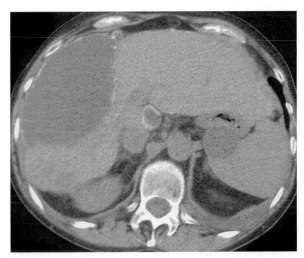

Figure 4.16   A

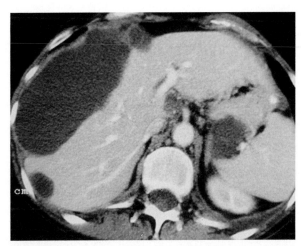

Figure 4.16   B

Findings: Axial NECT (A) and CECT (B) images demonstrate a cystic mass involving the anterior surface of the spleen. Similar lesions, some with peripheral calcifications, are seen along the liver surface.

Differential Diagnosis: Hydatid cyst, pancreatic pseudocyst, abscess, hematoma, infarct.

Diagnosis: Splenic ovarian metastasis.

Discussion: A cystic lesion within the spleen is a nonspecific finding. Note, however, that a large portion of the lesion extends outside the expected confines of the spleen and that similar lesions are present adjacent to the liver. This is the key to the diagnosis in this case. It is crucial to recognize that this lesion is not an intraparenchymal lesion but is a serosal metastasis compressing on the splenic parenchyma. Serosal implants are commonly seen in malignancies that spread by intraperitoneal seeding, such as ovarian and gastric carcinomas. The presence of soft tissue components in the cystic lesion would make a hydatid cyst and pancreatic pseudocyst unlikely. Hematomas and infarcts tend to be predominantly intraparenchymal. A large abscess would be another diagnostic consideration, but calcifications are uncommon in abscesses and correlation with clinical history would be important.

Clinical History: 44-year-old man post partial splenic embolization after motor vehicle accident.

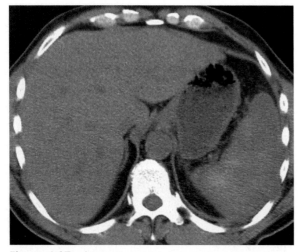

Figure 4.17 A

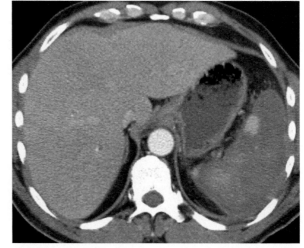

Figure 4.17 B

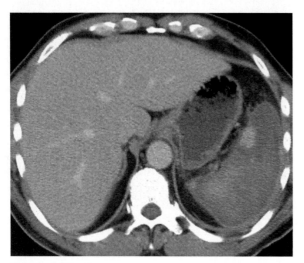

Figure 4.17 C

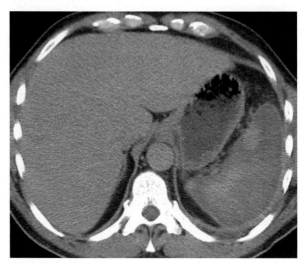

Figure 4.17 D

Findings: Axial NECT (A) and multiphasic CECT images (B–D) demonstrate spontaneous hyperdensity of the spleen and lack of enhancement, except a small island in the anterolateral aspect of the spleen. Also note capsular splenic enhancement.

Differential Diagnosis: Splenic laceration, fracture.

Diagnosis: Iatrogenic subtotal splenic infarction.

Discussion: There are multiple causes for splenic infarcts including emboli, hematologic diseases, and iatrogenic causes. In patients younger than 40 years, hemoglobinopathies are the most common cause of splenic infarction. Infarcts can have a variety of CT appearances ranging from the classic peripheral wedge-shaped defect to focal round lesions and ill-defined areas of low attenuation. These lesions are best demonstrated on a CECT. During the acute stage, infarcts are ill defined and heterogeneously hyperdense due to areas of hemorrhage within them. As an infarct begins to fibrose, it will appear better demarcated and may cause contraction of the surrounding normal spleen. When serial CT scans demonstrate progressive liquefaction and necrosis with outward extension, developing subcapsular hemorrhage, and free peritoneal hematoma, the possibility of impending rupture or superimposed infection should be considered.

Case images courtesy of Dr. Giovanni Artho, McGill University Health Center, Montreal, Canada.

CASE 4-18

Clinical History: 44-year-old woman with abdominal pain, nausea, and vomiting.

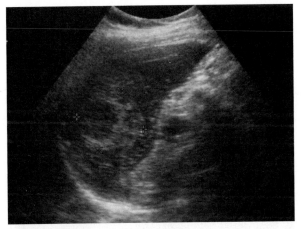

Figure 4.18   A

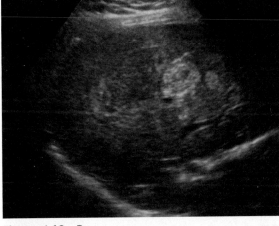

Figure 4.18   B

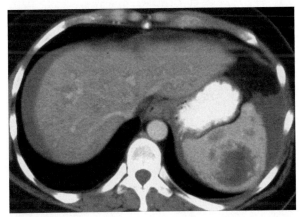

Figure 4.18   C

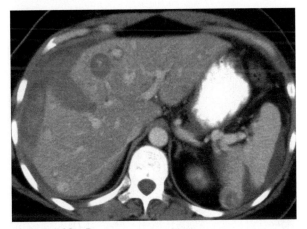

Figure 4.18   D

Findings: Sonographic images of the spleen (A) and liver (B) show ill-defined masses of heterogeneous mixed echogenicity in the liver and spleen. Axial CECT images (C and D) demonstrate a peripherally enhancing mass in the spleen with satellite nodules. Also note numerous enhancing liver lesions and hyperdense peritoneal fluid originating from the liver.

Differential Diagnosis: Metastases, hemangiomas.

Diagnosis: Splenic angiosarcoma with liver metastases and hemoperitoneum.

Discussion: Although splenic angiosarcoma is exceedingly rare, it is the most common nonlymphoid primary malignant tumor of the spleen. Angiosarcoma of the spleen may present either as well-defined hemorrhagic nodules or as diffuse splenic involvement. As in this case, angiosarcoma is frequently (30%) complicated by spontaneous rupture with hemorrhage. Prognosis is very poor (20% survival rate at 6 months), with early and widespread metastases, most commonly to the liver. CT typically demonstrates an enlarged spleen with hypodense areas having irregular and poorly defined contours. Hyperdensity on NECT scans may represent hemorrhage or hemosiderin deposition. Enhancement of splenic angiosarcoma may simulate that of hepatic hemangioma, although the filling pattern is variable. Angiosarcomas of the spleen are most common in patients previously exposed to Thorotrast, a colloidal suspension of thorium dioxide used as a contrast agent until the 1950s.

Case images courtesy of Dr. Angela D. Levy, Armed Forces Institute of Pathology, Washington, DC.

Clinical History: 42-year-old man with known hepatitis C cirrhosis.

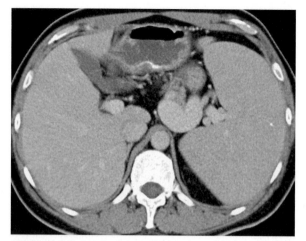

Figure 4.19   A

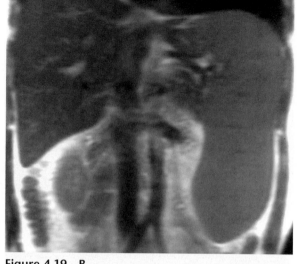

Figure 4.19   B

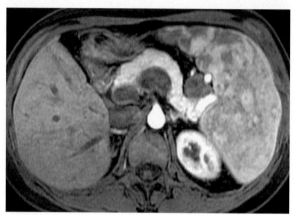

Figure 4.19   C

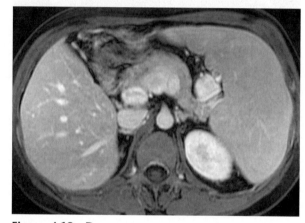

Figure 4.19   D

Findings: Axial CECT image (A) demonstrates a homogeneously enlarged spleen. Also note engorgement of the splenic vein. Coronal T2-WI (B) shows that the spleen measures 23.6 cm craniocaudally. Multiphasic gadolinium-enhanced, fat-suppressed axial T1-WI (C and D) show early heterogeneous enhancement with homogeneous enhancement on delayed images.

Differential Diagnosis: Lymphoma, leukemia.

Diagnosis: Splenomegaly due to portal hypertension.

Discussion: The spleen grows throughout childhood, reaching maximal size in adulthood. Normally, the splenic tip is visualized at the level or just below the lower pole of the left kidney on cross-sectional imaging studies. Standard splenic measurements have been determined, guiding the assessment of splenic size. Although normal standard splenic volume is related to the patient's body weight, the craniocaudal span of the normal spleen usually measures less than 13 cm. Splenomegaly occurs in numerous conditions and diseases, and in order to limit the differential diagnosis, it is important to evaluate, in addition to the size of the spleen, other diagnostic features. Splenomegaly associated with abnormal portal and splenic blood flow is typically caused by hepatic cirrhosis or congestive heart failure. Splenomegaly with or without morphologic abnormalities can be caused by hematologic disorders (e.g., early sickle cell anemia, leukemias, lymphomas, and nutritional anemias), infectious diseases (e.g., mononucleosis, acquired immunodeficiency syndrome [AIDS], cytomegalovirus [CMV], malaria, sepsis, subacute bacterial endocarditis), or miscellaneous conditions (e.g., rheumatoid arthritis, Felty syndrome, drug reactions).

Clinical History: 77-year-old woman with a history of renal cell carcinoma.

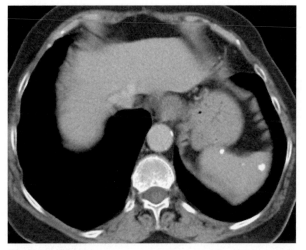

Figure 4.20 A

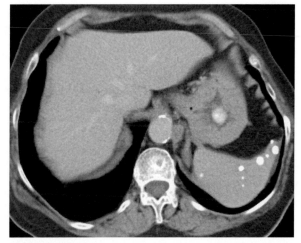

Figure 4.20 B

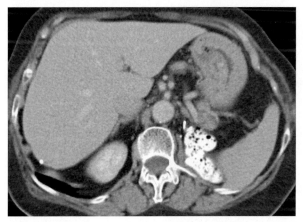

Figure 4.20 C

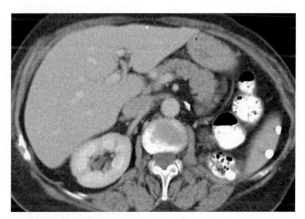

Figure 4.20 D

Findings: Axial CECT images demonstrate multiple calcifications of varying sizes in the spleen and liver.

Differential Diagnosis: Tuberculosis, treated fungal microabscesses.

Diagnosis: Splenic histoplasmosis.

Discussion: The central United States is an area where histoplasmosis is endemic. Since the onset of the AIDS epidemic, disseminated *Histoplasma capsulatum* infection has been reported with much greater frequency in both endemic and nonendemic areas. Most cases of histoplasmosis are associated with enlargement of mediastinal lymph nodes, which can calcify and cause mediastinal obstructive symptoms. Abdominal CT findings in patients with disseminated histoplasmosis include hepatomegaly (63%), splenomegaly (38%), diffuse splenic hypoattenuation (19%), bilateral adrenal enlargement, and enlarged lymph nodes (44%). Healed *Histoplasma capsulatum* infection is the most common cause of diffuse splenic calcification in the United States. Other causes of multiple splenic calcifications are healed tuberculosis, brucellosis, or *Pneumocystis* infections, hemangiomas, phleboliths, hemosiderosis, sickle cell anemia, and Gamna-Gandy bodies.

Clinical History: 30-year-old man presenting with hypotension after minor trauma.

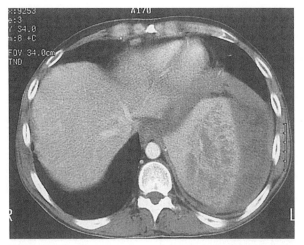

Figure 4.21   A

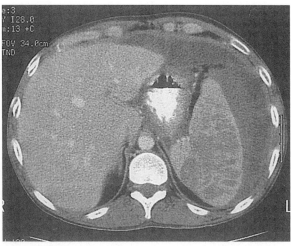

Figure 4.21   B

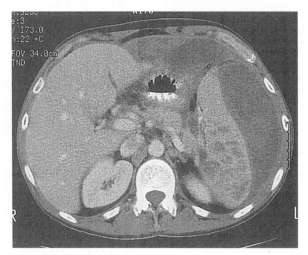

Figure 4.21   C

Findings: Axial CECT images demonstrate multiple, low-density, rounded lesions of varying sizes scattered throughout the spleen. Note a large associated perisplenic hematoma.

Differential Diagnosis: Metastases, abscesses, hemangiomatosis.

Diagnosis: Splenic peliosis.

Discussion: Peliosis is a rare disorder of the reticuloendothelial system that may involve the liver, spleen, and bone marrow; it is characterized by multiple blood-filled cysts (1–30 mm in diameter) scattered throughout the affected organ. Splenic peliosis may be associated with hematologic malignancy, infection (e.g., tuberculosis, *Bartonella* infections, HIV), and anabolic steroids or oral contraceptives. Histologically, the cystic areas consist of irregular blood-filled lakes ranging from less than 0.1 cm to greater than 1 cm in diameter. Microscopically, the lesions consist of irregular cystic spaces with or without endothelial lining. Peliosis is usually found incidentally or at autopsy but can present with hemoperitoneum due to rupture of a blood-filled cystic space. Imaging findings consist of hepatosplenomegaly and multiple small hepatosplenic lesions. On ultrasound (US), multiple hypoechoic or hyperechoic areas with irregular margins may be seen. On CECT, some lesions may not enhance, probably due to thrombosis, while others may present the "target" appearance, with central enhancing foci. The CT appearance can be similar to metastases, abscesses, and hemangiomatosis, especially if there is an associated hemangiomatosis. In the present case, the large amount of hemorrhage out of proportion to the trauma as well as the multiple lesions in the spleen suggest an underlying disorder. Peliosis was discovered at surgery.

Clinical History: 48-year-old man with a history of splenectomy presenting with abdominal pain.

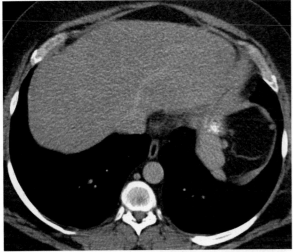

Figure 4.22   A

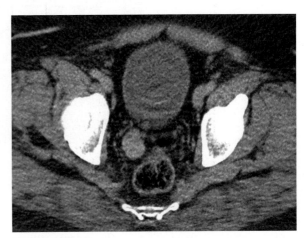

Figure 4.22   B

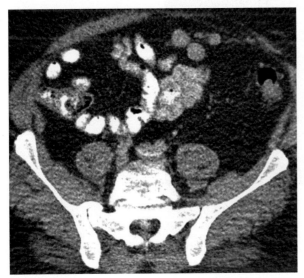

Figure 4.22   C

Figure 4.22   D

Findings: Axial CECT images through the abdomen and pelvis demonstrate small round soft tissue masses posterior to the stomach in the region of the splenic bed and similar lesions in the omentum and mesorectal space.

Differential Diagnosis: Lymph nodes, metastases.

Diagnosis: Splenosis nodules.

Discussion: Splenosis results from autotransplantation of splenic tissue from a prior trauma to the spleen or splenectomy, which leads to implantation of splenic tissue anywhere in the peritoneal cavity. The blood supply to these implants is typically from small perforating vessels; the lesions will demonstrate enhancement similar to that of a normal spleen. Splenosis can develop several years after an injury and will be discovered incidentally because patients are asymptomatic. The CT appearance of splenosis involves numerous (a few to 400) small (rarely >3 cm) enhancing nodules of varying size and shape. No hilum is identified, and most lesions are sessile in location. They can be found intra- or extraperitoneally, even in the chest after penetrating trauma. Without a history of splenic trauma, it would be difficult to distinguish splenosis from peritoneal metastases and lymph nodes. Nuclear medicine with the use of technetium-labeled, heat-damaged erythrocytes or sulfur colloid is very sensitive and specific to diagnose splenosis.

Clinical History: 60-year-old pedestrian struck by a car.

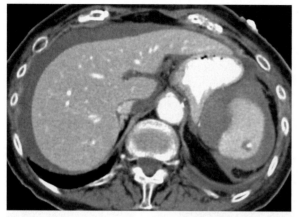

Figure 4.23 A

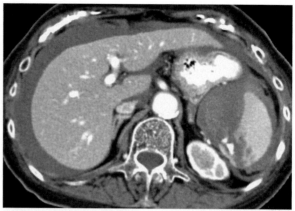

Figure 4.23 B

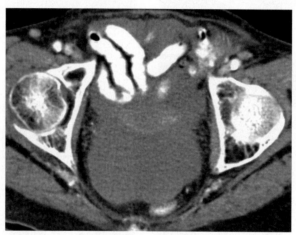

Figure 4.23 C

Findings: Axial CECT images demonstrate a linear low-attenuation lesion through the medial portion of the spleen with active contrast extravasation in the splenic hilum. Note the associated perisplenic, perihepatic, and pelvic hemoperitoneum.

Differential Diagnosis: None.

Diagnosis: Splenic rupture.

Discussion: The spleen is the most commonly injured organ after blunt trauma to the abdomen. This can be due to motor vehicle accidents, falls, or direct blows. Other injuries to the spleen include penetrating trauma and iatrogenic causes. The sensitivity of CT for detecting splenic trauma exceeds 90%, but the utility of CT for predicting outcome has been poor. Several CT grading systems for splenic trauma have been devised, but the accuracy of these systems is questionable. Ranging from best to worst prognosis, most systems incorporate the findings of a subcapsular hematoma, extracapsular fluid, laceration with or without involvement of major vessels, and a shattered spleen. Despite the discrepancy in the accuracy of predicting outcome, two common factors indicate poor prognosis: hemodynamic instability and injuries to other organs. A shattered spleen with involvement of major vessels is usually associated with a large hemoperitoneum, which can lead to hypotension, cardiac decompensation, and shock. A subcapsular hematoma or a splenic fracture not involving the hilum will typically have a small amount of hemorrhage, and the patient will be clinically stable. In this example, the fracture involved a large portion of the spleen with major vessel injuries and acute contrast extravasation. This patient was hemodynamically unstable and treated successfully with urgent surgery. Percutaneous embolization may have been an adequate alternative to surgery.

CASE 4-24

Clinical History: 31-year-old man presenting with intermittent low back pain for several months in duration.

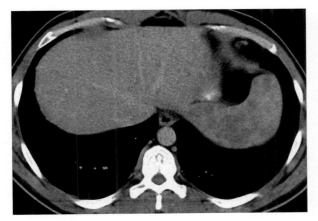

Figure 4.24 A

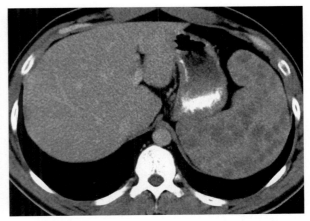

Figure 4.24 B

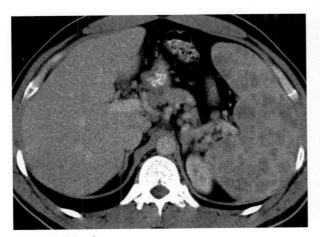

Figure 4.24 C

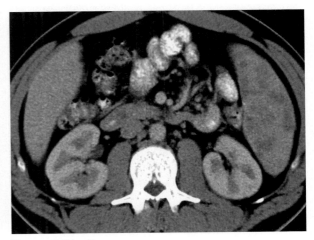

Figure 4.24 D

Findings: Axial CECT images demonstrate multiple small hypodense lesions within the spleen and liver. Note presence of splenomegaly.

Differential Diagnosis: Metastases, abscesses, lymphoma, multiple hemangiomas or lymphangiomas.

Diagnosis: Splenic sarcoidosis.

Discussion: Sarcoidosis is a systemic disease of unknown etiology that primarily affects the mediastinal and hilar lymph nodes, lung parenchyma, skin, and eyes. It is characterized by the presence of noncaseating granulomas that can affect almost any organ. Abdominal sarcoidosis is common, and splenic involvement is microscopically demonstrated in approximately 24% to 59% of patients, but its clinical significance is uncertain, and splenic dysfunction is rare. Mild splenomegaly occurs in 11% to 42% of patients with sarcoidosis. The radiologic features in the abdomen are nonspecific, and most often, the diagnosis is made by biopsy of peripheral nodes, liver, or skin. On CT, splenic sarcoidosis is usually not detected or abdominal involvement appears as nonspecific hepatospenomegaly and retroperitoneal lymphadenopathy. Multiple low-density intrasplenic lesions are present in 11% to 33% of cases, ranging in size from 1 to 30 mm. When nodules increase in size, a more coalescent hypodense nodular pattern is seen.

Clinical History: 23-year-old asymptomatic woman being evaluated for a left lower quadrant mass.

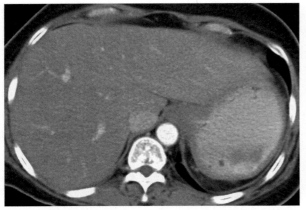

Figure 4.25 A

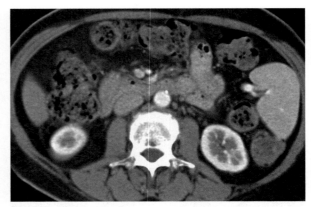

Figure 4.25 B

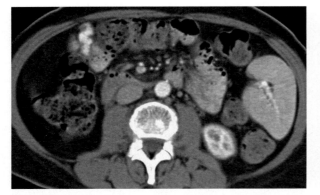

Figure 4.25 C

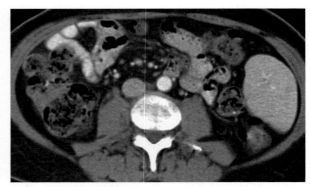

Figure 4.25 D

Findings: Axial CECT images demonstrate absence of a spleen in the left upper quadrant. A large well-defined soft tissue mass is noted anterior to the left kidney and extends into the left pelvis.

Differential Diagnosis: None.

Diagnosis: Wandering spleen.

Discussion: Wandering or ectopic spleen occurs where there is laxity of the ligaments that fix the spleen in the left upper quadrant, leading to a mobile spleen. One theory on the etiology of a wandering spleen is that it is due to a congenital fusion abnormality of the ligaments, which leads to hypermobility. Another theory suggests that it may be acquired from the effects of hormones. Although most patients are asymptomatic, a complication of a wandering spleen includes torsion that results in acute or chronic intermittent abdominal pain. This can lead to venous congestion and splenic infarcts. Chronic torsion can produce omental and peritoneal adhesions that can form a thick capsule around the spleen. Diagnosis can be made by the absence of the spleen in the normal location and the presence of a mass similar in appearance to a normal spleen but in an abnormal location. Diagnosis can be confirmed with a nuclear medicine sulfur colloid scan. Treatment consists of splenectomy in patients with symptoms of intermittent torsion.

Clinical History: 24-year-old man with history of leukemia presenting with fever.

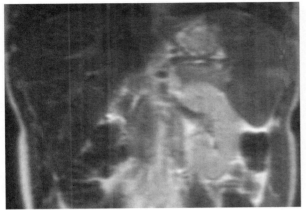

Figure 4.26 A

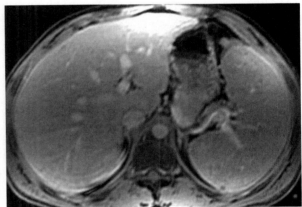

Figure 4.26 B

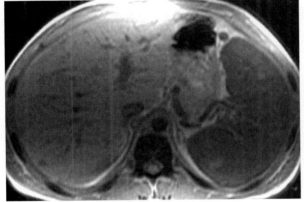

Figure 4.26 C

Figure 4.26 D

Findings: Coronal (A) and axial (B) T2-WI shows several small hyperintense lesions within the liver and spleen. Unenhanced (C) and gadolinium-enhanced, fat-suppressed axial T1-WI (D) show the lesions to be hyperintense and rim enhancing, respectively. Note abnormal low signal of liver, spleen, and bone marrow due to transfusional iron overload (hemosiderosis).

Differential Diagnosis: Leukemia, lymphoma.

Diagnosis: Splenic fungal microabscesses.

Discussion: Fungal abscesses have been reported to represent up to 26% of splenic abscesses. The most common pathogen is *Candida albicans* and is usually diagnosed in immunocompromised patients on therapy for leukemia. Other fungi that may cause splenic abscesses include *Aspergillus* and *Cryptococcus*. Histologically, concentric rings with central necrotic hyphae can be seen; these rings are surrounded by viable hyphae and a rim of peripheral inflammation. Grossly, the entire spleen may demonstrate multiple small (<5 mm in size) fungal deposits. On CT, multiple small lesions of relatively low attenuation, typically ranging from a few millimeters to 2 cm in diameter, are seen. Occasionally, a central area of higher attenuation or a "wheel-within-a-wheel" pattern may be demonstrated. At MRI, splenic fungal abscesses appear as multiple small lesions, which are hypointense on T1-WI and hyperintense on T2-WI. The use of fat saturation with T2-WI may improve detection of these small lesions, as well as the use of gadolinium. Rim enhancement is typically present after gadolinium administration.

Clinical History: 48-year-old woman presenting with left upper quadrant pain.

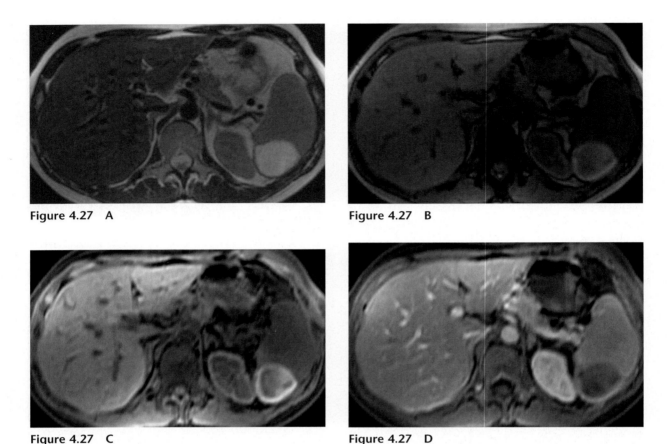

Figure 4.27   A

Figure 4.27   B

Figure 4.27   C

Figure 4.27   D

Findings: Axial T2-WI (A), out-of-phase T1-WI (B), and unenhanced (C) and gadolinium-enhanced (D) fat-suppressed axial T1-WI demonstrate a 6-cm subcapsular splenic nonenhancing lesion, which displaces the spleen anteriorly. The lesion is high in signal on T1-WI due to the paramagnetic effect of methemoglobin.

Differential Diagnosis: Pyogenic abscess, hydatid cyst.

Diagnosis: Subcapsular splenic hematoma.

Discussion: CT has definitely become the imaging modality of choice in the evaluation of patients with suspected splenic trauma. Splenic injuries can be classified on CT scans as subcapsular or intraparenchymal hematomas, lacerations, fractures, or vascular pedicles injuries. Intrasplenic hematomas typically appear as hypodense areas within the spleen after administration of contrast medium, but in some cases, they may be nearly isodense. Subcapsular hematomas usually appear as crescentic or round fluid collection along the lateral aspect of the spleen, which may be difficult to distinguish from perisplenic fluid. MRI is seldom employed in the acute setting of splenic trauma, although it has high sensitivity for the detection of blood and blood breakdown products. The signal intensity of hematomas depends on the age of the extravascular blood. During the first 48 hours following extravasation, blood undergoes transformation into deoxyhemoglobin and other paramagnetic products. Deoxyhemoglobin within red blood cells may be identified on T2-WI within a few hours after trauma. Subacute hematomas are of high signal on T1-WI because of the paramagnetic effect of the extracellular methemoglobin, which shortens the T1 relaxation time.

Clinical History: 57-year-old woman presenting with epigastric pain.

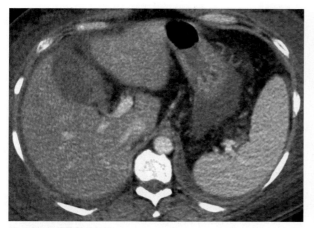

Figure 4.28   A

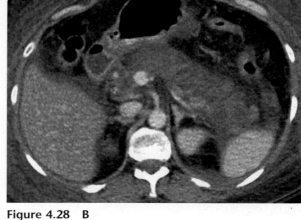

Figure 4.28   B

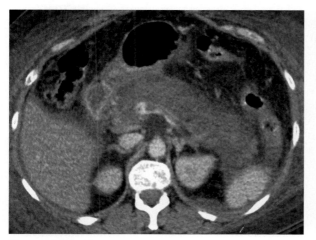

Figure 4.28   C

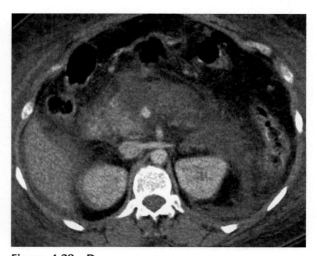

Figure 4.28   D

Findings: Axial CECT images show subtotal pancreatic necrosis and acute fluid collections in the retroperitoneum due to acute pancreatitis. A linear filling defect is identified within the splenic vein.

Differential Diagnosis: None.

Diagnosis: Splenic vein thrombosis.

Discussion: The pathophysiology of splenic vein thrombosis includes compression, encasement, and inflammation of the splenic vein. In most cases, thrombosis is related to pancreatic carcinoma or pancreatitis, but it is also seen in cirrhosis of the liver, after liver transplantation, and after splenectomy, or it is due to idiopathic causes. Splenic vein thrombosis causes development of gastric varices. In acute thrombosis of the splenic vein, NECT scan may demonstrate an intraluminal, high-density filling defect. After contrast administration, as shown in this case, this filling defect does not enhance. Chronic splenic vein thrombosis is characterized by the presence of a nonenhancing attenuated or absent splenic vein, with presence of varices. On MRI, the thrombosed splenic vein shows hyperintensity on T2-WI, and the gastric varices are seen as multiple, tortuous structures with a signal void on T2-WI.

Clinical History: 47-year-old woman with HIV presenting with diarrhea, fever, and left upper quadrant pain.

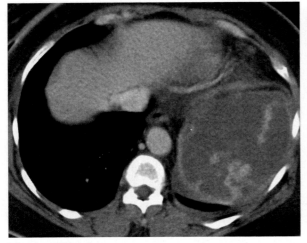

Figure 4.29   A

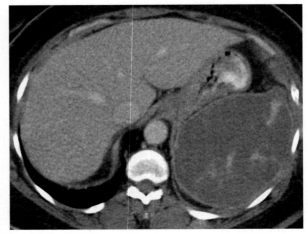

Figure 4.29   B

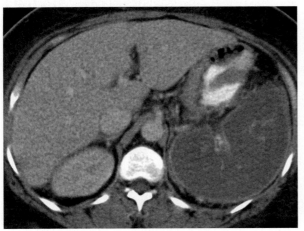

Figure 4.29   C

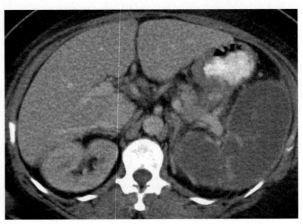

Figure 4.29   D

Findings: Axial CECT images show near complete cystic change of the spleen with presence of some preserved islands of normal enhancing splenic tissue. Note enhancement of the splenic capsule.

Differential Diagnosis: Splenic infarct, splenic cyst, lymphoma, hematoma.

Diagnosis: Pyogenic splenic abscess.

Discussion: Splenic pyogenic abscesses are uncommon, with a reported incidence less than 1% in large autopsy series. However, their frequency is growing as a result of an increasing number of immunosuppressed or chronically debilitated patients because of aggressive chemotherapy treatments, hematologic disorders, diabetes, and AIDS. Immuno-suppressed patients account for 25% of patients with splenic abscess. The most common pathogens are *Streptococci*, *Staphylococci*, and *Salmonella*, but every pyogenic organism may be involved. CT may show the presence of focal low-attenuating, well-defined lesion, with an attenuation ranging from 20 to 40 Hounsfield units (HU). Minimal peripheral contrast enhancement may be present when a capsule has developed, although it is less common in splenic than in hepatic abscesses. The presence of gas is usually diagnostic; unfortunately, only a minority of splenic abscesses contain gas. CT is very sensitive in detecting splenic abscesses but is not specific. There are several differential diagnoses including splenic infarct, cysts, tumors, and hematomas, so fine-needle aspiration may be useful to confirm the diagnosis in the appropriate clinical setting.

CASE 4-30

Clinical History: 59-year-old man presenting with jaundice.

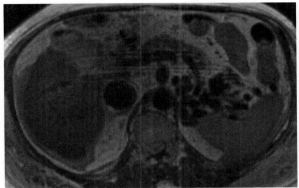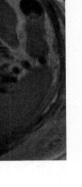

Figure 4.30   A

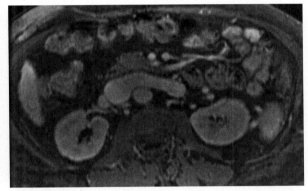

Figure 4.30   B

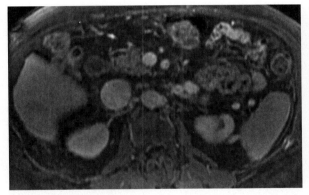

Figure 4.30   C

Figure 4.30   D

Findings: Axial T2-WI (A) shows liver cirrhosis and ascites, and numerous rounded flow voids in the splenic hilum. Gadolinium-enhanced, fat-suppressed axial T1-WI (B–D) show enhancement of the tubular structures near the splenic hilum, of a large vessel lateral to the left upper renal pole, and of a dilated left renal vein.

Differential Diagnosis: None.

Diagnosis: Splenic varices with splenorenal shunt due to portal hypertension.

Discussion: The differential diagnosis of left upper quadrant varices includes portal hypertension and portal vein thrombosis. The identification of an enlarged left gastroepiploic vein without a recanalized paraumbilical vein suggests venous thrombosis rather than portal hypertension. On CT, splenic varices are seen as multiple enhancing nodular structures in the left upper quadrant. On MRI, varices are seen as multiple, tortuous structures with a signal void on T2-WI that are enhancing following gadolinium administration. Development of a splenorenal shunt is a spontaneous adaptation of the body to overcome the increased pressure in the portal venous system due to cirrhosis. Typically, patients with a spontaneous splenorenal shunt will show a normal sized spleen (as the pressure is shunted away from the spleen), tortuous vessels connecting the splenic vein with the left renal vein, a dilated left renal vein, and sometimes reversed flow in a dilated left gonadal vein.

Clinical History: 43-year-old woman presenting with diffuse abdominal pain.

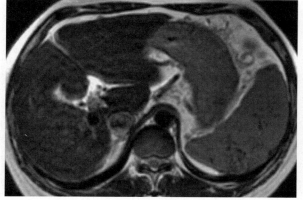

Figure 4.31   A

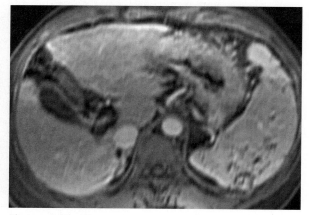

Figure 4.31   B

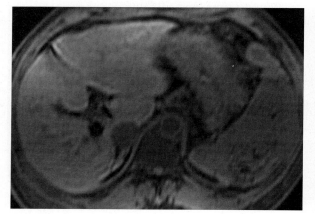

Figure 4.31   C

Figure 4.31   D

Findings: Axial T2-WI (A), flow-sensitive T2*-WI (B), and unenhanced (C) and gadolinium-enhanced (D) fat-suppressed axial T1-WI demonstrate ill-defined small areas of signal void scattered within an enlarged spleen. Also note presence of hepatic cirrhosis and presence of a transjugular intrahepatic portosystemic shunts (TIPS) in the right hepatic lobe (D).

Differential Diagnosis: Calcified granulomas (tuberculosis, histoplasmosis, brucellosis).

Diagnosis: Gamna-Gandy bodies.

Discussion: Portal hypertension causes enlargement of the splenic vein, formation of perisplenic collaterals and splenomegaly, and eventually, small areas of intrasplenic hemorrhage. The remnants of these tiny foci of hypertensive bleeding, which are composed of hemosiderin, fibrous tissue, and calcium, are referred to as siderotic nodules or Gamna-Gandy bodies. They vary in size but are usually less than 1 cm. On CT, noncalcified foci may appear as multiple, punctate, low-attenuation areas. Calcified foci may appear as multiple high-density lesions. On MRI, they can be seen as multiple, punctate, low signal intensity lesions on T1-WI, T2-WI, and gradient-echo sequences. The blooming artifact on gradient-echo images is pathognomonic for this entity because these sequences are more sensitive to detect the superparamagnetic effect of hemosiderin.

CASE 4-32

Clinical History: 60-year-old man with longstanding history of Crohn disease.

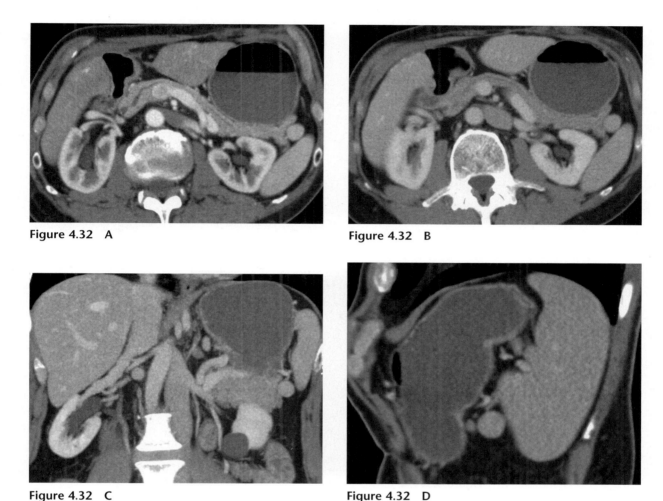

Figure 4.32 A

Figure 4.32 B

Figure 4.32 C

Figure 4.32 D

Findings: Axial late arterial (A) and portal venous (B) CECT images and coronal (C) and sagittal (D) portal venous phase reformatted images show the presence of a small, well-defined, round soft tissue nodule adjacent to the main spleen. Note that the enhancement of the nodule parallels that of the main spleen.

Differential Diagnosis: Splenosis nodule, lymph node, peritoneal implant.

Diagnosis: Accessory spleen.

Discussion: Accessory spleens, also known as supernumerary spleens or splenunculi, are congenital foci of normal splenic tissue that are separate from the main body of the spleen. They arise from failure of fusion of the splenic anlage, located in the dorsal mesogastrium, during the fifth week of fetal life. Accessory spleens are relatively common, as they

are described in 10% to 30% of cases at autopsy. Although usually asymptomatic and incidentally discovered, they are clinically important in some patients. First, accessory spleen may mimic lymphadenopathy and tumors in other abdominal organs, such as pancreas, adrenal gland, and kidney. Second, they occasionally may become symptomatic due to torsion, spontaneous rupture, hemorrhage, and cyst formation. Third, a surgeon's awareness of their presence may be important when the intention is to remove all functional splenic tissue (e.g., hematologic disorders). The majority of accessory spleens have a characteristic appearance on CT. Typically, they are well-marginated, homogeneously enhancing, round masses that are smaller than 2 cm. Their most frequent location is posteromedial to the spleen. When smaller than 1 cm, the may appear hypodense relative to the spleen.

Clinical History: 56-year-old woman with a history of acute myelogenous leukemia evaluated for fever.

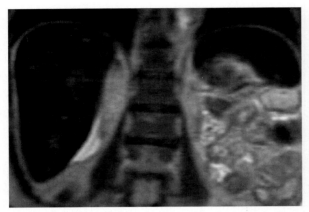

Figure 4.33   A

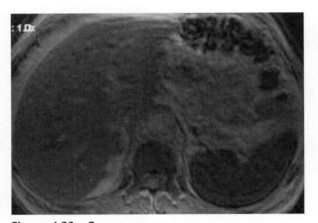

Figure 4.33   B

Figure 4.33   C

Findings: Axial (A) and coronal (B) single-shot T2-WI show decreased signal intensity of both liver and spleen. Axial gradient-echo T1-WI (C) shows the signal intensity of the liver, spleen, and bone marrow to be lower than spinal muscle.

Differential Diagnosis: Primary hemochromatosis.

Diagnosis: Hemosiderosis.

Discussion: Iron overload diseases consist of two different groups of disorders depending on the location of iron deposition. Primary hemochromatosis is a common inherited autosomal recessive disorder, consisting of abnormal parenchymal iron deposition, which occurs mainly in the hepatocytes but also in the pancreas, heart, and synovium. This parenchymal iron deposition may cause damage and organ dysfunction, such as cirrhosis of the liver and development of hepatocellular carcinoma. Hemosiderosis is the term used for iron deposition in the reticuloendothelial system of the liver, spleen, lymph nodes, and bone marrow; it most commonly develops after multiple blood transfusions (transfusional iron overload) and has little clinical significance. MRI is a sensitive and specific method to detect iron deposition because of the magnetic-susceptibility effect caused by the accumulated iron. This demonstrates a markedly decreased signal intensity (compared with that seen in skeletal muscle) in involved organs on T2-WI, especially on gradient-echo T2*-WI. In hemochromatosis, a low signal intensity on T2-WI and T2*-WI is found in the liver, pancreas, myocardium, and endocrine glands, but the spleen remains normal. In hemosiderosis, spleen, liver, and bone marrow reveal decreased intensity on MRI studies, and the pancreas tends to be spared.

Clinical History: 26-year-old woman with recent travel to Sierra Leone presenting with fever and anemia.

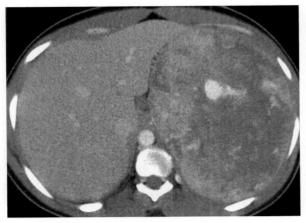

Figure 4.34   A

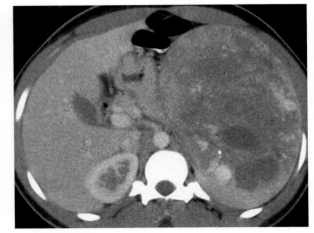

Figure 4.34   B

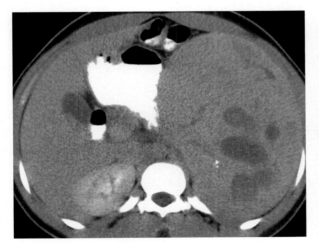

Figure 4.34   C

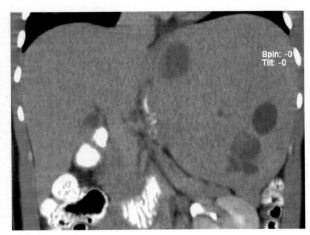

Figure 4.34   D

Findings: Axial and coronal CECT images obtained during the arterial phase (A and B) and delayed phase (C and D) show a large heterogeneous mass nearly replacing the entire spleen. Areas of arteriovenous shunting and necrosis are present.

Differential Diagnosis: Angiosarcoma, epithelioid vascular tumors, hemangiopericytoma.

Diagnosis: Splenic spindle cell sarcoma.

Discussion: Nonlymphoid primary malignant neoplasms of the spleen are rare, and those of vascular origin constitute the majority, with angiosarcoma, hemangiopericytoma, and epithelioid neoplasms being the tumors most frequently encountered. Hemangiopericytomas are rare vascular tumors of parenchymal origin that are especially aggressive. Histologically, hemangiopericytomas consist of numerous capillary channels lined with epithelium and surrounded by and enclosed by nests and masses of spindle cells, which occasionally can be ovoid or even round. On CT scan, reported findings include the presence of a large mass with polylobular contour, along with numerous other smaller lesions disseminated throughout the entire spleen. Hyperattenuation of the solid portions and areas of autoinfarction and necrosis due to rapid growth, shown best after contrast medium administration, reflect the hypervascularity and aggressiveness of this tumor.

Clinical History: 36-year-old man presenting with dysuria and bloody penile discharge.

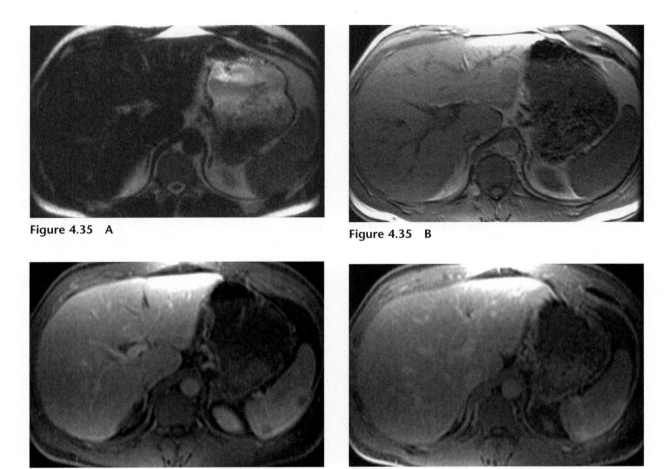

Figure 4.35   A

Figure 4.35   B

Figure 4.35   C

Figure 4.35   D

Findings: Axial T2-WI (A) and T1-WI (B) and gadolinium-enhanced, fat-suppressed axial T1-WI in the arterial phase (C) and delayed phase (D) demonstrate small nodules in the spleen that are hypointense on T2-WI and show delayed enhancement.

Differential Diagnosis: Abscesses, tuberculosis, lymphoma.

Diagnosis: Splenic sarcoidosis.

Discussion: Sarcoidosis is a chronic multisystem disease of unknown etiology characterized by accumulation of T-cell lymphocytes and mononuclear phagocytes and formation of noncaseating granulomas in different organs. Any age group can be affected, but most patients present between 20 and 40 years of age. The prevalence is 10 to 40 in 100,000 individuals, and the disease is more common in African American females. Histologically, sarcoidosis is characterized by noncaseating granulomas frequently less than 2 mm in size that consist of aggregates of Langerhans type giant cells surrounded by necrotic or fibrotic tissues. MRI may demonstrate splenomegaly, contour irregularity, nodularity, and diffuse heterogeneity with decreased signal intensity on T2-WI, suggestive of iron overload. Splenic sarcoidosis lesions are small (<1 cm) and hypovascular and, therefore, hypointense on T1-WI and T2-WI. Low signal intensity on T2-WI is a differential diagnostic feature used to differentiate nodular sarcoidosis lesions from acute infections.

Clinical History: 76-year-old woman with anemia.

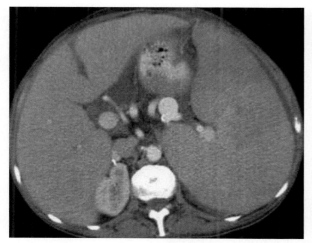

Figure 4.36   A

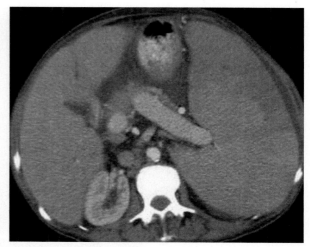

Figure 4.36   B

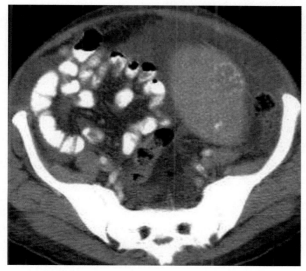

Figure 4.36   C

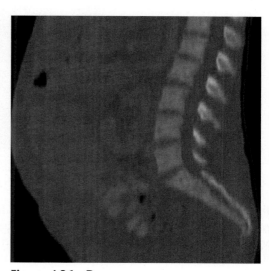

Figure 4.36   D

Findings: Axial CECT images (A–C) show splenomegaly with heterogeneous enhancement. Note presence of small calcifications in the lower pole. Sagittal reformatted CECT image displayed in bone window (D) shows diffuse increased density of the bone.

Differential Diagnosis: Leukemia, lymphoma, sickle cell disease (acute phase).

Diagnosis: Myelofibrosis.

Discussion: Myelofibrosis is a myeloproliferative disorder, with defects of the bone marrow matrix and myeloid metaplasia (proliferation of the neoplastic myeloid stem cells) occurring primarily in the spleen and liver. Fibrosis of the bone marrow may represent the ultimate histologic stage of a number of different bone marrow actions. The spleen appears markedly enlarged. On section, it is firm and red to gray; multiple subcapsular infarcts may be present. Histologically, there is proliferation affecting normoblast, granulocyte precursors, and megakaryocytes. Sometimes, disproportional activity of any one of the three major cell lines is seen. Initially, the extramedullary hematopoiesis is confined to the sinusoids, but later, it may extend to involve the cords. CT may demonstrate splenomegaly with homogeneous enhancement. Hemosiderosis resulting from repeated transfusion can sometimes be seen together with infarction and hemorrhage.

Clinical History: 37-year-old man presenting with weight loss and fever.

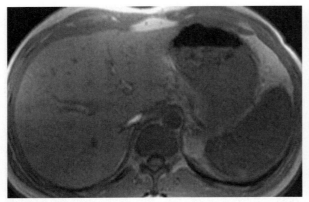

Figure 4.37 A

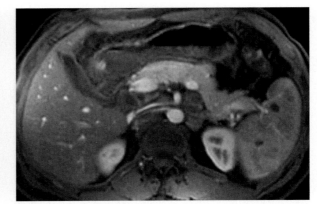

Figure 4.37 B

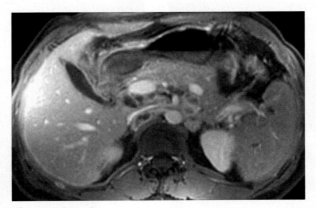

Figure 4.37 C

Findings: Axial T1-WI (A) shows two small, ill-defined, hyperintense splenic lesions. Gadolinium-enhanced, fat-suppressed axial T1-WI in the early arterial (B) and portal venous (C) phase show faint peripheral enhancement around the lesions.

Differential Diagnosis: Sarcoidosis, brucellosis, leukemia, fungal microabscesses.

Diagnosis: Splenic tuberculosis.

Discussion: Tuberculosis (TB) is a chronic bacterial infection caused by *Mycobacterium tuberculosis* and characterized by the formation of granulomas in infected tissues and by cell-mediated hypersensitivity. The usual site of disease is the lung, but other organs may be involved. The rate of extrapulmonary involvement has increased with the onset of the HIV epidemic. Splenic TB is extremely common in patients with disseminated disease; however, it is not usually identified at initial presentation. When present, there usually is miliary hepatosplenic dissemination in association with miliary pulmonary TB. On CT, tiny, low-density foci scattered throughout the spleen may be seen; when the lesions are larger, they may appear as small, focal splenic nodules of low attenuation. In the macronodular form, occurring less commonly, the disease appears on CT as a diffuse splenic enlargement containing multiple, low-density, 1- to 3-cm, round lesions or a single mass. This feature may evolve to an abscess with single or multiple low-density, septated, or "honeycomblike" lesions. These lesions have irregular, ill-defined margins and show minimal or slight central enhancement after intravenous contrast medium administration.

Case images courtesy of Dr. Adelard De Backer, St.-Lucas Hospital, Ghent, Belgium.

Clinical History: 38-year-old man presenting with left upper quadrant fullness.

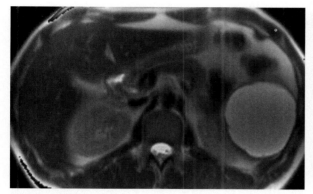

Figure 4.38 A

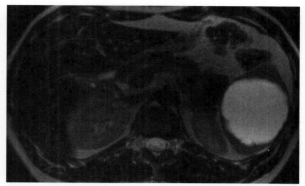

Figure 4.38 B

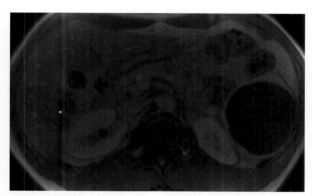

Figure 4.38 C

Findings: Axial T2-WI (A) and heavily T2-WI (B) show a well-defined, 9-cm cystic lesion in the spleen. Small peripheral septations are seen. Gadolinium-enhanced axial T1-WI (C) shows no enhancement of the cystic lesion.

Differential Diagnosis: Posttraumatic cyst, hydatid cyst, abscess, cystic hemangioma.

Diagnosis: Splenic epidermoid cyst.

Discussion: Cysts of the spleen may be divided into primary (or true) cysts, which possess a cellular lining, and secondary (or false) cysts, which are without a cellular lining. Primary cysts are either parasitic (echinococcal) or nonparasitic (epithelial). Nonparasitic epithelial-lined cysts of the spleen (typically epidermoid) account for 10% to 25% of all cystic lesions and may be a manifestation of a genetic defect of mesothelial migration. On CT, both true and false cysts appear as thin-walled, unilocular, spherical intrasplenic masses of fluid density, without rim enhancement after contrast material administration. Cyst wall trabeculations or peripheral septations may be found in either type of cyst, but rim calcification is more common in false cyst. Debris or high-density material may be noted in either type of cyst secondary to intracystic hemorrhage or in the case of a false cyst due to resolving hematoma. MRI shows a well-defined, rounded mass with high signal intensity on T2-WI and a variable intensity on T1-WI depending on the protein or hemorrhagic component of the cystic fluid. Peripheral rim of hypointensity may be caused by the presence of a calcified wall or hemosiderin deposits in the cyst wall.

Clinical History: 34-year-old woman presenting with left flank pain.

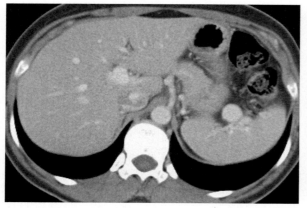

Figure 4.39   A

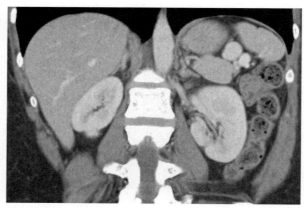

Figure 4.39   B

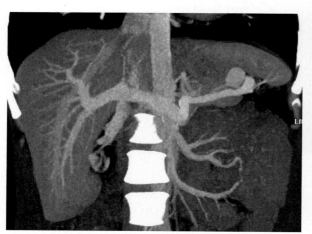

Figure 4.39   C

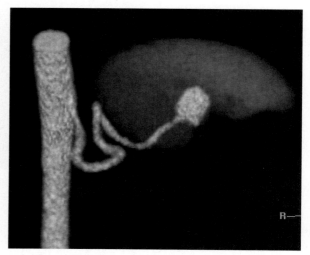

Figure 4.39   D

Findings: Axial (A) and coronal (B) CECT images show an enhancing nodule, isodense to the aorta, in the splenic hilum. Coronal maximum-intensity projection (C) and three-dimensional, volume-rendered (D) images show that the nodule connects to the splenic artery.

Differential Diagnosis: None.

Diagnosis: Splenic artery aneurysm.

Discussion: Splenic artery aneurysm is the most common abdominal visceral artery aneurysm, representing approximately 60% of visceral arterial aneurysms. Various causes and predisposing conditions may lead to splenic artery aneurysm, including portal hypertension, pregnancy and history of multiparity, pancreatitis, arteriosclerotic disease, penetrating gastric ulcer, trauma, and vasculitis. Splenic aneurysms are most often saccular, and over 75% occur at the distal third of the splenic artery. They are multiple in 20% of cases and range in size from less than 1 cm to 3 cm. Splenic artery aneurysms are usually diagnosed by the presence of ring calcification in the left upper quadrant on plain film, CT, or US. On NECT, splenic aneurysm appears as a well-defined, low-density mass with or without calcifications; after intravenous contrast medium administration, marked and early arterial enhancement within the residual patent lumen may be demonstrated. On MRI, splenic aneurysm may demonstrate a well-defined ring of low signal intensity at the periphery, corresponding to the aneurysm wall, whereas the signal intensity within the aneurysm depends on the presence and the velocity of flowing blood and the presence and age of the thrombus. Fast-flowing blood within the patent lumen usually produces a signal void, which persists on all spin-echo sequences.

Clinical History: 66-year-old woman with chronic pancreatic duct leak following acute pancreatitis.

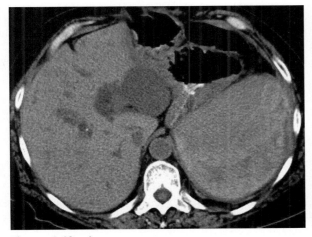

Figure 4.40   A

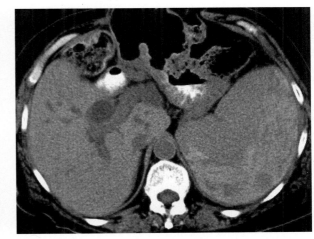

Figure 4.40   B

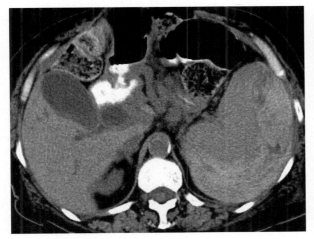

Figure 4.40   C

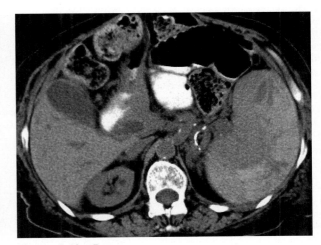

Figure 4.40   D

Findings: Axial NECT images show a large crescentic-shaped heterogeneous hyperdense collection adjacent to the spleen. Note compression of the splenic parenchyma.

Differential Diagnosis: Abscess.

Diagnosis: Splenic subcapsular hematoma.

Discussion: The spleen is known to be the most frequently injured intraperitoneal organ in cases of blunt abdominal trauma. Other less common causes include iatrogenic etiologies (e.g., abdominal surgery), penetrating abdominal trauma, spontaneous rupture, and pancreatitis. The main concern following trauma of the spleen is the possibility of splenic rupture, which is associated with mortality in more than 75% of cases if surgery is not performed promptly. In adults, the incidence of splenic involvement in blunt abdominal trauma is 25% of cases, whereas in penetrating abdominal trauma, it accounts for approximately 7% of cases. Injuries that result in parenchymal/subcapsular hematomas with an intact capsule are less common than was originally believed but may account for the 1% to 2% incidence of delayed splenic rupture. Delayed splenic rupture is defined as bleeding occurring more than 48 hours after trauma in previously hemodynamically stable patients. Its reported frequency varies between 1% and 14%, with mortality rates higher than in acute splenic injury (5–15% vs. 1%, respectively).

SUGGESTED READINGS

NEOPLASMS

- Barrier A, Lacaine F, Callard P, et al. Lymphangiomatosis of the spleen and 2 accessory spleens. *Surgery* 2002;131:114–116.

- Bezzi M, Spinelli A, Pierleoni M, et al. Cystic lymphangioma of the spleen: US-CT-MRI correlation. *Eur Radiol*. 2001;11:1187–1190.

- Dachman AH, Buck JL, Krishnan J, et al. Primary non-Hodgkin's splenic lymphoma. *Clin Radiol*. 1998;53:137–142.

- Dachman AH, Ros PR, Olmsted WW, et al. Nonparasitic splenic cysts: a report of 52 cases with radiologic-pathologic correlation. *Am J Roentgenol*. 1986;147:537–542.

- Fernandez-Canton G, Capelastegui A, Merino A, et al. A typical MRI presentation of a small splenic hamartoma. *Eur Radiol*. 1999;9:883–885.

- Ferrozzi F, Bova D, Draghi F, et al. CT findings in primary vascular tumors of the spleen. *Am J Roentgenol*. 1996;166:1097–1101.

- Fishman EK, Kuhlman JE, Jones RJ. CT of lymphoma: spectrum of disease. *Radiographics* 1991;11:647–669.

- Ha HK, Kim HH, Kim BK, et al. Primary angiosarcoma of the spleen: CT and MR imaging. *Acta Radiol*. 1994;35:455–458.

- Hahn PF, Weissleder R, Stark DD, et al. MR imaging of focal splenic tumors. *Am J Roentgenol*. 1988;150:823–827.

- Karakas HM, Demir M, Ozyilmaz F, et al. Primary angiosarcoma of the spleen: in vivo and in vitro MRI findings. *Clin Imaging*. 2001;25:192–196.

- Mortele KJ, Mergo PJ, Kunnen M, et al. Tumoral pathology of the spleen. In: De Shepper AM, Vanhoenacker F, eds. *Medical imaging of the spleen*. 1st ed. Berlin: Springer; 2000:101–122.

- Rabushka LS, Kawashima A, Fishman EK. Imaging of the spleen: CT with supplemental MR examination. *Radiographics* 1994;14:307–332.

- Ramani M, Reinhold C, Semelka RC, et al. Splenic hemangiomas and hamartomas: MR imaging characteristics of 28 lesions. *Radiology* 1997;202:166–172.

- Rao BK, AuBuchon J, Lieberman LM, et al. Cystic lymphangiomatosis of the spleen: a radiologic-pathologic correlation. *Radiology* 1981;141:781–782.

- Ros PR, Moser RP, Dachman AH, et al. Hemangioma of the spleen: radiologic-pathologic correlation in ten cases. *Radiology* 1987;162:73–77.

- Rose SC, Kumpe DA, Manco-Johnson ML. Radiographic appearance of diffuse splenic hemangiomatosis. *Gastrointest Radiol*. 1986;11:342–345.

- Shirkoda A, Freeman J, Armin AR, et al. Imaging features of splenic epidermoid cysts with pathologic correlation. *Abdom Imaging*. 1995;20:449–451.

- Strijk SP, Wagener DJT, Bogman MJJT, et al. The spleen in Hodgkin disease: diagnostic value of CT. *Radiology* 1985;154:753–757.

- Urrutia M, Mergo, PJ, Ros PR, et al. Cystic masses of the spleen: radiologic-pathologic correlation. *Radiographics* 1996;16:107–129.

INFECTION

- Callen PW, Filly RA, Marcus FS. Ultrasonography and computed tomography in the evaluation of hepatic microabscesses in the immunosuppressed patient. *Radiology* 1980;136:433–434.

- Chew FS, Smith PL, Barboriak D. Candidal splenic abscesses. *Am J Roentgenol*. 1981;156:474.

- Drevelengas A. The spleen in infectious disorders. In: De Shepper AM, Vanhoenacker F, eds. *Medical imaging of the spleen*. 1st ed. Berlin: Springer; 2000:67–80.

- Franquet T, Montes M, Lecumbern FJ, et al. Hydatid disease of the spleen: imaging findings in nine patients. *Am J Roentgenol*. 1990;154:525–528.

- Pierkarski J, Federle MP, Moss AA, et al. Computed tomography of the spleen. *Radiology* 1980;135:683–689.

- Shirkhoda A. CT findings in hepatosplenic and renal candidiasis. *J Comput Assist Tomogr*. 1987;11:795–798.

TRAUMA

- Do HM, Cronan JJ. CT appearance of splenic injuries managed nonoperatively. *Am J Roentgenol*. 1991;157:757–760.

- Emery KH. Splenic emergencies. *Radiol Clin North Am*. 1997;35:831–843.

- Gavant ML, Schurr M, Flick PA, et al. Predicting clinical outcome of non-surgical management of blunt splenic injury; using CT to reveal abnormalities of splenic vasculature. *Am J Roentgenol*. 1997;168:207–212.

- Jeffrey RB, Laing FC, Federle MP, et al. Computed tomography of splenic trauma. *Radiology* 1981;141:729–732.

- Malangoni MA, Cue JI, Fallat ME, et al. Evaluation of splenic injury by computed tomography and its impact on treatment. *Ann Surg*. 1990;211:592–599.

- Mirvis SE, Whitley NO, Gens DR. Blunt splenic trauma in adults: CT-based classification and correlation with prognosis and treatment. *Radiology* 1981;171:33–39.

- Naylor R, Coln D, Shires GT. Morbidity and mortality from injuries to the spleen. *J Trauma*. 1974;14:773–778.

- Umlas SL, Cronan JJ. Splenic trauma: can CT grading systems enable prediction of successful nonsurgical treatment? *Radiology* 1991;178:481–487.

- Wolfman NT, Bechtold RE, Scharling ES, et al. Blunt upper abdominal trauma: evaluation by CT. *Am J Roentgenol*. 1992;158:492–501.

MISCELLANEOUS

- Allen KB, Gay BB, Skandalakis JE. Wandering spleen: anatomic and radiologic considerations. *South Med J*. 1992;85:976–984.

- Balcar I, Seltzer SE, Davis S, et al. CT patterns of splenic infarction: a clinical and experimental study. *Radiology* 1984;151:723–729.

- Darling JD, Flickinger FW. Splenosis mimicking neoplasm in the perirenal space: CT characteristics. *J Comput Assist Tomogr*. 1990;14:839–841.

- Folz SJ, Johnson CD, Swensen SJ. Abdominal manifestations of sarcoidosis in CT studies. *J Comput Assist Tomogr*. 1995;19:573–579.

- Freeman JL, Jafri SZH, Roberts JL, et al. CT of congenital and acquired abnormalities of the spleen. *Radiographics* 1993;13:597–610.

- Gentry LR, Brown JM, Lindgren RD. Splenosis: CT demonstration of heterotopic autotransplantation of splenic tissue. *J Comput Assist Tomogr*. 1982;6:1184–1187.

- Gorden DH, Burell MI, Levin DC, et al. Wandering spleen—the radiological and clinical spectrum. *Radiology* 1977;125:39–46.

- Hoeffel C, Bokemeyer C, Hoeffel JC, et al. CT hepatic and splenic appearances with sarcoidosis. *Eur J Radiol*. 1996;23:94–96.

- Ito K, Mitchell DG, Honjo K, et al. MR imaging of acquired abnormalities of the spleen. *Am J Roentgenol*. 1997;168:697–702.

- Jaroch MT, Broughan TA, Hermann RE. The natural history of splenic infarction. *Surgery* 1986;100:743–749.

- Kessler A, Mitchell DG, Israel HL, et al. Hepatic and splenic sarcoidosis: ultrasound and MR imaging. *Abdom Imaging*. 1993;18:159–163.

- Magid D, Fishman EK, Charache S, et al. Abdominal pain in sickle cell disease: the role of CT. *Radiology* 1987;163:325–328.

- Magid D, Fishman EK, Seigelman SS. Computed tomography of the spleen and liver in sickle cell disease. *Am J Roentgenol*. 1984;143:245–249.

- Mortele KJ, Mortele B, Silverman SG. CT features of the accessory spleen. *Am J Roentgenol*. 2004;183:1653–1657.

- Mortele KJ, Praet M, Van Vlierberghe H, et al. Splenic and perisplenic involvement in acute pancreatitis: determination of prevalence and morphological helical CT features. *J Comput Assist Tomogr*. 2001;25:50–54.

- Shiels WE, Johnson JF, Stephenson SR, et al. Chronic torsion of the wandering spleen. *Pediatr Radiol*. 1989;19:465–467.

- Torres GM, Terry NL, Mergo PJ, et al. MR imaging of the spleen. *Magn Reson Imaging Clin North Am*. 1995;3:39–50.

- Tsuda K, Nakamura H, Murakami T, et al. Peliosis of the spleen with intraperitoneal hemorrhage. *Abdom Imaging*. 1993;18:283–285.

CHAPTER FIVE

MESENTERY, OMENTUM, AND PERITONEUM

VINCENT PELSSER,
PABLO R. ROS,
AND KOENRAAD J. MORTELE

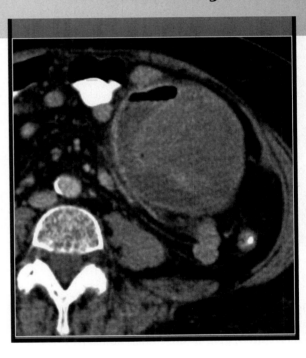

Clinical History: 49-year-old woman who underwent recent surgery for left ovarian cyst.

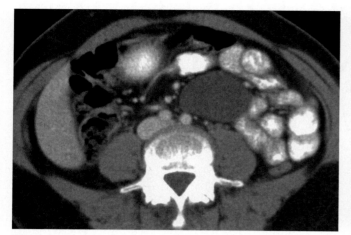

Figure 5.1   A

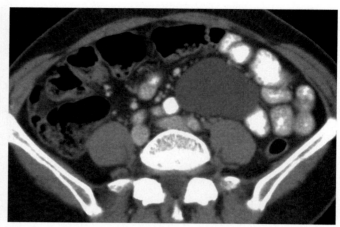

Figure 5.1   B

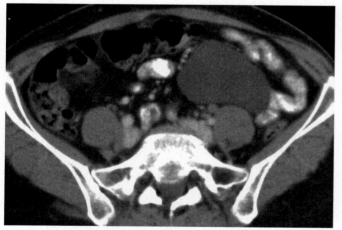

Figure 5.1   C

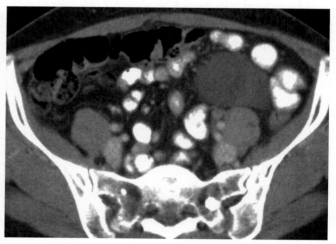

Figure 5.1   D

Findings: Axial contrast-enhanced CT (CECT) images demonstrate a homogeneous 7.2 × 5.3 cm fluid collection with imperceptible wall in the jejunal mesentery.

Differential Diagnosis: Duplication cyst, pancreatic pseudocyst, lymphangioma, ovarian cyst.

Diagnosis: Mesenteric cyst.

Discussion: Mesenteric cysts can be lined by either epithelial (duplication cyst and enteric cyst subtypes), endothelial (lymphangioma), or mesothelial (mesothelial cyst subtype) cells. If there is absence of a lining in a cyst of the mesentery, it is classified as a pseudocyst (nonpancreatic). Mesenteric cysts,

regardless of the histologic subtype, are typically filled with either serous (duplication, enteric, or mesothelial cyst), fatty or chylous (lymphangioma), hemorrhagic (pseudocyst), or purulent fluid (pseudocyst). Mesenteric cysts are usually unilocular (except lymphangioma, which is usually multilocular) and thin walled (except duplication cyst and pseudocyst, which usually have a thick wall). Lymphangioma is intimately attached to the bowel wall because it originates from it and, therefore, is one of the cyst subtypes that will require bowel resection to remove it. For the same reason, lymphangiomas may produce bowel dilatation and obstruction.

Clinical History: 69-year-old man presenting with decreased oral intake, diffuse abdominal pain, and generalized weakness.

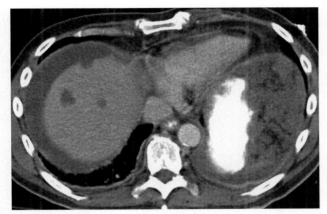

Figure 5.2   A

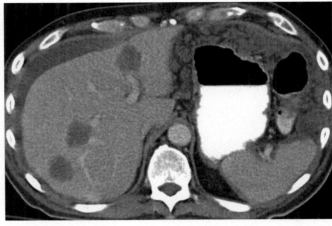

Figure 5.2   B

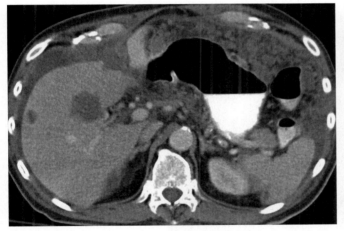

Figure 5.2   C

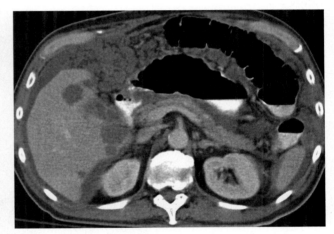

Figure 5.2   D

Findings: Axial CECT images demonstrate multiple soft tissue nodules in all peritoneal and omental compartments in the upper abdomen. Ascites and low-density liver lesions are also present.

Differential Diagnosis: Mesothelioma, tuberculosis, lymphoma.

Diagnosis: Peritoneal carcinomatosis from colon adenocarcinoma.

Discussion: Metastatic disease involving the peritoneum is commonly seen in patients with primary neoplasms of the ovary, colon, pancreas, and stomach. The metastases can have a variety of appearances. They can present as soft tissue nodules varying in size from a few millimeters to several centimeters, large plaquelike lesions along the peritoneum, and thickening of the mesentery. If the primary tumor is mucinous (ovary and colon adenocarcinoma), then the metastases can be cystic in appearance. These metastases can often be difficult to distinguish from normal unopacified or fluid-filled bowel loops. Good contrast opacification of the bowel is necessary to distinguish between normal bowel loops and metastases. Delayed imaging and decubitus scanning are often helpful.

Clinical History: 52-year-old man presenting with a palpable mass in the right abdomen.

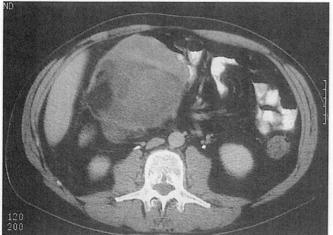

Figure 5.3   A

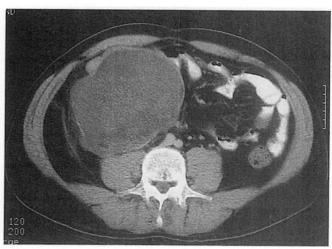

Figure 5.3   B

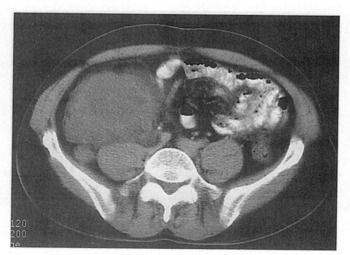

Figure 5.3   C

Findings: Axial CECT images demonstrate a large well-defined, 10-cm, solid, heterogeneously enhancing mass in the right mid abdomen arising from the mesentery. A fat attenuation area is present within the right side of the mass.

Differential Diagnosis: Teratoma.

Diagnosis: Liposarcoma.

Discussion: A large, well-defined, solid mass in the mesentery is typically due to a sarcoma, lymphoma, or ovarian neoplasm metastasis. If the mass is of fluid attenuation, abscess or hemorrhage is likely. Lymphoma tends to have homogeneous enhancement rather than heterogeneous enhancement, as seen in this case. The presence of fat narrows the differential diagnosis to a liposarcoma or teratoma. Mesenteric teratomas are extremely rare and are typically seen in the pediatric population (85% of patients are younger than 1 year of age). A large, well-defined, fat-containing lesion in the mesentery is highly suggestive of a liposarcoma. However, most abdominal liposarcomas originate in the retroperitoneum.

Clinical History: 43-year-old man presenting with abdominal pain and inability to tolerate oral intakes.

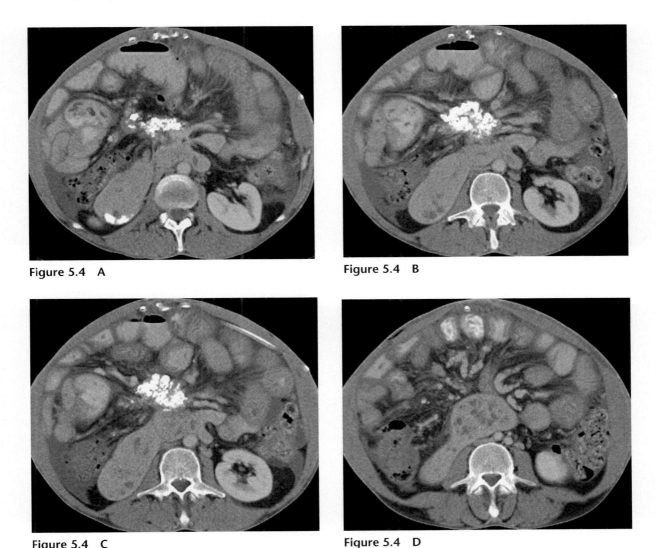

Figure 5.4   A

Figure 5.4   B

Figure 5.4   C

Figure 5.4   D

Findings: Axial CECT images demonstrate a 6.0 × 3.5 cm calcified soft tissue mass infiltrating the mesentery and causing engorgement of the mesenteric vessels. There is wall thickening of some small bowel loops anteriorly. Ascites is also present.

Differential Diagnosis: Carcinoid, metastasis, lymphoma, sarcoma.

Diagnosis: Sclerosing mesenteritis (retractile mesenteritis).

Discussion: Sclerosing mesenteritis is a disorder of unknown etiology that results in chronic inflammation and fibrosis. Depending on the predominant tissue type within the mass, sclerosing mesenteritis can be subgrouped as: (a) mesenteric panniculitis (inflammation); (b) mesenteric lipodystrophy (fat necrosis); or (c) retractile mesenteritis (fibrosis), as seen in this case. This disorder is usually confined to the mesentery and can occasionally calcify. By CT, retractile mesenteritis presents as a soft tissue mass that can contain fat and calcifications extending from the root of the mesentery towards the small bowel. This can lead to retraction and kinking of the bowel, resulting in crampy abdominal pain. The bowel wall thickening in this case is due to venous or lymphatic congestion. Carcinoid tumor arising in the small bowel can have mesenteric metastasis causing desmoplastic reaction, calcifications, and bowel kinking similar to retractile mesenteritis. This would be the best differential diagnosis in this example. Other entities that can involve the mesentery include lymphoma, metastases, and sarcomas. These do not usually calcify or cause bowel obstruction.

Clinical History: 10-year-old boy presenting with acute right-sided abdominal pain.

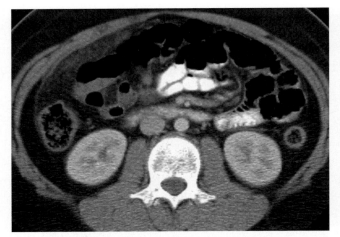

Figure 5.5   A

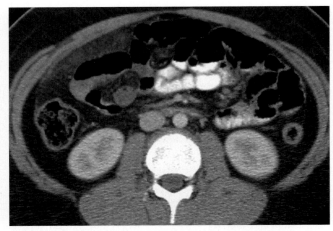

Figure 5.5   B

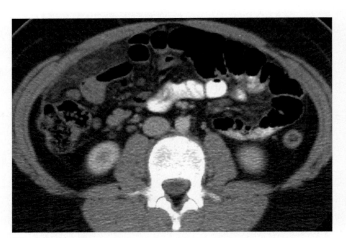

Figure 5.5   C

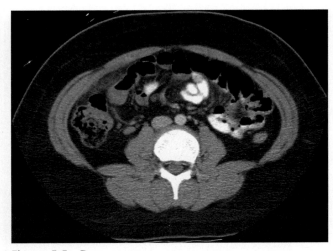

Figure 5.5   D

Findings: Axial CECT images demonstrate fat stranding anterior to the ascending colon associated with peritoneal thickening anteriorly. Adjacent bowel loops have normal wall thickness. Small regional mesenteric lymph nodes are noted.

Differential Diagnosis: Epiploic appendagitis, lymphoma, tuberculosis, metastasis.

Diagnosis: Omental infarct.

Discussion: Omental infarct is seen more frequently in males, and obesity, as seen in this case, appears to be a predisposing factor. Patients typically present with acute lower quadrant pain. The infarct may be due to torsion of the omentum, adhesions, precarious blood supply, or prior surgery. On CT, focal infiltration of the affected omentum by soft tissue stranding is seen, but a more masslike lesion mimicking a fat-containing neoplasm, such as liposarcoma, may be encountered. Clinically, an omental infarct may mimic acute appendicitis, epiploic appendagitis, or diverticulitis. Making the diagnosis by imaging is important because the treatment for this condition is symptomatic relief without surgical intervention. Spontaneous and complete resolution of the symptoms is typically observed within 2 weeks. Epiploic appendagitis is a fatty lesion on the antimesenteric side of the colon surrounded by a hyperdense rim and may have a central dot representing a thrombosed vessel. Omental lymphoma is exceedingly rare without any other involved region. Tuberculous peritonitis does not usually present acutely but could have the same CT appearance. Omental metastases are very uncommon in children.

Clinical History: 63-year-old man with a history of elevated prostate-specific antigen (PSA).

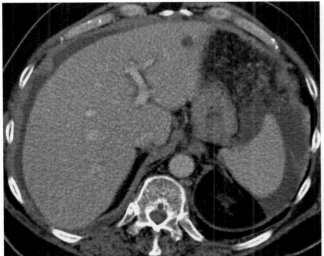
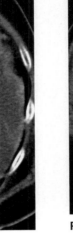

Figure 5.6   A

Figure 5.6   B

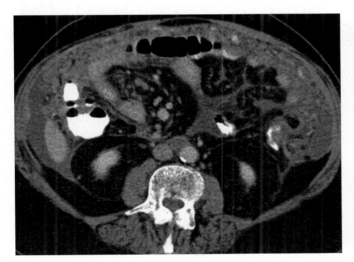

Figure 5.6   C

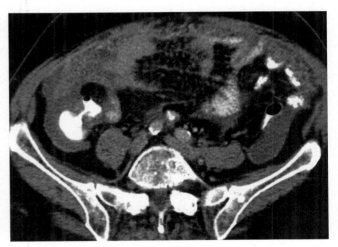

Figure 5.6   D

Findings: Axial CECT images demonstrate plaquelike and nodular soft tissue thickening of the greater omentum. Nodular thickening of peritoneal surfaces and ascites are also noted.

Differential Diagnosis: Tuberculosis, mesothelioma, lymphoma.

Diagnosis: Metastatic "omental caking" in a patient with prostate cancer.

Discussion: Omental caking is a term used to describe peritoneal metastases or other processes, such as tuberculosis, that replace the normal fat of the greater omentum. The greater omentum extends caudally from the transverse colon and is located just deep to the anterior abdominal wall. Metastases in this fat plane can thicken or replace the fatty density of the omentum with a soft tissue density, as seen in this case. The most common primary neoplasms presenting with peritoneal metastases include GI tract and ovarian malignancies. Other entities that can simulate peritoneal metastases are lymphoma, tuberculosis, and mesothelioma. Prostate carcinoma is a rare cause of omental caking, and other causes of omental thickening need to be excluded. Image-guided biopsy can easily be performed through the anterior abdominal wall, if necessary.

Clinical History: 24-year-old man with multiple abdominal surgeries for gunshot wounds presenting with hematocrit drop.

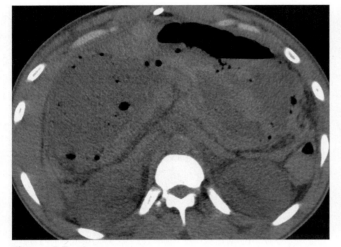

Figure 5.7   A

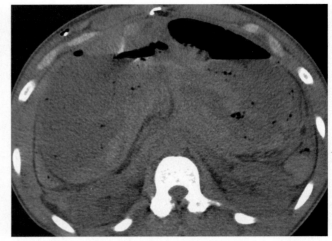

Figure 5.7   B

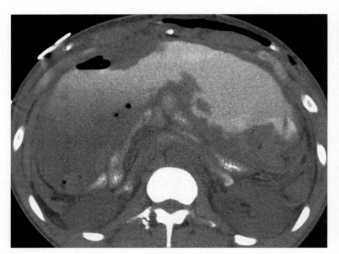

Figure 5.7   C

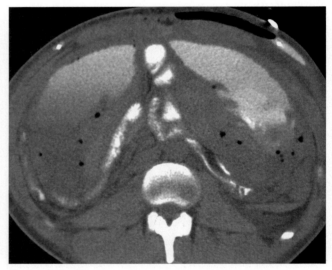

Figure 5.7   D

Findings: Nonenhanced CT (NECT) images (A and B) demonstrate a large low-attenuation mass containing multiple gas bubbles and hyperdense material (suggesting hemorrhage) encompassing most of the anterior abdominal cavity. NECT images after oral contrast administration (C and D) show contrast extravasation within the mass. Anterior pneumoperitoneum (A and B) and subcutaneous areas containing gas and contrast (D) are also present.

Differential Diagnosis: None.

Diagnosis: Peritoneal abscess secondary to perforated viscus.

Discussion: Without oral contrast, this case is difficult to correctly diagnose because of the large size of the abscess

and its anterior location. This abscess could easily be confused with a dilated stool-filled colon, as is seen in institutionalized patients. The colon, however, is displaced posteriorly by this large abscess, and no identifiable bowel wall is seen surrounding it. Pneumoperitoneum, which appears contiguous with the fluid, confirms the diagnosis of a large intra-abdominal abscess. Most of the time, abscesses can easily be drained percutaneously. The presence of pneumoperitoneum and mottled air within the lesion excludes pseudomyxoma peritonei and simple ascites.

Clinical History: 34-year-old woman presenting with increasing abdominal girth and abdominal tenderness.

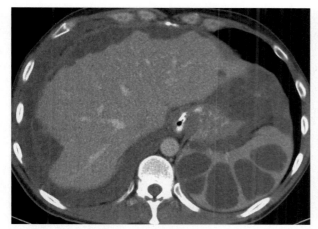

Figure 5.8   A

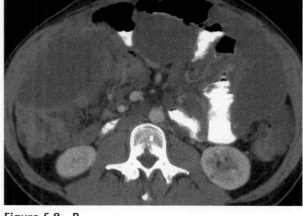

Figure 5.8   B

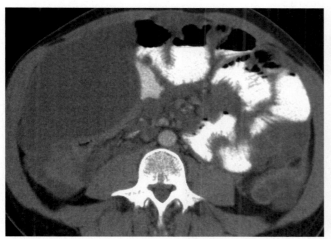

Figure 5.8   C

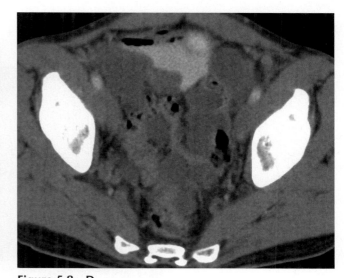

Figure 5.8   D

Findings: Axial CECT images demonstrate multiple, large, loculated fluid collections within the peritoneal cavity, including the omentum, mesentery, and serosal surface of the liver, scalloping its contour. Low-density lesions are present in the spleen.

Differential Diagnosis: Ascites, omental cyst, cystic mesothelioma, ovarian cystadenoma.

Diagnosis: Pseudomyxoma peritonei.

Discussion: Pseudomyxoma peritonei is the result of diffuse spread of mucinous material throughout the abdomen due to a mucinous neoplasm, either benign or malignant. This is most commonly due to an appendiceal or ovarian tumor but, less commonly, can be due to urachal or endometrial neoplasm. Patients present with a slow increase in abdominal girth and abdominal pain. By CT imaging, pseudomyxoma peritonei can present as a single or multiple large fluid density mass or masses compressing and scalloping adjacent organs. Occasionally, the hepatic or splenic surface implants can invade the underlying parenchyma, as seen in the spleen in this case. Septations and, rarely, calcifications can occur within pseudomyxoma peritonei. Pseudomyxoma peritonei can be localized and simulate loculated ascites. Implants can be found in peritoneal recesses where ascites or cells tend to collect, such as on the serosal surface of the liver, omentum, mesentery, subhepatic space, and pouch of Douglas.

Clinical History: 59-year-old woman presenting with abdominal pain.

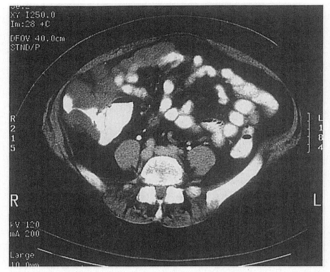

Figure 5.9   A

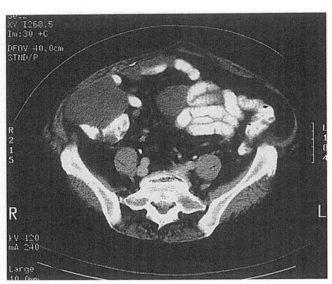

Figure 5.9   B

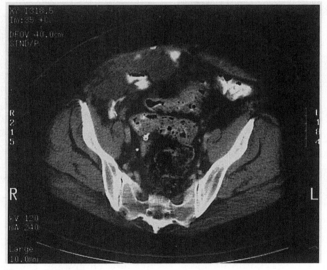

Figure 5.9   C

Findings: Axial CECT images demonstrate multiple loculated fluid collections surrounding small and large bowel loops and the anterior peritoneal surface. No bowel obstruction is seen.

Differential Diagnosis: Mesothelial cysts, cystic metastases, duplication cysts, pseudomyxoma peritonei.

Diagnosis: Cystic mesothelioma.

Discussion: Cystic mesothelioma is an uncommon primary peritoneal tumor. It is more commonly seen in females between 30 and 45 years of age, and local recurrence is common after treatment. It is, however, unrelated to malignant peritoneal mesothelioma and asbestos exposure. By CT imaging, there are multiple loculated cystic lesions found on the bowel surface, mesentery, and peritoneal surfaces, as seen in this case. Although these lesions surround and demonstrate mass effect on the bowel, obstruction is rare. The cysts in cystic mesothelioma are filled with clear fluid and are of water density by CT. Multiple cystic lesions in the abdomen can be due to cystic metastases, such as from ovarian or appendiceal primaries. Pseudomyxoma peritonei can have a similar appearance. Multiple duplication cysts and mesothelial cysts are extremely rare and would be unlikely in this case.

CASE 5-10

Clinical History: 55-year-old woman presenting with nausea and vomiting.

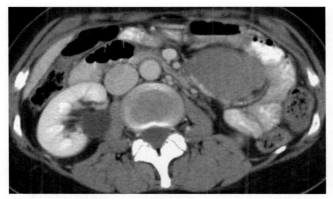

Figure 5.10   A

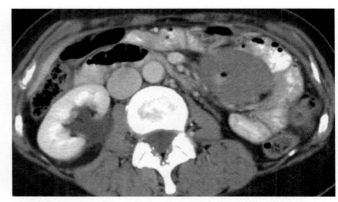

Figure 5.10   B

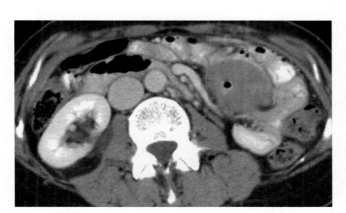

Figure 5.10   C

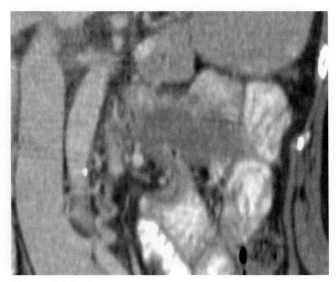

Figure 5.10   D

Findings: Axial CECT images (A–C) demonstrate a 5-cm, left-sided, homogeneous, solid mesenteric mass containing a central gas bubble and high-density material (oral contrast). The coronal reformatted CT image (D) shows a fistula between the mass and an adjacent small bowel loop.

Differential Diagnosis: Gastrointestinal stromal tumor, schwannoma, lymphoma, metastasis.

Diagnosis: Desmoid tumor.

Discussion: Desmoid tumor, a benign lesion included in the fibromatosis group, is composed entirely of fibrous tissue. It most commonly occurs in women in the third and fourth decades of life and is associated with trauma, estrogen

therapy, and pregnancy. In the abdomen, desmoid tumors most commonly involve the small bowel mesentery and represent the most common primary tumors in this location. They may also arise in the abdominal wall or in the retroperitoneum. Although benign, they can be locally aggressive, as evidenced by invasion of adjacent structures, such as in this case, which is why they are often confused with a malignant process. Desmoid tumors present as a well-circumscribed and homogeneous masses, but infiltrative margins or heterogeneity may be seen. On MRI, lesions are isointense to muscle on T1-weighted images (WI) and variable in signal intensity on T2-WI. Despite complete excision, the recurrence rate after surgery may be as high as 77%.

Clinical History: 59-year-old man with previous Billroth II surgery presenting with acute left upper quadrant pain.

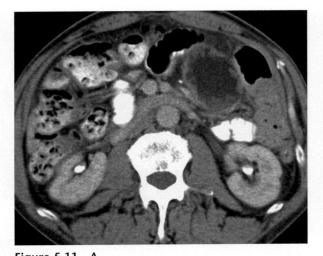

Figure 5.11   A

Figure 5.11   B

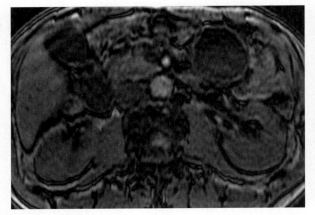

Figure 5.11   C

Figure 5.11   D

Findings: Axial CECT image (A) shows a 6.4 × 4.5 cm, fat-containing mesenteric mass with dependent debris surrounded by a nodular rim of soft tissue density. MRI shows a fat-fluid level within the mass with nondependent bright fluid on the in-phase axial T1-WI (B) that suppresses on the out-of-phase axial T1-WI (C). Gadolinium-enhanced, fat-suppressed axial T1-WI (D) shows a rim-enhancing unilocular cyst.

Differential Diagnosis: Liposarcoma, lipoma, teratoma, lymphangioma, duplication cyst, abscess, pancreatic pseudocyst.

Diagnosis: Chylous cyst (nonpancreatic pseudocyst).

Discussion: A chylous cyst is a rare type of mesenteric cyst, classified as a nonpancreatic pseudocyst. It contains chyle in various quantities, which accounts for the fat attenuation identified on CT. A fat-fluid level, the less dense fat being nondependent, is thought to be almost diagnostic of lesions containing chyle. On MRI, the liquid composed of microscopic fat would appear bright on T1-WI, and the intensity of that liquid would suppress on the out-of-phase T1-WI. The dependent debris identified on CT and the thick walls in this case are likely related to internal hemorrhage because multiple abnormal blood vessels were identified around the cyst at pathology. A lymphangioma or a teratoma would be the best differential diagnosis in this case. Lymphangiomas may contain chyle and thus have negative attenuation values, but they are often multilocular. Teratomas may have an identical appearance to chylous cysts. Identification of calcifications or of a hairball is helpful to allow the diagnosis of a teratoma. Liposarcomas and lipomas are solid fat-containing lesions and would not have a fat-fluid level. This is the same for duplication cysts, abscesses, and pancreatic pseudocysts that are also thick-walled cysts in a mesenteric location and typically do not contain fat.

Clinical History: 9-month-old boy presenting with a palpable abdominal mass.

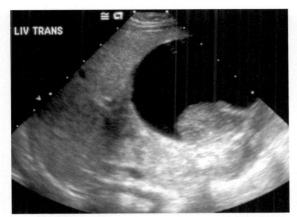

Figure 5.12   A

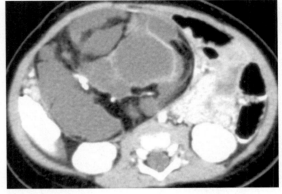

Figure 5.12   B

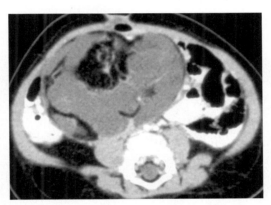

Figure 5.12   C

Findings: Sonographic axial image (A) through the right upper quadrant demonstrates a large cystic, well-defined lesion with a dependent echogenic nodule, causing mass effect on the liver. Axial CECT images (B and C) show that the mesenteric mass is composed of fluid and fat attenuation areas, with coarse calcifications and multiple septations. A thin dense peripheral rim is seen in some segments of the mass.

Differential Diagnosis: Lipoblastoma, liposarcoma, lipoma, hibernoma.

Diagnosis: Mesenteric teratoma.

Discussion: Nongonadal abdominal teratomas are extremely rare, occurring once in every million births. Nearly all nongonadal abdominal teratomas are encountered in the pediatric age group. Most teratomas in the pediatric population, however, occur in a sacrococcygeal location. Teratomas are usually derived from all three germinal layers and frequently contain skin appendages, cartilage, bone, teeth, and adipose tissue. The imaging characteristics of teratomas, reflecting the histologic features of the lesion, are all present in this case and consist of multiple cystic areas of varying sizes, coarse calcifications, fat areas that are peripherally located, and a capsule that is responsible for the well-marginated appearance of the mass. Sonography is very valuable to assess the cystic portions of the mass, while CT depicts with great specificity the fat areas and calcifications. Prognosis after complete surgical excision is excellent. Lipoblastomas are rapidly growing, benign mesenchymal tumors almost always seen before the age of 10 years; however, these tumors occur most commonly in the superficial soft tissues of the extremities. A lipoblastoma is a well-defined lesion, but when infiltrative, it is called lipoblastomatosis. Lipoblastomas are composed of fat and soft tissue areas but do not contain cystic spaces or calcifications, which is key to differentiating them from teratomas. Similarly, hibernomas (which most frequently occur in adults) and lipomas do not have cystic spaces. Liposarcomas are extremely rare under the age of 10 years (only 2 cases in 2500 in the Armed Forces Institute of Pathology series) and unheard of under the age of 2 years.

Case images courtesy of Dr. Angela D. Levy, Armed Forces Institute of Pathology, Washington, DC.

Clinical History: 75-year-old man presenting with weight loss and a palpable abdominal mass.

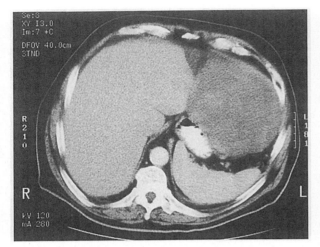

Figure 5.13   A

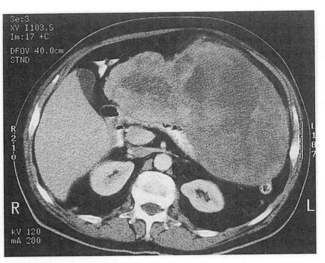

Figure 5.13   B

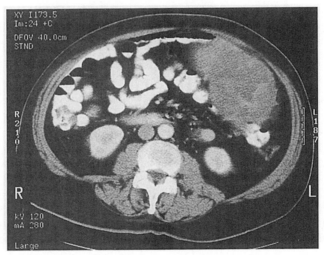

Figure 5.13   C

Findings: Axial CECT images demonstrate a large 30-cm, well-defined heterogeneous enhancing mass in the left abdomen originating near the diaphragm and extending caudally to the pelvis.

Differential Diagnosis: Metastasis, lymphoma, desmoid tumor (fibromatosis).

Diagnosis: Malignant fibrous histiocytoma.

Discussion: Malignant fibrous histiocytoma (MFH) is a soft tissue sarcoma that most commonly arises in the proximal portions (e.g., thigh, arm) of the extremities followed by the retroperitoneum. Rarely MFH arises from the mesentery, as seen in this case. As with most sarcomas, MFH tends to appear by CT as a well-defined, large mass. MFHs are hypervascular and enhance with contrast administration. Other solid masses in the mesentery can be due to lymphoma, metastases, and fibromatosis. There is no adenopathy to suggest lymphoma, and metastases tend to be smaller, multiple masses. Pancreatic pseudocyst and mesenteric cyst are excluded due to the solid nature of this lesion, confirmed by central enhancement. Fibromatosis and one of the various sarcomas are the best differential diagnostic possibilities in this case.

CASE 5-14

Clinical History: 28-year-old man presenting with marked abdominal distension, diffuse abdominal pain, and fatigue. A testicular mass was detected on physical exam.

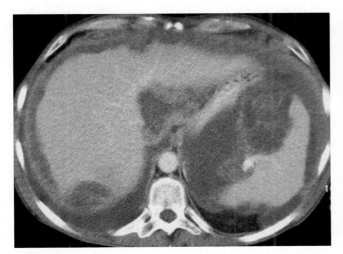

Figure 5.14   A

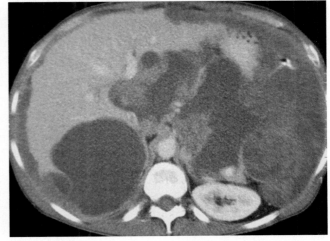

Figure 5.14   B

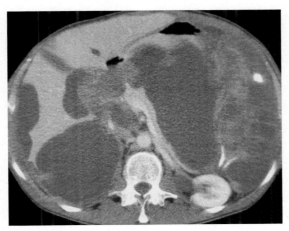

Figure 5.14   C

Findings: Axial CECT images show involvement of the peritoneal cavity by fluid density material that is seen indenting the liver and the spleen and compressing the stomach and the colon. Several loops of bowel, the stomach, and the pancreas are displaced. Liver scalloping is noted. The retroperitoneum appears uninvolved.

Differential Diagnosis: Tuberculosis peritonitis, peritoneal carcinomatosis, peritoneal lymphangiomatosis, pseudomyxoma peritonei.

Diagnosis: Metastatic choriocarcinoma.

Discussion: Choriocarcinoma is a very rare neoplasm in men but can occur in the context of a mixed germ cell tumor of the testis with predominance of the choriocarcinoma element. Metastases from choriocarcinomas into the peritoneal cavity are, in addition, extremely rare. By imaging, they are characterized by massive involvement of the peritoneal cavity with cystic masses producing scalloping of the liver and other solid organs and mimicking the appearance of pseudomyxoma peritonei, which is the main differential diagnosis. In this case, the history of a testicular mass may suggest the diagnosis. Prognosis of metastatic choriocarcinoma to the peritoneum in men is very poor. Testicular germ cell tumors present in approximately 50% of patients with metastases. These metastases can occur in the liver, lung, brain, and rarely the peritoneum. Beta subunit of human chorionic gonadotropin (HCG) would be very elevated due to the large tumor burden. Peritoneal tuberculosis is a possibility, but the massive involvement and lack of omental caking and adenopathy would make this diagnosis less likely.

Clinical History: 35-year-old woman post gastric bypass surgery.

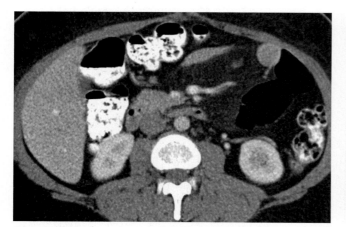

Figure 5.15 A

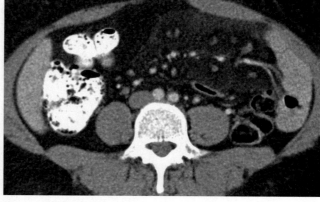

Figure 5.15 B

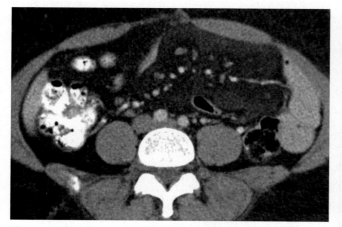

Figure 5.15 C

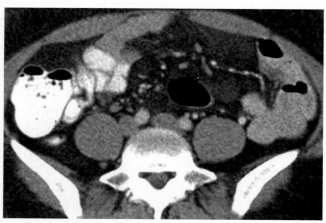

Figure 5.15 D

Findings: Axial CECT images demonstrate a large mass, with a density slightly higher than the retroperitoneal fat and causing mass effect on adjacent bowel loops. A hypodense fatty halo surrounds the multiple small mesenteric nodules. The mesenteric veins are engorged.

Differential Diagnosis: Lymphoma, lipoma, liposarcoma, peritoneal carcinomatosis.

Diagnosis: Sclerosing mesenteritis (mesenteric panniculitis).

Discussion: Sclerosing mesenteritis is a disorder of unknown etiology that results in chronic inflammation and eventually fibrosis. When the predominant process is inflammatory, it is subcategorized as mesenteric panniculitis. It is associated with other autoimmune processes such as retroperitoneal fibrosis, sclerosing cholangitis, Riedel thyroiditis,

and orbital pseudotumor. An association with malignancies, such as lymphoma, melanoma, and breast, lung, and colon cancer, has been described in up to 69% of patients. CT features are discrete fat stranding in the mesenteric fat, which may have a masslike appearance; a left-sided orientation; scattered, less than 5-mm, soft tissue nodules; a hypodense fatty halo (called "fat ring sign") surrounding the nodules and vessels; and a hyperattenuating stripe surrounding the mass. The constellation of these features is quite unique to mesenteric panniculitis and, when present, allows a more confident diagnosis. These imaging characteristics would not be present in lymphoma, lipoma, liposarcoma, or peritoneal carcinomatosis. Lymphoma may be the hardest to differentiate from mesenteric panniculitis, but the fat ring sign, not seen in cases of lymphoma, would be a key distinguishing feature.

Clinical History: 61-year-old woman presenting with intermittent abdominal pain.

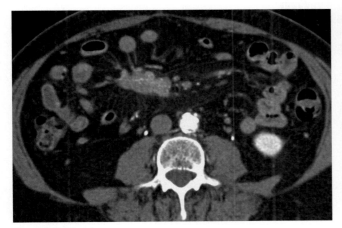

Figure 5.16   A

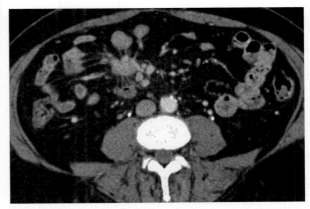

Figure 5.16   B

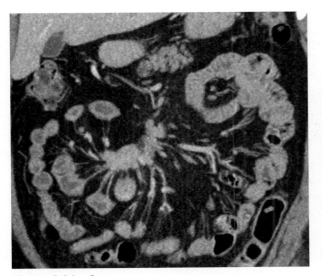

Figure 5.16   C

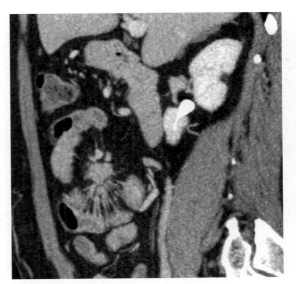

Figure 5.16   D

Findings: Axial (A and B), coronal (C), and sagittal reformatted (D) CECT images demonstrate a 4.5 × 2.2 cm mesenteric mass in the right lower abdomen with punctate central calcifications and desmoplastic reaction tethering the surrounding small bowel loops.

Differential Diagnosis: Retractile mesenteritis, desmoid tumor, lymphoma, sarcoma, metastasis.

Diagnosis: Mesenteric metastasis from carcinoid tumor.

Discussion: Carcinoid tumors are neuroendocrine neoplasms categorized as apudomas because they arise from the amine precursor uptake and decarboxylation cells (APUD cells). Presenting symptoms are vague, such as intermittent abdominal pain, and the diagnosis is often delayed until the patient develops the carcinoid syndrome, which consists of flushing and diarrhea, due to release of vasoactive substances from hepatic metastases. The most common sites of origin of carcinoid tumors are the appendix, the terminal ileum, and the rectum. The tumor originates in the bowel submucosa. Histologic differentiation between benign and malignant carcinoid tumors can be impossible. The probability of metastasis is directly related to the size of the primary tumor. The primary tumors are often difficult to localize on CT due to their small size. However, CT is excellent to demonstrate mesenteric or hepatic metastases. The appearance of mesenteric metastasis is typical, consisting of a mass with central calcifications in 70% of cases. The surrounding desmoplastic reaction can be intense and produces vascular encasement that may lead to bowel ischemia. Retractile mesenteritis may mimic every aspect of mesenteric carcinoid, and the only distinguishing features for differentiating it with a carcinoid tumor would be the lack of a bowel nodule or of liver metastasis in cases of retractile mesenteritis.

Clinical History: 80-year-old woman presenting with recurrent episodes of epigastric pain.

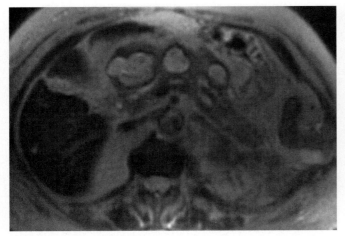

Figure 5.17   A

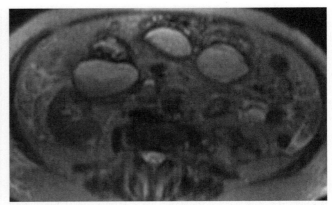

Figure 5.17   B

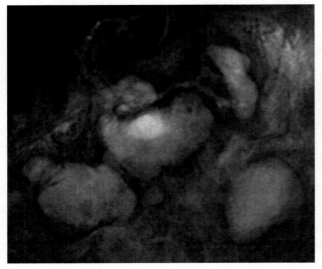

Figure 5.17   C

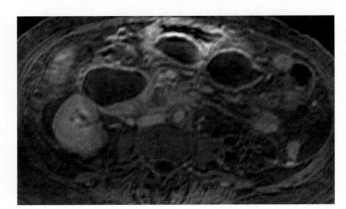

Figure 5.17   D

Findings: Axial T2-WI shows several thick-walled, fluid-filled cysts anterior to the pancreas (A) and in the mesentery (B). The most right-sided cyst contains dependent hypointense debris. Projective coronal, oblique, thick-slab magnetic resonance cholangiopancreatography (MRCP) image (C) shows cysts around the pancreatic duct and more inferiorly in the mesentery. Gadolinium-enhanced, fat-saturated axial T1-WI (D) demonstrates enhancement of the cyst walls.

Differential Diagnosis: Abscess, pancreatic cystic neoplasm, enteric duplication cyst.

Diagnosis: Pancreatic pseudocysts.

Discussion: Pancreatic pseudocyst is one of the most common complications of acute pancreatitis. The exudate and pancreatic fluid released at the time of the acute attack can dissect in virtually any peritoneal or retroperitoneal space, organ, or even extraperitoneal or thoracic regions. The fluid may become walled-off by adjacent organs or by fibrous tissue. The resultant cyst is termed pseudocyst because it does not have a true epithelial lining. The cyst may contain fluid or debris. Typically, a semirecent episode ($\geq$6 weeks) of acute pancreatitis is elicited and helps in making the correct diagnosis. A primary pancreatic cystic neoplasm may have thick walls but would be solitary and not multiple, as in this case. The only other mesenteric cyst that has a thick wall is an enteric duplication cyst, but this cyst is also solitary. Unless gas is present within the fluid, an infected fluid collection (pancreatic abscess) cannot be reliably differentiated from a noninfected collection by imaging, and percutaneous needle aspiration is often needed to confirm the presence of infection.

Clinical History: 25-year-old woman presenting with right upper quadrant pain.

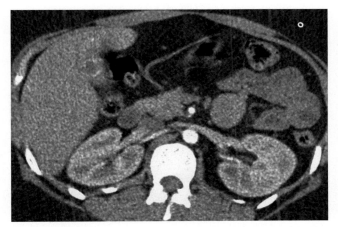

Figure 5.18 A

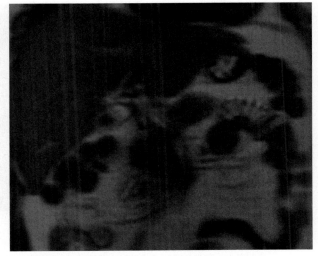

Figure 5.18 B

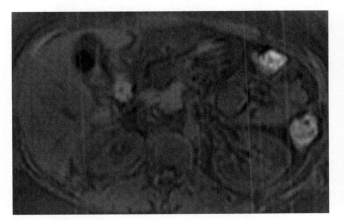

Figure 5.18 C

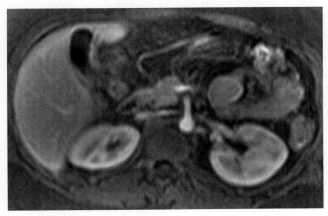

Figure 5.18 D

Findings: Axial CECT image (A) shows a 2.8 × 2.6 cm, well-defined mass in the mesentery. The mass is homogenous and isointense to muscle on coronal T2-WI (B) and fat-saturated axial T1-WI (C) and demonstrates marked enhancement on the gadolinium-enhanced, fat-saturated axial T1-WI (D).

Differential Diagnosis: Desmoid tumor (fibromatosis), lymphoma, metastasis, gastrointestinal stromal tumor.

Diagnosis: Castleman disease, hyaline-vascular type.

Discussion: Castleman disease is also known as benign giant lymph node hyperplasia or angiofollicular hyperplasia. Two histologic subtypes have been described: (a) the hyaline vascular type, which accounts for 90% of cases and is most commonly solitary; and (b) the plasma cell type, which accounts for the remaining 10% of cases and can be either solitary or multifocal. Occasionally, a mixed form may be encountered. The hyaline vascular subtype occurs in patients younger than 30 years old in 70% of cases and is usually asymptomatic. Castleman disease involves the abdomen in 12% of cases, with most lesions being located in the retroperitoneum and pelvis, but it is also encountered in the mesentery or porta hepatis. Smaller lesions present as well-circumscribed homogeneous masses that may contain calcifications, whereas larger lesions can be heterogeneous. They are typically isointense to muscle on T1-WI and hyperintense on T2-WI. Hypervascularity of the mass is characteristic on postcontrast images; this feature allows differentiation with lymphoma, which is usually hypovascular. A connection to bowel is usually present in cases of gastrointestinal stromal tumor; such a sign was not seen in this case.

Clinical History: 33-year-old man with acquired immunodeficiency virus (AIDS) presenting with fever.

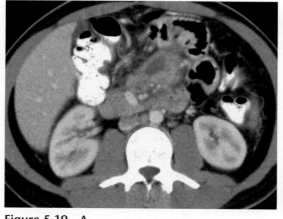

Figure 5.19   A

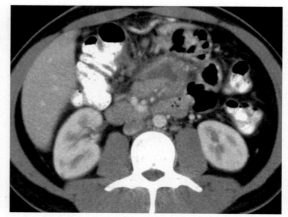

Figure 5.19   B

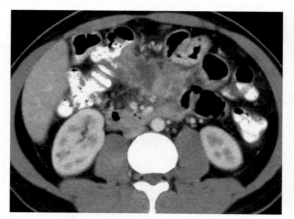

Figure 5.19   C

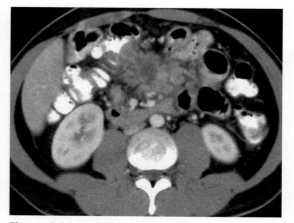

Figure 5.19   D

Findings: Axial CECT images demonstrate an ill-defined, 3.3 × 2.2 cm mesenteric mass with central hypodensity. Note surrounding fat stranding and smaller satellite nodules.

Differential Diagnosis: *Mycobacterium tuberculosis* infection, abscess, metastasis, lymphoma, Kaposi sarcoma, celiac disease, Whipple disease.

Diagnosis: *Mycobacterium avium-intracellulare* lymphadenopathy.

Discussion: Human immunodeficiency virus (HIV) infection eventually results in reduction in the number of CD4 lymphocytes, which leads to significant immunosuppression, predisposing affected individuals to both malignancies and opportunistic infections. *Mycobacterium avium-intracellulare* (MAI) infection usually develops when the CD4 count falls below 100 cells μL^{-1}, whereas *Mycobacterium tuberculosis* (MTB) infection is more prevalent when the CD4 is above 200 cells μL^{-1}. This patient's CD4 count was 32 cells μL^{-1}. There is significant overlap in the abdominal radiologic findings of both MTB and MAI; lymphadenopathy, hepatomegaly,

splenomegaly, and focal hepatic, splenic, and renal lesions are features common to both. However, necrotic lymph nodes are much more frequent in MTB but can also be seen with MAI. Another distinguishing feature between MAI and MTB is the location of potential small bowel involvement, which is proximal in MAI and distal in MTB. Infection with cytomegalovirus producing severe colitis or with *Pneumocystis carinii* producing small low-attenuation splenic and hepatic lesions with calcification can also be observed in patients with AIDS. AIDS patients are also prone to infection by many other organisms. Visceral involvement by Kaposi sarcoma is almost always preceded by skin lesions; lymph nodes are typically hypervascular following contrast administration. Lymphoma presents as bulky lymphadenopathy, which may be necrotic in AIDS patients. In patients with cavitating mesenteric lymph node syndrome in celiac disease or low-density lymph nodes in Whipple disease, symptoms of or a history of these diseases are almost always present. Percutaneous biopsy is often needed, as was performed in this case, to correctly diagnose the cause of the lymphadenopathy.

Clinical History: 68-year-old man presenting with dyspepsia.

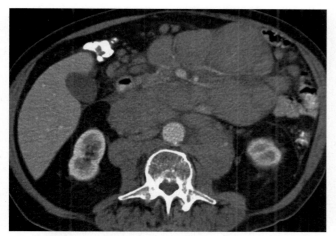

Figure 5.22   A

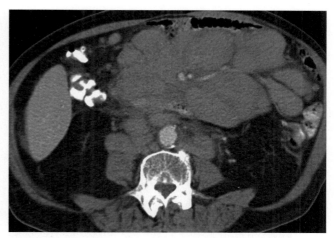

Figure 5.22   B

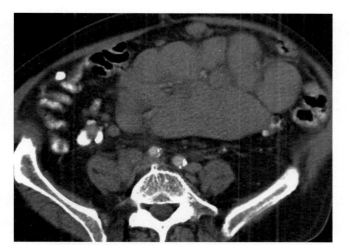

Figure 5.22   C

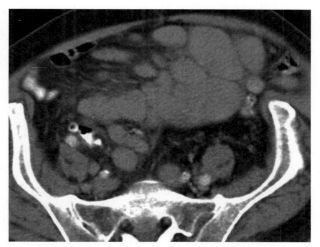

Figure 5.22   D

Findings: Axial CECT images demonstrate homogeneous, large, confluent, predominantly mesenteric but also retroperitoneal masses with well-defined borders.

Differential Diagnosis: Metastasis, mesenteric panniculitis, desmoid tumor.

Diagnosis: Lymphoma.

Discussion: Lymphoma is a common cause of massive lymphadenopathy in the abdomen. Most commonly, non-Hodgkin lymphoma is identified at pathology. Lymph nodes in all nodal stations can be involved. The characteristic appearance of untreated lymphoma is a homogeneous mass even when it is large. Rarely, untreated lymphoma may have central necrosis. Treated lymphoma may have decreased central density on CECT or surrounding mesenteric stranding.

Knowledge of the treatment status is important when interpreting the CT study in order to not confuse treated lymphoma with other causes of necrotic lymph node, such as tuberculosis or metastasis. Percutaneous biopsy is the method of choice to establish the correct diagnosis. The most easily accessible mass, which may not necessarily be abdominal, should be targeted for biopsy. Large-needle biopsy is required to adequately subtype the lymphoma. Metastasis may be indistinguishable from lymphoma and would be the best differential diagnosis in this case. There are too many masses for this process to represent desmoid tumors. In mesenteric panniculitis, the mesenteric nodules are smaller, typically less than 5 mm, and are surrounded by a hypodense fatty halo.

Clinical History: 36-year-old man with congenital hydrocephalus presenting with nausea.

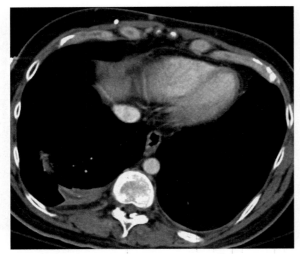

Figure 5.23　A

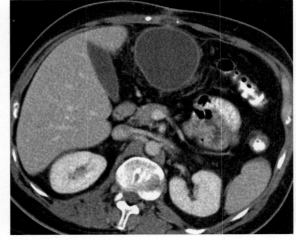

Figure 5.23　B

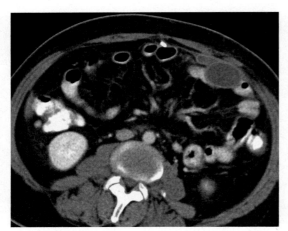

Figure 5.23　C

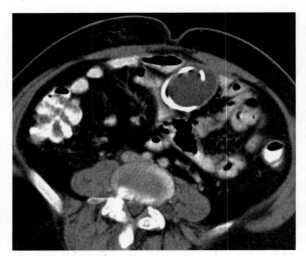

Figure 5.23　D

Findings: Axial CECT images demonstrate several thin-walled cysts within the peritoneal space. A catheter courses craniocaudally through the abdominal wall with its distal end curled in one of the mesenteric cysts.

Differential Diagnosis: Pancreatic pseudocyst, duplication cysts, metastasis.

Diagnosis: Cerebrospinal fluid nonpancreatic pseudocyst.

Discussion: Cerebrospinal fluid (CSF) pseudocysts are commonly referred to as "CSFomas." They represent rare complications of ventriculoperitoneal shunting, occurring in 0.7% to 10% of cases. Formation of these cysts is thought to be related to peritoneal inflammatory response to CSF proteins, prior surgery with adhesions, and sequela of infection, which has been suggested as the leading cause. Presenting symptoms are mainly abdominal in adults, whereas in children, they may be either abdominal or related to increased intracranial pressure. Other abdominal complications of ventriculoperitoneal shunts include tube fracture, bowel obstruction, and perforation and blockage of the catheter tip. CSF pseudocysts are thin-walled cystic lesions typically surrounding the shunt tip. Identification of the shunt is key to the diagnosis. The absence of a history of acute pancreatitis makes a pancreatic origin unlikely. Sometimes, metastasis seeding the abdomen from the brain through the shunt may present as cystic masses, but the cyst walls would be thick, irregular, and nodular. Duplication cysts are often solitary and not associated with a catheter, as in this case. Treatment of CSF pseudocysts classically consists of shunt externalization and antibiotic therapy followed by shunt revision and internalization.

Clinical History: 57-year-old man status post aortic valve replacement presenting with diffuse abdominal pain of 3 days in duration.

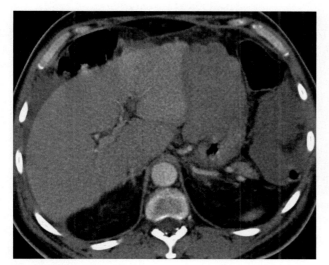

Figure 5.24   A

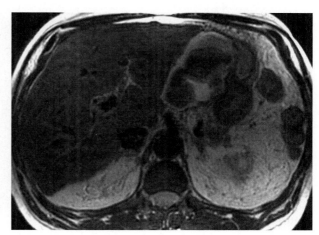

Figure 5.24   B

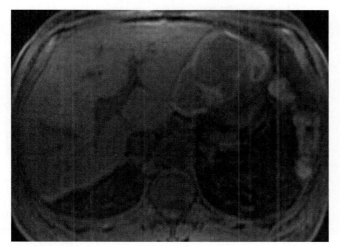

Figure 5.24   C

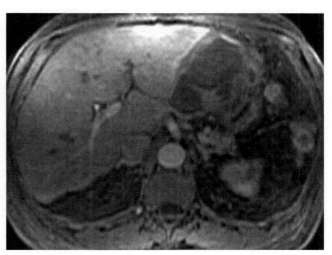

Figure 5.24   D

Findings: Axial CECT image (A) shows a hyperdense 10 × 8 cm mass in the gastrohepatic ligament associated with ascites. Axial T2-WI (B) shows the mass to be partly cystic with central hypointensity. Unenhanced fat-saturated axial T1-WI (C) shows high signal intensity areas within the mass. No enhancement is seen on the gadolinium-enhanced, fat-saturated axial T1-WI (D).

Differential Diagnosis: Metastasis, abscess, sarcoma.

Diagnosis: Hematoma.

Discussion: A key element in this case is the history of prior aortic valve replacement. After valvular replacement, patients are placed on warfarin (Coumadin). Patients on warfarin can have spontaneous hematomas in the retroperitoneum as well as in the peritoneal cavity. Spontaneous hematoma in the gastrohepatic ligament is uncommon. Hematomas in this location, although rare, can occur due to ruptured aneurysms of the hepatic artery or the superior mesenteric artery. The high attenuation of this mass on CECT, the lack of enhancement after gadolinium administration, and the signal intensity of the contents of this mass by MRI are all diagnostic clues for a hematoma. The lack of enhancement and of history of a primary tumor diminishes the possibility of a metastatic deposit in the gastrohepatic ligament. The history also does not match that of an abscess. Primary sarcoma of the lesser omentum is possible, but again, the lack of enhancement by MRI also makes this diagnosis unlikely.

Clinical History: 20-year-old woman presenting with an enlarging abdominal mass.

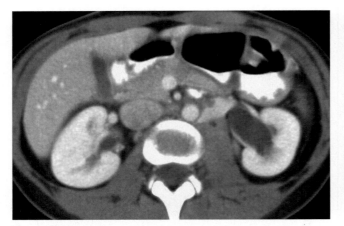

Figure 5.25   A

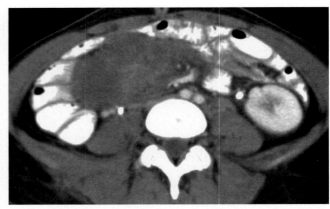

Figure 5.25   B

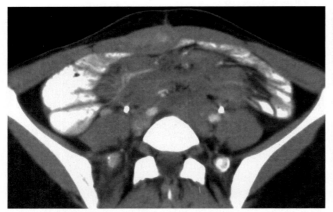

Figure 5.25   C

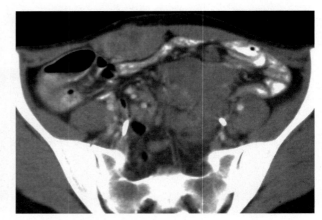

Figure 5.25   D

Findings: CECT images demonstrate a large heterogeneous mesenteric mass that has ill-defined margins. A smaller heterogeneous mass is present in the right rectus abdominis muscle. Note also the absence of the entire colon.

Differential Diagnosis: Metastasis, sarcoma.

Diagnosis: Desmoid tumors in a patient with familial adenomatous polyposis syndrome.

Discussion: Familial adenomatous polyposis syndrome (FAPS) is an autosomal dominant disease in which hundreds of adenomatous polyps originate from the colonic mucosa. Colon cancers develop in virtually 100% of affected patients, and therefore, prophylactic total colectomy at a young age is recommended. The absence of the colon in a young patient, such as in this case, is an important clue to the correct diagnosis. Desmoid tumors are common extracolonic abdominal findings in patients with FAPS and are among the leading cause of morbidity and mortality in these patients. Desmoid tumors typically present as well-circumscribed, homogeneous, noncalcified masses, but infiltrative margins or heterogeneity may be seen. They can invade or cause compression on adjacent structures, such as the ureter or bowel. Medical therapy is initially favored because the recurrence rate after surgical resection is very high. Polyps involving the remainder of the gastrointestinal tract from the stomach to the ileum and carcinomas in the periampullary region, pancreas, gallbladder, and bile ducts are other abdominal manifestations of FAPS.

Clinical History: 70-year-old man complaining of two episodes of melena in the last 14 months.

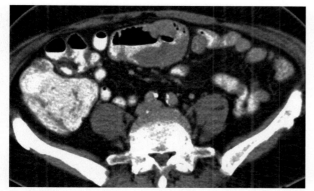

Figure 5.26   A

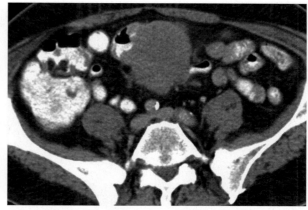

Figure 5.26   B

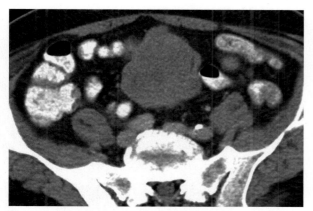

Figure 5.26   C

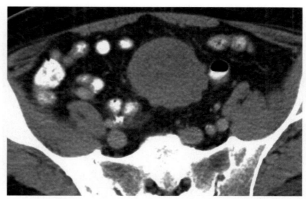

Figure 5.26   D

Findings: Axial CECT images show an 8.2 × 7.4 cm, mesenteric mass displacing and invading a loop of small bowel. There are pockets of gas within the mass and a contrast-filled track.

Differential Diagnosis: Metastasis, desmoid tumor (fibromatosis), lymphoma, malignant fibrous histiocytoma, neural tumor.

Diagnosis: Gastrointestinal stromal tumor.

Discussion: Gastrointestinal stromal tumor (GIST) is a mesenchymal spindle cell (80%) or epithelioid (20%) neoplasm. GIST is a relatively new entity because, in the past, most of these tumors were diagnosed pathologically as leiomyomas, leiomyoblastomas, or leiomyosarcomas. The histologic diagnosis is based on a positive C-kit stain. GISTs occur most often in the stomach (60–70%), followed by the small bowel, the colon/rectum, and, least likely, the esophagus (<5%). The majority of GISTs are benign, but up to 30% can be malignant. The factors that increase the likelihood of malignancy include an extragastric location, size greater than 5 cm, central necrosis, extension into adjacent organs, and distant metastases (most commonly in the liver and peritoneum). GIST can grow in different patterns. This case exhibits an exoenteric growth pattern, with the bulk of the tumor placed in the small bowel mesentery. This is the most common growth pattern (65% of cases) in small bowel GIST. Other growth patterns include intramural and intraluminal. Exoenteric GISTs, like this one, are discovered later than endoenteric GISTs. They are not discovered until they attain a large size and present as a palpable mass or bleed into the lumen due to tumoral excavation, as in this case. Lymphoma may present with a similar appearance, but the lack of adenopathy and the exoentric bowel involvement in this case make lymphoma less likely. Melanoma or breast metastasis may have the same appearance, but there is no history for such a primary. Other sarcomas, such as malignant fibrous histiocytoma, will typically have a faster evolution and be larger with marked central necrosis. Neural tumors will not erode into the lumen, such as in this case.

CASE 5-27

Clinical History: 22-year-old man presenting with abdominal pain and tenderness.

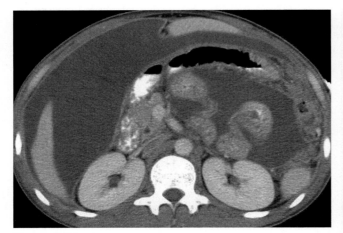

Figure 5.27   A

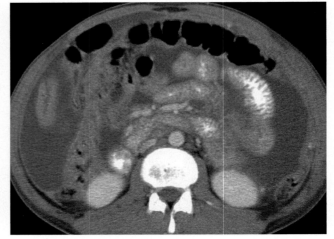

Figure 5.27   B

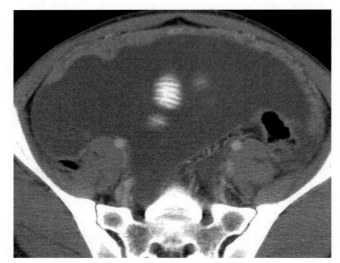

Figure 5.27   C

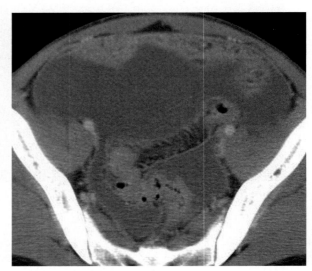

Figure 5.27   D

Findings: Axial CECT images demonstrate high-density ascites as well as a thick enhancing peritoneum. There are also omental and retroperitoneal lymph nodes.

Differential Diagnosis: Peritoneal carcinomatosis, malignant mesothelioma.

Diagnosis: Tuberculosis peritonitis and omentitis.

Discussion: Although tuberculosis is unusual in Western countries, there has been an increased incidence of tuberculosis due to the larger number of chronically immunosuppressed patients due to transplantation, HIV infection, and other causes. Extrapulmonary tuberculosis has proportionally also increased, reaching up to 15% of new cases of tuberculosis documented in the United State. Furthermore,

in only 15% of cases of abdominal tuberculosis, there is pulmonary disease. Ascites due to tuberculosis has high attenuation (20–45 HU) due to the high protein and cellular contents. CT also demonstrates peritoneal thickening, enhancement, and sometimes nodularity corresponding to the tuberculomas present in it. Omental caking can be seen in up to 82% of patients with abdominal tuberculosis. Peritoneal carcinomatosis is very difficult to distinguish from tuberculous peritonitis except for the fact that, in the latter, there is history of a known malignancy. Peritoneal mesothelioma can also produce some of the findings seen in tuberculous peritonitis, but the peritoneal thickening is much more pronounced, and the ascites is less massive than in tuberculosis.

Clinical History: 45-year-old man presenting with loss of consciousness.

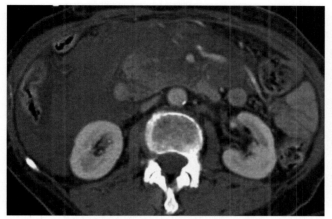

Figure 5.28   A

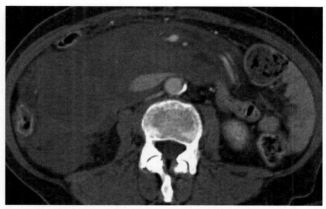

Figure 5.28   B

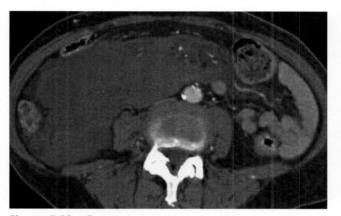

Figure 5.28   C

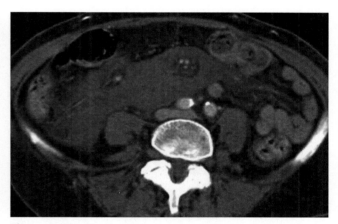

Figure 5.28   D

Findings: CECT images demonstrate a very large mesenteric mass extending to the right anterior pararenal space. It is heterogeneous with hyperdense areas, and some of its borders are ill defined.

Differential Diagnosis: Lymphoma, desmoid tumor.

Diagnosis: Hematoma.

Discussion: Mesenteric hematoma can be iatrogenic, due to trauma or anticoagulation. The clinical history can often elicit the cause. Rarely, a hematoma can be idiopathic, as in this case, and an underlying lesion that bled should be excluded. Depending on the age of the blood, it may be hyperdense to muscle on CT when it is acute, and it becomes isodense to hypodense as it progressively liquefies.

The spontaneous hyperdensity of blood can be difficult to detect on CECT, and this can lead to diagnostic errors. In the absence of a relevant history, it can be easily confused with an infiltrative neoplasm, and patients may be referred for percutaneous biopsy, which would yield only blood. If there is radiologic suspicion that a lesion may be hemorrhagic, MRI may be performed to target any enhancing component at the time of the biopsy. A positron emission tomography (PET) scan would show no metabolic activity in case of a hematoma and may be helpful in selected cases. Lymphoma is usually of homogeneous density despite its large size. A desmoid tumor would be the best differential diagnosis in this case.

Clinical History: 30-year-old man post recent abdominal sarcoma resection presenting with fever and mild abdominal pain.

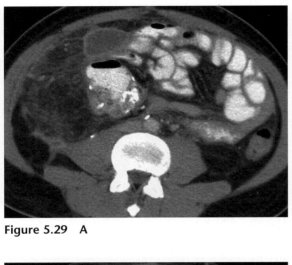

Figure 5.29   A

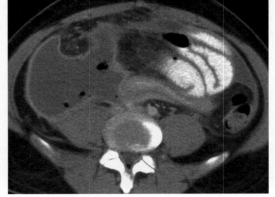

Figure 5.29   B

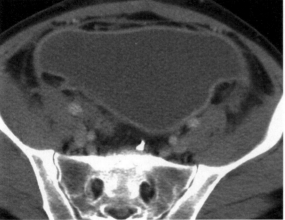

Figure 5.29   C

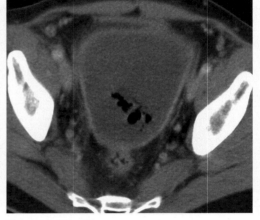

Figure 5.29   D

Findings: Axial CECT images demonstrate a large 18 × 8 cm, fluid density, space-occupying lesion located in the right lower quadrant and pelvis, surrounded by fat stranding. This lesion also contains several pockets of gas and has rim enhancement. Note the presence of a small amount of ascites.

Differential Diagnosis: Intraperitoneal hematoma, cystic mesothelioma, mesenteric cyst.

Diagnosis: Intraperitoneal abscess.

Discussion: A large majority of intraperitoneal abscesses are a sequela of an intra-abdominal surgical procedure. There are other causes, such as perforated diverticulitis or appendicitis and pelvic inflammatory disease. Intraperitoneal abscess, if unrecognized and untreated, continues to be a dangerous process, with a mortality rate of up to 30%. The advent of percutaneous drainage of intra-abdominal and pelvic abscesses offers patients with intraperitoneal abscesses a minimally invasive and expeditious treatment. In many cases, patients can ultimately avoid surgery or postpone it after the acute inflammatory phase has passed. The key for the accurate diagnosis in this case includes, first of all, an appropriate history of prior intra-abdominal surgery. In addition, the fluid density of the mass, the rim enhancement, and the presence of gas bubbles highly suggest the diagnosis of intraperitoneal abscess. Intraperitoneal hematomas will not have gas bubbles if not infected, and the attenuation would be higher due to the presence of blood products. Cystic mesothelioma will also have no gas bubbles if no previous intervention has occurred and typically will be multiloculated. Finally, mesenteric cysts would also be devoid of gas bubbles, and their morphology would be more spheric than that seen in this case, which adapts to the shape of the peritoneal space.

CASE 5-30

Clinical History: 58-year-old man with a remote history of removal of a mole on his back presenting with abdominal pain and distention.

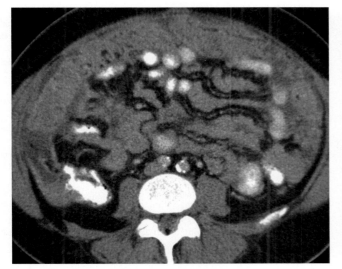

Figure 5.30   A

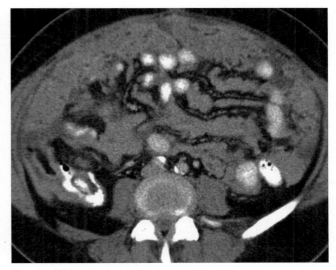

Figure 5.30   B

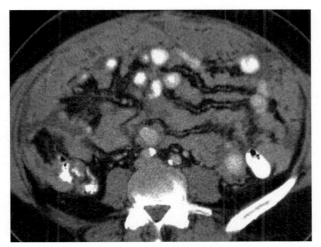

Figure 5.30   C

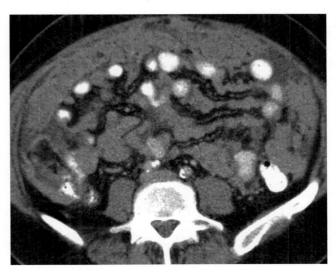

Figure 5.30   D

Findings: Axial CECT images show omental caking with replacement of the normal fatty attenuation of the omentum by soft tissue attenuation. There is also soft tissue thickening between the mesenteric leaves and ascites.

Differential Diagnosis: Tuberculosis, malignant mesothelioma.

Diagnosis: Melanoma metastases.

Discussion: Malignant melanoma is a common malignancy with an increasing prevalence due to, among other factors, increased sun exposure. It represents up to 3% of cancers in the United States. Melanoma metastases in the gastrointestinal tract and mesentery have traditionally connoted a very poor prognosis. Metastases can be seen as serosal implants, mesenteric masses of variable size, and replacement of the omentum by metastases (called omental caking). Melanoma metastases produce little or no desmoplastic reaction, and therefore, bowel kinking, dilatation, and obstruction are rare. The differential diagnosis includes peritoneal tuberculosis, where omental caking and mesenteric thickening is likely. However, there is no evidence of large adenopathy or appropriate clinical history. Lymphoma is also a possibility because, as in melanoma metastases, there is no desmoplastic reaction. However, the absence of adenopathy would not favor lymphoma.

SUGGESTED READINGS

- Akhan O, Pringot J. Imaging of abdominal tuberculosis. *Eur Radiol.* 2002;12:312–323.

- Bowen B, Ros PR, McCarthy MJ, et al. Gastrointestinal teratomas: CT and US appearance with pathologic correlation. *Radiology* 1987;162: 431–433.

- Bui-Mansfield LT, Kim-Ahn G, O'Bryant LK. Multicystic mesothelioma of the peritoneum. *Am J Roentgenol.* 2002;178:402.

- Busch JM, Kruskal JB, Wu B. Best cases from the AFIP: malignant peritoneal mesothelioma. *Radiographics* 2002;22:1511–1515.

- Coley BD, Shiels II WE, Elton S, et al. Sonographically guided aspiration of cerebrospinal fluid pseudocysts in children and adolescents. *Am J Roentgenol.* 2004;183:1507–1510.

- Crim JR, Seeger LL, Yao L, et al. Diagnosis of soft-tissue masses with MR imaging: can benign masses be differentiated from malignant ones? *Radiology* 1992;185:581–586.

- Daskalogiannaki M, Voloudaki A, Prassopoulos P, et al. CT evaluation of mesenteric panniculitis: prevalence and associated diseases. *Am J Roentgenol.* 2000;174:427–431.

- Debatin JF, Spritzer CE, Dunnick R. Castleman disease of the adrenal gland: MRI imaging features. *Am J Roentgenol.* 1991;157:781–783.

- Dowe MF, Shanmuganathan K, Mirvis SE, et al. CT findings of mesenteric injury after blunt trauma: implications for surgical intervention. *Am J Roentgenol.* 1997;168:425–428.

- Faria SC, Iyer RB, Rashid A, et al. Desmoid tumor of the small bowel and the mesentery. *Am J Roentgenol.* 2004;183:118.

- Fisher MF, Fletcher BD, Dahms BB, et al. Abdominal lipoblastomatosis: radiographic, echographic, and computed tomographic findings. *Radiology* 1981;138:593–596.

- Fishman EK, Kuhlman JE, Schuchter LM, et al. CT of malignant melanoma in the chest, abdomen, and musculoskeletal system. *Radiographics* 1990;10:603–620.

- Fleck RM, Schade RR, Kowal CD, et al. Testicular choriocarcinoma with metastasis to gastric mucosa. *Gastrointest Endosc.* 1984;30:188–189.

- Fujita N, Noda Y, Kobayashi G, et al. Chylous cyst of the mesentery: US and CT diagnosis. *Abdom Imaging.* 1995;20:259–261.

- Garcia P, Garcia-Giannoli H, Meyran S, et al. Primary dissecting aneurysm of the hepatic artery: sonographic, CT and angiographic findings. *Am J Roentgenol.* 1996;166:1316–1318.

- Ha HK, Jung JI, Lee MS, et al. CT differentiation of tuberculous peritonitis and peritoneal carcinomatosis. *Am J Roentgenol.* 1996;167: 743–748.

- Hamed RK, Buck JL, Olmsted WW, et al. Extracolonic manifestations of the familial adenomatous polyposis syndromes. *Am J Roentgenol.* 1991; 156:481–485.

- Horton KM, Kamel I, Hofman L, et al. Carcinoid tumors of the small bowel: a multitechnique imaging approach. *Am J Roentgenol.* 2004;182: 559–567.

- Horton KM, Lawler LP, Fishman EK. CT findings in sclerosing mesenteritis (panniculitis): spectrum of disease. *Radiographics* 2003;23: 1561–1567.

- Hui GC, Amaral J, Stephens D, et al. Gas distribution in intraabdominal and pelvic abscesses on CT is associated with drainability. *Am J Roentgenol.* 2005;184:915–919.

- Huppert BJ, Farrell MA. Case 60: cavitating mesenteric lymph node syndrome. *Radiology* 2003;228:180–184.

- Koh DM, Langroudi B, Padley SPG. Abdominal CT in patients with AIDS. *Imaging* 2002;14:24–34.

- Korobkin M, Silverman PM, Quint LE, et al. CT of the extraperitoneal space: normal anatomy and fluid collections. *Am J Roentgenol.* 1992; 159:933–941.

- Levy AD, Cantisani V, Miettinen M. Abdominal lymphangiomas: imaging features with pathologic correlation. *Am J Roentgenol.* 2004;182: 1485–1491.

- Levy AD, Remotti HE, Thompson WM, et al. Gastrointestinal stromal tumors: radiologic features with pathologic correlation. *Radiographics* 2003;23:283–304.

- McDermott VG, Low VH, Keogan MT, et al. Malignant melanoma metastatic to the gastrointestinal tract. *Am J Roentgenol.* 1996;166: 809–813.

- McLeod AJ, Zornoza J, Shirkhoda A. Leiomyosarcoma: computed tomographic findings. *Radiology* 1984;152:133–136.

- Meador TL, McLarney JK. CT features of Castleman disease of the abdomen and pelvis. *Am J Roentgenol.* 2000;175:115–118.

- Miller FH, Keppke AL, Dalal K, et al. MRI of pancreatitis and its complications: part 1, acute pancreatitis. *Am J Roentgenol.* 2004;183: 1637–1644.

- Murphey MD, Carroll JF, Flemming DJ, et al. From the archives of the AFIP: benign musculoskeletal lipomatous lesions. *Radiographics* 2004; 24:1433–1466.

- Pannu HK, Bristow RE, Montz FJ, et al. Multidetector CT of peritoneal carcinomatosis from ovarian cancer. *Radiographics* 2003;23:687–701.

- Pereira JM, Madureira AJ, Vieira A, et al. Abdominal tuberculosis: imaging features. *Eur J Radiol.* 2005;55:173–180.

- Pereira JM, Sirlin CB, Pinto PS, et al. CT and MR imaging of extrahepatic fatty masses of the abdomen and pelvis: techniques, diagnosis, differential diagnosis, and pitfalls. *Radiographics* 2005;25:69–85.

- Pernas JC, Catala J. Case 72: pseudocyst around ventriculoperitoneal shunt. *Radiology* 2004;232:239–243.

- Pickhardt PJ, Bhalla S. Primary neoplasms of peritoneal and subperitoneal origin: CT findings. *Radiographics* 2005;25:983–995.

- Ros PR, Yuschok TJ, Buck JL, et al. Peritoneal mesothelioma: radiologic appearances correlated with histology. *Acta Radiol.* 1991;32:355–358.

- Sheth S, Horton KM, Garland MR, et al. Mesenteric neoplasms: CT appearances of primary and secondary tumors and differential diagnosis. *Radiographics* 2003;23:457–473.

- Stoupis C, Ros PR, Abbitt PL, et al. Bubbles in the belly: imaging of cystic mesenteric or omental masses. *Radiographics* 1994;14:729–737.

- Sulkin TV, O'Neill H, Amin AI, et al. CT in pseudomyxoma peritonei: a review of 17 cases. *Clin Radiol.* 2002;57:608–613.

- Suzuki S, Furui S, Kohtake H, et al. Isolated dissection of the superior mesenteric artery: CT findings in six cases. *Abdom Imaging.* 2004;29: 153–157.

- van Breda Vriesman AC, Puylaert JBCM. Omental infarction: a self-limiting disease *Am J Roentgenol.* 2005;185:280–281.

- Walensky RP, Venbrux AC, Prescott CA, et al. Pseudomyxoma peritonei *Am J Roentgenol.* 1996;167:471–474.

- Wong WL, Johns TA, Herlihy WG, et al. Best cases from the AFIP: multicystic mesothelioma. *Radiographics* 2004;24:247–250.

- Yang ZG, Min PQ, Sone S, et al. Tuberculosis versus lymphoma in the abdominal lymph nodes: evaluation with contrast-enhanced CT. *Am J Roentgenol.* 1999;172:619–623.

- Yeh HC, Chahinan AP. Ultrasonography and computed tomography of peritoneal mesothelioma. *Radiology* 1980;135:705–712.

CHAPTER SIX

KIDNEY, URETER, AND BLADDER

VINCENT PELSSER,
KOENRAAD J. MORTELE,
AND PABLO R. ROS

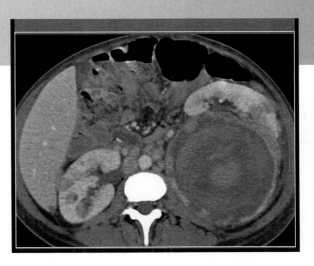

Clinical History: 43-year-old man presenting with chest soreness.

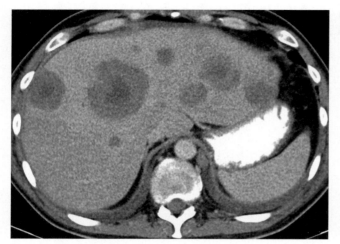

Figure 6.1 A

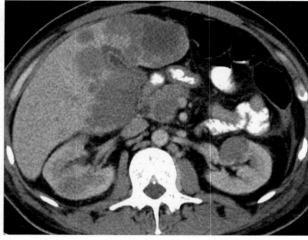

Figure 6.1 B

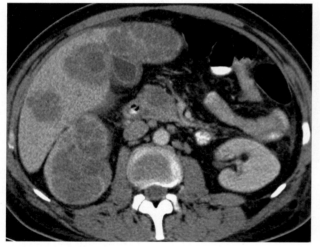

Figure 6.1 C

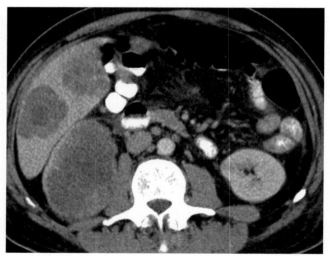

Figure 6.1 D

Findings: Axial contrast-enhanced CT (CECT) images demonstrate multiple low-attenuation, rim-enhancing lesions in the liver. Bilateral soft tissue renal masses are present, and the one on the right is infiltrative. Note a pancreatic head mass and a nodule along the serosal surface of a left upper quadrant small bowel loop.

Differential Diagnosis: Lymphoma, abscess.

Diagnosis: Lung cancer metastases.

Discussion: Metastases to the kidneys are commonly seen at time of autopsy, being nearly four times more common than a primary renal neoplasm. Typically there is widespread metastatic disease when renal metastases are present. The most common primary malignancies to metastasize to the kidneys include melanoma, lung, breast, and colon cancer. Patients are usually asymptomatic from the renal metastases but can occasionally have hematuria if there is invasion of the collecting system. There is a limited differential diagnosis for multiple solid renal masses. This includes metastases, lymphoma, multiple renal cell carcinomas, and abscesses. Lymphoma is usually part of a generalized process, and widespread lymphadenopathy is usually present. Multiple renal cell carcinomas are rare and are typically seen in patients with von Hippel-Lindau disease. The presence of other lesions in the liver, pancreas, and peritoneum makes metastatic disease the best diagnosis.

Clinical History: 53-year-old man presenting with a right groin mass.

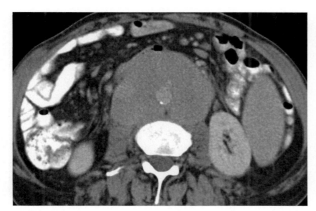

Figure 6.2   A

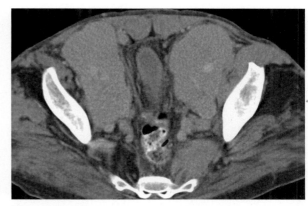

Figure 6.2   B

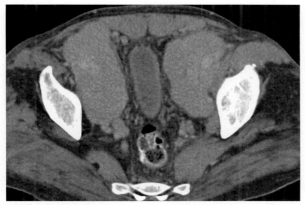

Figure 6.2   C

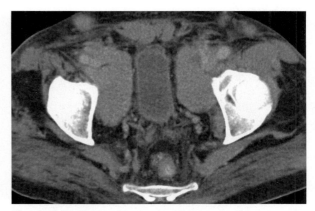

Figure 6.2   D

Findings: Axial CECT images demonstrate splenomegaly and bulky retroperitoneal adenopathy. Pelvic images demonstrate an elongated bladder due to surrounding soft tissue masses along the iliac vessels.

Differential Diagnosis: Pelvic lipomatosis, pelvic hematoma, pelvic tumor, iliopsoas hypertrophy.

Diagnosis: Pelvic lymphoma producing a teardrop-shaped bladder.

Discussion: A pear- or teardrop-shaped bladder by plain film can be due to multiple etiologies including pelvic lipomatosis, pelvic hematoma or abscess, pelvic neoplasm, and iliopsoas hypertrophy. These causes can be easily differentiated by CT imaging. The presence of fat surrounding the bladder is diagnostic of pelvic lipomatosis. Pelvic lipomatosis is seen commonly in asymptomatic black men in their fourth decade. Pelvic hematomas are associated with pelvic fractures secondary to trauma, with high-density fluid often present. A soft tissue mass in the pelvis compressing the bladder can be due to a pelvic tumor (e.g., uterine, prostatic, ovarian) or from adenopathy in patients with lymphoma. In this case, the presence of splenomegaly with the homogeneous retroperitoneal and pelvic adenopathy is diagnostic of lymphoma.

Clinical History: 52-year-old woman with history of right renal mass.

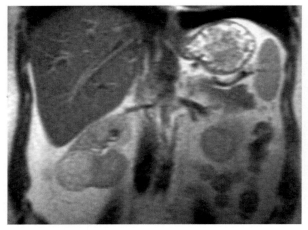

Figure 6.3   A

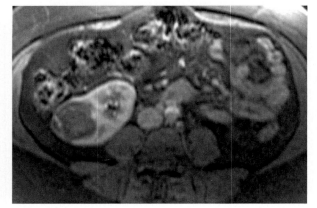

Figure 6.3   B

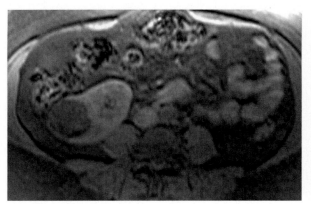

Figure 6.3   C

Figure 6.3   D

Findings: Coronal T2-weighted image (WI) (A) demonstrates a hyperintense, exophytic, 3.7 × 4.5 cm mass in the right lower renal pole. Axial T1-WI (B) shows the mass has predominantly hyperintense signal. Fat-suppressed axial T1-WI before (C) and after (D) gadolinium administration show the mass has predominantly hypointense signal with few linear areas of enhancement.

Differential Diagnosis: None.

Diagnosis: Angiomyolipoma.

Discussion: An angiomyolipoma (AML) is a benign renal mass that is composed of fat, smooth muscle, and abnormal blood vessels. Those tissues are present in variable quantity within the mass, such that approximately 95% of AMLs will have fat components detectable by imaging. CT and MRI are often diagnostic due to their ability to detect fat with high specificity. On CT, the fat-containing portions of the lesion will measure less than −10 Hounsfield units (HU) on both nonenhanced CT (NECT) and CECT, a threshold that is considered diagnostic for fat. On MRI, the fat in the lesion will follow the signal intensity of the adjacent retroperitoneal subcutaneous fat. In addition, fat suppression techniques are required for absolute confirmation of fat within a lesion. However, the ability of MRI to detected fat within a lesion using either fat-suppression techniques or in- and out-of-phase images depends on the quantity of fat present within each voxel imaged. Enhancement is usually pronounced because of the abnormal vessels present in AML.

Clinical History: 43-year-old woman presenting with frequent urinary tract infections.

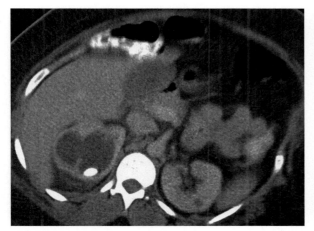

Figure 6.4   A

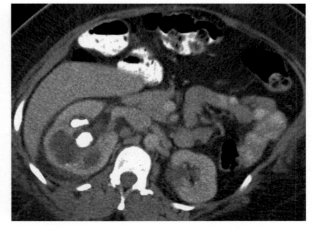

Figure 6.4   B

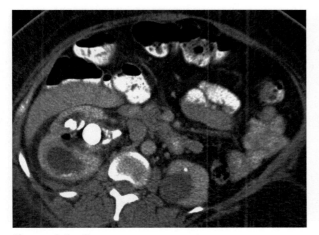

Figure 6.4   C

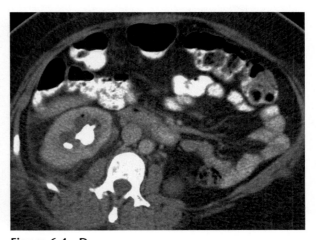

Figure 6.4   D

Findings: Axial CECT images demonstrate multiple large calcifications in the right renal collecting system and renal pelvis, resulting in severe calyceal dilatation. Note gas in the right collecting system, left renal calcification, and cysts.

Differential Diagnosis: Xanthogranulomatous pyelonephritis.

Diagnosis: Severe right hydronephrosis due to renal calculi.

Discussion: Causes for hydronephrosis are numerous and can be divided into endoluminal causes (such as stone or blood clot), wall lesions (such as urothelial neoplasm or fibrosis), and extrinsic causes (such as lymphadenopathy or retroperitoneal fibrosis). The most common locations for obstruction from a stone are the ureterovesical junction, ureteropelvic junction, and pelvic inlet. Acute hydronephrosis can lead to urinary stasis and infection. CT findings of hydronephrosis include dilatation of the collecting system above the level of obstruction. NECT is useful for detecting an obstructing calculus in the ureter. CECT is useful for assessing perfusion and function of the kidney, which are often diminished in acute obstruction. However, because the density of iodine, especially when excreted in the collecting system, may appear similar to stones on standard soft tissue windows, renal stones can easily be missed if only CECT is performed and the images are not adequately windowed. The gas present in the collecting system in this case were related to recent urologic manipulation. They were not present prior, which would go against superimposed infection, such as in focal bacterial or xanthogranulomatous pyelonephritis.

Clinical History: 52-year-old man presenting with hematuria.

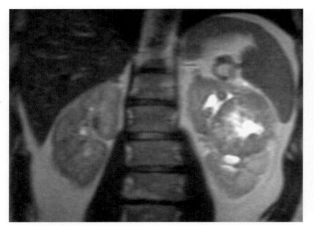

Figure 6.5   A

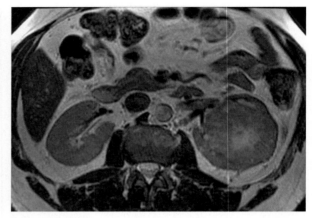

Figure 6.5   B

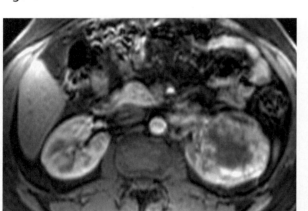

Figure 6.5   C

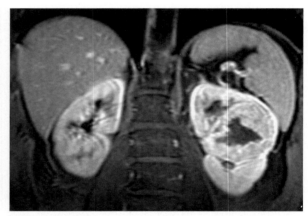

Figure 6.5   D

Findings: Coronal (A) and axial (B) T2-WI demonstrate a 6.6 × 7.2 × 6.6 cm, isointense left renal mass with areas of central necrosis. Gadolinium-enhanced, fat-suppressed axial (C) and coronal (D) T1-WI show heterogeneous enhancement of the periphery of the mass.

Differential Diagnosis: Oncocytoma, renal abscess, adenoma.

Diagnosis: Renal cell carcinoma.

Discussion: The use of MRI for renal cell carcinoma has been limited due to the success of CT. CT possesses better spatial resolution than MRI and is better tolerated by most patients. Renal cell carcinoma can be isointense to normal kidney on both T1-WI and T2-WI. For a small lesion, it can be difficult to separate the neoplasm from the normal renal parenchyma. Because renal cell carcinomas are hypervascular, the use of gadolinium is helpful in detecting these smaller lesions. Often a heterogeneous signal is seen in the tumor due to necrosis and hemorrhage, which is easily detected by MRI. MRI is useful in detecting tumor extension into the perirenal space, involvement of Gerota's fascia, and extension into the renal vein and inferior vena cava (IVC). Because of its multi-planar capabilities, MRI is also helpful in separating renal neoplasms from adrenal or perirenal neoplasms. This case demonstrates the typical findings of a large renal cell carcinoma. It is relatively isointense on T2-WI with areas of necrosis and has heterogeneous enhancement after gadolinium administration. An oncocytoma or renal adenoma may have a similar appearance. The predominantly solid appearance of the mass and lack of surrounding fat stranding make an abscess extremely unlikely.

Clinical History: 51-year-old man presenting with severe left flank pain.

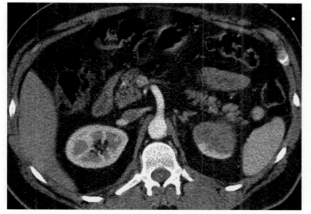

Figure 6.6   A

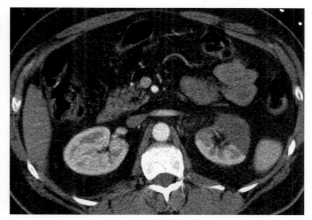

Figure 6.6   B

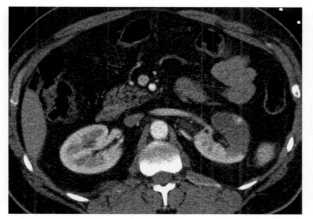

Figure 6.6   C

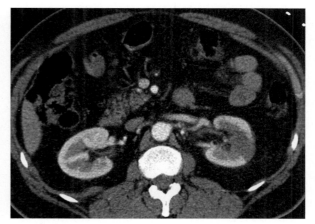

Figure 6.6   D

Findings: Axial CECT images demonstrate no enhancement of a large portion of the upper pole of the left kidney with sharp demarcation with the normally enhancing parenchyma.

Differential Diagnosis: Acute pyelonephritis.

Diagnosis: Renal infarct.

Discussion: Renal infarction may have various causes, the most common being thromboembolism from cardiovascular disease. Other causes include vasculitis, trauma, paraneoplastic syndrome, and hypercoagulable state. The latter was subsequently identified in the patient in this case: he had antiphospholipid antibody syndrome. As in this case, the most common clinical presentation is acute flank or back pain. CECT shows absent enhancement of the affected parenchyma, typically having a wedge-shape configuration. Subcapsular 2- to 4-mm thick cortical enhancement, called the cortical rim sign, is characteristic of vascular injuries to the kidney. The rim sign is produced by capsular collateral branches from the inferior adrenal artery or lumbar arteries that supply the peripheral-most cortex. Such a sign would not be seen in cases of acute pyelonephritis. In pyelonephritis, the affected parenchyma still enhances, although less than the normal renal parenchyma, as opposed to renal infarcts in which the parenchyma shows no enhancement; perinephric stranding is typically present in infections. Therapy for renal infarcts usually only consists of anticoagulation. More invasive intervention may be attempted in cases of bilateral renal infarcts, infarcts in a solitary kidney, or unilateral total renal infarcts.

Clinical History: 50-year-old woman presenting with hematuria.

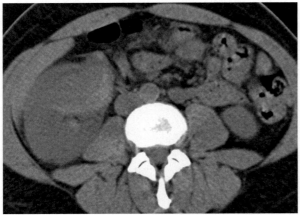

Figure 6.7   A

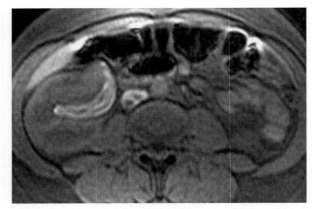

Figure 6.7   B

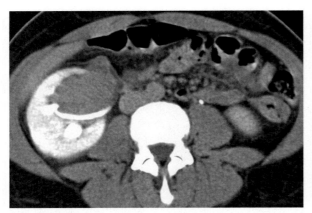

Figure 6.7   C

Figure 6.7   D

Findings: Axial NECT image (A) shows a 4.8 × 2.4 cm, soft tissue lesion in the anterior aspect of the right renal sinus, lined posteriorly by a 5.3 × 1.2 cm, hyperdense, crescentic-shaped structure. Axial CECT image in the corticomedullary phase (B) shows enhancement of the lesion but not of the hyperdense structure posterior to it. Axial CECT in the excretory phase (C) shows excreted contrast along the posterior aspect of the renal pelvis. On the fat-suppressed axial T1-WI (D), the enhancing lesion has soft tissue attenuation, and the posterior structure is hyperintense.

Differential Diagnosis: Renal cell carcinoma.

Diagnosis: Transitional cell carcinoma with hemorrhage.

Discussion: There are many different etiologies associated with transitional cell carcinoma (TCC). These include cigarette smoking, cyclophosphamide therapy, analgesic use (phenacetin), and industrial chemicals (aromatic amines). TCC can be single or multiple and is bilateral in approximately 2% of cases. When the upper tracts are involved by TCC, a synchronous or metachronous TCC will develop in 40% of cases. Treatment is usually radical nephroureterectomy. A filling defect in the collecting system can be due to many causes including stone, blood clot, fungus ball, polyp, neoplasm (TCC or polyp), or sloughed papilla in papillary necrosis. In this case, the presence of a soft tissue mass in the renal pelvis limits the differential diagnosis to neoplasm, blood clot, sloughed papilla, and fungus ball. The soft tissue lesion demonstrates enhancement, which eliminates the latter three choices. The hyperdense, nonenhancing, posterior, crescentic-shaped structure represents blood clot in the renal pelvis. A renal cell carcinoma, which can enhance, rarely invades the collecting system.

Clinical History: 14-year-old girl with longstanding renal insufficiency.

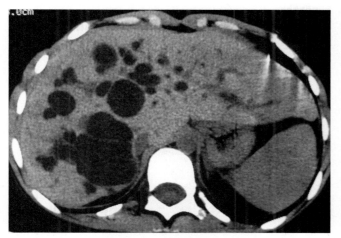

Figure 6.8   A

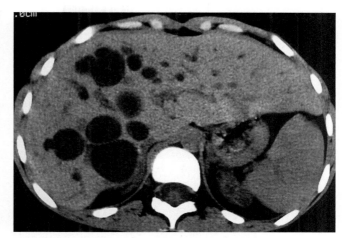

Figure 6.8   B

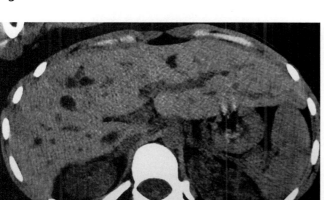

Figure 6.8   C

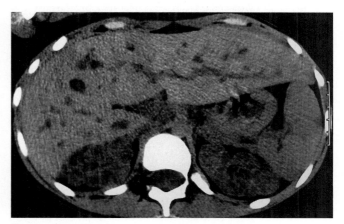

Figure 6.8   D

Findings: Axial NECT images demonstrate multiple hepatic cystic lesions, some of which are branching. Note the presence of multiple low-density renal lesions.

Differential Diagnosis: None.

Diagnosis: Autosomal recessive polycystic kidney disease.

Discussion: Autosomal recessive polycystic kidney disease (ARPKD) constitutes a spectrum of liver and renal abnormalities that can present either in the newborn period or in childhood. The degree of hepatic and renal involvement is inversely proportional. If ARPKD manifests itself in the newborn, the predominant abnormality is the renal disorder, which leads to death in the first few days of life from renal insufficiency and/or secondary pulmonary hypoplasia. If ARPKD manifests in childhood or adolescence, it has a milder renal disease, with hepatic disease being the predominant abnormality. Liver disease consists of bile duct dilatation due to ductal plate malformation (as seen in Caroli disease) and fibrosis along the portal tracts. The liver parenchyma itself is normal. These older patients tend to die from complications of portal hypertension, such as gastrointestinal bleeds. In ARPKD, the kidneys are enlarged but typically function poorly. There are innumerable small cysts (1–2 mm) found primarily in the medullary portion of the kidneys. These small cysts do not enhance with contrast administration. Tubular ectasia is also present, which can lead to contrast stasis, giving the kidneys a typically striated appearance. The presence of severe bile duct dilatation and enlarged kidneys containing multiple small cysts, as seen in this case, is virtually diagnostic of ARPKD.

Case images courtesy of Dr. Susan A. Connolly, Children's Hospital Boston, Boston, MA.

Clinical History: 58-year-old woman presenting with suprapubic pain.

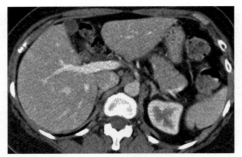

Figure 6.9   A

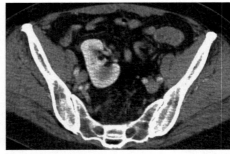

Figure 6.9   B

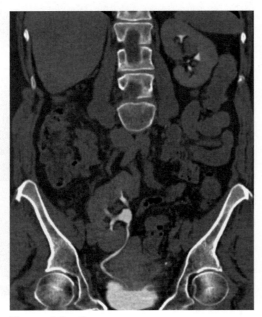

Figure 6.9   C

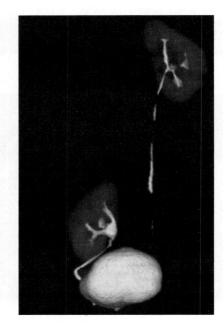

Figure 6.9   D

Findings: Axial CECT images (A and B) demonstrate absence of the right kidney in the renal fossa and presence of a normally located right adrenal gland. The kidney is noted on the right side of the pelvis. Curved multiplanar reformatted (MPR) (C) and three-dimensional, volume-rendered (D) images confirm the pelvic location of the right kidney. Note the normally positioned left kidney in the upper abdomen.

Differential Diagnosis: None.

Diagnosis: Pelvic kidney.

Discussion: The kidney normally migrates cephalad from the pelvis to the upper abdomen. Initially, the kidney receives its blood supply from the iliac artery and then the aorta. If there is an abnormality in the spine or blood supply to the kidney, then cephalad migration will be halted. The most common form of renal ectopy is a pelvic kidney. Pelvic kidney is often associated with hydronephrosis and vesicoureteral reflux, which can lead to repeated infections. Other congenital abnormalities are also associated with a pelvic kidney, including genitourinary malformations (ureteropelvic junction obstruction, cryptorchidism, hypospadias, and vaginal agenesis), gastrointestinal malformations (malrotation and imperforate anus), and cardiac malformations (septal defects). Contralateral urinary (such as agenesis or ectopia) or genital (such as Müllerian fusion anomalies, hypospadias, or undescended testis) abnormalities are frequently associated. Ultrasound and CT are typically diagnostic, obviating further workup. Pelvic kidneys are malrotated: early in embryology, the renal sinus faces anteriorly; with renal ascent, it progressively rotates 90 degrees medially; thus, ectopic kidneys always have an associated degree of malrotation. The adrenal gland on the ipsilateral side of the pelvic kidney is normally in the upper abdomen.

CASE 6-10

Clinical History: 20-year-old woman presenting with abdominal pain and fever.

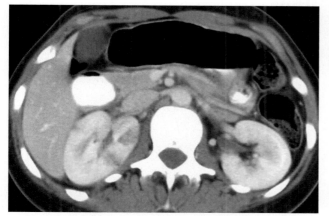

Figure 6.10   A

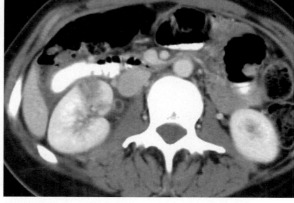

Figure 6.10   B

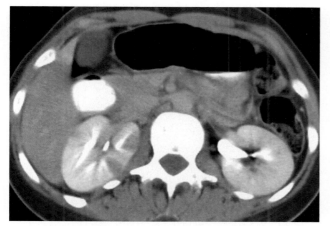

Figure 6.10   C

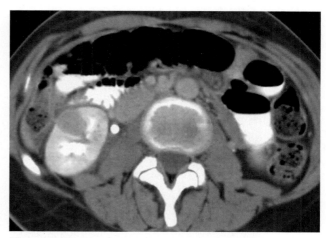

Figure 6.10   D

Findings: Axial CECT images in the nephrographic (A and B) and excretory phase (C and D) demonstrate multiple wedge-shaped areas of hypoenhancement in the right renal parenchyma. Note right urothelial thickening, perinephric fat stranding, and mild renal enlargement.

Differential Diagnosis: Renal infarct, renal trauma.

Diagnosis: Acute bacterial pyelonephritis.

Discussion: Acute pyelonephritis is the most common infection involving the kidney. It is usually the result of an ascending infection from the bladder, most commonly by *Escherichia coli*. Colonization of the ureter by *E. coli* results in loss of peristalsis and stasis of urine within the ureter. This allows the infection to reach the kidney in a retrograde manner. Acute pyelonephritis remains a clinical diagnosis; imaging is only indicated after nonresponse to antibiotic therapy for 36 to 48 hours to search for complications. By CECT, typical wedge-shaped or rounded areas of decreased enhancement in the renal parenchyma are seen. The affected kidney is enlarged from edema. Late parenchymal staining and delayed excretion into the collecting system can be seen. The degree of contrast enhancement delay is directly proportional to the degree of renal inflammation. This case nicely demonstrates decreased enhancement of the affected parenchyma seen in pyelonephritis. Renal trauma can have a similar CECT appearance with wedge-shaped areas of delayed enhancement, but in this case, the urothelial thickening points to an inflammatory process. In renal infarcts, the affected renal parenchyma can also be wedge shaped but should demonstrate no enhancement, except of the subcapsular cortex.

Clinical History: 56-year-old man presenting with urinary frequency, urgency, and dysuria.

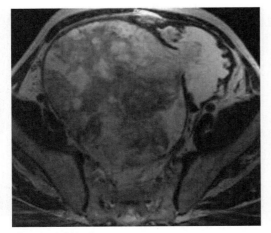

Figure 6.11   A

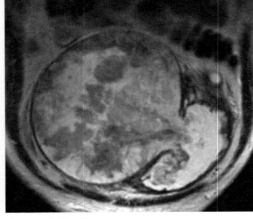

Figure 6.11   B

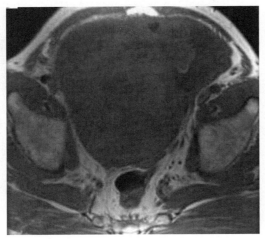

Figure 6.11   C

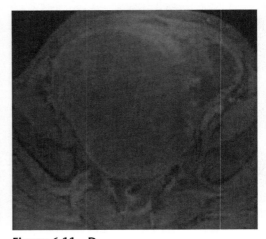

Figure 6.11   D

Findings: Axial (A) and coronal (B) T2-WI and axial T1-WI (C) demonstrate a 16-cm outpouching off the right lateral portion of the bladder, which is displaced to the left. A lesion of heterogeneous intensity fills the outpouching and extends into the bladder. Gadolinium-enhanced, fat-suppressed axial T1-WI (D) shows patchy and poor enhancement of the soft tissue lesion.

Differential Diagnosis: Urachal diverticulum.

Diagnosis: Transitional cell carcinoma originating in a bladder diverticulum.

Discussion: Bladder diverticula are most commonly due to bladder outlet obstruction rather than a congenital anomaly. The congenital diverticulum or "Hutch" diverticulum results from a musculature defect near the ureterovesical junction. Bladder outlet obstruction can be due to a prostatic

disorder (e.g., prostatitis, prostate cancer, prostatic hypertrophy), a urethral stricture or cancer, or neurologic dysfunction. Bladder diverticula can be single or multiple and typically arise from the lateral bladder wall. Bladder diverticula can give rise to complications. If the neck of the diverticulum is narrow, urinary stasis can develop, leading to stone formation and infection. Approximately 2% of epithelial bladder carcinomas arise from a bladder diverticulum, as in this case. They can be either transitional cell carcinoma (since the diverticulum is lined with urothelium) or squamous cell carcinoma (from chronic infection). A urachal diverticulum, although much less common, is another possibility. However, urachal diverticula occur at the superior and anterior portion of the bladder, and adenocarcinoma is usually the subtype of tumor originating from the urachus.

Clinical History: 67-year-old woman presenting with digital clubbing.

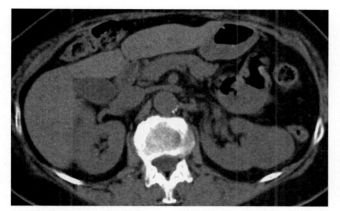

Figure 6.12 A

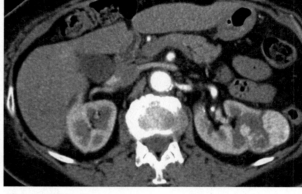

Figure 6.12 B

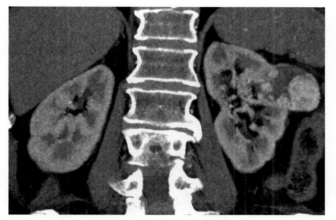

Figure 6.12 C

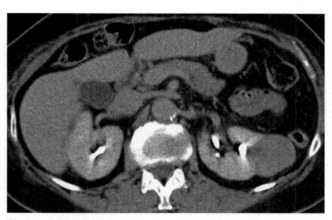

Figure 6.12 D

Findings: Axial NECT image (A) and axial (B) and coronal (C) CECT images in the corticomedullary phase and axial CECT image in the excretory phase (D) demonstrate a 6.5 × 4.4 × 3.5 cm, exophytic, heterogeneously enhancing mass in the upper pole of the left kidney.

Differential Diagnosis: Oncocytoma, renal adenoma, metastasis.

Diagnosis: Renal cell carcinoma.

Discussion: Renal cell carcinoma is the most common primary malignancy of the kidney. It arises from the proximal convoluted tubules, and approximately 50% of patients present with hematuria. Other signs include a palpable flank mass and flank pain from stretching of the renal capsule. Renal cell carcinoma typically appears as a heterogeneously enhancing solid tumor of the kidney; 10% to 20% of cases will have calcifications that tend to be amorphous and centrally located. Areas of necrosis can be seen, as in this case. The digital clubbing of the patient in this case was caused by a coexistent primary lung adenocarcinoma. A solid mass in the kidney can also be due to an oncocytoma, adenoma, metastasis, or angiomyolipoma. An oncocytoma is considered benign, but differentiation from a well-differentiated oncocytic renal cell carcinoma requires histologic evaluation of the entire tumor. An adenoma is considered premalignant. Therefore, resection is recommended for most solid tumors of the kidney.

Clinical History: 32-year-old man presenting with acute left flank pain and syncope.

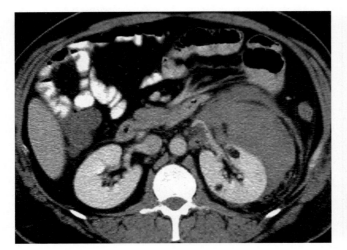

Figure 6.13   A

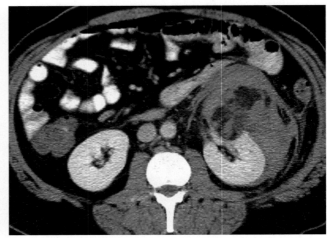

Figure 6.13   B

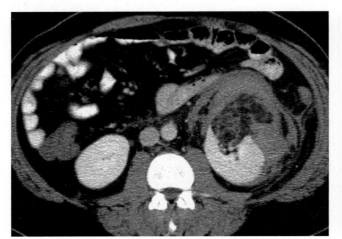

Figure 6.13   C

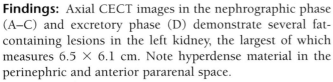 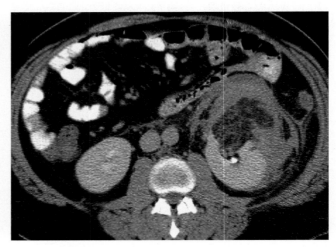

Figure 6.13   D

Findings: Axial CECT images in the nephrographic phase (A–C) and excretory phase (D) demonstrate several fat-containing lesions in the left kidney, the largest of which measures 6.5 × 6.1 cm. Note hyperdense material in the perinephric and anterior pararenal space.

Differential Diagnosis: Retroperitoneal liposarcoma.

Diagnosis: Hemorrhage from an angiomyolipoma.

Discussion: Angiomyolipoma (AML) is a benign mesenchymal hamartoma of the kidney containing variable amounts of fat, muscle, and blood vessels. Most of these lesions are found sporadically (80%), but there is a high association of AMLs with tuberous sclerosis. When the lesion is sporadic, it is typically found in middle-age women. The lesion is usually solitary and found incidentally except when hemorrhage from the lesion occurs, as in this case, producing flank pain. The risk of hemorrhage from an AML is significantly greater when the mass measures 4 cm or more; between 50% and 60% of AMLs above this size bleed spontaneously. CT imaging is usually diagnostic due to the presence of fat within the lesion. The absence of fat, however, does not exclude an AML because variable amounts of each mesenchymal component can be present. If the AML arises from the cortical surface, it can be difficult to distinguish from other retroperitoneal fat-containing tumors, such as liposarcoma. Therefore, it is crucial to find the organ of origin of the fatty mass. In this example, the lesion is shown to arise from the renal parenchyma, confirming the diagnosis of AML.

Clinical History: 50-year-old woman presenting with incidental renal mass discovered after hernia repair.

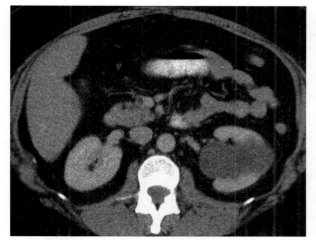

Figure 6.14   A

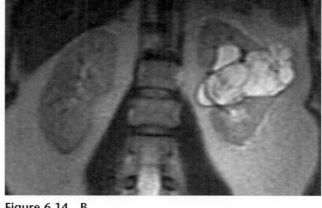

Figure 6.14   B

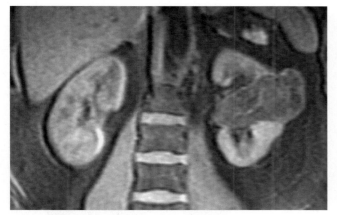

Figure 6.14   C

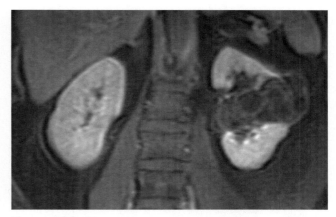

Figure 6.14   D

Findings: Axial CECT image (A) shows an 8.3 × 5.0 cm cystic lesion arising from the left kidney, with suggestion of internal septations. Coronal T2-WI (B) and unenhanced (C) and gadolinium-enhanced (D) fat-suppressed T1-WI confirm the cystic nature of this lesion. Many more internal septations are visualized than on the CECT. Note protrusion in the renal sinus and enhancement of the thin septations.

Differential Diagnosis: Cystic renal cell carcinoma, multiloculated renal cyst.

Diagnosis: Cystic nephroma.

Discussion: Multilocular cystic renal tumor is a term that includes two histologically distinct entities: cystic nephroma and cystic partially differentiated nephroblastoma (CPDN). Cystic nephroma is identical to CPDN on imaging and gross pathology; the only difference is that the septa in cystic nephroma do not contain blastemal cells. Multilocular cystic renal tumors are rare nonhereditary congenital lesions.

They typically occur in children younger than 4 years of age, with approximately 70% being in males. A second peak occurs in women older than 30 years of age. Patients are usually asymptomatic, but they can occasionally present with hematuria. Multilocular cystic renal tumors are large cystic lesions with multiple noncommunicating cysts separated by septations. The lesions are well circumscribed due to a thick fibrous capsule. The cysts contain clear serous fluid and do not usually hemorrhage. They are commonly found in the lower pole of the kidney without left or right side predilection. Although a nonspecific finding that can also be seen with renal cell carcinoma, the tumor has a tendency to herniate into the renal pelvis. The CT finding of a multiloculated large cystic lesion is characteristic of a multilocular cystic renal tumor but cannot be differentiated from a cystic renal cell carcinoma. Biopsy or aspiration is inconclusive, and frequently, local excision or nephrectomy is required for definitive diagnosis and curative treatment.

Clinical History: 69-year-old man presenting with gross hematuria.

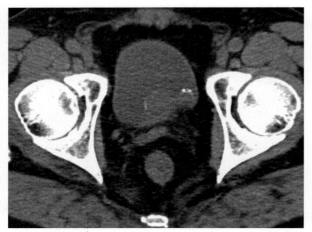

Figure 6.15   A

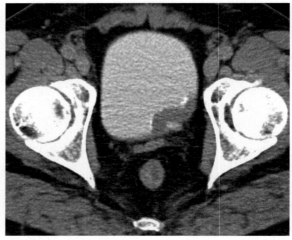

Figure 6.15   B

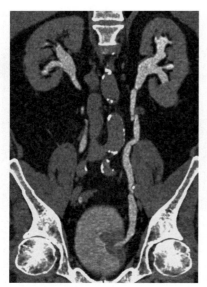

Figure 6.15   C

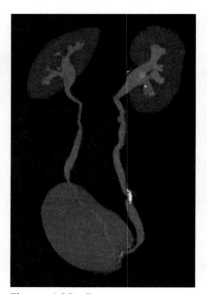

Figure 6.15   D

Findings: Axial NECT (A) and delayed CECT (B) images demonstrate a 4.7 × 2.0 × 3.3 cm papillary mass along the left bladder base wall, with peripheral calcifications. Curved MPR (C) and three-dimensional, volume-rendered (D) images confirm the mass is centered at the left ureterovesical junction. It causes mild left hydronephrosis.

Differential Diagnosis: Primary neoplasm of the bladder (squamous cell carcinoma, adenocarcinoma), schistosomiasis, tuberculosis, hematoma, metastasis.

Diagnosis: Transitional cell carcinoma.

Discussion: Transitional cell carcinoma of the bladder occurs most commonly in males in the sixth decade of life. These carcinomas make up 85% to 90% of bladder tumors, followed by squamous cell carcinoma and adenocarcinoma. Transitional cell carcinoma most commonly presents as an intraluminal mass with a broad base. They can be single or multiple and, although infrequent, may contain calcifications. Hydronephrosis is not frequently seen in transitional cell carcinoma of the bladder unless the ureteral orifice is obstructed, as in this case. An intraluminal mass is a nonspecific finding and can be due to any bladder neoplasm or, occasionally, to an infection, such as tuberculosis or schistosomiasis. CT is excellent in evaluating for lymphadenopathy and invasion of adjacent organs. MRI is superior to evaluate the depth of wall invasion or extravesical extension by the tumor.

CASE 6-16

Clinical History: 72-year-old woman with recent duodenal surgery presenting with abdominal distention.

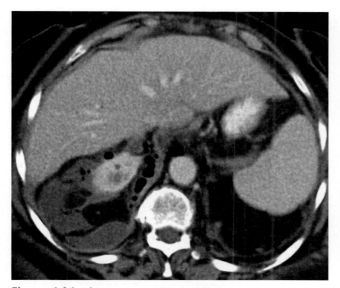

Figure 6.16   A

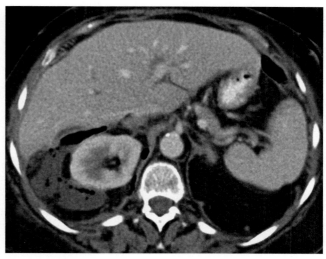

Figure 6.16   B

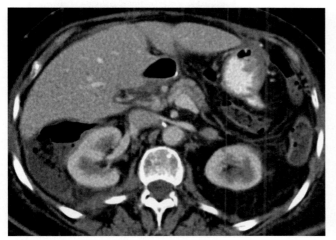

Figure 6.16   C

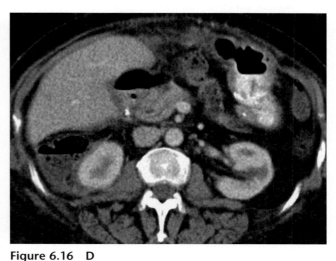

Figure 6.16   D

Findings: Axial CECT images in the corticomedullary phase demonstrate several collections with air-fluid levels, gas bubbles, and fat stranding in the right perinephric and pararenal space.

Differential Diagnosis: Trauma, instrumentation.

Diagnosis: Perirenal abscess.

Discussion: Air in the perirenal space originates either from gas-forming organisms or is introduced into the perirenal space from either penetrating trauma (e.g., stab wound, gunshot) or instrumentation (e.g., biopsy, surgery). Air from the latter two causes does not necessarily imply infection. A perirenal abscess, however, requires antibiotics and drainage either percutaneously or surgically. Given the history of recent surgery in this case, the abscesses were a surgical complication. Pyelonephritis with extension through the renal capsule, forming a perirenal abscess, is a common cause of perirenal abscess. Acute obstruction with a ruptured fornix can also lead to a perirenal abscess, but in this case, there is no evidence of renal calculi or collecting system obstruction to suggest this diagnosis. The lack of air in the renal parenchyma excludes emphysematous pyelonephritis.

Chapter 6: Kidney, Ureter, and Bladder   **307**

Clinical History: 43-year-old man with severe left flank pain that has recently improved.

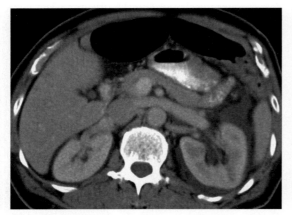

Figure 6.17 A

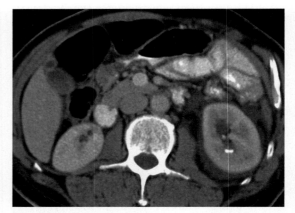

Figure 6.17 B

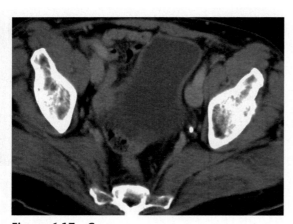

Figure 6.17 C

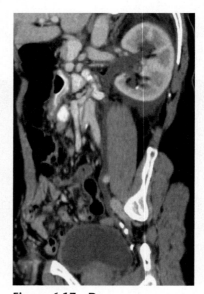

Figure 6.17 D

Findings: Axial CECT images in the nephrographic phase (A–C) show left renal enlargement and delay of enhancement of the parenchyma. Moderate amount of fluid is present in the perinephric space. Two nonobstructive left lower pole calyceal stones and a stone in the left side of the pelvis are seen. Curved MPR image (D) shows mild left hydronephrosis due to three distal ureteral stones.

Differential Diagnosis: Perinephric abscess, trauma.

Diagnosis: Ruptured fornix due to obstructive ureteral stones.

Discussion: Acute obstruction of the collecting system is most commonly due to an obstructing calculus. Plain films are sensitive for detecting most stones because 85% to 90% are radiopaque. The problem arises in small stones, stones obscured by bowel gas, stones overlying bony structures, and radiolucent stones. Ultrasound is limited in the evaluation of the ureter. A NECT is very sensitive in detecting stones in the kidney and ureter, even those that are radiolucent by plain film. Uric acid stones, which are common less dense stones, measure approximately 125 to 300 HU, which makes them easily detectable by CT. Complications of acute obstruction include loss of renal function and forniceal or renal pelvis rupture, as in this case. Forniceal rupture leads to the formation of subcapsular and perinephric fluid. These patients typically describe relief in the flank pain corresponding to decompression of the calyceal system after forniceal or pelvic rupture. This can be misinterpreted clinically as passage of a stone. If the urine is infected, forniceal rupture can lead to a perirenal abscess.

Clinical History: 74-year-old woman with a history of chronic myelogenous leukemia presenting with septic shock.

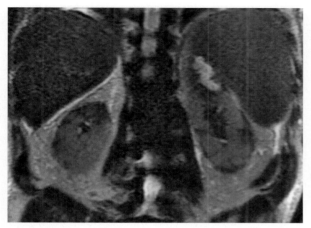

Figure 6.18   A

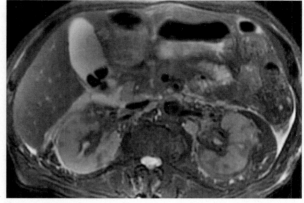

Figure 6.18   B

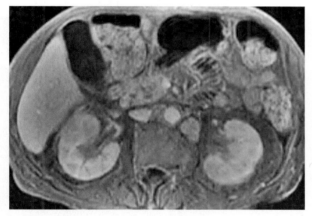

Figure 6.18   C

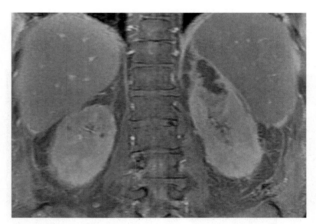

Figure 6.18   D

Findings: Coronal T2-WI (A) demonstrates a 2.8 × 4.8 × 3.4 cm, exophytic, left upper pole, hyperintense, thick-walled lesion. Fat-suppressed axial T2-WI (B) shows wedge-shaped areas of decreased signal intensity. Gadolinium-enhanced, fat-suppressed axial (C) and coronal (D) T1-WI show enhancement of the irregular wall of the left upper pole cystic lesion and wedge-shaped areas of decreased enhancement of the renal parenchyma. Note left interpolar renal scarring, cholelithiasis, and para-aortic lymph node.

Differential Diagnosis: Renal cell carcinoma, necrotic metastasis, leukemic infiltration.

Diagnosis: Renal abscess complicating pyelonephritis.

Discussion: Renal abscesses are commonly the result of obstruction from calculi, tumors, or strictures resulting in an ascending infection. Hematogenous spread can also occur from infection of the skin or endocarditis, as seen in intravenous drug abusers, which result in microabscesses that can coalesce and form a large abscess. The most common

infecting organisms are *Escherichia coli* and *Proteus mirabilis*. Renal abscesses can be single or multiple. Multiple abscesses are more commonly due to hematogenous spread. By CT or MRI, the lesion is typically of fluid attenuation (10–20 HU) or signal intensity with a thick wall that can demonstrate enhancement. There can be spread of inflammation outside the kidney, with thickening of Gerota's fascia. The presence of air within the fluid is pathognomonic of a renal abscess. The wedge-shaped areas present in the kidneys, as seen in this case, suggest pyelonephritis, although renal leukemic infiltration may present similarly. A simple cyst would not have a thick wall or fluid of high attenuation. The appearance of this lesion is indistinguishable from a cystic renal cell carcinoma, although a neoplasm was excluded by observing resolution on subsequent imaging. Clinical symptoms can usually help differentiate the two entities, as in this case.

Case images courtesy of Dr. Caroline Reinhold, McGill University Health Center, Montreal, Canada.

Clinical History: 36-year-old woman presenting with right flank discomfort.

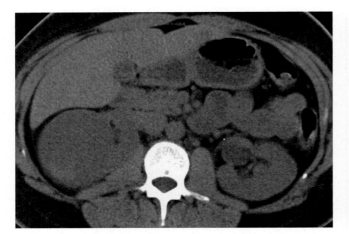

Figure 6.19   A

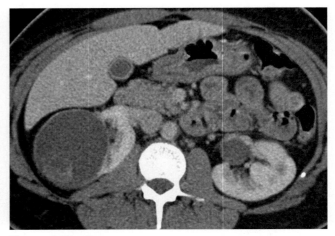

Figure 6.19   B

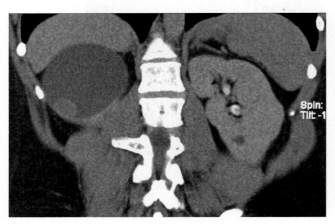

Figure 6.19   C

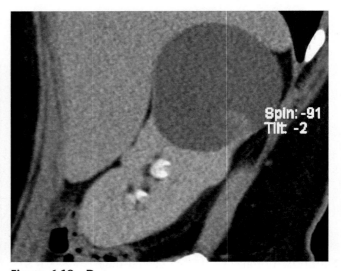

Figure 6.19   D

Findings: Axial NECT (A), CECT in the nephrographic phase (B), and coronal (C) and sagittal (D) CECT images in the excretory phase demonstrate a large exophytic cystic lesion in the right kidney. It has wall enhancement and an enhancing mural nodule.

Differential Diagnosis: Abscess.

Diagnosis: Cystic renal cell carcinoma.

Discussion: Renal cell carcinoma can occur in a wall of a cyst, as in this case, or have central necrosis, resulting in a cystic, complex lesion. It is critical to closely evaluate a cystic lesion for signs of malignancy. A simple cyst by CT should be round and well defined with a thin wall. The fluid should be of water density and not enhance with contrast. Thin septations or thin peripheral calcifications can also be seen in benign cysts. Thick and irregular walls or septations, thick calcifications, and a tumor nodule are all suggestive of a malignancy. The lesion in this case demonstrates an enhancing nodule (Bosniak category IV). This finding is strongly suggestive of a malignancy, and a cystic renal cell carcinoma was found at surgery. A well-organized abscess would not have a dominant mural nodule, as seen in this case. Clinical history is helpful to differentiate the two entities.

Clinical History: 36-year-old woman being evaluated for infertility.

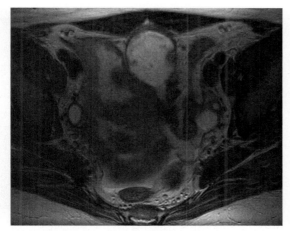

Figure 6.20   A

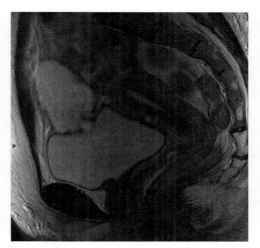

Figure 6.20   B

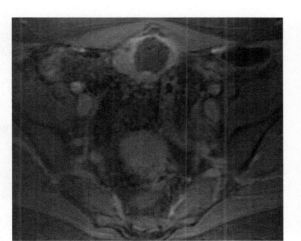

Figure 6.20   C

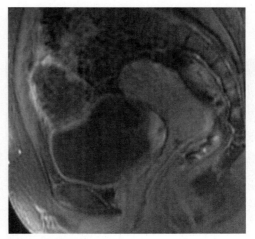

Figure 6.20   D

Findings: Axial (A) and coronal (B) T2-WI demonstrate a 5.4 × 3.7 × 2.3 cm cystic lesion with nodular wall located superiorly to the bladder dome at the midline level. Gadolinium-enhanced, fat-suppressed axial (C) and sagittal (D) T1-WI show enhancement of the nodular wall. Note absence of communication of the lesion with the bladder lumen.

Differential Diagnosis: Abscess, urachal cyst, transitional cell carcinoma in a bladder diverticulum.

Diagnosis: Urachal carcinoma.

Discussion: The urachus is a vestigial remnant of the cloaca and allantoid. It extends over the midline from the umbilicus to the anterior superior surface of the bladder. The transitional epithelium of the urachus can undergo metaplasia and dysplasia and even become malignant and convert to a mucin-producing adenocarcinoma. This accounts for almost 70% of the malignancies in the urachus. They are commonly cystic with septations. Because of the mucin produced, these urachal adenocarcinomas often have stippled or granular calcifications, which are best assessed by CT. The presence of a cystic mass at the superior anterior surface of the bladder at the midline level is highly suggestive of a urachal mucinous adenocarcinoma. Other malignancies of the urachus include sarcomas, transitional cell carcinoma, and squamous cell carcinoma; these malignancies are less commonly seen but can arise either from the urachus or the bladder. Urachal abscess may be indistinguishable from a urachal mucinous adenocarcinoma by imaging, and only the clinical history may help to differentiate the two. A communication with the bladder lumen was not present in this case, which excludes a bladder or urachal diverticulum. An uncomplicated urachal cyst should have smooth walls.

Clinical History: 44-year-old woman with recent bone marrow transplantation for leukemia presenting with fever.

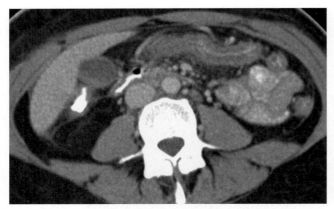

Figure 6.21   A

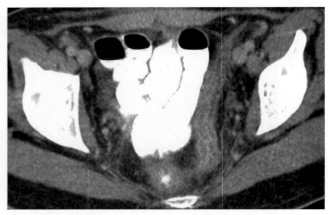

Figure 6.21   B

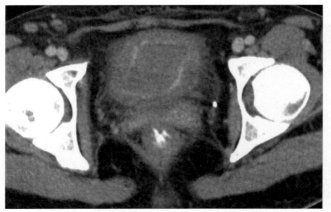

Figure 6.21   C

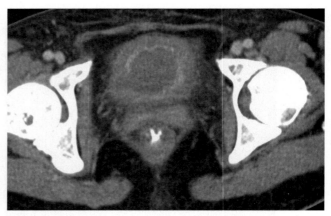

Figure 6.21   D

Findings: Axial CECT images show colonic and bladder wall thickening with mucosal hyperenhancement. Note surrounding fat stranding, which is more pronounced around the bladder.

Differential Diagnosis: Radiation cystitis, infectious cystitis, cyclophosphamide cystitis.

Diagnosis: Graft-versus-host disease of the bladder.

Discussion: Graft-versus-host disease (GVHD) occurs when the donor lymphoid cells damage organs of the recipient. Involvement occurs in 30% to 50% of allogeneic transplantation recipients within the first 100 days of the transplantation. The most commonly involved organs are the skin, liver, and bowel. In this case, the bladder mucosa was also involved. Gastrointestinal involvement is often nonspecific; bowel wall thickening is most commonly present. The bladder wall thickening in this case was also caused by GVHD. A biopsy of the involved organ is necessary to establish the diagnosis. Cancer patients receiving cyclophosphamide may develop hemorrhagic cystitis, but this drug would not directly cause bowel toxicity and bowel wall thickening observed in this case. The immunosuppressive regimen patients are exposed to prior to bone marrow transplantation puts them at increased risk for opportunistic infections, which should be excluded in this case. Exclusion of an infectious etiology is crucial because patients with GVHD are treated with immunosuppressive agents, which would be contraindicated in case of infectious enterocolitis. In the absence of small bowel pathology, radiation cystitis and colitis is unlikely because small bowel loops would have been included in the radiation field given the extent of colonic disease.

Clinical History: 37-year-old woman with history of seizures and recurrent pneumothoraces.

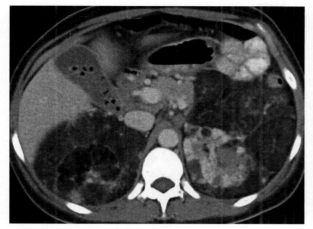

Figure 6.22   A

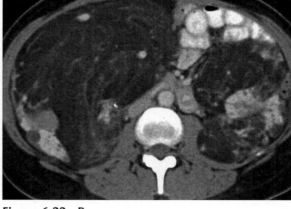

Figure 6.22   B

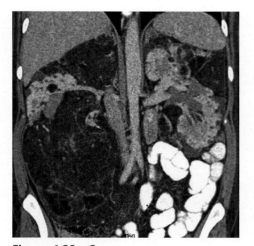

Figure 6.22   C

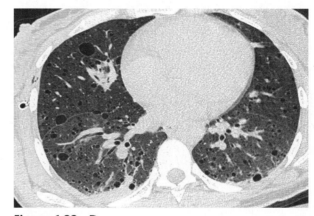

Figure 6.22   D

Findings: Axial (A and B) and coronal (C) CECT images demonstrate multiple fat-containing masses with enlarged blood vessels in both kidneys, with the largest one on the right measuring 18.0 × 9.9 cm. Several renal cysts are also present. Axial CECT image (D) shows multiple thin-walled lung cysts. Note the chest tube in the right subcutaneous tissues and cholelithiasis.

Differential Diagnosis: None.

Diagnosis: Angiomyolipomas in a patient with tuberous sclerosis.

Discussion: Angiomyolipoma (AML) of the kidneys can be found incidentally in asymptomatic patients as an isolated lesion or as part of tuberous sclerosis. Tuberous sclerosis is an autosomal dominant neuroectodermal disorder characterized by a classic clinical triad of mental retardation, seizures, and facial adenoma sebaceum. Multiple bilateral renal cysts may be encountered. Approximately 80% of patients with tuberous sclerosis have renal AMLs that are commonly multiple and bilateral. In tuberous sclerosis, the AMLs can become very large, involving the entire retroperitoneum and deforming the kidney parenchyma, as in this case. Besides the fatty component, a large amount of muscle and/or vascular tissue is also present. AMLs are sometimes hard to distinguish from other retroperitoneal sarcomas and specifically from liposarcomas. The key to the diagnosis is to recognize that the fatty lesions arise from the kidney and not the surrounding tissues. The presence of multiple, bilateral, fat-containing lesions within the kidney ensures the diagnosis of tuberous sclerosis with AMLs. An important clue to the correct diagnosis is also the presence of multiple lung cysts; these cause recurrent pneumothoraces, which is why the patient in this case has a chest tube. In tuberous sclerosis, AMLs may also be present in the liver.

Clinical History: 67-year-old man presenting with anemia and abdominal pain.

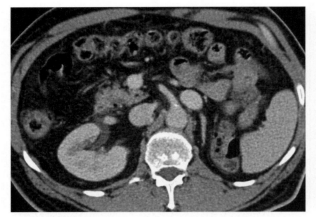

Figure 6.23   A

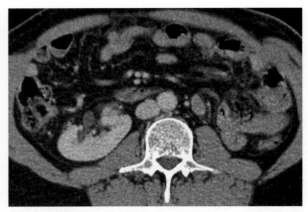

Figure 6.23   B

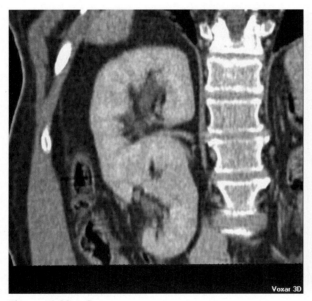

Figure 6.23   C

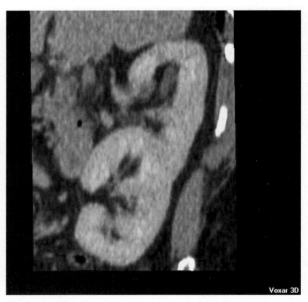

Figure 6.23   D

Findings: Axial CECT images (A and B) demonstrate two renal pelves originating in the right renal fossa. No kidney is present in the left renal fossa. Coronal (C) and sagittal (D) curved MPR images show fusion of the two kidneys. Note malrotation of the caudal kidney.

Differential Diagnosis: None.

Diagnosis: Crossed fused renal ectopia.

Discussion: Crossed ectopy occurs when the kidney lies on the side opposite of the ureteral insertion into the bladder. The ureteral insertion is typically normal, and the incidence of associated congenital anomalies is low. The crossed kidney usually lies inferior to the normally positioned kidney, and partial fusion is present in 90% of the cases. Males are more commonly affected than females. The left kidney is more commonly ectopic than the right. The etiology is uncertain but may be related to an abnormal umbilical artery, which inhibits the normal cephalad migration of the kidney. These patients are typically asymptomatic, with only a slightly higher incidence of stones and urinary tract infections, which are thought to be related to urinary stasis. CT imaging is usually diagnostic, and further workup is unnecessary.

Clinical History: 35-year-old man with acute left lower quadrant pain.

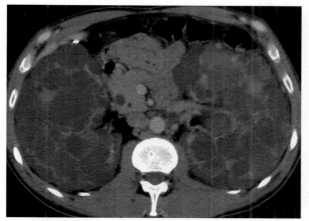

Figure 6.24   A

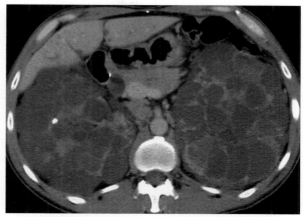

Figure 6.24   B

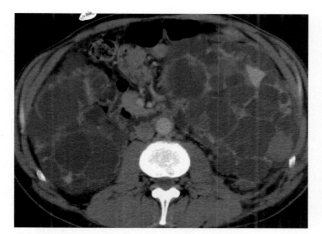

Figure 6.24   C

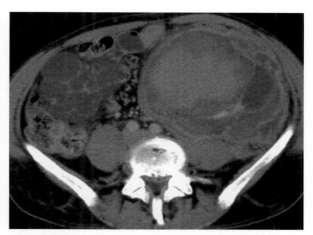

Figure 6.24   D

Findings: Axial CECT images demonstrate markedly enlarged kidneys almost completely replaced by multiple cysts, some of which have increased attenuation. A large heterogeneous lesion with central hyperdensity is present in the lower pole of the left kidney.

Differential Diagnosis: None.

Diagnosis: Autosomal dominant polycystic kidney disease with acute hemorrhage in a cyst.

Discussion: Autosomal dominant polycystic kidney disease (ADPKD) commonly presents in the third and fourth decades of life. Patients often complain of hypertension, flank pain, and palpable abdominal masses. All patients will eventually develop some degree of renal failure, which may require either dialysis or renal transplantation. Approximately 20% of these patients have berry aneurysms in the circle of Willis, which is one of the leading causes of death in these patients. Diagnosis of ADPKD is usually not difficult and can be made by family history, CT, or ultrasound. CT is often used to follow these patients to identify renal stones, which develop in 20% of cases, and hemorrhagic cysts. A hyperdense cyst on NECT can be secondary to hemorrhage, proteins, or infection, which can lead to acute flank pain. Chronic pain is usually due to enlargement of the cysts, causing stretching of the renal capsule. This case nicely demonstrates the bilateral innumerable cysts of varying density in enlarged kidneys, diagnostic of ADPKD. A large cyst containing a hyperdense retracted clot from acute hemorrhage is present in the left lower pole.

Clinical History: 79-year-old man presenting with dysuria and hematuria.

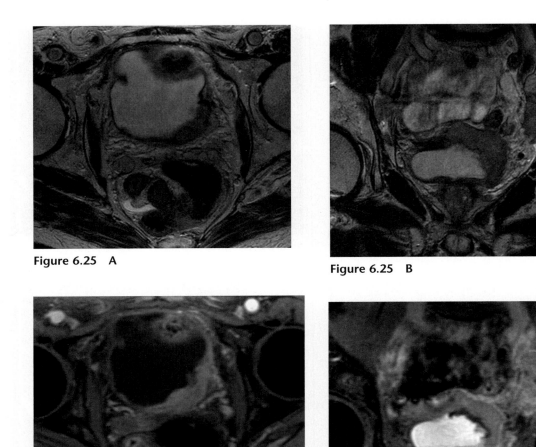

Figure 6.25   A

Figure 6.25   B

Figure 6.25   C

Figure 6.25   D

Findings: Axial (A) and coronal (B) T2-WI demonstrate a 4.8 × 2.4 × 1.7 cm mass of intermediate signal intensity in the left bladder wall, causing interruption of the hypointense muscular layer of the bladder. Portions of the mass and spiculations originating from it extend into the perivesical fat. Note the 3.5 × 2.0 cm left obturator lymphadenopathy and dilated ureter medial to it. Gadolinium-enhanced, fat-suppressed axial (C) and coronal (D) T1-WI show marked enhancement of the bladder wall mass and lymphadenopathy.

Differential Diagnosis: Other primary bladder neoplasm (squamous cell carcinoma, adenocarcinoma), metastasis.

Diagnosis: Transitional cell carcinoma of the bladder.

Discussion: MRI is an excellent modality for evaluating bladder neoplasms. MRI allows visualization of the tumor in multiple planes, which aids in evaluating involvement of adjacent organs, such as ureter, prostate, seminal vesicles, rectum, and pelvic sidewall. Lymphadenopathy is also easily detected with MRI. Perivesical extension is critical in the staging of transitional cell carcinoma of the bladder. Perivesical extension changes the tumor staging from a stage B (within the bladder muscle) to a stage C (extension through the bladder muscle and into perivesical tissue). This can be detected with MRI due to the high water content of the tumor (hyperintense on T2-WI compared to the bladder wall) and its marked enhancement with gadolinium. Full thickness disruption of the normally hypointense muscularis propria of the bladder by tumor on T2-WI is indicative of extravesical extension. The use of fat saturation allows even better contrast resolution between enhancing tumor and perivesical fat.

Clinical History: 7-day-old boy with a palpable mass in the right flank.

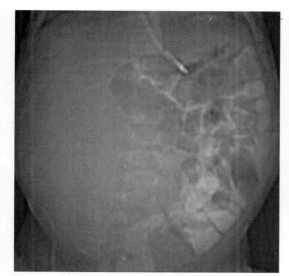

Figure 6.26   A

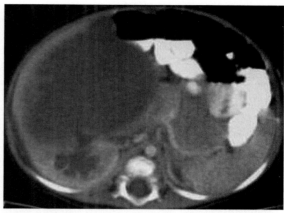

Figure 6.26   B

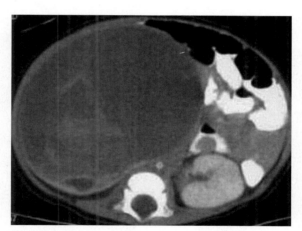

Figure 6.26   C

Findings: Abdominal radiograph (A) demonstrates a large right abdominal mass displacing the bowel to the left. Axial CECT images (B and C) show a large low-attenuation heterogeneous mass involving the right kidney. Normal parenchyma can be seen surrounding the mass posteriorly. The mass causes hydronephrosis.

Differential Diagnosis: Hydronephrosis, Wilms tumor, neuroblastoma.

Diagnosis: Mesoblastic nephroma.

Discussion: Mesoblastic nephroma is the most common solid renal neoplasm in a newborn. However, hydronephrosis is the most common cause of a palpable flank lesion in the neonate. Mesoblastic nephroma is a benign tumor that has also been called benign congenital Wilms tumor or fetal renal hamartoma. The tumor arises from renal connective tissue and very rarely undergoes sarcomatous transformation. Patients are typically asymptomatic, and the mass is usually found incidentally by prenatal ultrasound or after birth by the parents. By CT imaging, the mass is usually solid but may have multiple cystic spaces due to hemorrhage or necrosis. It may replace a large portion of the renal parenchyma. It can be mistaken for hydronephrosis, so care must be taken to identify the renal collecting system. An adrenal mass, such as a neuroblastoma, can displace the kidney and mimic a renal mass. The presence of a claw sign by the renal parenchyma at the edges of the mass, as seen in this case, ensures the renal origin of the lesion. Treatment is surgical resection, and prognosis is typically excellent.

Case images courtesy of Dr. Jeannette M. Perez-Rossello, Children's Hospital Boston, Boston, MA.

Clinical History: 77-year-old man presenting with gross hematuria.

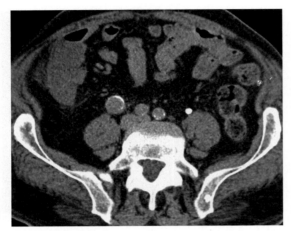

Figure 6.27   A

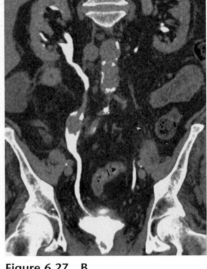

Figure 6.27   B

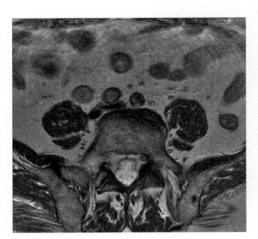

Figure 6.27   C

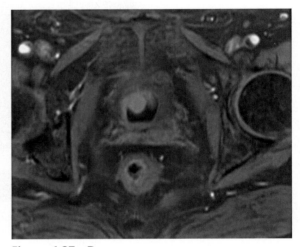

Figure 6.27   D

Findings: Axial (A) and curved MPR (B) CECT images in the excretory phase demonstrate a 2.0 × 2.2 × 5.8 cm soft tissue mass in the right mid ureter, surrounded by excreted contrast. Axial T2-WI (C) shows the intermediate signal intensity of the mass anterior to the right psoas muscle. Gadolinium-enhanced, fat-suppressed T1-WI (D) shows a 1.7 × 1.4 cm enhancing nodule along the anterior bladder wall.

Differential Diagnosis: Primary neoplasm (squamous cell carcinoma, adenocarcinoma, papilloma), metastasis, tuberculosis.

Diagnosis: Transitional cell carcinoma of the ureter and bladder.

Discussion: Transitional cell carcinoma (TCC) of the ureter is frequently associated with involvement of other areas of the collecting system. This is thought to be due to the greater amount of urothelial surface present in the bladder and renal pelvis in comparison to the ureter. In approximately 25% to 30% of patients with ureteral TCC, there is a synchronous lesion in the collecting system. TCCs of the ureter can be single or multiple. When multiple, they can be difficult to distinguish from inflammatory conditions such as malako-plakia, leukoplakia, or ureteritis cystica. Cystoscopy and histologic correlation are often necessary to make the diagnosis. Occasionally, periureteral fat stranding may be seen at the level of the mass, and this may be due to inflammation or periureteral extension of tumor, which are indistinguishable from each other by CT.

CASE 6-28

Clinical History: 68-year-old man with history of renal calculi presents with fevers and left flank pain.

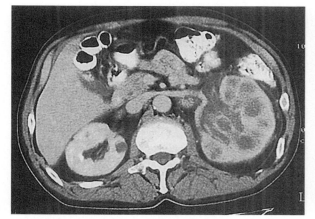

Figure 6.28   A

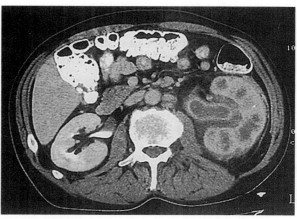

Figure 6.28   B

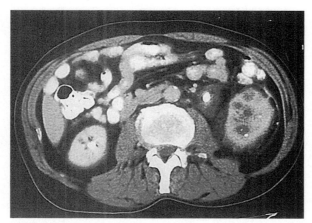

Figure 6.28   C

Findings: Axial CECT images demonstrate an enlarged, poorly perfused left kidney. The renal pelvis and calyces are dilated and irregular in appearance. There is stranding in the renal sinus and perinephric space. Note multiple low-density lesions in the renal parenchyma. The renal pelvis is dilated due to a proximal ureteral obstructing calculus.

Differential Diagnosis: Transitional cell carcinoma, lymphoma.

Diagnosis: Xanthogranulomatous pyelonephritis.

Discussion: Xanthogranulomatous pyelonephritis (XGP) is a chronic suppurative granulomatous infection of the kidney secondary to obstruction of the collecting system. As the kidney becomes chronically obstructed, the calyces dilate and fill with purulent material and debris, and the kidney

itself enlarges. Typically there is an obstructing calculus or a staghorn calculus. XGP is much more commonly diffuse (90%) than focal (10%). On CECT, the affected renal parenchyma is nonfunctioning and diffusely enlarged, with dilated calyces filled with pus. Low-density masses, which may measure fat density, are typically present in the renal parenchyma. An obstructing stone or staghorn calculus is almost always seen, as in this example. Treatment consists of nephrectomy. Simple hydronephrosis would not account for the inflammatory changes around the kidney. An infiltrating malignant process, such as transitional cell carcinoma or lymphoma, can diffusely infiltrate the kidney and globally enlarge it. A dilated collecting system is not commonly seen in these cases unless the tumor involves the ureter.

Clinical History: 69-year-old man with a history of mild chronic renal failure presenting with malaise and fatigue.

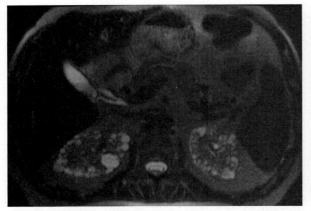

Figure 6.29   A

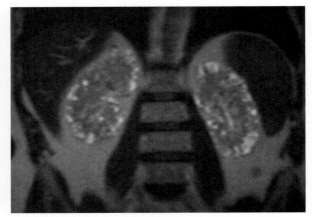

Figure 6.29   B

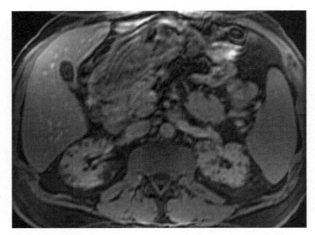

Figure 6.29   C

Findings: Axial (A) and coronal (B) T2-WI demonstrate innumerable small cortical-based cystic lesions in normal-sized kidneys. The cysts show no enhancement on the gadolinium-enhanced, fat-suppressed axial T1-WI (C).

Differential Diagnosis: Chronic lithium nephropathy, autosomal dominant polycystic kidney disease, acquired cystic disease.

Diagnosis: Glomerulocystic kidney disease.

Discussion: Glomerulocystic kidney disease is a rare form of cystic renal disease characterized histologically by cystic dilatation of Bowman's capsule. Therefore, the cysts are only cortical in location. Most cases occur in neonates and children who may have mild renal failure. Few cases have been reported in adult patients. The cysts may be undetected on NECT given their small size and appear as small hypodense cortical lesions on CECT. On MRI, the lesions have the typical signal of cysts, being hypointense on T1-WI and hyperintense on T2-WI and showing no enhancement following intravenous gadolinium injection. The main differential diagnosis in this case would be chronic lithium nephropathy, which may have an identical appearance. Only the clinical information of lithium intake would be useful to determine the correct diagnosis. In autosomal dominant polycystic kidney disease, the cysts affect both the cortex and the medulla, and the kidneys are enlarged. In acquired cystic disease, in which a history of chronic renal failure needs to be present, the kidneys are often atrophied and have cortical and medullary cysts.

Clinical History: 30-year-old man presenting with hematuria and burning sensation with urination.

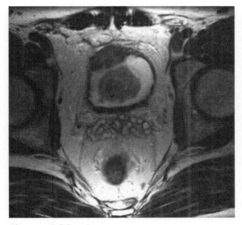

Figure 6.30   A

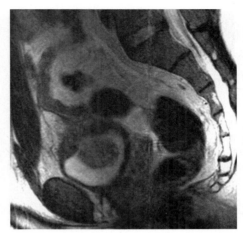

Figure 6.30   B

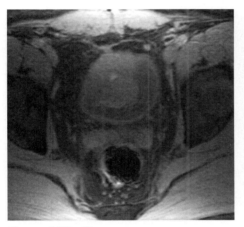

Figure 6.30   C

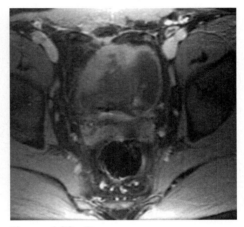

Figure 6.30   D

Findings: Axial (A) and sagittal (B) T2-WI show a 5.1 × 3.1 × 3.0 cm solid mass along the bladder wall at the dome, centered to the right of midline. An intraluminal lesion is also present within the bladder. Fat-suppressed axial T1-WI before (C) and after (D) gadolinium administration demonstrate enhancement of the bladder wall mass but no enhancement of the intraluminal lesion.

Differential Diagnosis: Transitional cell carcinoma, squamous cell carcinoma.

Diagnosis: Urachal carcinoma with intraluminal hematoma.

Discussion: Urachal malignancies account for 0.5% of all bladder cancers. The most common histology of urachal cancer is adenocarcinoma. Although the urachus is lined by squamous epithelium, adenomatous transformation is thought to be due to columnar metaplasia prior to malignant transformation. Most urachal tumors arise in the juxtavesical urachal ligament and then extend to the bladder or towards the umbilicus. Urachal tumors are usually present at the midline, but deviation to the left or right of the midline may be present due to fusion of the urachus with an obliterated umbilical artery, which was present in this case. The first diagnostic consideration in this case is a transitional cell carcinoma, but the young age of the patient is atypical. The location of the tumor near the dome should raise concern for a urachal neoplasm. Squamous cell carcinoma of the bladder wall occurs in the setting of chronic inflammation. Urachal cancers can be solid or partly cystic due to mucin produced by some tumors. Psammomatous calcifications may be identified by CT in 50% to 70% of cases. In this case, the nonenhancing intraluminal lesion in the bladder is a blood clot; absence of attachment of this abnormality to the bladder wall is an important diagnostic clue.

Clinical History: 57-year-old man presenting with weight loss, abdominal pain, and progressive difficulty passing stools.

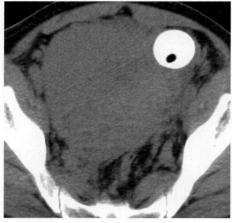

Figure 6.31   A

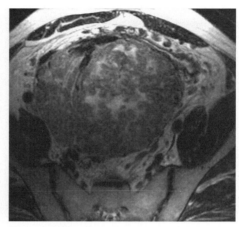

Figure 6.31   B

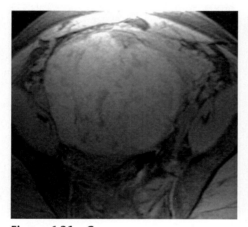

Figure 6.31   C

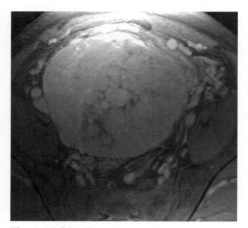

Figure 6.31   D

Findings: Axial NECT image (A) shows a 13-cm mass inseparable from the bladder wall. The bladder, which contains a contrast-filled Foley catheter balloon, is displaced to the left. Axial T2-WI (B) demonstrates that the large mass contains areas of bright signal (suggesting necrosis). Intact internal bladder lining is identified. The mass is more hyperintense than muscle on the unenhanced, fat-suppressed axial T1-WI (C) and shows heterogeneity on the gadolinium-enhanced, fat-suppressed axial T1-WI (D).

Differential Diagnosis: Transitional cell carcinoma, adenocarcinoma, squamous cell carcinoma, sarcoma.

Diagnosis: Solitary fibrous tumor of the bladder.

Discussion: Solitary fibrous tumors are either of mesothelial or fibroblast/primitive mesenchymal cell origin. The most common locations for these tumors are the pleura and mediastinum. Other reported locations include the abdominal cavity, parotid gland, pericardium, ovary, liver, intestine, lung, orbit, upper respiratory tract, bladder, and periosteum. The unifying characteristic of solitary fibrous tumors is positive staining for CD34, resulting from the spindle cells. Cases have been reported in patients from 9 to 86 years of age (average age, 57 years) and appear to be nearly evenly distributed between males and females. It is often difficult to assess the organ of origin of a very large mass. Multiplanar imaging is helpful to identify whether a fat plane is present between the mass and an adjacent structure; if such a finding is present, it indicates the mass displaces the structure and does not originate from it. Given the large size of the mass, a pelvic sarcoma is the best differential diagnosis in this case. The mass does not disrupt the urothelial lining of the bladder, best seen on the T2-WI, which excludes bladder transitional cell carcinoma, adenocarcinoma, and squamous cell carcinoma.

Clinical History: 54-year-old man who is renal transplantation candidate evaluated with MRI for a prominent pancreatic head.

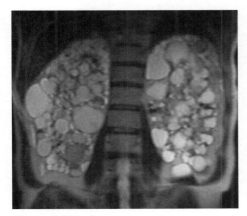

Figure 6.32   A

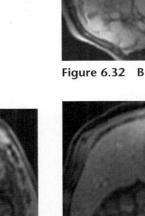

Figure 6.32   B

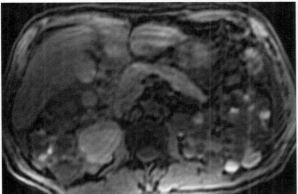

Figure 6.32   C

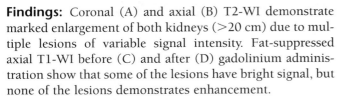

Figure 6.32   D

Findings: Coronal (A) and axial (B) T2-WI demonstrate marked enlargement of both kidneys (>20 cm) due to multiple lesions of variable signal intensity. Fat-suppressed axial T1-WI before (C) and after (D) gadolinium administration show that some of the lesions have bright signal, but none of the lesions demonstrates enhancement.

Differential Diagnosis: Multiple renal cysts, acquired cystic kidney disease, von Hippel-Lindau disease.

Diagnosis: Autosomal dominant polycystic kidney disease.

Discussion: Autosomal dominant polycystic kidney disease (ADPKD) is due to a mutation on chromosome 16. It results in renal cysts in 100% (penetrance) of affected patients but with wide variation in expressivity. Cysts can be present in many other organs, most commonly in the liver

(up to 88%). Cerebral aneurysms (20% of patients), mitral valve prolapse, and renal stones are associated abnormalities. The majority of the cysts are hypointense on T1-WI and hyperintense on T2-WI. Proteinaceous or hemorrhagic cysts will typically be hyperintense on both T1-WI and T2-WI. No enhancement associated with the cysts should be present. In fact, there is no increased risk of renal cell carcinoma in patients with ADPKD. A family history of polycystic renal disease is usually not present in patients with multiple renal cysts, and the cysts in these patients tend to be less diffuse. In acquired cystic kidney disease, the kidneys are small, and end-stage renal failure has to be present. Patients with von Hippel-Lindau disease will have a constellation of findings, including cerebral hemangioblastomas.

Clinical History: 63-year-old man presenting with right flank pain and hematuria.

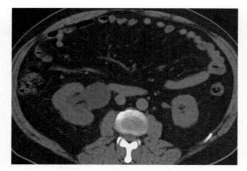

Figure 6.33   A

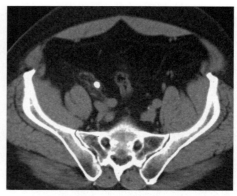

Figure 6.33   B

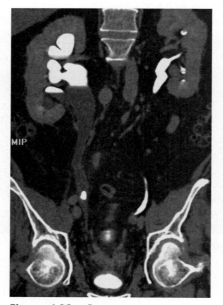

Figure 6.33   C

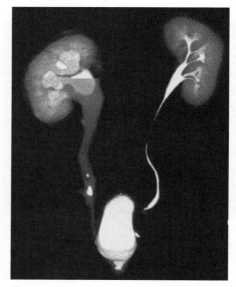

Figure 6.33   D

Findings: Axial NECT images (A and B) show right hydronephrosis and, adjacent to the iliac vessels, an 8-mm, high-density focus surrounded by a thin rim of soft tissue and fat stranding. Curved maximum-intensity projection (MIP) (C) and three-dimensional, volume-rendered (D) CECT images in the excretory phase confirm the ureteral location of the high-density focus and show delay in contrast excretion by the right kidney.

Differential Diagnosis: None.

Diagnosis: Obstructive ureterolithiasis.

Discussion: NECT is now the diagnostic test of choice to evaluate obstructive uropathy due to a renal stone. Every renal calculus is hyperdense on CT, except the rare unmineralized matrix stones and stones caused by indinavir (Crixivan), an HIV medication. On CT, in addition to identification of the stone in the ureter, secondary signs may be present, including hydronephrosis, hydroureter, perinephric and periureteral fat stranding, renal enlargement, and delay in function. In the early hours after passage of a stone in the ureter, when secondary signs have not developed, a helpful sign to ascertain that a high-density focus is in fact in the ureter is the rim sign; a peripheral rim of soft tissue surrounding a calcification indicates that the calcification is intraureteral. The soft tissue represents the inflamed ureteral wall. This sign would not be present if the calcification is a phlebolith, which may be confused for a ureteral calculus. Phleboliths may have a lucent center, which is another differentiating sign from a stone. Also, the "comet tail" sign has been described in association with phleboliths; the comet tail sign is a linear or curvilinear band of soft tissue extending from a calcification.

Clinical History: 31-year-old man with a history of ureteral stone 3 years prior presenting with right flank pain.

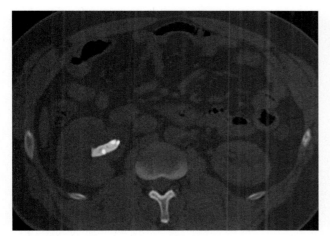

Figure 6.34   A

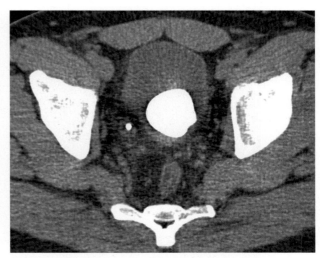

Figure 6.34   B

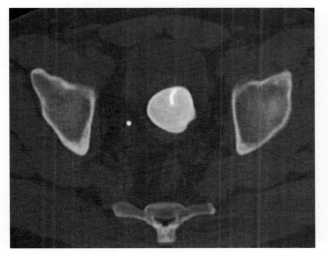

Figure 6.34   C

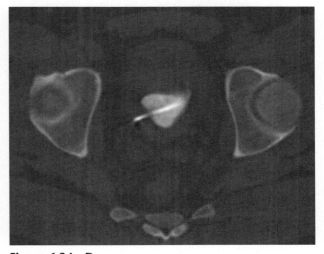

Figure 6.34   D

Findings: Axial NECT in bone (A, C, and D) and soft tissue (B) windows show a 3.6 × 3.9 cm calcification around the distal end of a double-J ureteral stent. Smaller calcification around the proximal end is also seen. Note marked right hydronephrosis.

Differential Diagnosis: None.

Diagnosis: Ureteral stent encrustation.

Discussion: In the United States, bladder stones are most commonly associated with bladder outlet obstruction. They are usually composed of calcium oxalate and calcium phosphate. Stones may also develop in a diverticulum due to stasis. Diverticular stones may eventually extend into the bladder, at which time they will have a dumbbell configuration. Vesical foreign bodies, such as Foley catheters, ureteral stents, or suture material, may serve as a nidus for stone formation, referred to as encrustation. In this case, the patient was lost to follow-up after treatment of a ureteral stone, and the ureteral stent remained in place for 3 years. Schistosomiasis is the most common worldwide cause of bladder wall calcifications. Transitional cell carcinomas calcify in 0.5% of cases. An enlarged calcified prostate protruding in the bladder base may also be a cause of bladder calcification. Other causes of bladder wall calcifications are urachal carcinomas, tuberculosis infection, radiation therapy, cyclophosphamide treatment, and amyloidosis.

Clinical History: 63-year-old woman presenting with left flank pain.

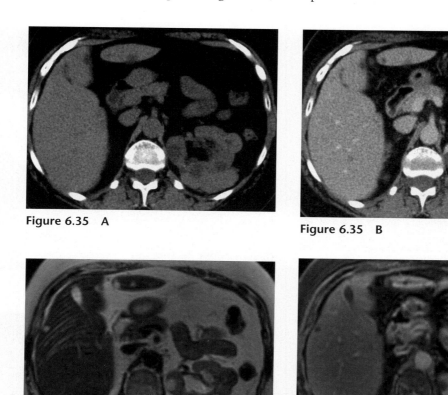

Figure 6.35   A

Figure 6.35   B

Figure 6.35   C

Figure 6.35   D

Findings: Axial NECT image (A) shows a 6.2 × 2.5 cm, hyperdense, homogeneous mass originating from the posterior portion of the left kidney. It demonstrates homogeneous enhancement on the axial CECT image (B). On the axial T2-WI (C), it is of darker signal intensity than the renal parenchyma and again has homogeneous enhancement on the gadolinium-enhanced, fat-suppressed axial T1-WI (D). Another solid left renal mass containing fat (angiomyolipoma) is seen. Note several hepatic and left renal cysts.

Differential Diagnosis: Renal cell carcinoma, leiomyoma of the renal capsule.

Diagnosis: Lipid-poor angiomyolipoma.

Discussion: An angiomyolipoma (AML) is a benign renal mass that is composed of fat, smooth muscle, and abnormal blood vessels. The vast majority of AMLs contain fat detectable at imaging, usually optimally identified with thin-section (3–5 mm) CT. Identification of fat on NECT is considered diagnostic. However, 4% to 5% of AMLs do not have

fat detectable by imaging and are termed lipid-poor AMLs. These lesions are typically hyperdense compared to the renal parenchyma on NECT due to the smooth muscle content and have marked homogeneous enhancement following contrast administration because of the abnormal blood vessels. On MRI, they can have signal intensity lower than the parenchyma on T2-WI. All these findings were present in this case. The most important differential diagnosis is a papillary or clear cell renal cell carcinoma (RCC). RCCs are usually heterogeneous masses, even if some portions of the mass are hyperdense due to hemorrhage. The enhancement pattern of RCCs is also very heterogeneous, especially with the larger clear cell variants. A papillary RCC may be homogeneous, hyperdense, and darker than the renal parenchyma on T2-WI but shows poor enhancement, as opposed to AMLs, which have marked enhancement. Leiomyomas of the renal capsule are exceedingly rare. To avoid surgical or ablative therapy, if a lipid-poor AML is suspected at imaging, the mass can be biopsied percutaneously to confirm its benign nature, as was performed in this case.

Clinical History: 75-year-old woman who underwent treatment for a renal mass.

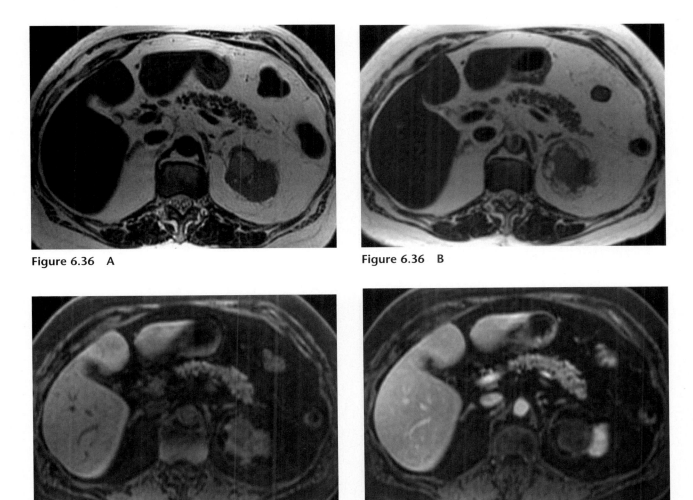

Figure 6.36   A

Figure 6.36   B

Figure 6.36   C

Figure 6.36   D

Findings: Pretreatment axial T2-WI (A) demonstrates a slightly hyperintense, 3.0 × 2.5 × 2.4 cm, left upper pole renal lesion. Ten months after treatment, axial T2-WI (B) shows a similar-appearing mass. Unenhanced (C) and gadolinium-enhanced (D) fat-suppressed axial T1-WI after treatment show no enhancement within the mass. A cuff of surrounding renal parenchyma is also not enhancing. Perinephric fat surrounding the mass is seen, bordered by a thin nonenhancing rim.

Differential Diagnosis: Angiomyolipoma.

Diagnosis: Cryoablated renal cell carcinoma.

Discussion: Numerous small solid renal masses are now discovered incidentally. This has led to advances in minimally invasive treatment techniques. Thermal ablation of small renal tumors can be performed using either radiofrequency ablation or cryoablation. This renal mass was biopsied prior to cryoablation and was proven to be a renal cell carcinoma. Follow-up imaging studies are performed to document regression of the tumor and also absence of residual enhancement in the lesion. Portions of the renal parenchyma are usually included in the ablation zone to ensure the tumor has been entirely covered. The ablation zone also usually extends, as in this case, into the perinephric fat. The border of the ablation zone is delimited by a thin nonenhancing rim seen in the perinephric fat, as seen on the posttreatment images. Knowledge of the prior cryoablation of a renal cancer is critical to avoid interpreting the rim in the perinephric fat as the border of a fat-containing lesion and, therefore, to avoid wrongfully diagnosing an angiomyolipoma.

Clinical History: 42-year-old woman who recently noted a lump in her abdomen.

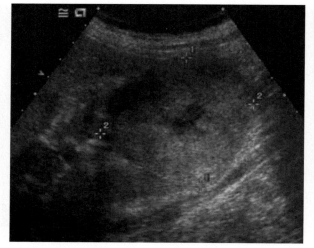

Figure 6.37   A

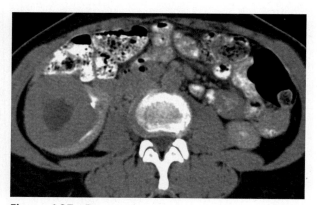

Figure 6.37   B

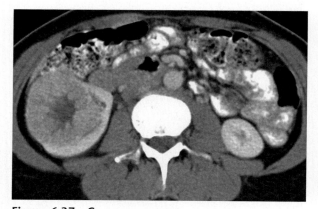

Figure 6.37   C

Figure 6.37   D

Findings: Sonographic sagittal image (A) through the right kidney shows a 6.1 × 7.2 cm exophytic mass off the lower pole of the right kidney. It is homogeneous except for a central area of decreased echogenicity. Axial NECT (B) and axial CECT in the nephrographic (C) and excretory (D) phases demonstrate a homogeneously enhancing solid mass with stellate central hypodensity.

Differential Diagnosis: Renal cell carcinoma, metanephric adenoma, metastasis, lymphoma.

Diagnosis: Oncocytoma.

Discussion: Oncocytomas are uncommon benign renal neoplasms, representing 3% to 6% of all primary renal tumors. They usually occur in patients in the sixth or seventh decade of life. Oncocytomas originate in the proximal tubular epithelium. Three percent are bilateral, and 5% are multifocal in the same kidney. The majority of these neoplasms are asymptomatic and found incidentally. They appear homogeneous on imaging and are well defined. In 30% of cases, especially in lesions over 3 cm in size, a central stellate scar is identified due to infarction and hemorrhage after the tumor has outgrown its blood supply. Percutaneous biopsy is often unreliable in differentiating an oncocytoma from an oncocytic renal cell carcinoma. Surgical resection, with nephron-sparing surgery if possible, is indicated. When they attain a large size, renal cell carcinomas almost invariably have more heterogeneous enhancement than what is seen in this case. Metanephric adenomas have little enhancement, can be homogeneous, and may even have an area of central hypodensity. Metastases usually have an infiltrative growth pattern, are often multiple, and occur late in the context of a known primary malignancy, which was not present in this case. Untreated secondary renal lymphoma has an entirely homogeneous appearance, and retroperitoneal lymphadenopathy usually accompanies renal lymphoma.

Clinical History: 24-year-old man with a history of chest pain.

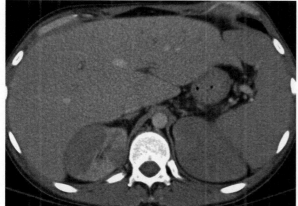

Figure 6.38   A

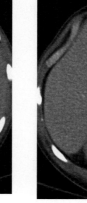

Figure 6.38   B

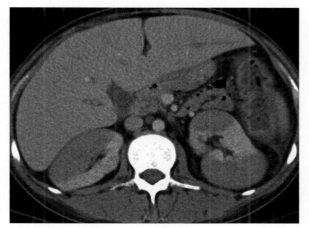

Figure 6.38   C

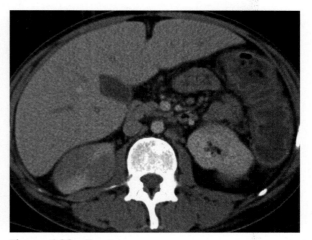

Figure 6.38   D

Findings: Axial CECT images show multiple well-defined, hypovascular, homogeneous renal parenchymal lesions, some having wedge-shape configuration and others causing renal contour deformity. Also note the periportal edema and colonic wall thickening with mucosal hyperenhancement.

Differential Diagnosis: Pyelonephritis, metastases, renal cell carcinomas.

Diagnosis: Renal lymphoma.

Discussion: Renal involvement by lymphoma is present in 30% to 60% of cases at autopsy. Primary renal lymphoma is rare; renal lymphomatous involvement is almost always secondary due to contiguous extension from retroperitoneal disease or hematogenous spread. It is much more commonly seen with non-Hodgkin disease. The kidneys are involved in one of the following five patterns: (a) multiple masses, which is the most common pattern (60%); (b) single mass; (c) contiguous extension from retroperitoneal disease; (d) perirenal

disease; and (e) diffuse infiltration. In the case of multiple masses, the disease may be unilateral or bilateral, and the masses typically range from 1 to 3 cm in size. The lesions in untreated cases are of homogeneous soft tissue density and mildly enhance after administration of intravenous contrast, as seen in this case. Associated retroperitoneal lymphadenopathy is present in approximately 50% of cases. The absence of perinephric inflammatory changes and the masslike appearance of some lesions make pyelonephritis unlikely. Metastases could have an identical appearance, but the lack of a known primary malignancy essentially eliminates that possibility. Renal cell carcinomas can be multifocal but are often heterogeneous in appearance. This patient presented with a pulmonary consolidation that was initially treated as a pneumonia but proven later to be lymphoma. He subsequently developed pseudomembranous colitis due to antibiotic therapy.

Clinical History: 34-year-old woman presenting with left lower quadrant pain.

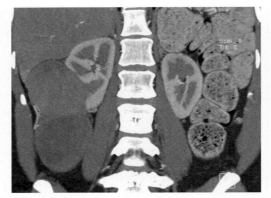

Figure 6.39   A

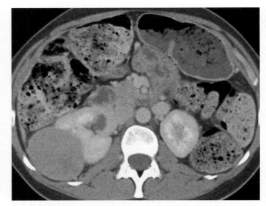

Figure 6.39   B

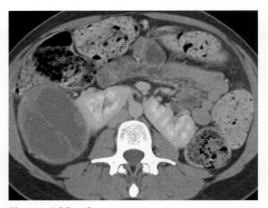

Figure 6.39   C

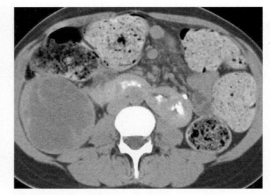

Figure 6.39   D

Findings: Coronal reformatted CECT image in the corti-comedullary phase (A) and axial CECT images in the nephrographic (B and C) and excretory (D) phases demonstrate a 12 × 5.7 × 6.2 cm, bilobed, exophytic right renal mass. The cranial solid component shows enhancement, and the caudal component is cystic with thick enhancing wall and septations. Note the fusion of the lower renal poles at the midline.

Differential Diagnosis: Renal cell carcinoma, lymphoma, metastasis, oncocytoma.

Diagnosis: Primary renal carcinoid in a horseshoe kidney.

Discussion: During normal embryology, the kidneys develop anterior to the sacrum and then progressively ascend to reach their adult position. If the metanephric buds fuse early during development, usually at the lower poles, a horseshoe kidney will form, and the ascent will be blocked by the root of the inferior mesenteric artery. Horseshoe kidneys occur 1 to 4 times per every 1000 births and are associated with vesicoureteral reflux and ureteropelvic junction obstruction. Primary carcinoid tumors of the kidney are extremely rare neoplasms; only approximately 30 cases have been reported in the English literature. They occur between 60 and 85 times more commonly in horseshoe kidneys than in normal kidneys. They occur in patients in the second to seventh decades of life. Renal carcinoids may be solid or cystic in appearance. An interesting described appearance is that of a bilobed mass, with one component being solid and the other one cystic, as seen in this case. Preoperative diagnosis is usually not made because most solid renal masses are presumed to be renal cell carcinomas until proven otherwise. Metastasis would be unlikely in the absence of a known primary tumor. Renal lymphoma presents as a mass of homogeneous soft tissue density. Oncocytomas, when large, may have a classic appearance of a homogeneous mass, occasionally with a central stellate scar.

Clinical History: 46-year-old man presenting with acute left flank pain.

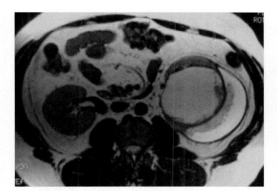

Figure 6.40   A

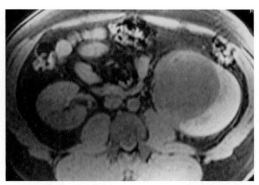

Figure 6.40   B

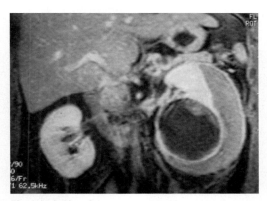

Figure 6.40   C

Findings: Axial T2-WI (A) shows an 8.5 × 8.9 × 8.7 cm left renal cystic mass with thick walls and mural nodularity. A 15 × 10.5 × 3.7 cm predominantly hyperintense crescentic abnormality is present adjacent to the mass. Fat-suppressed axial T1-WI before (B) and coronal T1-WI after (C) gadolinium administration show that the cystic mass has low signal intensity with nodular wall enhancement; the crescentic lesion is of high signal intensity before contrast and shows only smooth peripheral enhancement.

Differential Diagnosis: Abscess.

Diagnosis: Cystic renal cell carcinoma with perinephric hematoma.

Discussion: The Bosniak classification of cystic renal lesions was introduced to characterize these lesions and help in patient management. Category I lesions are simple cysts with no internal structure, wall thickening, or enhancement. They are entirely benign and do not have malignant potential. Category II lesions may have hairline septa, minimal thin calcification, or minimal perceived but not measurable enhancement. Hyperdense cysts smaller than 3 cm are considered category II lesions. Category IIF lesions require follow-up imaging; this category includes renal cysts that have an increased number of thin septa, minimal smooth septal or wall thickening, and thick or nodular calcifications but no measurable enhancing soft tissue components. Hyperdense cysts that are 3 cm or larger are considered category IIF lesions. Category III lesions are indeterminate lesions; they have thick and irregular septations or walls in which measurable enhancement is present. These lesions are malignant in 31% to 100% of cases. Category IV lesions are cystic renal cell carcinomas; they have enhancing soft tissue components that are adjacent to, but independent of, the walls or septa. Category IV lesions are malignant in 67% to 100% of cases. Category III and IV lesions require surgical treatment. The cystic renal mass in this case was classified as category IV and was surgically excised. The crescentic abnormality adjacent to it is a hematoma from prior tumoral hemorrhage. The nodular wall enhancement is more suggestive of a neoplasm than an abscess. A clinical history of infection was also not present.

Clinical History: 30-year-old woman being evaluated for renal transplantation.

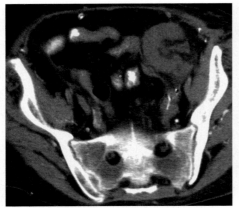

Figure 6.41   A

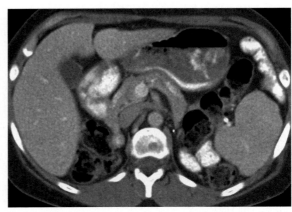

Figure 6.41   B

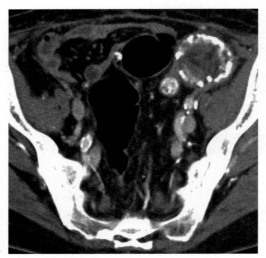

Figure 6.41   C

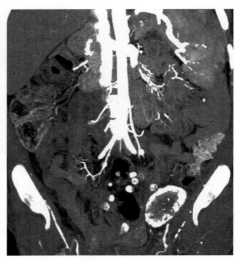

Figure 6.41   D

Findings: Axial NECT image (A) shows a left iliac fossa kidney. Axial CECT images (B and C) and coronal MIP image (D) obtained 2 years later demonstrate a 6.0 × 4.7 × 4.1 cm ovoid mass in the left lower quadrant with peripherally located coarse calcifications and central areas of fat attenuation. Note absence of native kidneys in the upper abdomen.

Differential Diagnosis: Sarcoma, pelvic kidney.

Diagnosis: Chronic renal transplantation rejection.

Discussion: Renal transplantation is the treatment of choice for patients with end-stage renal failure because survival is much longer than with peritoneal dialysis or hemodialysis. Transplanted kidneys are usually placed extraperitoneally in the right iliac fossa. Despite more effective immunosuppression, chronic rejection is the most common cause of late graft loss. It develops months to years after transplantation surgery. In the early stage of chronic rejection, the graft is enlarged and has increased cortical thickness. Later, cortical thinning, mild hydronephrosis, atrophy, and cortical nephrocalcinosis develop. In this case, knowledge of the history of previous renal transplantation and identification of the absence of the native kidneys are key to establish the correct diagnosis. Otherwise, the renal graft may be mistaken for a soft tissue sarcoma, and the patient may be referred for a biopsy. The lateral orientation of the renal sinus in this case makes a congenitally ectopic kidney less likely. In the early embryology, the renal sinus faces anteriorly and progressively rotates medially as the kidney ascends; it almost never faces laterally when the kidney remains in the pelvis.

Clinical History: 68-year-old man with a history of lung cancer.

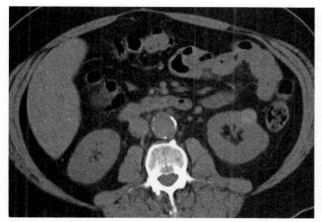

Figure 6.42   A

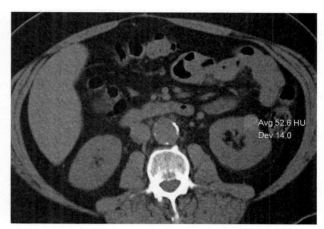

Figure 6.42   B

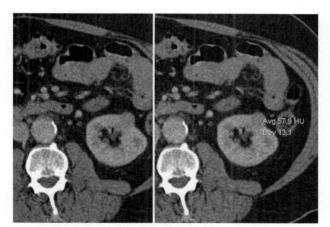

Figure 6.42   C

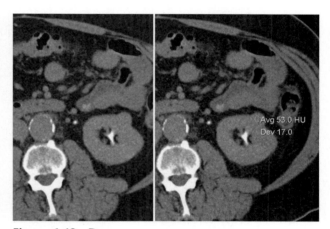

Figure 6.42   D

Findings: Axial NECT images (A and B) show a 1.6 × 1.9 cm, exophytic, left lower pole renal lesion measuring 52.6 HU. On the axial CECT image in the nephrographic phase (C), the mass measures 57.9 HU. On the axial CECT image in the excretory phase (D), the mass measures 53.0 HU.

Differential Diagnosis: Lipid-poor angiomyolipoma, papillary renal cell carcinoma, oncocytoma.

Diagnosis: Benign hyperdense cyst.

Discussion: A benign cyst can be hyperdense, and this is most often because of proteinaceous fluid accumulation within the cyst. For a lesion to be diagnosed as a hyperdense cyst, it has to meet specific criteria: it should be small (≤3 cm), well margined, homogeneously hyperdense, and nonenhancing. At least one fourth of the periphery of the lesion must contact the perinephric fat so that smoothness of the wall can be assessed. If the attenuation of a lesion increases by 10 HU or less after contrast administration, it is considered nonenhancing. An increase in attenuation by 20 HU or more after contrast administration is considered to be diagnostic of enhancement. An increase in density between 10 and 20 HU after contrast administration is equivocal for enhancement. In this case, the attenuation of the lesion increased by 5.3 HU between the NECT and the CECT in the nephrographic phase, indicating that the lesion is not enhancing. The vast majority of angiomyolipomas (AMLs) contain fat detectable at imaging, but 4% to 5% of AMLs do not and are termed lipid-poor AMLs. A hyperdense renal lesion other than a cyst would have some enhancement, and MRI could be helpful in distinguishing between the different solid renal masses.

Clinical History: 79-year-old woman with diabetes presenting with abdominal pain, nausea, and vomiting.

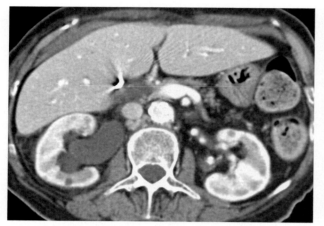

Figure 6.43   A

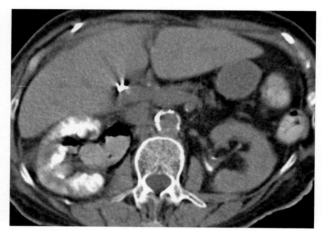

Figure 6.43   B

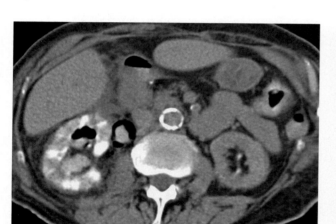

Figure 6.43   C

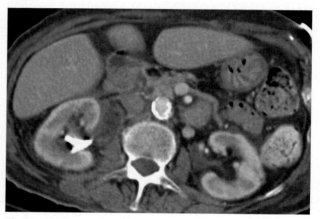

Figure 6.43   D

Findings: Axial CECT image (A) shows dilatation of the right renal collecting system. On the axial NECT images (B and C) obtained 1 day later, intraluminal and intramural gas is present in the collecting system and ureter, which also contain dense material. Note patchy persistent retained contrast in the right renal parenchyma. Axial CECT image (D) obtained 5 days later after nephrostomy tube placement demonstrates resolution of the gas and only minimal delay in enhancement compared to the left kidney.

Differential Diagnosis: Gas reflux from bladder, renogastrointestinal fistula.

Diagnosis: Emphysematous pyelitis.

Discussion: Emphysematous pyelitis is associated with gas limited to the wall of the renal collecting system. Women are more commonly affected than men (female-to-male ratio of 3:1), and 50% of the patients are diabetic.

Pyuria is almost always present upon urine analysis, and *Escherichia coli* is the most commonly identified bacteria. At imaging, gas is either present in the collecting system or outlines it. Dilatation and obstruction of the collecting system are almost always present, as seen in this case. This and the parenchymal inflammation explain the persistent delayed enhancement of the right kidney. This patient was successfully treated with percutaneous nephrostomy tube placement and antibiotic therapy. At times, intravesical gas, usually due to a Foley catheter, may reflux up the ureter, but in such a case, gas would not be present in the wall of the collecting system. Other causes of gas in the collecting system are due to fistula with gas-containing structures, such as bowel; in this case, no fistula could be identified. If gas is present in the renal parenchyma because of infection, it is termed emphysematous pyelonephritis.

Clinical History: 82-year-old woman on warfarin (Coumadin) presenting with left lower quadrant pain following hip surgery.

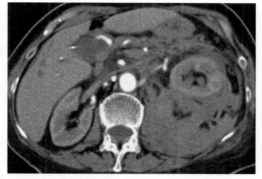

Figure 6.44   A

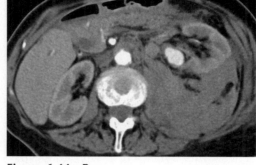

Figure 6.44   B

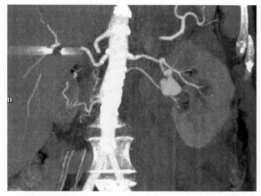

Figure 6.44   C

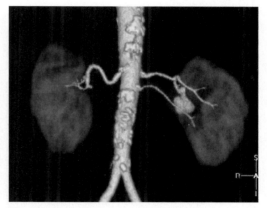

Figure 6.44   D

Findings: Axial CECT images (A and B) show a 2.0 × 1.4 cm hyperdense area medial to the left renal sinus. A large amount of left retroperitoneal hyperdense material (blood) is noted. Coronal MIP (C) and three-dimensional, volume-rendered images (D) demonstrate a bilobed structure in continuity with a branch of the dominant left renal artery.

Differential Diagnosis: Bleeding arteriovenous malformation.

Diagnosis: Ruptured renal artery aneurysm.

Discussion: A renal artery aneurysm is present in 0.01% to 0.1% of the population, and its discovery if often incidental. Renal artery aneurysms represent 22% of all visceral aneurysms. True aneurysms are most commonly caused by atherosclerotic disease, but fibromuscular dysplasia, pregnancy, and neurofibromatosis or Ehlers-Danlos syndrome are other possible etiologies. They can be classified into four types: (a) saccular, usually occurring at the first arterial bifurcation due to atherosclerosis; (b) fusiform secondary to medial fibroplasias; (c) dissecting; and (d) intrarenal, usually associated with arteritis, such as polyarteritis nodosa or Wegener granulomatosis. On NECT, rim calcification may be seen associated with a soft tissue density mass. On CECT, the patent enhancing lumen is usually isodense to the aorta, but the enhancing portion is variable depending on the amount of mural thrombus present. Aneurysms smaller than 2 cm with well-calcified rims in a normotensive patient usually require no treatment except in females who are pregnant or contemplating surgery because the risk of bleeding is significantly increased in this population. Although more aneurysms are treated percutaneously, surgery still represents the standard therapy for growing aneurysms or those with mural thrombus causing distal embolism. In this case, given the emergency of the situation, the patient's age, and the coexistent hematoma that might have obscured surgical visibility, percutaneous coiling was performed successfully. An arteriovenous malformation may show significant dilatation of involved vessels, but dilated or early draining veins can usually be identified, which were not present in this case.

Clinical History: 64-year-old man presenting with left lower quadrant pain.

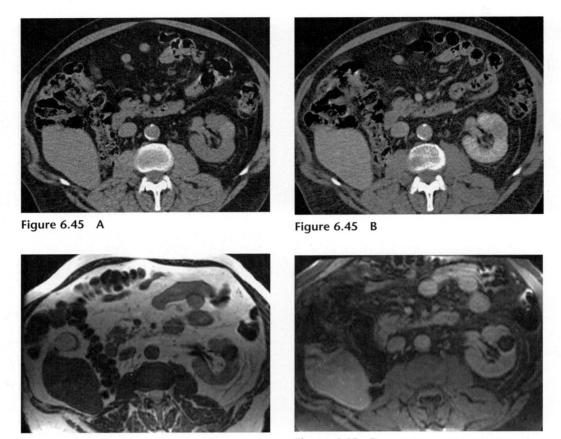

Figure 6.45   A

Figure 6.45   B

Figure 6.45   C

Figure 6.45   D

Findings: Axial NECT image (A) shows a 2.6 × 2.5 cm mass that has a density of 75 HU. On the axial CECT image in the nephrographic phase (B), the lesion has an attenuation of 95 HU. Axial T2-WI (C) shows the decreased signal intensity of the mass compared to the renal parenchyma. Gadolinium-enhanced, fat-suppressed axial T1-WI (D) shows marked hypointensity of the lesion.

Differential Diagnosis: Clear cell renal carcinoma, lipid-poor angiomyolipoma.

Diagnosis: Papillary renal carcinoma.

Discussion: Papillary renal carcinoma is the second most common (15–20%) pathologic subtype of primary renal neoplasm; clear cell carcinoma (conventional) is the most common (70%). The 5-year survival rate is also much better with the papillary subtype (80–90%) compared to the conventional type (55–60%). Although papillary renal cancer may be hyperdense on NECT, the attenuation value of the mass on NECT is not a reliable differentiating factor.

However, on CECT, papillary renal carcinoma enhances less than the clear cell subtype. Tumors that enhance more than 84 HU in the corticomedullary phase are more likely to be of the clear cell variant. Papillary renal carcinomas are considered hypovascular, as seen in this case. Calcifications in a renal mass are also more common in the papillary variant (32%) than in the conventional type (11%). On T2-WI, the signal intensity of the papillary subtype tends to be less than that of the renal parenchyma. On the gadolinium-enhanced, gradient-echo sequence, the papillary tumors may appear hypointense, as seen in this case, which is likely due to artifacts caused by hemosiderin within the mass. The subtype of renal cell carcinoma can be suggested based on imaging characteristics, but histologic confirmation is often needed to diagnose the correct subtype. A lipid-poor angiomyolipoma may be hyperdense on NECT and hypointense on T2-WI, but it is expected to markedly enhance following contrast administration.

Clinical History: 47-year-old man presenting with left flank pain.

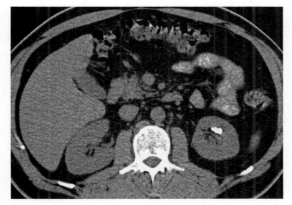

Figure 6.46   A

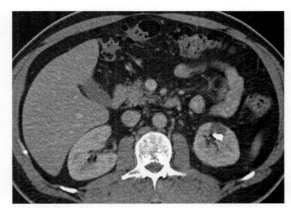

Figure 6.46   B

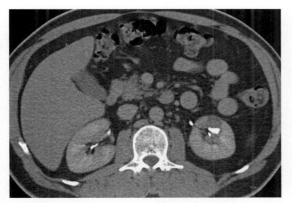

Figure 6.46   C

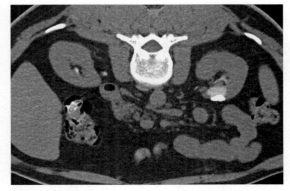

Figure 6.46   D

Findings: Axial NECT (A) and CECT in the nephrographic (B) and excretory (C) phases demonstrate a 1.9 × 2.1 cm cystic lesion in the left upper pole renal parenchyma. Dependent stones are present within the lesion. Axial CECT in the excretory phase (D), which was obtained with the patient in the prone position, shows filling of the cystic lesion by excreted contrast. The stones fall dependently.

Differential Diagnosis: Renal cyst, cystic renal cell carcinoma.

Diagnosis: Calyceal diverticulum.

Discussion: Calyceal diverticulum is a urine-filled cystic lesion within the renal parenchyma. It is most often congenital, but a lesion of similar appearance may occur after infection when a communication between the pyelocalyceal system and an abscess cavity persists or because of focal calyceal dilatation due to scarring. Two types of diverticulum have been described; type I, which is the most common, communicates with a minor calyx, whereas type II communicates directly with the renal pelvis or a major calyx. Up to 39% of diverticula contain layering stones or milk of calcium secondary to urine stasis because of a narrow diverticular neck. By CECT, the diverticular lumen gradually fills with excreted contrast, with the density within the lumen increasing with time; this should not be misinterpreted as enhancement of a solid lesion. As in this case, positional changes of the patient may be necessary to demonstrate a communication between the diverticulum and the collecting system. Because no solid enhancing component was present in this lesion, a renal cell carcinoma was excluded. Both renal cell carcinomas and renal cysts do not communicate with the pyelocalyceal system.

Clinical History: 39-year-old woman being evaluated for breast cancer staging.

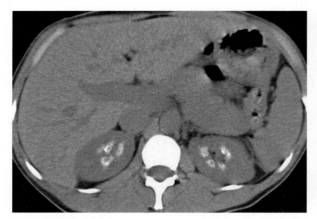

Figure 6.47 A

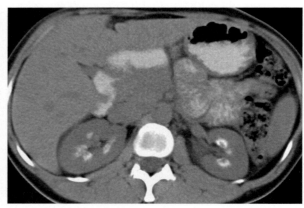

Figure 6.47 B

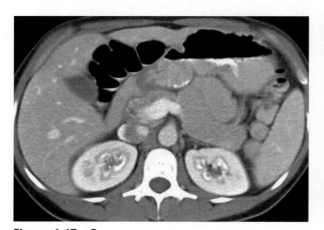

Figure 6.47 C

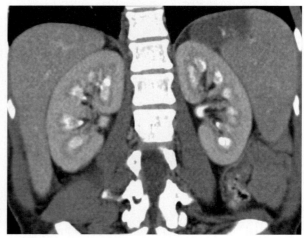

Figure 6.47 D

Findings: Axial NECT images (A and B) and axial (C) and coronal (D) CECT images in the corticomedullary phase show curvilinear calcifications in the pyramids of both kidneys.

Differential Diagnosis: None.

Diagnosis: Medullary nephrocalcinosis.

Discussion: Nephrocalcinosis is characterized by calcium deposition in the kidneys and is classified as medullary or cortical depending on the involved area. Medullary nephrocalcinosis is the most common form. The list of possible underlying etiologies is lengthy but primarily includes hyperparathyroidism (40%), distal renal tubular acidosis (20%), medullary sponge kidney (20%), and papillary necrosis. When it is caused by hyperparathyroidism or distal renal tubular acidosis, the calcifications are uniform in the medulla. When medullary sponge kidney is the cause, stones tend to form at the tip of the pyramids. Cortical nephrocalcinosis is due to, among other causes, chronic glomerulonephritis, cortical necrosis, acquired immunodeficiency syndrome (AIDS)-related nephropathy, and rejected renal transplantation (see Case 46).

Clinical History: 39-year-old man with a history of neurogenic bladder presenting with hematuria.

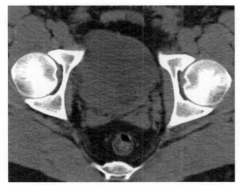

Figure 6.48   A

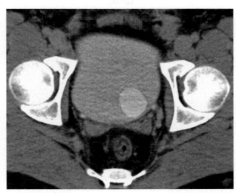

Figure 6.48   B

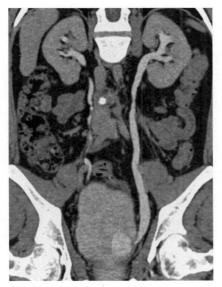

Figure 6.48   C

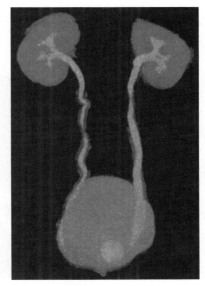

Figure 6.48   D

Findings: Axial NECT image (A) shows a 2.9 × 2.4 cm lesion of slightly lower density than urine protruding into the bladder lumen. Axial CECT (B), curved MPR (C), and three-dimensional, volume-rendered (D) images acquired in the excretory phase demonstrate filling of this lesion with excreted contrast. The lesion is centered on the left ureterovesical junction. Note mild dilatation of the left collecting system.

Differential Diagnosis: Ectopic ureterocele, cystitis cystica, hydatid cyst.

Diagnosis: Orthotopic ureterocele.

Discussion: Ureteroceles represent dilation of the submucosal segment of the distal ureter. The outer wall is made of the bladder urothelium, and the inner wall is composed of ureteral epithelium, with interposed fibrous and muscular tissue in between. Orthotopic ureteroceles (also termed simple) result, in young patients, from congenital meatal stenosis and, in adults, from inflammatory or neoplastic strictures. In congenital or inflammatory strictures, the walls of the ureterocele are smooth and thin. In neoplastic narrowing, the walls will be nodular or thick, typically over 2 mm. On imaging, orthotopic ureteroceles are cystic lesions in continuity with the normally implanted, dilated ureter. They will fill with contrast following intravenous injection and classically have a "cobra head" appearance. In ectopic ureteroceles, it is the distal end of the ureter draining the upper pole moiety of a duplicated collecting system that will be dilated. The ureter in such a case inserts more medially and inferiorly than the normally anatomically implanted lower moiety ureter. In the present case, only one ureter drains the left kidney, and the left ureterovesical junction is normally located at the bladder trigone, which excludes an ectopic ureterocele. Other causes of cystic bladder wall lesion will not fill with excreted contrast.

Clinical History: 55-year-old woman presenting with hematuria.

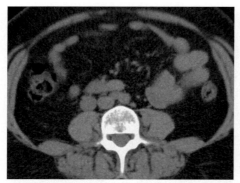

Figure 6.49   A

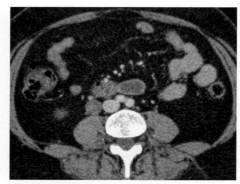

Figure 6.49   B

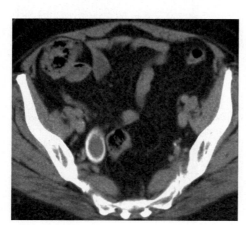

Figure 6.49   C

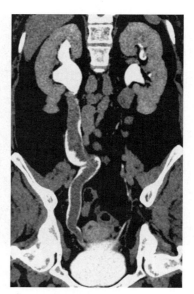

Figure 6.49   D

Findings: Axial NECT (A), axial CECT in nephrographic (B) and excretory (C) phases, and coronal curved reformatted image (D) show a 7.2 cm–long enhancing mass in the proximal third of the right ureter. The more distal ureter is filled with nonenhancing material. Note the marked dilatation of the right ureter.

Differential Diagnosis: Transitional cell carcinoma, hematoma.

Diagnosis: Fibroepithelial polyp.

Discussion: Primary neoplasms of the pelvicaliceal system are either of epithelial (the prototype being transitional cell carcinoma [TCC]) or of mesodermal origin. Mesodermal tumors are rarely encountered entities in the urinary tract, and the most common lesion in this category is a fibroepithelial polyp. Other tumors of mesodermal origin are angiomatous polyps, hemangiomas, leiomyomas, neurofibromas, and lymphangiomas. Fibroepithelial polyp usually occurs in patients between 20 and 40 years of age. Presenting symptoms are typically hematuria or nonspecific flank pain. Because the fibrous stalk of the polyp is covered by normal urothelium, urine cytology analysis is of very limited value in the diagnosis. On CT, an enhancing mass in the collecting system will be seen. As for gastrointestinal polyps, peristalsis may elongate the lesion over many years. The major differential diagnosis is a TCC, and differentiation may be difficult. Both tumors enhance and are intraluminal masses with mural attachment. Identification of the pedunculated nature of the mass may be the only clue that the lesion is a polyp. Because treatment of a fibroepithelial polyp consists of simple excision, whereas nephroureterectomy is preferred for upper tract TCC, correct preoperative diagnosis, which is sometimes impossible to make by imaging, is crucial. As for a hematoma, it should not enhance. In this case, the nonenhancing material in the distal ureter proved to be a clot.

Clinical History: 63-year-old man with recent bladder cancer resection presenting with lower abdominal pain.

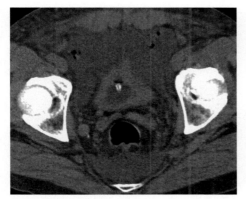

Figure 6.50   A

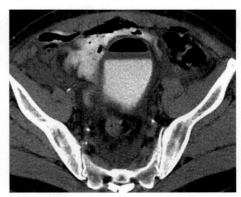

Figure 6.50   B

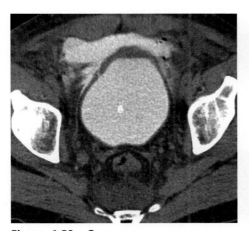

Figure 6.50   C

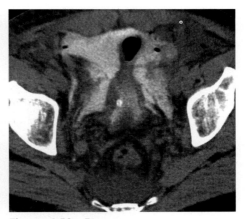

Figure 6.50   D

Findings: Axial NECT image (A) shows perivesical fluid containing gas bubbles and presacral fluid. A Foley catheter is in place in the bladder. CT cystogram images (B–D) demonstrate extravasation of contrast forming streaks in the perivesical fat.

Differential Diagnosis: None.

Diagnosis: Extraperitoneal bladder rupture.

Discussion: CT cystogram is a very sensitive method to diagnose and subtype bladder injuries. However, it requires adequate distention of the bladder with instillation of a minimum of 300 mL of a diluted solution of contrast (50 mL of Hypaque 60 in 450 mL of saline). With bladder underdistention, some injuries may be missed. Extraperitoneal bladder rupture is the most common type of major bladder injury, representing 80% to 90% of cases. It is usually caused by direct penetrating trauma, laceration due to bony fragments from pelvic trauma, or accidental surgical laceration. The extravasated contrast is close to the bladder and may have a flame-shaped appearance, with irregular but sharp margins. Extraperitoneal bladder rupture is treated with catheter diversion. Intraperitoneal bladder rupture represents 10% to 20% of major bladder injuries. It typically results from blunt trauma in the setting of a full bladder; the sudden increase in bladder pressure causes rupture of the dome, which is the mechanically weakest point. The extravasated contrast then collects in the peritoneal spaces. The treatment for intraperitoneal bladder rupture is immediate surgery. Other types of bladder traumatic injuries have been described, as follows: (a) bladder contusion consists of a partial tear of the mucosa, in which case CT cystography is typically normal; (b) interstitial injury is a partial-thickness tear with intact serosa; CT cystography demonstrates intramural contrast without extravasation; and (c) combined rupture.

Clinical History: 65-year-old woman with previous pelvic radiation therapy presenting with total incontinence.

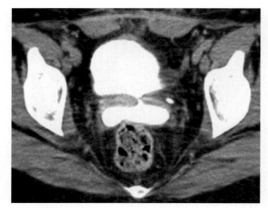

Figure 6.51 A

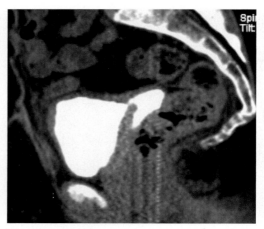

Figure 6.51 B

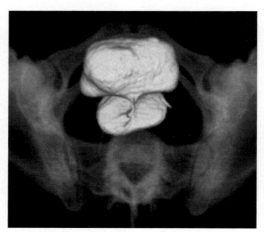

Figure 6.51 C

Findings: Axial (A) and sagittal reformatted (B) CECT images in the excretory phase demonstrate thickening of the anterior vaginal wall. Excreted contrast in the bladder extends through a short tract into the vagina. Three-dimensional, volume-rendered image (C) depicts the communication between the bladder and the upper vagina.

Differential Diagnosis: None.

Diagnosis: Vesicovaginal fistula.

Discussion: Acquired vesicovaginal fistulas may have various etiologies, such as obstetrical complications, iatrogenic or traumatic causes, pelvic malignancy, or radiation therapy.

Vaginal fistulas are reported to occur in 1% to 10% of patients following radiotherapy, especially for cervical cancer. Vaginal fistulas are difficult to delineate whether cystography, barium study, vaginography, or CT is used. The CT technique should be tailored to the type of the clinically suspected fistula; to evaluate a potential vesicovaginal communication, ideally only intravenous contrast should be used. Delayed views are often necessary because the fistulous tract may only be evident at that time. Identification of the tract and of contrast in the vagina is diagnostic. Contrast media may spill into the vagina in incontinent patients or patients who voided before the final images were acquired.

CASE 6-52

Clinical History: 55-year-old woman with low cardiac ejection fraction and renal failure after recent surgery for ischemic bowel.

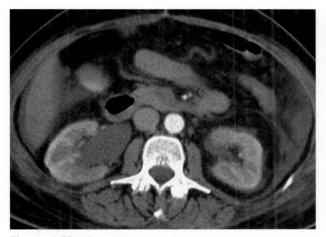

Figure 6.52   A

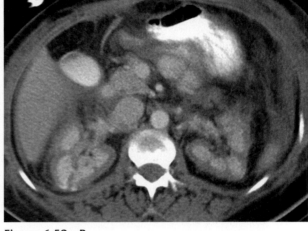

Figure 6.52   B

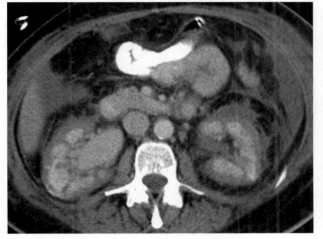

Figure 6.52   C

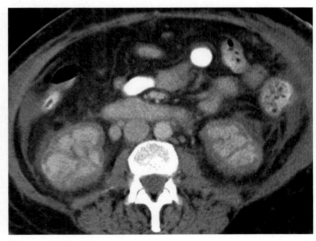

Figure 6.52   D

Findings: Early postoperative CECT image (A) shows normal enhancement of both kidneys in the corticomedullary phase. CECT images obtained 2 days later (B–D) demonstrate absent enhancement of the renal cortex and columns of Bertin bilaterally. The medulla and segments of subcapsular cortex are, however, enhancing normally. Note opacification of the right renal collecting system (from prior CT), perinephric stranding, and ascites.

Differential Diagnosis: Renal infarct.

Diagnosis: Acute cortical necrosis.

Discussion: Acute cortical necrosis is a rare form of acute renal failure. It results from ischemia due to vasospasm, toxic damage to glomerular capillary endothelium, and primary intravascular thrombosis. It is most often due to pregnancy-related complications, such as abruptio placentae, septic abortion, and placenta previa. Many other causes, including dehydration in children, hemolytic uremic syndrome, shock, and sepsis, have also been implicated. The kidneys are usually diffusely and bilaterally affected, but the involvement may be multifocal. Characteristic CECT findings are present in this case and consist of enhancement of the medulla but no enhancement of the cortex. Capsular or peripheral-most cortical enhancement may be observed due to capsular collateral vessels; a similar finding can be seen in renal infarction, but true renal infarcts do not spare the medulla. Progressive renal atrophy ensues, and rim or "tramline" cortical calcification may develop as early as 1 to 2 months after the injury.

Clinical History: 21-year-old man presenting with abdominal pain after a fall from a bicycle.

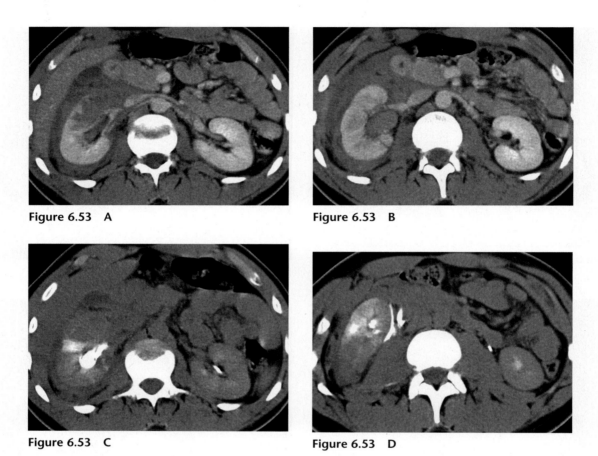

Figure 6.53   A

Figure 6.53   B

Figure 6.53   C

Figure 6.53   D

Findings: Axial CECT images in the nephrographic (A and B) and excretory (C and D) phases demonstrate an ill-defined (A) and linear (B) area of hypodensity (A) in the renal parenchyma. Contrast extravasation is present on the excretory phase. Persistent areas of parenchymal hyperenhancement are noted on the delayed images (C–D). Note soft tissue density in the perinephric space and high-density material in the renal sinus (B).

Differential Diagnosis: Pyelonephritis.

Diagnosis: Renal trauma.

Discussion: CECT is the imaging modality of choice to evaluate acute traumatic renal injuries. It can depict contusions, infarctions, lacerations, hematomas, active hemorrhage, and urine extravasation. Contusions may be seen as ill-defined or well-defined areas of decreased attenuation compared to the normal renal parenchyma. Contusions are differentiated from infarctions by the absence of enhancement in the latter.

Renal contusions result in hypofunction of the affected parenchyma, which accounts for the persistent focal hyperenhancement seen in this case on the images acquired in the nephrographic phase. Lacerations appear as linear areas of decreased density. Acute hematomas will have an attenuation between 40 and 90 HU. On the other hand, extravasation of contrast material, either from blood vessels or from the collecting system, will have much higher attenuation, ranging from 80 to 370 HU. Most cases are treated with conservative management. Percutaneous embolization can be performed in cases of active bleeding. Surgical intervention is often needed if: (a) over 50% of the renal parenchyma has been devitalized; (b) urine extravasation persists despite ureteral stenting or nephrostomy tube placement; or (c) arterial thrombosis is present. In pyelonephritis, a striated nephrogram due to areas of renal hypofunction may be seen, but perinephric hematoma or contrast extravasation is not expected.

Clinical History: 60-year-old man presenting with left lower quadrant pain.

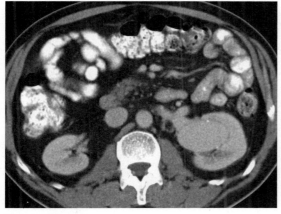

Figure 6.54 A

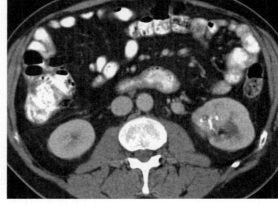

Figure 6.54 B

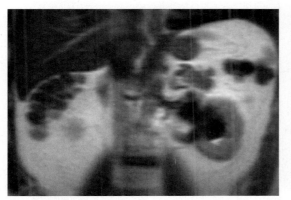

Figure 6.54 C

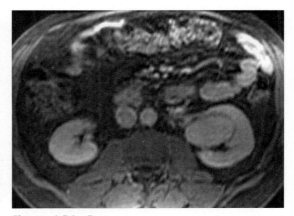

Figure 6.54 D

Findings: Axial CECT images (A and B) show a 5.5 × 3.7 cm, homogeneous, ovoid mass in the left renal sinus of density similar to the aorta. Note associated tubular structures immediately adjacent to this mass, some of which show curvilinear calcifications. Coronal T2-WI (C) demonstrates flow void in the mass, with adjacent round and tubular flow-void structures. Gadolinium-enhanced, fat-suppressed axial T1-WI (D) shows a homogeneous enhancement of the mass, which is isointense to the aorta.

Differential Diagnosis: Renal artery aneurysm.

Diagnosis: Arteriovenous malformation.

Discussion: Arteriovenous communications are of two types: arteriovenous malformations (AVMs) and arteriovenous fistulas (AVFs). AVMs can be either congenital or acquired, secondary to trauma, a rupture of an aneurysm, or a very vascular tumor. They are often asymptomatic and are more common in men. AVMs consist of multiple communications between segments of interlobar arteries and veins, usually of normal caliber. AVMs are typically located adjacent to the renal collecting system, as seen in this case. AVFs are more common than AVMs, representing 70% to 80% of arteriovenous communications; they can result from trauma, surgery, tumors, or rupture of an aneurysm into a vein. AVFs typically have a single feeding artery and draining vein, which are usually enlarged. Most close on their own. Fifty percent of symptomatic AVFs will cause high-output heart failure. On imaging, arteriovenous communications will demonstrate prompt early filling of the draining vein. In case of an AVM, a vascular mass and curvilinear calcifications may be seen. Therapy consists of percutaneous intravascular treatment, surgery, or a combination of percutaneous intravascular treatment and surgery. This case does not represent a simple renal artery aneurysm because multiple abnormal surrounding vessels are present, indicating a more complex vascular anomaly.

Clinical History: 29-year-old man presenting with left flank pain and microscopic hematuria.

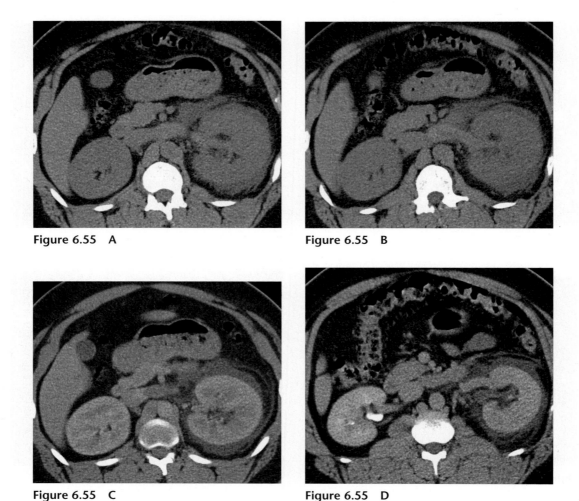

Figure 6.55 A

Figure 6.55 B

Figure 6.55 C

Figure 6.55 D

Findings: Axial NECT images (A and B) demonstrate an enlarged left kidney with fluid in the perinephric space. Note also the subtle hyperdensity along the course of the left renal vein. Axial CECT image (C) shows normal symmetrical enhancement in the corticomedullary phase and thrombus in the left renal vein as it enters the IVC; delayed excretion (D) is present on the left.

Differential Diagnosis: None.

Diagnosis: Acute left renal vein thrombosis.

Discussion: The most common cause of bland thrombus in a renal vein in adults is membranous glomerulonephritis, which this patient turned out to have. In children, dehydration is often the cause. Other etiologies are hypercoagulable states (e.g., nephrotic syndrome, lupus, inherited hypercoagulable state), trauma, neoplasm (e.g., renal cell carcinoma, Wilms tumor, adrenal carcinoma), abscess, adrenal hematoma, and extension of thrombus from the left gonadal vein. The left renal vein is more commonly involved than the right renal vein, and this is thought to be related to the left vein's longer length. The presenting symptoms are typically gross hematuria, flank pain, and loss of renal function. On CT, the kidney will appear enlarged. Perinephric or hilar edema, stranding or hemorrhage, and thickening of Gerota's fascia may be seen. On NECT, these findings can be nonspecific unless spontaneous hyperdense acute thrombus is identified in the vein. On CECT, pericapsular collateral veins, prolonged corticomedullary enhancement, striated nephrogram delayed or absent renal contrast excretion, and, most specifically, contrast outlining the clot in the renal vein can be seen. It is important to assess well the renal parenchyma to exclude an underlying mass. Identification of the renal vein thrombus in this case is the key finding to make the correct diagnosis.

Clinical History: 68-year-old woman with a history of colon cancer presenting with weight loss and malaise.

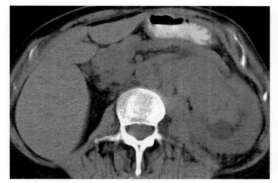

Figure 6.56   A

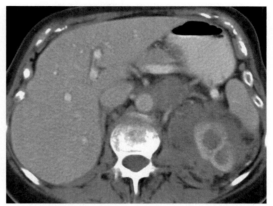

Figure 6.56   B

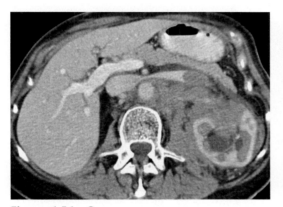

Figure 6.56   C

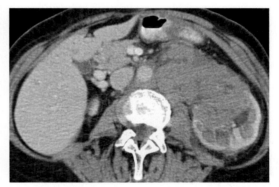

Figure 6.56   D

Findings: Axial NECT image (A) shows a 9.6 × 5.2 cm lobulated mass extending from the left para-aortic region into the left renal sinus. It has a slightly higher density than the renal parenchyma. Axial CECT images (B–D) demonstrate homogeneous enhancement of the mass. The mass extends into the perirenal space and invades the renal vein. Note presence of left hydronephrosis.

Differential Diagnosis: Transitional cell carcinoma, sarcoma, metastasis.

Diagnosis: Renal lymphoma.

Discussion: This case shows a typical example of one of the renal lymphoma imaging patterns: contiguous extension from retroperitoneal disease. It represents the second most common pattern observed on imaging (25–30%); the most common pattern is multiple renal masses (60%).

The attenuation of the mass is homogeneous, and the slightly higher density than the renal parenchyma on NECT is due to a high nuclear-to-cytoplasmic ratio. Vascular invasion is a rare finding in cases of lymphoma, and renal cell carcinoma, adrenal carcinoma, and Wilms tumor are much more likely to produce tumor thrombus in a renal vein. Lymphoma is considered a soft tumor, and this leads to encasement but not obliteration of blood vessels; in contrast, adenocarcinomas tend to be hard and cause vessel obstruction. Transitional cell carcinoma with hilar nodal metastasis would be the best differential diagnosis and may have an identical appearance. A primary retroperitoneal sarcoma, when large, would have heterogeneous density. Metastasis, especially from testicular cancer if the patient were a male, should also be considered.

Clinical History: 5-year-old boy presenting with fussiness, fever, and a palpable abdominal mass.

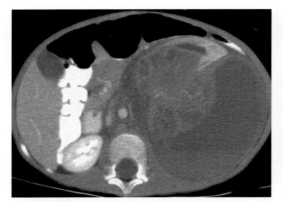

Figure 6.57   A

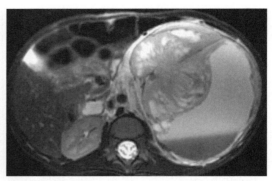

Figure 6.57   B

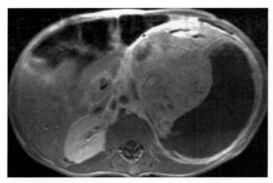

Figure 6.57   C

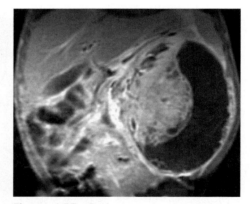

Figure 6.57   D

Findings: Axial CECT image (A) shows a 6.9 × 6.3 cm, heterogeneously enhancing mass invading the left kidney, with an associated 11.6 × 7.1 cm fluid density crescentic component containing dependent layering debris. Note that portions of the normal left renal parenchyma are displaced anteriorly. Axial fat-suppressed T2-WI (B) demonstrates heterogeneous high signal intensity in the mass and the layering low-intensity debris in the cystic component. Gadolinium-enhanced, fat-suppressed axial (C) and coronal (D) T1-WI show enhancement of the solid mass and nodular enhancement of the wall of the cystic component. Note intermediate signal intensity of the layering material on T1-WI.

Differential Diagnosis: Nephroblastomatosis, renal cell carcinoma, mesoblastic nephroma, clear cell sarcoma, rhabdoid tumor.

Diagnosis: Wilms tumor with hemorrhage.

Discussion: Wilms tumor is the most common renal mass in the pediatric population. The peak incidence is between the ages of 3 and 4 years; 80% of tumors present before the age of 5 years. Bilateral lesions occur in 4% to 13% of cases. Wilms tumor is associated with cryptorchidism, hemihypertrophy, hypospadia, and sporadic aniridia. The most common presentation is a palpable mass. Hypertension will be present in 25% of patients due to renin production by the tumor. Wilms tumor spreads by direct extension and displaces adjacent structures rather than encasing them (encasement is associated with neuroblastoma and is a key distinguishing feature). Metastases occur most commonly in the lungs, liver, and regional lymph nodes. Vascular extension in the renal vein, IVC, and even right atrium, which is better depicted by MRI, may be present. On imaging studies, Wilms tumor is heterogeneous in appearance due to the presence of fat, calcifications, hemorrhage, and necrosis. Treatment consists of surgical resection and adjuvant chemotherapy. Nephroblastomatosis is a focus of persistent metanephric blastema and presents as a poorly enhancing homogeneous mass. Renal cell carcinomas are rare in the first decade of life, with Wilms tumors outnumbering them 30 to 1. Other rare pediatric renal masses that may mimic Wilms tumor include mesoblastic nephroma (which is the most common neonatal renal mass), clear cell sarcoma, and rhabdoid tumor.

Case images courtesy of Dr. George A. Taylor, Children's Hospital Boston, Boston, MA.

Clinical History: 46-year-old man presenting with painless hematuria.

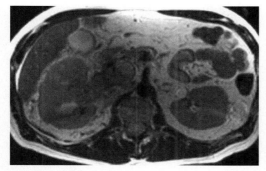

Figure 6.58   A

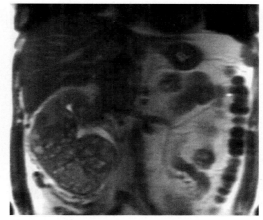

Figure 6.58   B

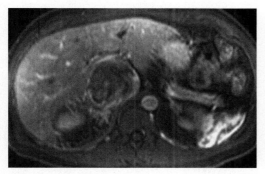

Figure 6.58   C

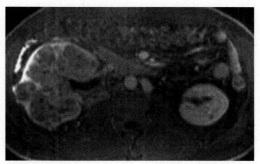

Figure 6.58   D

Findings: Axial and coronal T2-WI (A and B) show a 12.4 × 11.4 × 11.2 cm heterogeneous mass occupying the entire lower half of the right kidney. This mass extends into the right renal vein and IVC, which has a largest width of 7.2 cm in the infrahepatic segment. Gadolinium-enhanced, fat-suppressed axial T1-WI (C and D) demonstrate heterogeneous enhancement of the renal and intravenous mass.

Differential Diagnosis: Transitional cell carcinoma, Wilms tumor.

Diagnosis: Renal cell carcinoma with venous invasion.

Discussion: Venous thrombosis due to renal cell carcinoma is well evaluated by CECT in the nephrographic phase, but MRI is preferred to evaluate IVC extension. The thrombus may be bland or tumoral. Heterogeneous enhancement of the thrombus and direct continuity of the thrombus with the primary tumor suggest tumoral thrombus. If tumoral thrombus is present, the tumor will be staged according to the Robson classification as IIIB. The T stage of the tumor-node-metastasis (TNM) classification will vary according to the venous extent of the thrombus (T3b for renal vein invasion only, T3c for infradiaphragmatic invasion, and T4b for supradiaphragmatic invasion). Preoperative assessment of the extent of the tumor thrombus is essential because the surgical approach will differ depending on the level of superior involvement. If the thrombus remains in the renal vein or infrahepatic IVC, it can be resected through an abdominal incision. If it involves the retrohepatic IVC, a thoracoabdominal approach is necessary to access the IVC. Supradiaphragmatic or intracardiac extension will require cardiopulmonary bypass to facilitate the resection. If venous wall invasion is present, venous resection and reconstruction will be needed. In the present case, the mass involves the renal parenchyma and does not originate from the renal sinus, which makes transitional cell carcinoma unlikely. Wilms tumor can also invade the venous system, but Wilms tumor is exclusively seen in the pediatric population.

Clinical History: 64-year-old woman presenting with urinary frequency, urgency, and straining to void.

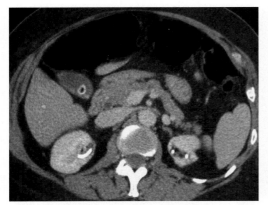

Figure 6.59   A

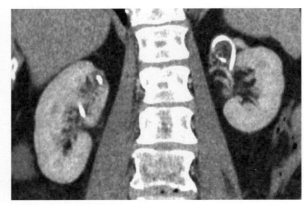

Figure 6.59   B

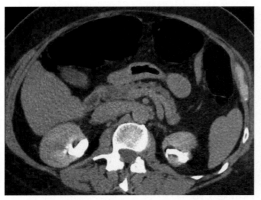

Figure 6.59   C

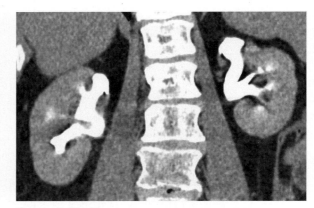

Figure 6.59   D

Findings: Axial and coronal oblique CECT images in the nephrographic phase (A and B) show severe parenchymal thinning of the upper pole of both kidneys. Axial and coronal oblique CECT images in the excretory phase (C and D) demonstrate dilation and blunting of the upper pole calyx of both kidneys. Note bilateral ureteral stents.

Differential Diagnosis: Pyelonephritis scar, postinfarction scar, postsurgery scar, analgesic nephropathy, postradiation scar.

Diagnosis: Reflux nephropathy.

Discussion: Ureterovesical reflux can lead to significant scarring of the renal parenchyma, called reflux nephropathy. The reflux-induced scarring may be caused by sterile or infected urine. Although the parenchymal damage occurs early in life, when the kidney is more vulnerable due to its immaturity, the atrophy may be detected at any point in life. Reflux nephropathy has a typical polar distribution, with relative sparing of the interpolar region. Normally, the openings of the ducts of Bellini are slitlike in configuration; these slit-like openings close with increasing pressure in the calyces,

preventing intraparenchymal reflux. However, some duct openings are circular, and such a shape is less effective at preventing intraparenchymal reflux. Circular openings are most commonly associated with compound calyces, which are usually present in the upper and lower poles of the kidneys. This explains the predominantly polar distribution of the reflux nephropathy, as seen in this case. The scarring may be unilateral or bilateral. The underlying calyces become dilated and blunted as a result of the scarring and the reflux. The symmetry and location of the scarring in this case are diagnostic clues to the correct diagnosis. Renal scarring may also be caused by pyelonephritis, renal infarcts, previous surgery, or analgesic nephropathy. Analgesic nephropathy is a bilateral process in which the underlying calyces are abnormal, but no polar predominance is present. Patients with lymphoma or upper abdominal malignancies may undergo radiotherapy, and the medial portions of the upper renal poles are often included in the radiation field; this may lead to atrophy localized to the upper poles, but a history of prior radiation therapy is present.

Clinical History: 32-year-old man presenting with left flank pain after a fall.

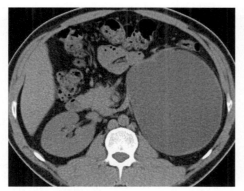

Figure 6.60 A

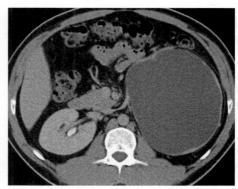

Figure 6.60 B

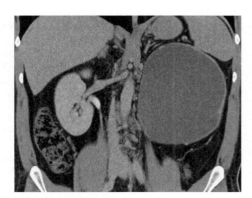

Figure 6.60 C

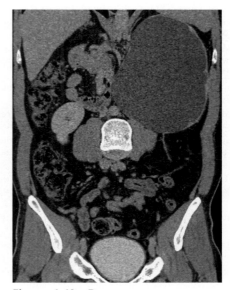

Figure 6.60 D

Findings: Axial NECT (A), axial CECT (B), and coronal (C) and curved (D) reformatted images show a 13.8 × 15.7 × 15.8 cm cystic lesion occupying the left renal fossa. A thin peripheral rim of soft tissue is present, except medially. Note absence of contrast excretion in the lesion.

Differential Diagnosis: Parapelvic cyst, cystic renal cell carcinoma.

Diagnosis: Ureteropelvic junction obstruction.

Discussion: Ureteropelvic junction obstruction (UPJO) results most commonly from intrinsic abnormalities due to excess collagen deposition and abnormal smooth muscle that result in an adynamic segment, leading to obstruction. Extrinsic causes can include crossing vessels or any other mass lesion. UPJO is bilateral in approximately 20% of cases and can be associated with other anomalies, such as vesicoureteral reflux or contralateral renal agenesis. Treatment aimed at relieving the obstruction would focus on preserving the residual renal function. Prior to endoscopic therapy, imaging should be obtained to document the presence or absence of crossing vessels of significant size. On imaging, dilatation of the renal pelvis and calyces would be present, with absence of ureteral dilatation. Later changes include decrease of renal function and parenchymal atrophy. In this case, correct identification of the thin soft tissue rim surrounding the cystic lesion as the markedly atrophied renal parenchyma should lead one to think that the cystic lesion is, in fact, the tremendously dilated collecting system. On occasion, a parenchymal cyst (termed a parapelvic cyst) may project into the renal sinus and cause obstruction of the collecting system. This would be the best differential diagnosis in this case. Absence of solid components associated with the cystic lesion excludes a cystic renal cell carcinoma.

SUGGESTED READINGS

NEOPLASMS

- Bosniak MA. The small (less than or equal to 3.0 cm) renal parenchymal tumor: detection, diagnosis, and controversies. *Radiology* 1991; 179:307–317.
- Browne RFJ, Meehan CP, Colville J, et al. Transitional cell carcinoma of the upper urinary tract: spectrum of imaging findings. *Radiographics* 2005;25:1609–1627.
- Choyke PL, White EM, Zeman RK, et al. Renal metastases: clinicopathologic and radiologic correlation. *Radiology* 1987;162:359–363.
- Ergen FB, Hussain HK, Caoili EM, et al. MRI for preoperative staging of renal cell carcinoma using the 1997 TNM classification: comparison with surgical and pathologic staging. *Am J Roentgenol.* 2004;182: 217–225.
- Hasegawa T, Matsuno Y, Shinoda T, et al. Extrathoracic solitary fibrous tumors: their histological variability and potentially aggressive behavior. *Hum Pathol.* 1999;30:1464–1473.
- Hopkins JK, Giles HW Jr, Wyatt-Ashmead J, et al. Best cases from the AFIP: cystic nephroma. *Radiographics* 2004;24:589–593.
- Israel GM, Bosniak MA. How I do it: evaluating renal masses. *Radiology* 2005;236:441–450.
- Israel GM, Hindman N, Bosniak MA. Evaluation of cystic renal masses: comparison of CT and MR imaging by using the Bosniak classification system. *Radiology* 2004;231:365–371.
- Jinzaki M, McTavish JD, Zou KH, et al. Evaluation of small (</= 3 cm) renal masses with MDCT: benefits of thin overlapping reconstructions. *Am J Roentgenol.* 2004;183:223–228.
- Jinzaki M, Tanimoto A, Narimatsu Y, at al. Angiomyolipoma: imaging findings in lesions with minimal fat. *Radiology* 1997;205:497–502.
- Kim JK, Kim TK, Ahn HJ, et al. Differentiation of subtypes of renal cell carcinoma on helical CT scans. *Am J Roentgenol.* 2002;178:1499–1506.
- Kundra V, Silverman PM. Imaging in the diagnosis, staging, and follow-up of cancer of the urinary bladder. *Am J Roentgenol.* 2003;180: 1045–1054.
- Kurl S, Rytkonen H, Farin P, et al. A primary carcinoid tumor of the kidney: a case report and review of the literature. *Abdom Imaging.* 1996;21:464–467.
- Laperriere J, Lafortune M. Case of the day. General. Oncocytoma of the right kidney. *Radiographics* 1990;10:1105–1107.
- Liu H, Cooke K, Frager D. Bilateral massive renal angiomyolipomatosis in tuberous sclerosis. *Am J Roentgenol.* 2005;185:1085–1086.
- Logue LG, Acker RE, Sienko AE. Best cases from the AFIP: angiomyolipomas in tuberous sclerosis. *Radiographics* 2003;23:241–246.
- Lowe LH, Isuani BH, Heller RM, et al. Pediatric renal masses: Wilms tumor and beyond. *Radiographics* 2000;20:1585–1603.
- Mariscal A, Mate JL, Guasch I, et al. Cystic transformation of a fibroepithelial polyp of the renal pelvis: radiologic and pathologic findings. *Am J Roentgenol.* 1995;164:1445–1446.
- Pickhardt PJ, Lonergan GJ, Davis CJ Jr, et al. From the archives of the AFIP: infiltrative renal lesions: radiologic-pathologic correlation. *Radiographics* 2000;20:215–243.
- Rafal RB, Markisz JA. Urachal carcinoma: the role of magnetic resonance imaging. *Urol Radiol.* 1991;12:184–187.
- Remer EM, Weinberg EJ, Oto A, et al. MR imaging of the kidneys after laparoscopic cryoablation. *Am J Roentgenol.* 2000;174:635–640.
- Scatarige JC, Sheth S, Corl FM, et al. Patterns of recurrence in renal cell carcinoma: manifestations on helical CT. *Am J Roentgenol.* 2001;177: 653–658.
- Sheth S, Scatarige JC, Horton KM, et al. Current concepts in the diagnosis and management of renal cell carcinoma: role of multidetector CT and three-dimensional CT. *Radiographics* 2001;21:S237–S254.
- Silverman SG, Lee BY, Seltzer SE, et al. Small (< or = 3 cm) renal masses: correlation of spiral CT features and pathologic findings. *Am J Roentgenol.* 1994;163:597–605.
- Tekes A, Kamel I, Imam K, et al. Dynamic MRI of bladder cancer: evaluation of staging accuracy. *Am J Roentgenol.* 2005;184:121–127.

- Urban BA, Fishman EK. Renal lymphoma: CT patterns with emphasis on helical CT. *Radiographics* 2000;20:197–212.
- Winalski CS, Lipman JC, Tumeh SS. Ureteral neoplasms. *Radiographics* 1990;10:271–283.
- Wong-You-Cheong JJ, Wagner BJ, Davis CJ Jr. Transitional cell carcinoma of the urinary tract: radiologic-pathologic correlation. *Radiographics* 1998;18:123–142.
- Zotalis G, Hicks DG. Solitary fibrous tumor of the soft tissues. *Arch Hellenic Pathol.* 1997;11:122–131.

INFECTION/INFLAMMATION

- Day DL, Carpenter DL. Abdominal complications in pediatric bone marrow transplant recipients. *Radiographics* 1993;13:1101–1112.
- Fan CM, Whitman GJ, Chew FS. Xanthogranulomatous pyelonephritis. *Am J Roentgenol.* 1995;165:1008.
- Kalantari BN, Mortelé KJ, Cantisani V, et al. CT features with pathologic correlation of acute gastrointestinal graft-versus-host disease after bone marrow transplantation in adults. *Am J Roentgenol.* 2003;181: 1621–1625.
- Kawashima A, Sandler CM, Goldman SM, et al. CT of renal inflammatory disease. *Radiographics* 1997;17:851–866.
- Kuhlman JE, Fishman EK. CT evaluation of enterovaginal and vesicovaginal fistulas. *J Comput Assist Tomogr.* 1990;14:390–394.
- Soulen MC, Fishman EK, Goldman SM. Sequelae of acute renal infections: CT evaluation. *Radiology* 1989;173:423–426.
- Talner L, Vaughan M. Nonobstructive renal causes of flank pain: findings on noncontrast helical CT (CT KUB). *Abdom Imaging.* 2003;28: 210–216.

CONGENITAL/DEVELOPMENTAL ANOMALIES

- Berrocal T, López-Pereira P, Arjonilla A, et al. Anomalies of the distal ureter, bladder, and urethra in children: embryologic, radiologic, and pathologic features. *Radiographics* 2002;22:1139–1164.
- Gay SB, Armistead JP, Weber ME, et al. Left infrarenal region: anatomic variants, pathologic conditions, and diagnostic pitfalls. *Radiographics* 1991;11:549–570.
- Hilpert PL, Friedman AC, Radecki PD, et al. MRI of hemorrhagic renal cysts in polycystic kidney disease. *Am J Roentgenol.* 1986;146: 1167–1172.
- Lonergan GJ, Rice RR, Suarez ES. Autosomal recessive polycystic kidney disease: radiologic-pathologic correlation. *Radiographics* 2000;20: 837–855.
- Segal AJ, Spataro RF. Computed tomography of adult polycystic disease. *J Comput Assist Tomogr.* 1982;6:777–780.
- Yu JS, Kim KW, Lee HJ, et al. Urachal remnant diseases: spectrum of CT and US findings. *Radiographics* 2001;21:451–461.

MISCELLANEOUS

- Dyer RB, Chen MY, Zagoria RJ. Abnormal calcifications in the urinary tract. *Radiographics* 1998;18:1405–1424.
- Farres MT, Ronco P, Saadoun D, et al. Chronic lithium nephropathy: MR imaging for diagnosis. *Radiology* 2003;229:570–574.
- Guest AR, Cohan RH, Korobkin M, et al. Assessment of the clinical utility of the rim and comet-tail signs in differentiating ureteral stones from phleboliths. *Am J Roentgenol.* 2001;177:1285–1291.
- Hann L, Pfister RC. Renal subcapsular rim sign: new etiologies and pathogenesis. *Am J Roentgenol.* 1982;138:51–54.
- Harris AC, Zwirewich CV, Lyburn ID, et al. CT findings in blunt renal trauma. *Radiographics* 2001;21:S201–S214.
- Hodson CJ. Neuhauser lecture. Reflux nephropathy: a personal historical review. *Am J Roentgenol.* 1981;137:451–462.
- Joseph RC, Amendola MA, Artze ME, et al. Genitourinary tract gas: imaging evaluation. *Radiographics* 1996;16:295–308.
- Katz DS, Lane MJ, Sommer FG. Unenhanced helical CT of ureteral stones: incidence of associated urinary tract findings. *Am J Roentgenol.* 1996;166:1319–1322.

- Kawashima A, Sandler CM, Ernst RD, et al. CT evaluation of renovascular disease. *Radiographics* 2000;20:1321–1340.
- Lawler LP, Jarret TW, Corl FM, et al. Adult ureteropelvic junction obstruction: insights with three-dimensional multi–detector row CT. *Radiographics* 2005;25:121–134.
- Oliva MRB, Hsing J, Rybicki FJ, et al. Glomerulocystic kidney disease: MRI findings. *Abdom Imaging.* 2003;28:889–892.
- Rathaus V, Konen O, Werner M, et al. Pyelocalyceal diverticulum: the imaging spectrum with emphasis on the ultrasound features. *Br J Radiol.* 2001;74:595–601.
- Sallomi DF, Yaqoob M, White E, et al. Case report: the diagnostic value of contrast-enhanced computed tomography in acute bilateral renal cortical necrosis. *Clin Radiol.* 1995;50:126–127.
- Sebastià C, Quiroga S, Boyé R, et al. Helical CT in renal transplantation: normal findings and early and late complications. *Radiographics* 2001;21:1103–1117.
- Vaccaro JP, Brody JM. CT cystography in the evaluation of major bladder trauma. *Radiographics* 2000;20:1373–1381.

CHAPTER SEVEN

PELVIS

Liesbeth J. Meylaerts,
Koenraad J. Mortele,
Vincent Pelsser,
and Pablo R. Ros

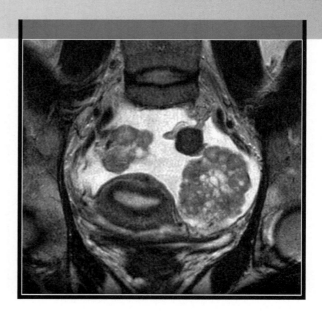

Clinical History: 20-year-old woman presenting with abdominal and lower back pain.

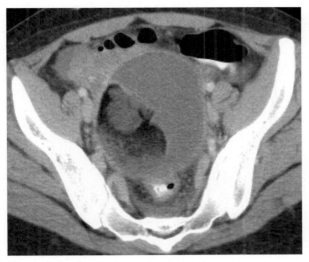

Figure 7.1   A

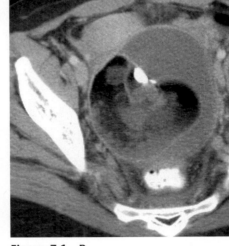

Figure 7.1   B

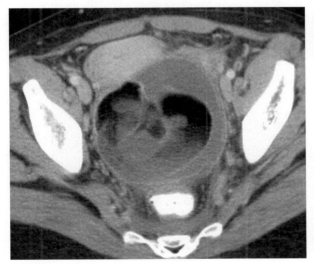

Figure 7.1   C

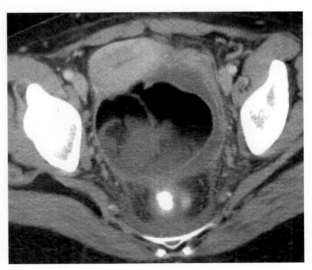

Figure 7.1   D

Findings: Axial contrast-enhanced CT (CECT) images show a 10-cm encapsulated mass within the cul-de-sac composed predominantly of fat and fluid; a smaller soft tissue protuberance attached to the wall and a punctate calcification (B) are seen. Note fat-fluid level within the mass.

Differential Diagnosis: Liposarcoma.

Diagnosis: Mature ovarian teratoma.

Discussion: Mature cystic teratoma (dermoid) is the most common incidentally encountered benign ovarian tumor (10–20% of all ovarian neoplastic lesions) in women; its peak incidence is between 20 and 29 years. In 10% to 15% of cases, it is bilateral. Ovarian dermoids are composed of well-differentiated derivates of the three germ cell layers (ectoderm, mesoderm, and endoderm) and tend to grow slowly. The diagnosis is easily made on CT due to the presence of fat, fluid (fat-fluid and/or fluid-fluid level occasionally), and calcifications. The presence of a characteristic Rokitansky nodule helps distinguish a dermoid from other fat-containing lesions, such as liposarcoma. It is defined as a dermoid plug projecting into the cavity. This protuberance contains a mixture of tissues, including bone, teeth, hair, and fat. Dermoids have an unusually high complication rate compared with other ovarian tumors. They are prone to torsion (3.2–16%), acute or chronic rupture inducing chemical peritonitis (1.2–3.8%), infection, and malignant transformation (1–2%).

Clinical History: 19-year-old woman presenting with subacute onset of severe abdominal pain that is worst in the right lower quadrant.

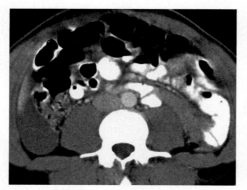

Figure 7.2   A

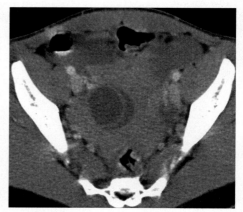

Figure 7.2   B

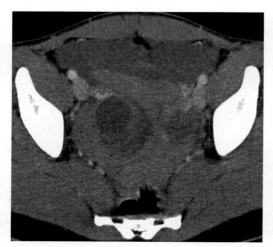

Figure 7.2   C

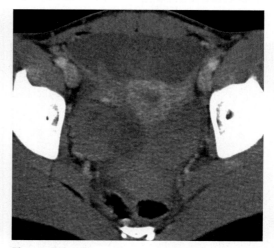

Figure 7.2   D

Findings: Axial CECT images show a large amount of high-density fluid within the right paracolic gutter (A) and pelvis (B–D), as well as bilateral heterogeneous cystic adnexal masses.

Differential Diagnosis: Tubo-ovarian abscesses, endometriomas, cystadenomas.

Diagnosis: Bilateral hemorrhagic ovarian cysts.

Discussion: Cystic masses in the adnexa include functional ovarian cysts, tubo-ovarian abscesses, endometriomas, and epithelial ovarian neoplasms. Functional ovarian cysts can be follicular cysts or corpus luteum cysts. Follicular cysts are unruptured follicles that enlarge due to continued hormonal stimulation. They are typically greater than 2.5 cm and can be multilocular in appearance. Debris is often seen inside the cyst from prior hemorrhage, which can result in sharp pelvic pain. In case of hemorrhage, a hematocrit level may be seen in the cyst, or frank peritoneal hemorrhage may be present, as seen in this case. Follicular cysts will usually regress after one or two menstrual cycles. Follow-up ultrasound 6 weeks following the initial examination is indicated to exclude an underlying tumor. The ultrasound should be performed preferably in the first week after menstruation to allow time for resolution of the cyst and avoid confusion with new physiologic cysts. The high-density fluid seen in the peritoneal space in this case suggests the diagnosis of ruptured hemorrhagic ovarian cysts or endometriomas.

Clinical History: 44-year-old woman with bladder outlet obstruction.

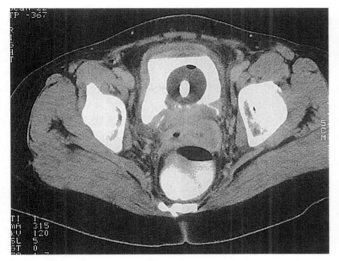

Figure 7.3   A

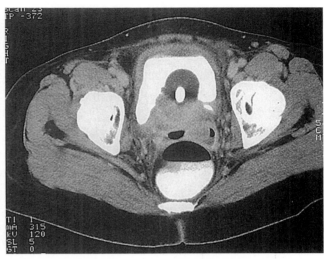

Figure 7.3   B

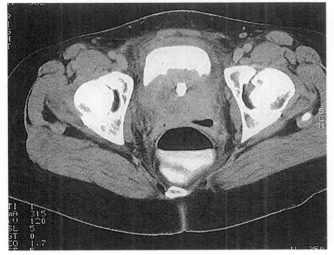

Figure 7.3   C

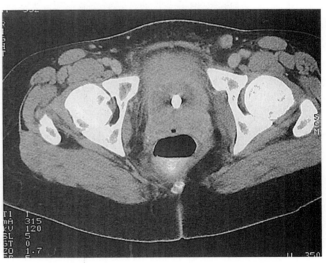

Figure 7.3   D

Findings: Axial CECT images demonstrate a large mass that involves the base of the bladder and extends distally surrounding a Foley catheter balloon. There is extension of the mass into the vagina.

Differential Diagnosis: Transitional cell carcinoma, sarcoma, metastasis.

Diagnosis: Urethral cancer (squamous cell carcinoma).

Discussion: Carcinoma of the urethra is much more common in females than in males. The most common histologic subtypes are squamous cell carcinoma followed by adenocarcinoma and transitional cell carcinoma. The peak age is in the sixth decade of life. The etiology is thought to be secondary to prior infections or trauma. Urethral cancers can be divided based on their location. Cancers arising from the distal urethra are typically low grade and have a good prognosis. The proximal urethral tumors, however, present later in life and are usually more advanced with a poorer prognosis. This case demonstrates an aggressive proximal urethral squamous cell carcinoma. This lesion involves the periurethral tissues and extends into the base of the bladder and the vagina. This lesion is similar in appearance to a transitional cell carcinoma arising from the bladder epithelium or an aggressive sarcoma. The key to the diagnosis is following the extent of the lesion distally into the perineum, which is suggestive of a urethral carcinoma.

Clinical History: 72-year-old woman post recent surgery for urine incontinence presenting with fever and foul-smelling vaginal discharge.

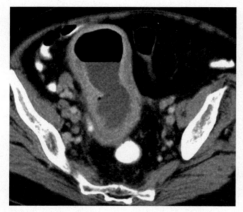

Figure 7.4 A

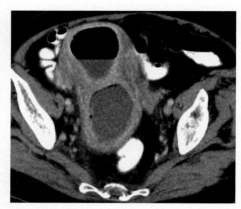

Figure 7.4 B

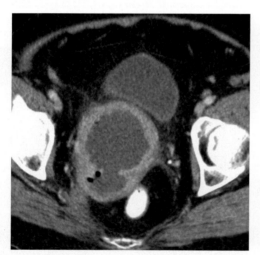

Figure 7.4 C

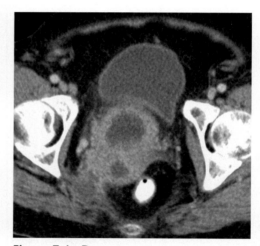

Figure 7.4 D

Findings: Axial CECT images demonstrate an enlarged and distended uterine cavity filled with fluid and air.

Differential Diagnosis: Hematometra, hydrometra.

Diagnosis: Pyometra.

Discussion: Fluid within the uterus can be due to several causes including pus (pyometra), sterile fluid (hydrometra), and blood (hematometra). Intrauterine fluid can be seen normally in menstruating and pregnant women. Larger fluid collections, as seen in this case, commonly occur in an obstructed uterus. In women of reproductive age, this can be due to cervical cancer, uterine leiomyoma, endometrial cancer, radiation therapy, or postsurgical scarring and stenosis.

In this case, the uterus was obstructed from cervical stenosis and postsurgical infection, resulting in pyometra with pus and air in the endometrial cavity. The infected fluid can escape from the uterus via the fallopian tubes into the peritoneal cavity. On MRI, differentiation between hydrometra and hematometra can be made based on the signal intensity of the fluid. Hematometra show increased signal intensity on T1-weighted images (WI) due to presence of blood products. The presence of a fluid-fluid level (hematocrit effect) may also be seen in hematometra. Both enhanced and unenhanced CT images have to be performed to differentiate fluid from tumor in the endometrial canal.

Clinical History: 27-year-old woman presenting with perineal pain.

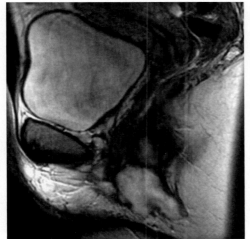

Figure 7.5   A

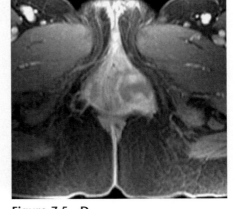

Figure 7.5   B

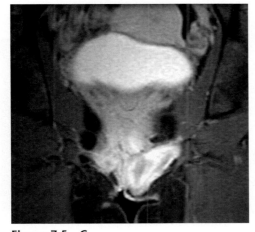

Figure 7.5   C

Figure 7.5   D

Findings: Sagittal T2-WI (A) demonstrates a heterogeneous hyperintense mass in the anterior perineum. Fat-suppressed coronal T1-WI (B) reveals a soft tissue mass in the left vulvar region isointense with musculature. Gadolinium-enhanced, fat-suppressed coronal (C) and axial (D) T1-WI show heterogeneous enhancement of the mass without obvious invasion of the adjacent structures.

Differential Diagnosis: Liposarcoma and infiltrating angiolipoma, myxoid peripheral nerve sheath tumor, myxoid smooth muscle tumor, angiomyofibroblastoma.

Diagnosis: Aggressive angiomyxoma.

Discussion: Aggressive angiomyxoma (AAM) is a rare, benign, soft tissue tumor that contains myxoid and vascular components. It is predominantly seen in women of childbearing age. The slow-growing tumor has a propensity to reach a large size within the pelvis, especially in the perineum. Although these tumors rarely show mitotic activity, the term aggressive refers to the locally infiltrative growth pattern and the high recurrence rate (36–72%) after surgery. The typical imaging features include a hypervascular tumor with indolent growth and local infiltration but no invasion of adjacent organs. On MRI, the tumor is isointense to muscle on T1-WI, and after contrast administration, it shows moderate enhancement. On T2-WI, the tumor has a swirled or layered appearance. The key features in differentiating AAM from the main differential considerations are the lack of fat content, the infiltrative but not invasive growth pattern, and the heterogeneous enhancement of the soft tissue mass in women of childbearing age. Long-term MRI follow-up is recommended because recurrence occurring several years after the initial excision has been reported.

Clinical History: 52-year-old woman presenting with abdominal discomfort.

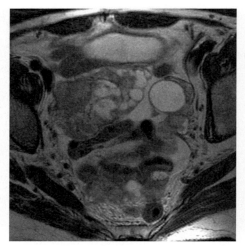

Figure 7.6   A

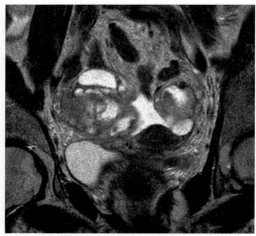

Figure 7.6   B

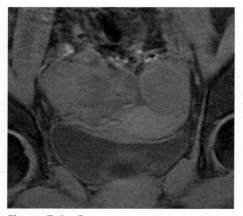

Figure 7.6   C

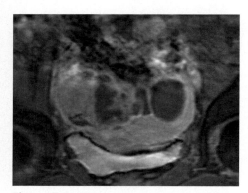

Figure 7.6   D

Findings: Axial (A) and coronal (B) T2-WI and unenhanced coronal (C) and gadolinium-enhanced (D) fat-suppressed axial T1-WI show bilateral cystic and solid ovarian masses with enhancement of the solid components. Note presence of ascites, and similar solid and cystic lesions in the cul-de-sac.

Differential Diagnosis: Mucinous cystadenocarcinoma, Krukenberg tumor, tubo-ovarian abscess.

Diagnosis: Serous cystadenocarcinoma.

Discussion: Epithelial ovarian tumors represent 85% of malignant ovarian neoplasms; 50% of them are serous cystadenocarcinomas. Their prevalence peaks in the sixth and seventh decades of life. Risk factors include early menarche, nulliparity, infertility, late menopause, and positive family history for ovarian cancer. In addition to imaging techniques, assessment of serum level of cancer antigen 125 (CA-125) is also of diagnostic use. However, the sensitivity of serum markers is low and depends on the tumor stage (50% in stage I disease). False-positive elevation of CA-125 can occur in endometriosis, uterine leiomyomas, pregnancy, pelvic inflammatory disease, and even in 1% of healthy women. The most important prognostic factors of serous cystadenocarcinoma are tumor grade and residual tumor after initial surgery. Patients with residual disease greater than 2 cm are not considered for further surgery. Staging according to the International Federation of Gynecology and Obstetrics (FIGO) guidelines is as follows: stage I, limited to the ovaries; stage II, involvement of the pelvis; stage III, tumor with intraperitoneal metastasis outside the pelvis and/or positive retroperitoneal nodes; and stage IV, distant metastasis or pleural effusion with positive cytology or hepatic metastasis. Features on imaging suggesting ovarian malignancy are large soft tissue masses, cyst wall thickness greater than 3 mm, enhancing papillary projections, presence of ascites, peritoneal implants, pelvic wall invasion, and adenopathy.

Clinical History: 48-year-old woman presenting with pelvic pain.

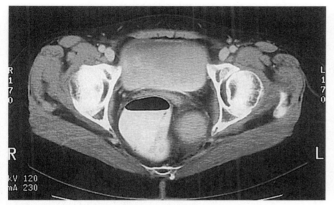

Figure 7.7 A

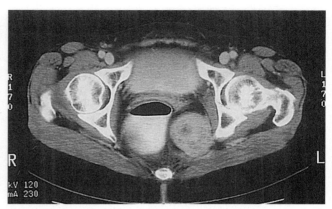

Figure 7.7 B

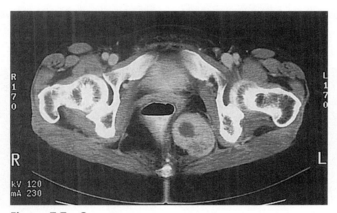

Figure 7.7 C

Findings: Axial CECT images demonstrate a 5-cm enhancing solid mass with small internal areas of low density located to the left of the rectum and displacing the rectum to the right.

Differential Diagnosis: Metastasis, sarcoma, lymphoma.

Diagnosis: Perirectal hemangiopericytoma.

Discussion: Hemangiopericytoma is a rare tumor arising from the capillary pericytes, which can be found in the lower extremities, retroperitoneum, and brain (dura). The lesion tends to be hypervascular with marked enhancement after intravenous contrast administration. As with other retroperitoneal and extraperitoneal masses, hemangiopericytoma can grow to be large (>10 cm) before being

detected. Symptoms usually do not occur until the lesion compresses an adjacent organ causing pain or decrease in function. A mass in the perirectal tissue is typically a neoplasm arising from the rectum. This lesion, however, appears to be separate from the rectum and uterus, making a rectal malignancy (e.g., adenocarcinoma, gastrointestinal stromal tumor, carcinoid, lymphoma) or pedunculated uterine leiomyoma unlikely. The tumor can also arise from the perirectal tissue. A mesenchymal tumor, such as a sarcoma, would be a good possibility in the differential diagnosis, along with lymphoma. Metastases, especially from an aggressive neoplasm such as melanoma, could have this appearance too.

Clinical History: 36-year-old woman presenting with pelvic pain, dyspareunia, and dysmenorrhea.

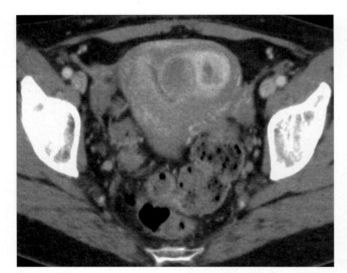

Figure 7.8   A

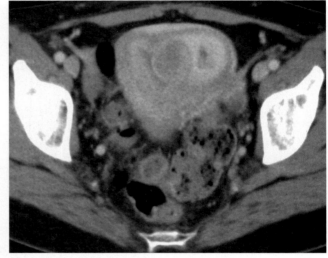

Figure 7.8   B

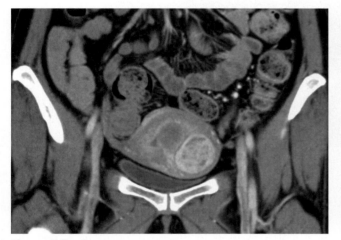

Figure 7.8   C

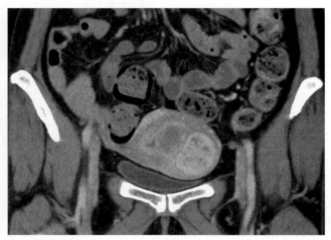

Figure 7.8   D

Findings: Axial (A and B) and coronal (C and D) CECT images demonstrate two well-demarcated heterogeneously enhancing myometrial masses. The smaller one indents the endometrial cavity.

Differential Diagnosis: Uterine leiomyosarcoma, endometrial polyp, adenomyosis.

Diagnosis: Uterine leiomyomas.

Discussion: Uterine leiomyoma, also known as myoma or fibroid, is the most common gynecologic neoplasm, occurring in 20% to 30% of women of reproductive age. According to their location in the myometrium, they are classified as intramural (most common), submucosal (most symptomatic, due to bleeding), or subserosal (if pedunculated, may simulate ovarian neoplasms). Acute pain can be a manifestation of acute degeneration, torsion of a pedunculated subserosal lesion, infarction during pregnancy, or prolapse of a submucosal leiomyoma. On CT, leiomyomas can be hypo-, iso-, or hyperdense relative to the normal uterus depending on the degree of internal hemorrhage and necrosis. They will commonly distort the uterine contour, displace the endometrial cavity, and show calcifications. On T2-WI, they appear as sharply marginated, low–signal intensity masses relative to the myometrium, often with a detectable high–signal intensity rim representing dilated lymphatics, veins, or edema. When leiomyomas are greater than 3 to 5 cm, they are often heterogeneous due to varying degrees of degeneration. Adenomyomas and leiomyosarcomas are typically ill defined; endometrial polyps arise from the endometrium, not the myometrium.

Clinical History: 70-year-old woman presenting with worsening abdominal pain.

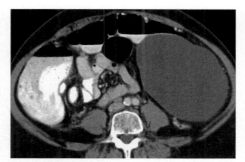

Figure 7.9   A

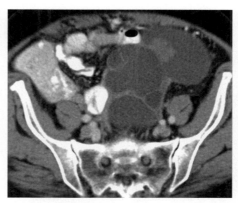

Figure 7.9   B

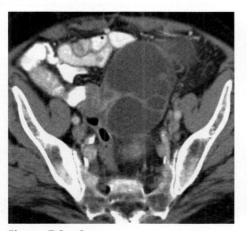

Figure 7.9   C

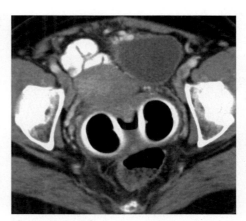

Figure 7.9   D

Findings: Axial CECT images demonstrate a multiloculated, cystic, left adnexal mass measuring 21 cm. Some internal septations are thick, and enhancing mural nodularity is present within the mass. Note presence of pessary (D).

Differential Diagnosis: Serous or mucinous cystadenoma or carcinoma, atypical mature teratoma, hydrosalpinx, tubo-ovarian abscess, cystic metastasis.

Diagnosis: Serous cystadenofibroma.

Discussion: Serous cystadenofibromas are benign epithelial ovarian masses. They are defined as serous cystadenomas consisting of more than 50% of fibrous tissue. Epithelial ovarian tumors represent 65% of all ovarian tumors. About 60% of all the serous ovarian neoplasms are smooth-walled benign cystadenomas, 15% are of low malignant potential (borderline tumors), and 25% are malignant. Serous cystadenomas manifest as a unilocular (more often) or multilocular cystic mass with homogeneous CT attenuation or MRI signal intensity of the locules, a thin regular wall or septum, and no endocystic or exocystic vegetations. Different attenuation and signal intensity of the locules of a multilocular cystic mass are more typical of mucinous tumors. Serous cystadenomas can reach 30 cm in size with a mean diameter of 10 cm; mucinous cystadenomas tend to be larger (reaching 50 cm in size). Diagnosis of a benign ovarian neoplasm should only be made if the following features (accuracy of 84%) are present: entirely cystic mass, wall thickness less than 3 mm, lack of internal structure, and absence of both ascites and invasive characteristics, such as peritoneal nodules or lymphadenopathy. After contrast administration, only the cyst wall and septations enhance.

Clinical History: 40-year-old woman presenting with menometrorrhagia and dysmenorrhea.

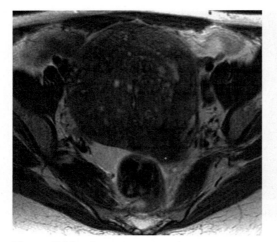

Figure 7.10   A

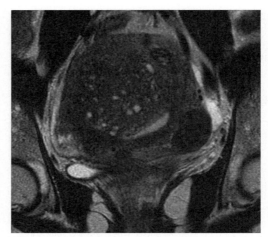

Figure 7.10   B

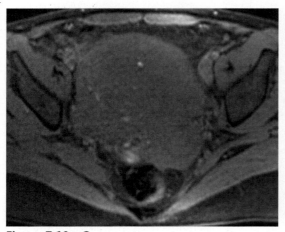

Figure 7.10   C

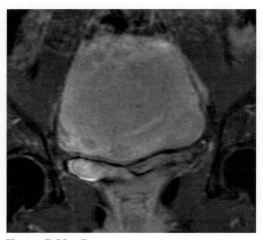

Figure 7.10   D

Findings: Axial (A) and coronal (B) T2-WI, fat-suppressed axial T1-WI (C), and gadolinium-enhanced, fat-suppressed axial T1-WI (D) demonstrate an ill-defined, Swiss cheese–like (hyperintense foci on T1-WI and T2-WI) mass in the uterine wall with loss of the zonal anatomy; the mass shows moderate enhancement compared to the normal myometrium. Note also two well-delineated T2 hypointense, T1 isointense, subserosal minimally enhancing nodules.

Differential Diagnosis: Myometrial contraction, muscular hypertrophy.

Diagnosis: Adenomyosis and two uterine leiomyomas.

Discussion: Adenomyosis is due to the presence of ectopic endometrial glands and stroma within the myometrium, often accompanied by myometrial hyperplasia. It affects women during their reproductive and perimenopausal years (40–60 years old). Symptoms include pelvic pain, menorrhagia, and

dysmenorrhea. Two morphologic forms are described: diffuse and, less frequently, local adenomyosis (so-called adenomyoma). Due to the predominance of endometrial zona basilaris, which is relatively refractive to the cyclic hormonal changes, adenomyosis does not typically undergo bleeding. MRI features characteristic for adenomyosis are focal or diffuse widening (>12 mm) of the low–signal intensity junctional zone, ill-defined margins, normal aspect of the endometrium, and high–signal intensity foci on T1-WI or T2-WI within a T2-WI hypointense mass (due to associated smooth muscle hyperplasia). The hyperintense foci represent small areas of hemorrhage, ectopic endometrium, and/or cystically dilated endometrial glands. Differentiation with diffuse muscular hypertrophy can be challenging; muscular hypertrophy also causes widening of the junctional zone, although milder, and is well defined compared to diffuse adenomyosis.

Clinical History: 45-year-old woman presenting with pelvic pain.

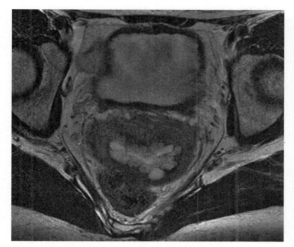

Figure 7.11 A

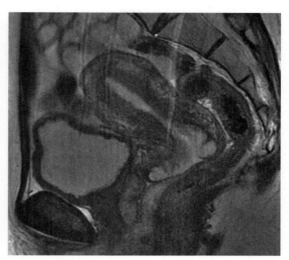

Figure 7.11 B

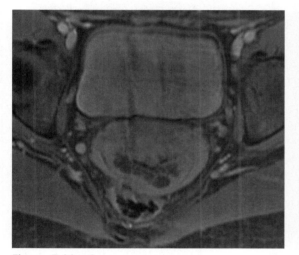

Figure 7.11 C

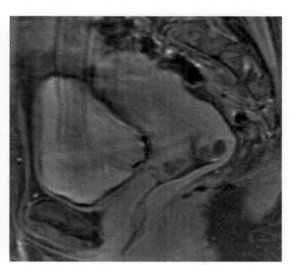

Figure 7.11 D

Findings: Axial (A) and sagittal (B) T2-WI reveal multiple irregularly margined hyperintense cystic lesions in the cervix extending into the cervical stroma. Gadolinium-enhanced, fat-suppressed axial (C) and sagittal (D) T1-WI show enhancement of the wall of the annular cystlike lesions and a solid component ventrolateral in the endocervix.

Differential Diagnosis: Nabothian cysts, florid endocervical hyperplasia, well-differentiated adenocarcinoma.

Diagnosis: Adenoma malignum.

Discussion: Adenoma malignum is a subtype of mucinous adenocarcinoma of the cervix with a prevalence of 3% of all cervical adenocarcinomas. Watery vaginal discharge can be an initial symptom. The prognosis is unfavorable because of the dissemination of adenoma malignum into the peritoneal cavity even in its early stages and because of its poor response to radiation and chemotherapy. Histopathologically, the tumor is composed of well-differentiated endocervical glands extending from the surface to the deeper portion of the cervical wall. They form an annular mass, with cystic mucin-filled spaces. Adenoma malignum is often associated with Peutz-Jeghers syndrome. Multicystic lesions in the endocervix with solid components characterize adenoma malignum on MRI. The possibility of differentiating adenoma malignum from other cervical lesions is still controversial. On histopathologic analysis, it is important to check for abnormalities deep in the endocervical stroma, which is a pathognomonic feature that differentiates it from a Nabothian cyst.

Clinical History: 54-year-old woman presenting with chronic pelvic pain and occasional vaginal bleeding.

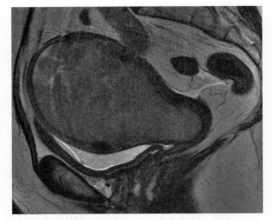

Figure 7.12   A

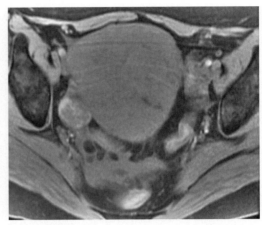

Figure 7.12   B

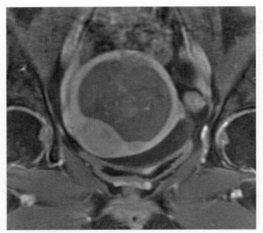

Figure 7.12   C

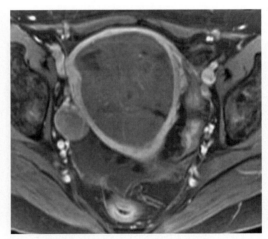

Figure 7.12   D

Findings: Sagittal T2-WI (A) demonstrates an 11-cm heterogeneously hypointense mass distending the endometrial canal and extending into the endocervix. There are multiple areas of myometrial invasion of greater than 50% of the myometrial thickness. On fat-suppressed axial T1-WI (B), the mass is heterogeneously isointense to the myometrium. There is also a heterogeneously hypointense enlarged right ovary. Gadolinium-enhanced, fat-suppressed coronal (C) and axial (D) T1-WI show the heterogeneous and minimally enhancing mass with myometrial invasion at its cranial pole.

Differential Diagnosis: Uterine fibroid, cervical cancer, pyometra, hematometra, mesenchymal uterine tumor.

Diagnosis: Endometrial cancer.

Discussion: Endometrial cancer is the most common invasive gynecologic malignancy in the United States, with its peak incidence between the sixth and seventh decades of life. It typically presents with postmenopausal uterine bleeding.

Risk factors for endometrial carcinoma include nulliparity, hormone replacement, late menopause, and obesity. Ninety percent of endometrial cancers are adenocarcinomas. Other histologic subtypes, such as papillary serous carcinoma and clear cell carcinoma, are less common and have a worse prognosis. On T2-WI, endometrial carcinoma is easily detected as a hyperintense mass compared with the T2 hypointense signal of the junctional zone. Myometrial invasion is suspected when the junctional zone is interrupted or presents an irregular interface with the endometrium. Endometrial adenocarcinomas are minimally enhancing masses compared with the normally enhancing uterine wall. Myometrial invasion of 50% or more results in a six- to sevenfold increased prevalence of pelvic and retroperitoneal lymph node metastases compared with myometrial invasion that is absent or less than 50%. Therefore, the preoperative assessment of myometrial invasion helps in planning the extent of lymphadenectomy.

Clinical History: 55-year-old woman presenting with severe vaginal bleeding.

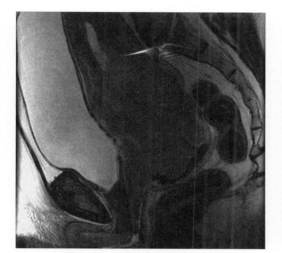

Figure 7.13   A

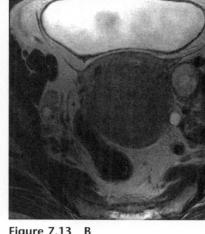

Figure 7.13   B

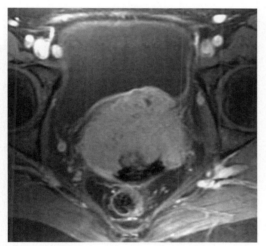

Figure 7.13   C

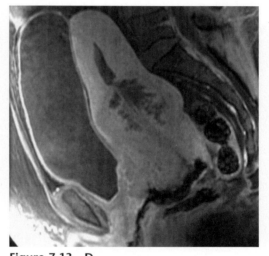

Figure 7.13   D

Findings: Sagittal T2-WI (A) shows an ill-defined, 9-cm cervical mass with protrusion into the anterior vaginal fornix. The lesion is isointense with the uterine myometrium. It demonstrates invasion into the bladder wall (disruption of the muscularis propria), into the upper one third of the anterior vaginal wall, and into the perimetrium (disruption of the low–signal intensity fibrous stroma of the cervix). Note the fluid-filled endometrial cavity. Axial T2-WI (B) reveals left-sided hydroureter and bilateral necrotic lymph nodes along the iliac vessels. Gadolinium-enhanced, fat-suppressed axial (C) and sagittal (D) T1-WI demonstrate enhancement of the mass and depict better the invasion into the adjacent organs.

Differential Diagnosis: Endometrial cancer.

Diagnosis: Cervical carcinoma (stage IV).

Discussion: MRI is the preferred imaging modality to stage cervical cancer, guide adequate treatment, determine prognosis, and assess response to radiochemotherapy (decrease in tumor volume and/or enhancement). Cervical cancer is staged according to the FIGO classification. Stage 0 is defined as a carcinoma in situ. Stage I is defined by tumor, which is confined to the cervix (stage IA, microinvasion; stage IB1, tumor size <4 cm; and stage IB2, tumor size >4 cm). Stage II is defined by tumor extension beyond the cervix, without involvement of pelvic sidewall or lower one third of the vagina. Stage III demonstrates involvement of the lower one third of the vagina or pelvic sidewall or ureter obstruction. Stage IV is defined by tumor extension outside the true pelvis or by invasion of bladder or rectum. Stages IB and IIA can be treated with either radical hysterectomy or radiation therapy. Intracavitary brachytherapy as an adjunct to surgery is used in patients with a tumor larger than 2 cm.

Clinical History: 36-year-old woman presenting with amenorrhea and a history of chemotherapy and radiotherapy treatment for leukemia.

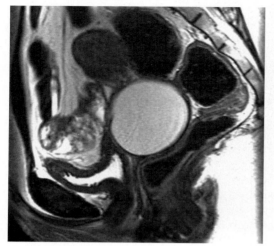

Figure 7.14   A

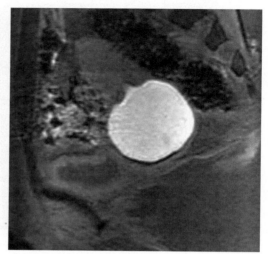

Figure 7.14   B

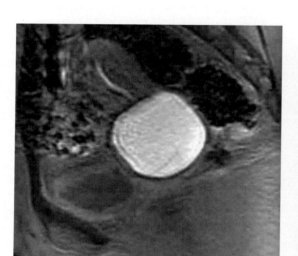

Figure 7.14   C

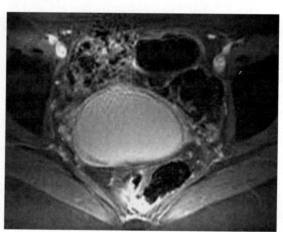

Figure 7.14   D

Findings: Sagittal T2-WI (A), fat-suppressed sagittal T1-WI (B and C), and gadolinium-enhanced, fat-suppressed axial T1-WI (D) demonstrate a large T1-WI and T2-WI hyperintense, nonenhancing, well-delineated mass in the upper third of the vagina extending into the endocervical canal.

Differential Diagnosis: Hematometros, Gartner duct cyst, endometriosis.

Diagnosis: Hematocolpos (secondary to radiation with resultant vaginal stenosis).

Discussion: Hematocolpos is defined by a markedly distended vagina with hemorrhagic debris demonstrating variable signal intensity on T1-WI and T2-WI, depending on the age of the blood products. Hematometros (hemorrhagic fluid distending the uterine cavity) should be differentiated from hematocolpos: the degree of dilatation of the endometrial cavity is usually less pronounced than the vagina because the muscular myometrium is less compliant than the thin wall of the distended vagina. Vaginal obstruction may be caused by Müllerian duct anomalies, which can be complicated by a transverse vaginal septum (in the upper third of the vagina), an imperforated hymen (lower third of the vagina), or secondary neoplasm, or be iatrogenic (radiotherapy), as seen in this case. Gartner duct cyst would be a well-defined structure and would not show extension in the uterine cervix. The finding of fluid extending into the endocervical canal from the vagina implies the abnormality is endoluminal.

Case images courtesy of Dr. Caroline Reinhold, McGill University Health Center, Montreal, Canada.

Clinical History: 32-year-old woman presenting with vaginal bleeding.

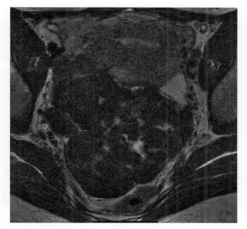

Figure 7.15　A

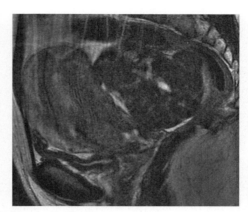

Figure 7.15　B

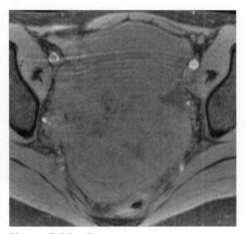

Figure 7.15　C

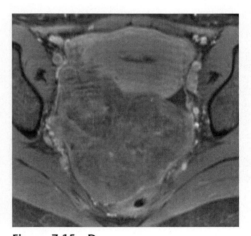

Figure 7.15　D

Findings: Axial (A) and sagittal (B) T2-WI demonstrate a multilobulated, heterogeneous, and hypointense mass in the cul-de-sac, with hyperintense foci centrally. Unenhanced (C) and gadolinium-enhanced (D) fat-suppressed axial T1-WI show minimal enhancement of the mass and surrounding capsule.

Differential Diagnosis: Pedunculated subserosal uterine or broad ligament leiomyoma, Brenner tumor.

Diagnosis: Ovarian fibroma/fibrothecoma.

Discussion: Fibromas, fibrothecomas, and thecomas represent approximately 4% of all ovarian tumors and 50% of sex cord stromal tumors. These benign tumors occur in the second and third decades of life. Fibromas are composed of collagen-producing spindle cells and are not hormonally active. They can be associated with two clinical syndromes. First, fibromas associated with ascites and pleural effusion are defined as Meigs syndrome (1% of all fibromas). Even in the absence of the syndrome, ascites is commonly associated with all, except small, fibromas. Second, fibromas can occur in the basal cell nevus syndrome and are typically bilateral, multinodular, and calcified. Fibrothecomas also contain a small amount of thecal cells, which have intracellular lipid and are often hormonally active. Thus, the latter can be associated with endometrial hyperplasia from hormonal stimulation. On MRI, fibromas and fibrothecomas are isointense on T1-WI and hypointense on T2-WI compared to skeletal muscle. In fibromas, edema and cystic degeneration can be present (hyperintense on T2-WI), especially in large lesions, as seen in this case. On gadolinium-enhanced images, they may demonstrate mild enhancement. Calcifications (hypointense foci on T1-WI and T2-WI) may be present. To differentiate ovarian fibromas/thecomas from uterine leiomyomas, the key feature is to depict "feeding vessels" from the uterus to the mass, which indicate the uterine origin of the lesion and thus suggest a uterine leiomyoma. Broad ligament fibroids and Brenner tumors may have a similar appearance.

Clinical History: 71-year-old man with a large mass at the base of the penis.

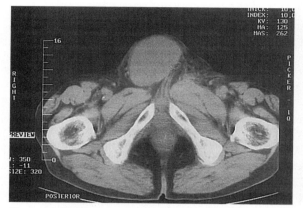

Figure 7.16   A

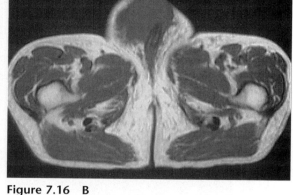

Figure 7.16   B

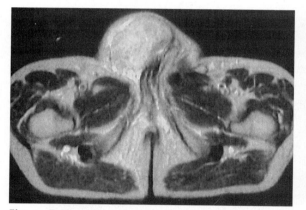

Figure 7.16   C

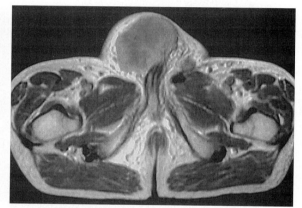

Figure 7.16   D

Findings: Axial NECT image (A) demonstrates an 8-cm, well-defined solid mass to the right of the base of the penis. It appears to be displacing the penile muscles to the left. Axial T1-WI (B) shows the mass to be isointense to muscle. The penile muscles are intact. Axial T2-WI (C) shows the mass to be hyperintense relative to muscle. Gadolinium-enhanced axial T1-WI (D) shows the mass to have heterogeneous enhancement.

Differential Diagnosis: Penile cancer, metastasis.

Diagnosis: Leiomyosarcoma of the spermatic cord.

Discussion: The key to the diagnosis in this case is to recognize that the large mass is displacing the penis rather than arising from it. A primary penile neoplasm, such as a squamous cell carcinoma, would tend to infiltrate the muscles and the skin of the penis. Inguinal adenopathy would probably be present with a penile neoplasm of this size. Instead, this mass arises from the spermatic cord. The most common neoplasm of the spermatic cord is a sarcoma, either malignant fibrous histiocytoma or leiomyosarcoma. This lesion appears to be separate from the testicle and is too medial to represent inguinal lymphadenopathy. Metastasis would also be a good diagnostic consideration.

CASE 7-17

Clinical History: 35-year-old woman presenting with pelvic pain and anemia.

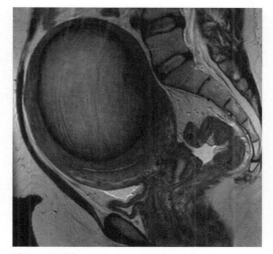

Figure 7.17   A

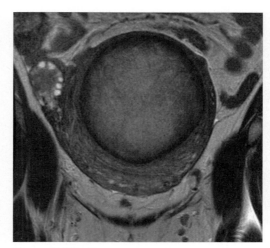

Figure 7.17   B

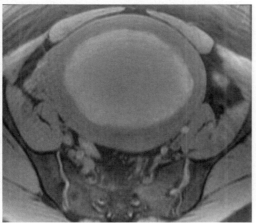

Figure 7.17   C

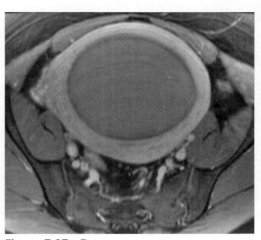

Figure 7.17   D

Findings: Sagittal (A) and coronal (B) T2-WI and unenhanced (C) and gadolinium-enhanced (D) fat-suppressed axial T1-WI show an intramural, well-demarcated, nonenhancing mass in the fundus of the uterus. The mass is predominantly hyperintense on T2-WI and T1-WI.

Differential Diagnosis: Hematometros.

Diagnosis: Hemorrhagic degeneration of a uterine leiomyoma.

Discussion: As leiomyomas enlarge, they may outgrow their blood supply and result in various types of degeneration. Hyalinization (>60%) is characterized by extensive replacement of smooth muscle cells by proteinaceous tissue; these fibroids typically show low signal intensity on T2-WI. Advanced hyaline degeneration may be accompanied by fatty degeneration. A second type of degeneration is the cystic type (~4%); large or small cystic spaces develop in the edematous,

acellular center. These cystic spaces appear as round, well-demarcated, nonenhancing areas that show typical fluid signal intensity on MRI. A third type is myxoid degeneration, which is relatively rare; cystic masses filled with gelatinous material are seen. The lesions enhance well except for the mucinous lakes, which are hyperintense on T2-WI. This type of degeneration can also be seen in leiomyosarcoma. A fourth type is the red or carneous degeneration, which involves hemorrhagic infarction due to obstruction of draining veins at the periphery. It occurs most often during pregnancy and is also associated with oral contraceptive use. Unlike the other types, red degeneration causes systemic symptoms. In this case, the entire lesion shows no enhancement, indicating complete interruption of the blood flow. Identification of the compressed endometrial cavity caudal to the mass excludes hematometros.

Clinical History: 46-year-old woman presenting with urinary dribbling.

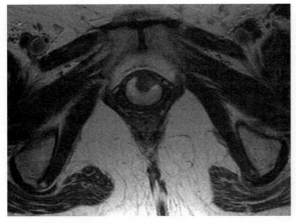

Figure 7.18   A

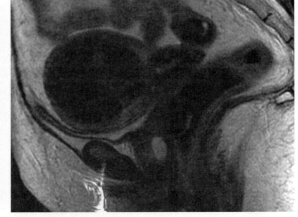

Figure 7.18   B

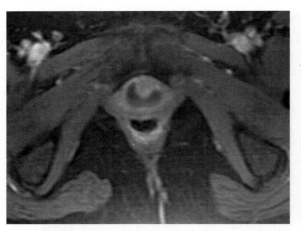

Figure 7.18   C

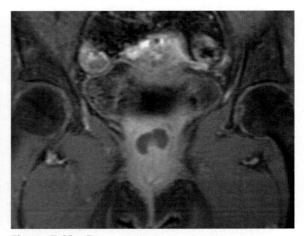

Figure 7.18   D

Findings: Axial (A) and coronal T2-WI (B) reveal a well-defined, homogeneous, bright, horseshoe-shaped lesion encasing the urethra. Gadolinium-enhanced, fat-suppressed axial (C) and coronal (D) T1-WI show enhancement of the smooth wall of the lesion. Note presence of uterine fibroid.

Differential Diagnosis: Periurethral collagen injection, Bartholin cyst.

Diagnosis: Urethral diverticulum.

Discussion: Urethral diverticula are saccular, bilobed, or circumferential ("horseshoe") outpouchings of obstructed small secretory glands in the wall of the mid urethra. The greatest number of these glands is located posteriorly in the urethral wall. It is important to identify the exact location of the neck of the diverticulum and the presence of other diverticula because surgery is often technically difficult. The lesions can be congenital or acquired. The acquired lesions are much more common in women and may occur after urethral infection, trauma, or prolonged transurethral catheterization. Unlike the congenital diverticula, the acquired lesions are not lined by epithelium. On T2-WI, a diverticulum appears as a bright focus with a well-defined border. Debris or calculi may be identified in the depending portions of the diverticulum. Gadolinium-enhanced, fat-suppressed T1-WI is indicated to detect the presence of granulation tissue or, uncommonly, carcinoma. Differentiation between granulation tissue and carcinoma is not possible based on the MRI findings.

CASE 7-19

Clinical History: 45-year-old woman presenting with left lower quadrant pain.

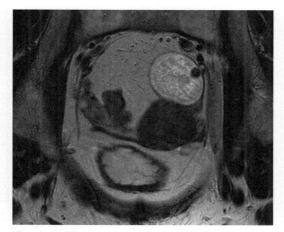

Figure 7.19   A

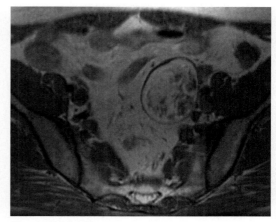

Figure 7.19   B

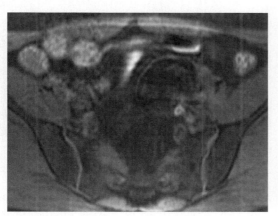

Figure 7.19   C

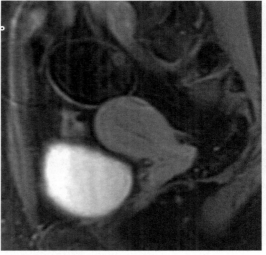

Figure 7.19   D

Findings: Coronal T2-WI (A) and axial T1-WI (B) reveal a thin-walled, predominantly hyperintense, 5-cm left ovarian mass, with a small hypointense nodule adjacent to the wall. Unenhanced axial (C) and gadolinium-enhanced sagittal (D) fat-suppressed T1-WI show heterogeneous signal drop of the lesion and no internal enhancement.

Differential Diagnosis: Hemorrhagic ovarian cyst.

Diagnosis: Mature ovarian teratoma.

Discussion: Fat-saturation MRI techniques are proven to be 100% specific and 96% accurate for the diagnosis of the most common germ cell tumor (99%), mature ovarian teratoma, due to depiction of the pathognomonic fat content of the lesion. Although hemorrhagic lesions can have T1 values similar to fat, they do not lose signal after fat suppression.

Presence of a dermoid plug projecting from the wall is known as the Rokitansky nodule; it is a nonenhancing nodular component, which represents solid fat, hair, and/or teeth. The lack of enhancement of the dermoid enables the differentiation from an ovarian carcinoma or the rare malignant transformation of a mature teratoma, also known as an immature teratoma. Immature teratoma occurs in the first two decades of life. It has a prominent solid component and may demonstrate hemorrhage and necrosis. Also in contrast with the mature teratoma, calcifications are rather scattered in immature teratoma. Immature teratoma is a rapidly growing tumor and frequently demonstrates local invasion. Elevated levels of serum CA 19-9 can be seen in all germ cell tumors; elevated alpha-fetoprotein is concerning for immature teratoma.

Clinical History: 44-year-old woman presenting with fever postpartum.

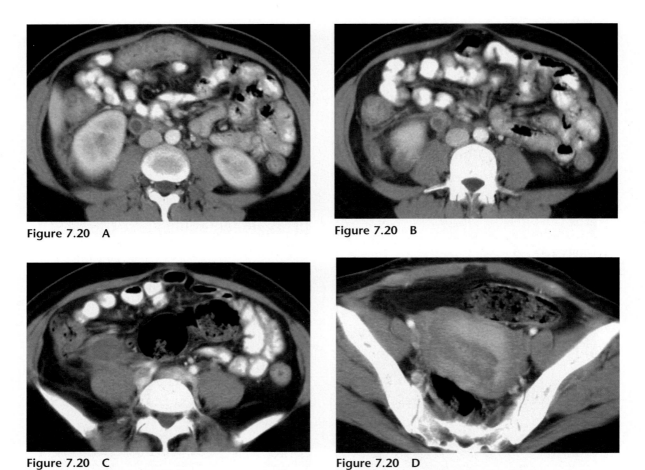

Figure 7.20 A

Figure 7.20 B

Figure 7.20 C

Figure 7.20 D

Findings: Axial CECT images show a low-density tubular structure with thin peripheral enhancement, surrounded by inflammatory changes, coursing anteriorly to the right psoas muscle. Note enlarged blood-filled uterus.

Differential Diagnosis: None.

Diagnosis: Ovarian vein thrombophlebitis.

Discussion: When thrombophlebitis is diagnosed in the postpartum period, it commonly is a septic thrombophlebitis involving the ovarian vein and is associated with endometritis in 67% of cases. Endometritis can occur after cesarean section or vaginal delivery. Since patients are in a hypercoagulable state during pregnancy and the early postpartum period, thrombosis may occur any time during these periods. Most commonly, it occurs in the first 3 days postpartum. The right ovarian vein is affected more frequently than the left. This case demonstrates the classic findings of ovarian vein thrombophlebitis. There is a postpartum uterus with a tubular structure in the location of the right ovarian vein, with a low-attenuation center representing the thrombus. Inflammatory changes are present around the vessel, and the vessel appears enlarged due to the thrombosis. The peripheral enhancement may be due to intraluminal contrast around a nonocclusive thrombus or contrast in the vasa vasorum. Many complications may arise from ovarian vein thrombosis including inferior vena cava or renal vein thrombosis, pulmonary embolism, sepsis, and septic emboli. Treatment is conservative, with administration of intravenous antibiotics and anticoagulation to avoid spread of the thrombus.

Clinical History: 39-year-old woman presenting with dyspareunia.

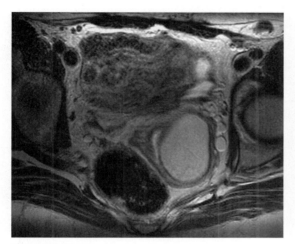

Figure 7.21 A

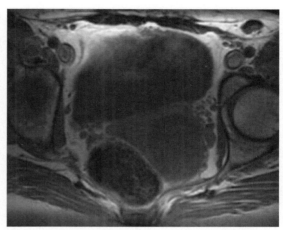

Figure 7.21 B

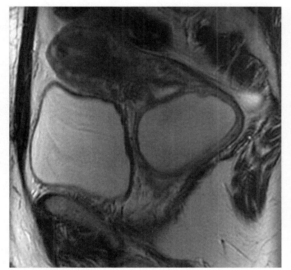

Figure 7.21 C

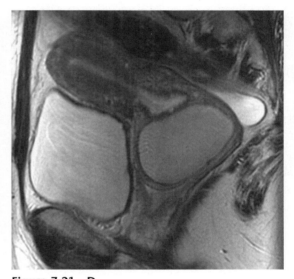

Figure 7.21 D

Findings: Axial T2-WI (A) and axial T1-WI (B) demonstrate a thin-walled, homogeneous, 8-cm cystic lesion in the left upper vagina. Sagittal T2-WI (C and D) show the location of the mass below the cervix in the upper portion of the vagina.

Differential Diagnosis: Nabothian cyst, hematocolpos, Bartholin gland cyst.

Diagnosis: Gartner duct cyst.

Discussion: A Gartner duct cyst is an embryologic remnant of the caudal end of the mesonephric/Wolffian duct. Occurring in 1% of women, Gartner duct cysts are the most common benign cystic lesions of the vagina. Associated anomalies can be seen in both the urinary tract (e.g., ectopic ureteral insertion, ipsilateral renal dysgenesis or agenesis, crossed fused renal ectopia) and genital tract (e.g., bicornuate uterus, didelphys uterus, ipsilateral Müllerian duct obstruction, diverticulosis of the fallopian tube). The cysts are located in the anterolateral vaginal wall or extend out into the ischiorectal fossa; they show no enhancement after contrast administration. When large, the cyst can cause pelvic pain and dyspareunia and/or interfere with the birth process. Symptomatic cysts are treated by marsupialization into the vagina. When the cyst originates in the posterolateral aspect of the vulvovaginal vestibule below the pelvic diaphragm, it needs to be differentiated from a Bartholin cyst. Nabothian cysts, which are located in the cervix itself, and hematocolpos, representing blood in the uterine endocavity and cervix, can easily be differentiated on imaging from Gartner duct cysts based on their respective locations.

Clinical History: 66-year-old man presenting with upper abdominal pain.

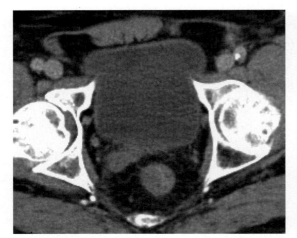

Figure 7.22 A

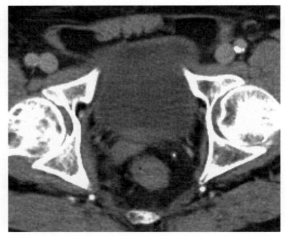

Figure 7.22 B

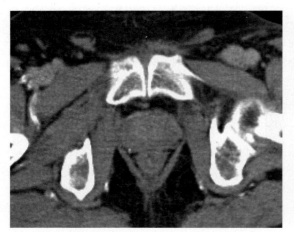

Figure 7.22 C

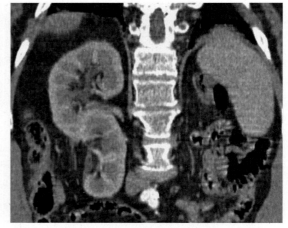

Figure 7.22 D

Findings: Axial CECT images (A–C) reveal absence of the left seminal vesicle (A). Coronal reformatted CECT image (D) demonstrates absence of a kidney in the left renal fossa and two kidneys that are fused in the right.

Differential Diagnosis: Renal agenesis, renal hypogenesis, renal ptosis, duplication anomaly.

Diagnosis: Seminal vesicle agenesis with crossed fused renal ectopia.

Discussion: Crossed renal ectopia is an uncommon congenital renal abnormality characterized by a kidney located on the opposite side of its ureterovesical junction. There is a male predominance, and the left kidney crosses the midline more commonly than the right kidney. The adrenal gland is typically in its normal place (in renal agenesis, the adrenal gland loses its characteristic V or Y shape and becomes elliptical). The ureters insert in their normal positions. The length of the ureter of the ectopic kidney must adjust itself to the position of the kidney. The arterial blood supply arises ectopically, usually from a major artery in the immediate vicinity of the malpositioned kidney (in renal ptosis, renal arteries arises from their normal sites). In decreasing order of frequency, crossed renal ectopia may occur with fusion, without fusion, or as a solitary kidney. One embryologic hypothesis is that both mesonephric ducts and ureteral buds stray from their normal course (which explains the typical absence of an ipsilateral seminal vesicle) and cause crossed ectopia. Associated anomalies involve the urinary tract (e.g., ureteropelvic junction obstruction, vesicoureteral reflux, uni- or bilateral duplicated collecting system), the gastrointestinal (GI) tract (e.g., anorectal or esophageal atresia, rectovaginal fistula, omphalocele), and other systems (e.g., cardiovascular, vertebral, neurologic, skeletal, and facial).

Clinical History: 75-year-old man presenting with elevated prostate-specific antigen (PSA).

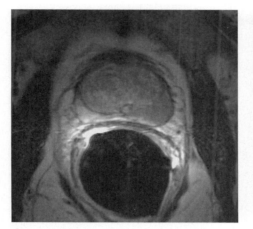
Figure 7.23   A

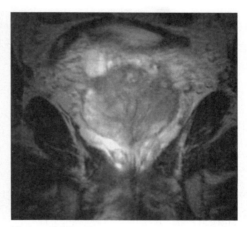
Figure 7.23   B

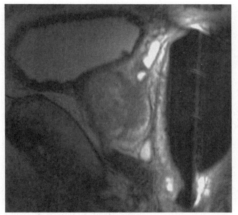
Figure 7.23   C

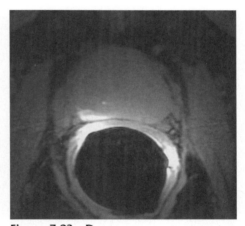
Figure 7.23   D

Findings: Axial (A), coronal (B), and sagittal (C) T2-WI demonstrate an area of hypointense signal in the posterior left side of the peripheral zone of the prostate. This area is hypointense on fat-suppressed axial T1-WI (D). The hyperintense area on T1-WI on the right in the peripheral zone represents hemorrhage from a recent biopsy.

Differential Diagnosis: Hyperplasia (fibrous, fibromuscular, muscular, and atypical adenomatous types), prostatitis, infarction, scar and hemorrhage after biopsy.

Diagnosis: Prostate cancer (adenocarcinoma).

Discussion: In the United States, prostate cancer is the most common malignancy in men and the second most common cause of cancer-related deaths after lung carcinoma. After the diagnosis of prostate cancer has been made (often after ultrasound-guided prostate biopsy), the staging of prostate cancer has important implications for treatment. The majority of prostate cancers arise from the peripheral zone (70%); a smaller number originate in the central gland. Tumors that extend outside the gland (stage T3a or C1 according to the Jewett-Whitmore staging system) and invade surrounding tissues (stage T3b or C2) have high rates of recurrence and morbidity. Therefore, an important staging threshold for treatment is between stages T2 or B (tumor confined to the prostate gland; treated with curative radical prostatectomy) and T3b or C (gross or bilateral extraglandular tumor; treated with external-beam radiation, hormonal therapy, or both). Research on stage T3a suggests that patients with microscopic extraglandular tumor can be candidates for surgery. Multiplanar MRI has a specificity of 90% to 95% in staging T2/B and T3/C prostate cancers. On T2-WI, the majority of prostate adenocarcinomas appear as focal areas of hypointensity in the normally hyperintense peripheral zone (acinar mucin). Hemorrhage after recent biopsy usually appears as a hyperintense area on T1-WI and as a hypointense area on T2-WI.

Clinical History: 31-year-old woman presenting with vaginal bleeding and pain 3 months after pregnancy termination.

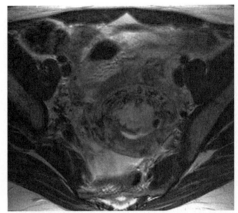

Figure 7.24   A

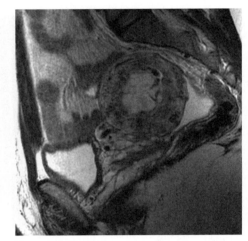

Figure 7.24   B

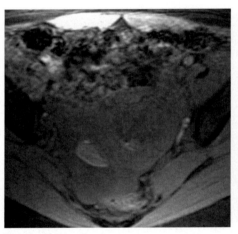

Figure 7.24   C

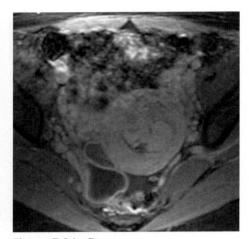

Figure 7.24   D

Findings: Axial (A) and sagittal (B) T2-WI demonstrate a heterogeneous hyperintense mass in the anterior uterine wall, with the bulk of the mass protruding in the uterine cavity. Note the interruption of the junctional zone. The mass is isointense to the myometrium on fat-suppressed axial T1-WI (C). After gadolinium administration (D), the mass shows homogeneous enhancement. Note the small amount of blood in the endometrial cavity.

Differential Diagnosis: Gestational trophoblastic disease, choriocarcinoma, endometrial proliferative disease, hydropic placental degeneration after incomplete abortion, myxoid or carneous degeneration of a leiomyoma, uterine arteriovenous malformation.

Diagnosis: Retained products of conception.

Discussion: Retained products of conception (RPOC) complicate nearly 1% of all pregnancies, more often after termination of pregnancy than after vaginal or cesarean delivery. Common symptoms are vaginal bleeding and abdominal or pelvic pain. The main differential diagnosis is gestational trophoblastic disease, in which the serum level of beta human chorionic gonadotropin (HCG) characteristically remains elevated; trophoblastic disease requires chemotherapy. Hormone levels fall to an undetectable level over 2 to 3 weeks in patients with RPOC. RPOC is treated with curettage or conservatively if endometritis coexists. Endometritis presents as fluid in the endometrial cavity, with diffuse enhancement and/or thickening of the endometrium. RPOC appear as an intracavitary soft tissue mass with variable amounts of enhancing tissue and with variable degrees of myometrial thinning and obliteration of the junctional zone. Frequently RPOC undergo necrosis with deposition of fibrin and may form so-called placental polyps. Development of arteriovenous fistulas within the placenta caused by necrosis of the chorionic villi may also be seen, and their presence is important for selecting the appropriate treatment (e.g., methotrexate therapy, hysterectomy, or embolization).

Clinical History: 42-year-old woman presenting with pelvic pain.

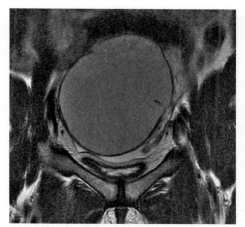

Figure 7.25   A

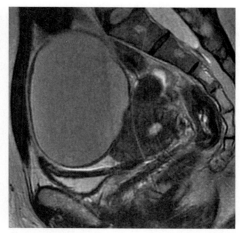

Figure 7.25   B

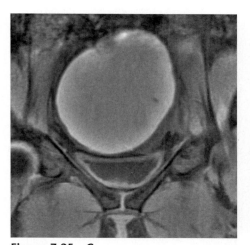

Figure 7.25   C

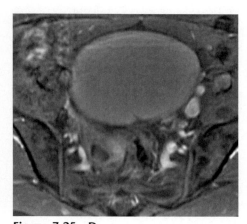

Figure 7.25   D

Findings: Coronal (A) and sagittal (B) T2-WI demonstrate a 10 × 7 cm cystic left ovarian mass with intermediate signal intensity, a thin wall, some septations, and a small amount of free fluid. Fat-suppressed coronal T1-WI (C) reveals homogeneous hyperintense content of the mass. No enhancement of the mass is seen on the gadolinium-enhanced, fat-suppressed axial T1-WI (D). The right ovary shows a rim-enhancing heterogeneous cystic lesion with a T1 hyperintense component in the dependent part.

Differential Diagnosis: Hemorrhagic ovarian cyst, teratoma, tubo-ovarian abscess.

Diagnosis: Endometriosis with an endometrioma.

Discussion: Endometriosis is defined as the presence of ectopic endometrial glands and stroma. Clinical presentations include dysmenorrhea; dyspareunia; chronic lower abdominal, pelvic, and back pain; irregular bleeding; and infertility. Approximately 15% of infertile women of reproductive age

have endometriosis. Common pathologic manifestations of endometriosis are development of endometriomas and adhesions resulting from fibrosis and endometrial implants. In descending order of frequency, the most common sites of these implants are the ovaries, uterine ligaments, cul-de-sac, serosal surface of the uterus, fallopian tubes, rectosigmoid colon, and bladder dome. Less common sites are the mesentery, bowel serosa, ureters, and along a prior caesarean section scar. Due to the presence of blood products, endometriomas are usually hyperintense on T1-WI (with and without fat suppression; differentiates it from teratoma) and hypointense on T2-WI. The typical appearance of heterogeneous low signal on T2-WI of endometriomas is termed "shading" and is due to the layering effect of blood products caused by the repeated bleeding within the lesion. This distinguishes an endometrioma from a hemorrhagic ovarian cyst. A rare complication of endometriosis is development of clear cell carcinomas.

Clinical History: 54-year-old woman presenting with hematuria.

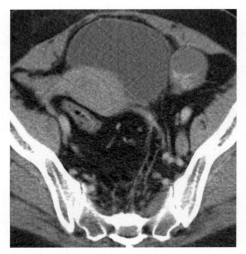

Figure 7.26   A

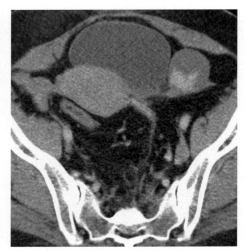

Figure 7.26   B

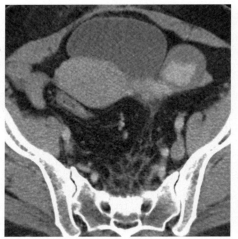

Figure 7.26   C

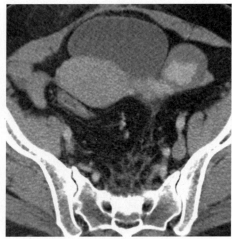

Figure 7.26   D

Findings: Axial CECT images demonstrate a left ovarian cystic mass measuring 4.5 × 4.3 cm with a nodular solid component.

Differential Diagnosis: Ovarian dermoid, epithelial ovarian neoplasm, ovarian metastasis, endometrioma, tubo-ovarian abscess.

Diagnosis: Malignant struma ovarii (papillary thyroid carcinoma, follicular variant).

Discussion: Approximately 20% of all ovarian tumors are germ cell tumors, and 95% of these tumors are mature cystic teratomas. Fifteen percent of all mature teratomas predominantly contain thyroid tissue on histology, the so-called struma ovarii. Malignant transformation occurs in less than 5% of all struma. The average age of presentation is 44 years in reported cases. Struma ovarii are usually unilateral and seldom present with clinical hyperthyroidism (5–8%). The tumor rarely metastasizes to regional pelvic and para-aortic lymph nodes or spreads directly to the omentum, the peritoneal cavity, or contralateral ovary. Hematologic dissemination to the bone, lung, liver, and brain has been reported. Malignant struma ovarii are, similar to thyroid cancers, histologically classified into three types: papillary carcinoma (44%), follicular carcinoma (30%), and a follicular variant of the papillary carcinoma (26%), as seen in this case. There is no standard treatment known for this rare tumor. Elevated thyroglobulin levels are believed to be key in the detection of recurrent tumor after therapy (after cervical thyroid ablation and struma ovarii resection). Thyroglobulin elevation has been demonstrated both in benign and malignant struma ovarii.

Clinical History: 54-year-old woman presenting with weight loss.

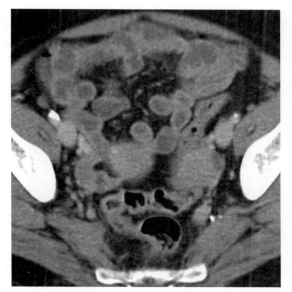

Figure 7.27 A

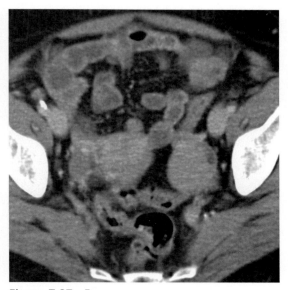

Figure 7.27 B

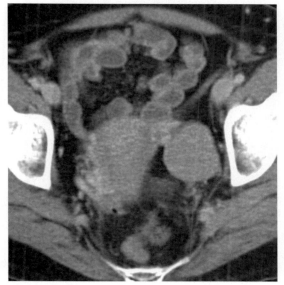

Figure 7.27 C

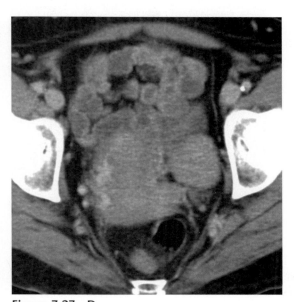

Figure 7.27 D

Findings: Axial CECT images demonstrate a 3.9 × 3.5 cm solid left ovarian mass.

Differential Diagnosis: Fibroma, fibrothecoma, malignant epithelial tumor.

Diagnosis: Brenner tumor.

Discussion: Brenner tumors are usually benign epithelial ovarian tumors, representing 2% to 3% of ovarian tumors. Brenner tumors are most often found in women between the fifth and seventh decades of life. They are composed of transitional cells in prominent fibrous connective tissue. Thirty percent are associated with epithelial ovarian neoplasms in the ipsilateral or contralateral ovary. Brenner tumors are usually small (<2 cm) and discovered incidentally, but affected patients may present with a palpable mass or pain. The solid components of these tumors show mild or moderate enhancement after contrast administration on CT or MRI. On MRI, the solid nodule is isointense to the myometrium on T1-WI and hypointense on T2-WI. Extensive amorphous calcifications may be noted within the nodule. Cystic areas usually represent a coexistent cystadenoma. The Brenner tumor is the exception to the rule that an enhancing soft tissue nodule in a cystic ovarian mass indicates malignancy.

Clinical History: 39-year-old woman presenting with urinary frequency and pelvic pain.

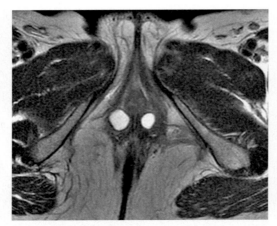

Figure 7.28   A

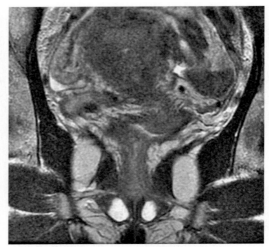

Figure 7.28   B

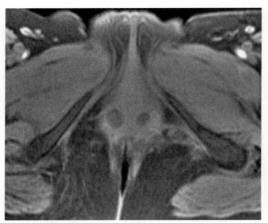

Figure 7.28   C

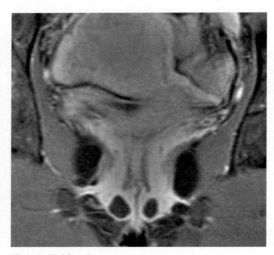

Figure 7.28   D

Findings: Axial (A) and coronal (B) T2-WI and fat-suppressed axial T1-WI (C) reveal bilateral, thin-walled, homogeneous, 1-cm cystic lesions in the posterolateral aspect of the vulvovaginal vestibule. Gadolinium-enhanced, fat-suppressed coronal T1-WI (D) shows thin regular enhancement of the wall of these lesions.

Differential Diagnosis: Gartner duct cysts, Nuck duct cysts.

Diagnosis: Bartholin gland cysts.

Discussion: Bartholin gland cyst is a cystic dilatation of the paired mucus-secreting glands confined in the posterolateral aspect of the vulvovaginal vestibule. Bartholin gland cysts usually range in size from 1 to 4 cm and are asymptomatic incidental findings. However, superinfection with abscess formation may result in severe vulvar pain. Large cysts may cause dyspareunia. Rarely adenocarcinoma or squamous cell carcinoma may arise from a Bartholin gland cyst. Bartholin gland cysts may show intense wall enhancement when superimposed infection is present or show enhancement of the solid nodular elements when a tumor arises in a cyst. Treatment of an infected cyst is marsupialization because it has fewer complications than cyst excision. Excision is preferred in postmenopausal females because of the possibility of coexistent tumor. Gartner duct cysts arise from the anterolateral aspect of the vaginal wall; Nuck duct cysts present as cystic lesions with a thin enhancing wall in the major labia or mons pubis.

Clinical History: 43-year-old man presenting with buttock and scrotal pain and subcutaneous edema.

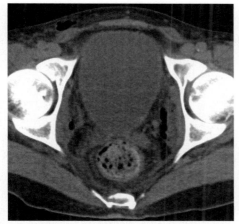

Figure 7.29   A

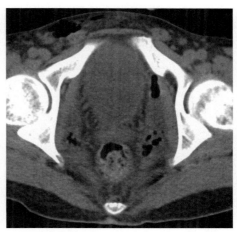

Figure 7.29   B

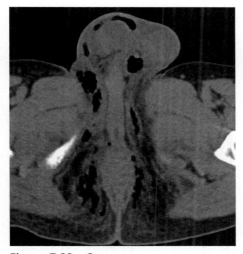

Figure 7.29   C

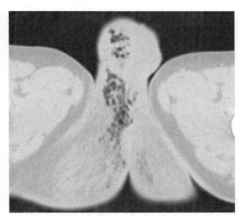

Figure 7.29   D

Findings: Axial nonenhanced CT (NECT) images (A–C) demonstrate multiple gas bubbles in the subcutaneous fat of the right groin along the fascia of Scarpa, along both internal obturator muscles, in the ischioanal fossa, in the perineum, and into the scrotal sac. Axial NECT image displayed in lung window (D) better shows the gas.

Differential Diagnosis: Postsurgical gas, penetrating injury.

Diagnosis: Fournier gangrene.

Discussion: Fournier gangrene is defined as a polymicrobial necrotizing fasciitis of the perineal, perirectal, or genital area. The severe subcutaneous infection begins adjacent to the site of origin, which may be urethral, rectal, or cutaneous. The testicles are commonly spared because of their separate blood supply directly from the aorta instead of the cutaneous and subcutaneous vessels. Fournier gangrene is a surgical emergency because the progression of fascial necrosis has been documented to be as much as 2 to 3 cm/hr. A mortality rate of 76% with a delay of 6 days and a mortality rate of only 12% with less than a 24-hour delay before surgical debridement have been reported. Most patients are between 50 and 70 years old. The symptoms begin insidiously with genital discomfort. The diagnosis of Fournier gangrene is based on clinical examination. However, to confirm, evaluate the extent, and detect the underlying cause, CT can be performed, demonstrating the subcutaneous gas bubbles, as seen in this case. The absence of a recent surgical history or of a penetrating injury makes Fournier gangrene the most likely diagnosis.

Clinical History: 35-year-old woman presenting with infertility.

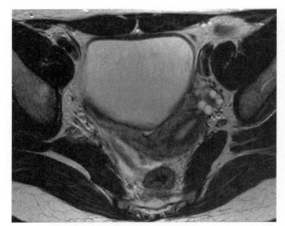

Figure 7.30   A

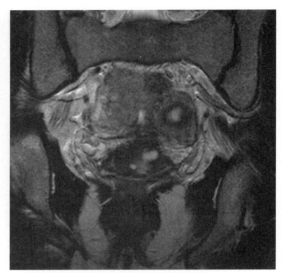

Figure 7.30   B

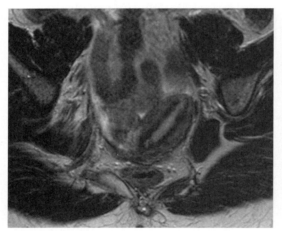

Figure 7.30   C

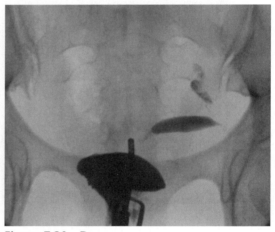

Figure 7.30   D

Findings: Axial (A), coronal (B), and oblique along the long axis of the uterine body (C) T2-WI demonstrate a curved and elongated ("banana-shaped") uterus with maintained zonal anatomy, which is shifted towards the left hemipelvis. Note a rudimentary horn without endometrium in the right hemipelvis. Hysterosalpingogram image (D) reveals no communication of the left portion of the uterus with the right rudimentary horn.

Differential Diagnosis: None.

Diagnosis: Noncavitary unicornuate uterus.

Discussion: Unicornuate uteri arise from hypoplasia or agenesis of one paramesonephric (Müllerian) duct, while the other duct develops normally. It represents approximately 20% of all uterine anomalies. If a rudimentary horn is present, it is subdivided into noncavitary, if no endometrial segment is seen in the rudimentary horn, or cavitary, if an associated endometrial segment is identified. A cavitary horn is further subdivided into noncommunicating if the endometrial segment is isolated and shows no connection to the endometrium of the dominant horn; if there is continuity between the endometrium of both horns, it is designated as communicating. When an endometrial segment is present in the rudimentary horn, surgical transabdominal resection of that horn is indicated because of associated dysmenorrhea, hematometria, and risk of pregnancy within the hypoplastic horn. Coexistent renal anomalies, if present (40%), are always ipsilateral to the rudimentary horn, with renal agenesis being the most common abnormality.

Clinical History: 73-year-old man presenting with penile swelling.

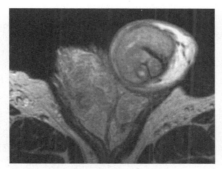

Figure 7.31 A

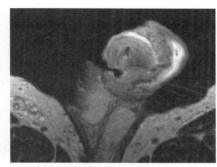

Figure 7.31 B

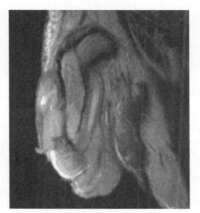

Figure 7.31 C

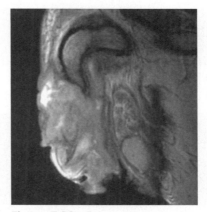

Figure 7.31 D

Findings: Axial (A and B) and sagittal (C and D) T2-WI demonstrate a 4.5 × 4.3 cm, ill-defined, solid C-shaped penile mass, originating from the skin, prepuce, and glans penis. It invades the tunica albuginea and right corpus cavernosum and abuts the corpus spongiosum.

Differential Diagnosis: Metastasis.

Diagnosis: Penile cancer (invasive squamous cell carcinoma).

Discussion: Penile cancers are relatively rare neoplasms in developed countries and typically occur in the sixth and seventh decades of life. Risk factors are the presence of fore-skin (3 times higher than circumcised men), poor hygiene, phimosis (present in 25% of penile cancer patients), chronic inflammatory conditions, smoking, treatment with ultraviolet A phototherapy, and human papilloma virus 16 and 18. More than 95% of primary penile neoplasms are squamous cell carcinomas; they are most commonly (48%) located in the glans penis. Less frequent primary neoplasms are sarcoma, melanoma, basal cell carcinoma, and lymphoma. Metastasis to the penis should be suspected in patients with a known primary (nearly 70% originating from the urogenital tract). The main prognostic factors for penile carcinoma are the degree of invasion by the primary tumor and the status of the draining lymph nodes. The 5-year survival rate is 0% in patients with pelvic nodal disease. Buck fascia, a fibrous layer surrounding the corpora cavernosa and tunica albuginea, acts as a barrier to corporal invasion and hematogenous spread. The lymphatic spread depends on the location of the lesion: cancer of the penile skin and prepuce drains into superficial inguinal nodes, cancer of the glans penis drains into the deep inguinal and external iliac nodes, and cancer of erectile tissue and penile urethra drains into the internal iliac nodes. On MRI, primary penile cancers are most often solitary, ill-defined, infiltrating masses. They are relatively hypointense to the corpora on both T1-WI and T2-WI and enhance less than the corpora cavernosa. Penile metastases present usually as multiple discrete masses in the corpora cavernosa and corpus spongiosum.

Clinical History: 51-year-old woman with known uterine adenomyosis and fibroids presenting with an enlarged cervix on clinical examination.

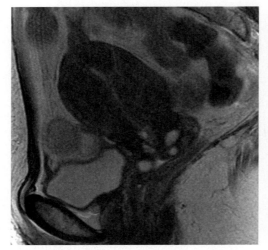

Figure 7.32 A

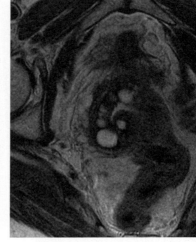

Figure 7.32 B

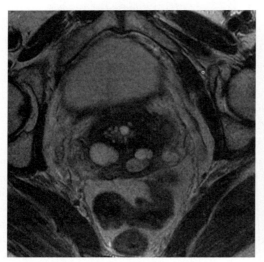

Figure 7.32 C

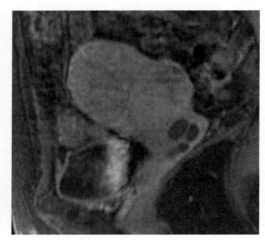

Figure 7.32 D

Findings: Sagittal (A) and axial (B and C) T2-WI demonstrate multiple smooth, thin-walled cysts in the uterine cervix. Gadolinium-enhanced, fat-suppressed sagittal T1-WI (D) reveals no enhancement of these cysts.

Differential Diagnosis: Adenomyosis, adenoma malignum.

Diagnosis: Nabothian cysts.

Discussion: Nabothian cysts (retention or endocervical gland cysts) are common, usually asymptomatic incidental findings on CT or MRI. The prevalence of Nabothian cysts increases with age, and they are seen in 8% of adult women and 13% of postmenopausal women. They are true cysts outlined by mucin-producing epithelium. It is believed that they result from squamous metaplasia obstructing the endocervical glands of the ectocervix; an association with cervicitis has been reported. The majority of cysts are small (<1cm); typically they are hypointense on T1-WI and hyperintense on T2-WI and do not enhance after contrast administration. Rarely, high signal intensity is seen in the cyst on T1-WI due to the mucinous content. In adenomyosis, the hyperintense foci on T2-WI are located in the uterine corpus rather than in the cervix. Adenoma malignum is distinguishable from Nabothian cysts because it has solid elements, and the cysts tend to be larger. However, it may be difficult to distinguish deep-seated Nabothian cysts from adenoma malignum.

Clinical History: 24-year-old man presenting with a painless right-sided scrotal mass.

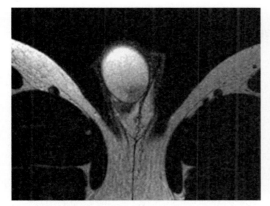

Figure 7.33   A

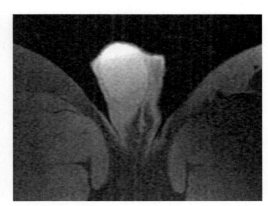

Figure 7.33   B

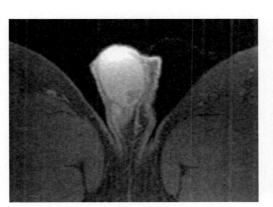

Figure 7.33   C

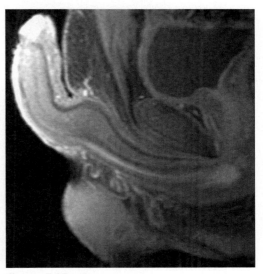

Figure 7.33   D

Findings: Axial T2-WI (A) reveals a heterogeneous hypointense focus within the posterior medial aspect of the right testis. This focus is also hypointense on the fat-suppressed axial T1-WI (B). Gadolinium-enhanced, fat-suppressed axial (C) and sagittal (D) T1-WI demonstrate rim enhancement of the lesion.

Differential Diagnosis: Infection, hemorrhage, infarction.

Diagnosis: Testicular cancer (nonseminomatous germ cell tumor).

Discussion: Testicular neoplasms can be primary or metastatic and are bilateral in 1% to 3% of cases. Primary testicular neoplasms are classified as germ cell (90–95%) or stromal (5–10%) tumors. Germ cell tumors are, in turn, grouped into seminomatous (40%), nonseminomatous (55%), and mixed (10–15%) lesions. Seminomas (peak incidence in the late 30s) are mildly heterogeneous and rarely visible on T1-WI.

On T2-WI, they are hypointense to the normally hyperintense testicular tissue. They rarely bleed or necrose centrally. Nonseminomas (peak incidence in the 20s and early 30s) are markedly heterogeneous and visible on T1-WI, which distinguishes them from seminomas. An enhancing fibrous tumor capsule can be seen as in our case. Hemorrhage of various ages (due to their high propensity to invade vessels) and islands of muscle or cartilage within the mass (teratomatous features) are characteristic. Stromal tumors (presenting between 20 and 60 years) are well circumscribed and rarely show hemorrhage or necrosis. Because they usually produce hormones, prepubertal boys can present with precocious puberty, and adults can present with gynecomastia. Testicular infection, hemorrhage, and infarction usually are associated with local or systemic symptoms and would not present as a painless mass.

Clinical History: 44-year-old woman presenting with urinary incontinence.

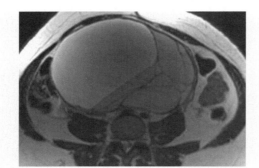

Figure 7.34   A

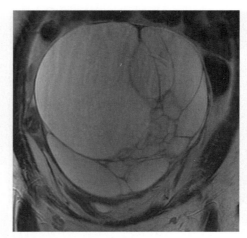

Figure 7.34   B

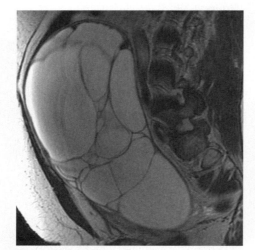

Figure 7.34   C

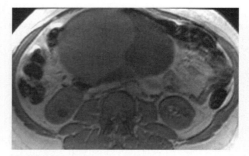

Figure 7.34   D

Findings: Axial (A), coronal (B), and sagittal (C) T2-WI and axial T1-WI (D) demonstrate a large multiloculated mass originating from the pelvis and extending into the upper abdomen. It contains innumerable thin septations, with cranially a hypointense thick septation representing a calcification. Note varying signal intensities in the different locules.

Differential Diagnosis: Serous cystadenoma (carcinoma), cystic teratoma, endometrioma.

Diagnosis: Mucinous cystadenoma.

Discussion: Mucinous cystadenomas/carcinomas are epithelial ovarian neoplasms. Of all mucinous ovarian neoplasms, 80% are smooth-walled benign cystadenomas, 10% to 15% are of low malignant potential, and 5% to 10% are

malignant. The latter account for 10% of all malignant ovarian neoplasms, and serous cystadenocarcinomas account for 50%. Compared to serous ovarian neoplasms, mucinous ovarian neoplasms tend to be larger, are multilocular with smaller cystic components (honeycomblike locules), and rarely show linear calcifications. The typical heterogeneous appearance of the individual locules may result from different degrees of hemorrhage or protein content. Imaging findings suggestive for malignancy are a thick, irregular wall, thick septations (both >3 mm), papillary projections, and a large soft tissue component with necrosis. Pelvic organ invasion, implants (mesenteric, omental, or peritoneal), ascites, and adenopathy are also indicative of malignancy. To characterize an adnexal mass, contrast-enhanced MRI allows better identification of solid portions in cystic lesions or necrosis in solid lesions.

Clinical History: 72-year-old man presenting with a painless perineal mass.

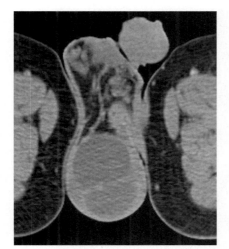

Figure 7.35 A

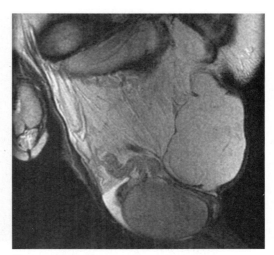

Figure 7.35 B

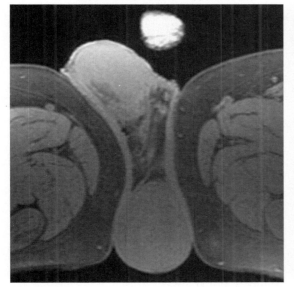

Figure 7.35 C

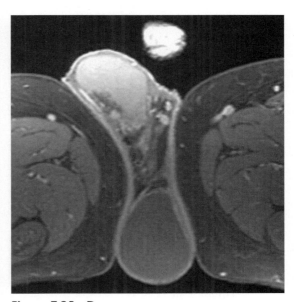

Figure 7.35 D

Findings: Axial CECT image (A) demonstrates a subcutaneous cystic mass located between the scrotum and anus, with faint enhancement of the thin wall. Sagittal T2-WI (B) shows the cystic nature of this extratesticular lesion. The mass has intermediate signal intensity on the fat-suppressed axial T1-WI (C). Note faint internal heterogeneity. On the gadolinium-enhanced, fat-suppressed axial T1-WI (D), only the thin wall reveals mild enhancement.

Differential Diagnosis: Teratoma, pilonidal cyst, seroma, abscess.

Diagnosis: Epidermal inclusion cyst.

Discussion: Epidermal inclusion cysts are benign solitary lesions of germ cell origin. Typically they are located in the testis, but as seen in this case, they can present in an extratesticular location. The tumor is lined by keratinizing, stratified, squamous epithelium supported by fibrous tissue and is filled with keratohyaline material. On MRI, the cysts are slightly darker than the testis on T1-WI and brighter than the testis on T2-WI. The key to the diagnosis is the presence of T1 bright and T2 dark linear structures within the lesion representing the keratohyaline material and the poorly enhancing fibrous wall. Treatment consists of excision. An abscess in this location would not present as a painless mass. Seromas are seen in postoperative patients or following trauma; no such history was present in this patient.

Clinical History: 19-year-old woman presenting with vaginal bleeding for 8 months.

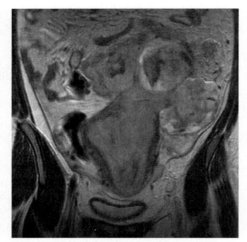

Figure 7.36　A

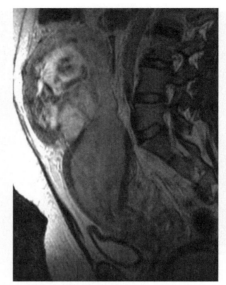

Figure 7.36　B

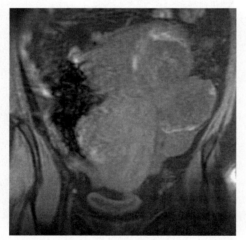

Figure 7.36　C

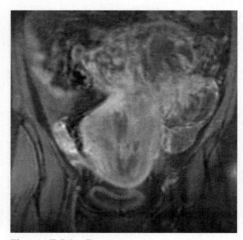

Figure 7.36　D

Findings: Coronal (A) and sagittal (B) T2-WI demonstrate a heterogeneous uterine mass invading through the fundal myometrium and extending into the peritoneal cavity. On the unenhanced coronal T1-WI (C), the mass is isointense to the myometrium, and the extrauterine component shows a thin hyperintense peripheral rim. Gadolinium-enhanced, fat-suppressed coronal T1-WI (D) shows heterogeneous enhancement of the mass.

Differential Diagnosis: Endometrial carcinoma, lymphoma, metastasis.

Diagnosis: Uterine carcinosarcoma.

Discussion: Uterine sarcoma is a rare (2–3%) uterine tumor and is classified into four subtypes (malignant mesodermal tumor, endometrial stromal sarcoma, carcinosarcoma, and leiomyosarcoma). Most of these tumors are diagnosed on histology after hysterectomy due to insufficient tissue sampling during endometrial biopsy. On imaging, an ill-defined infiltrative lesion is suggestive for malignancy. Although gadolinium-enhanced dynamic study appears to be able to differentiate uterine sarcoma (significant enhancement) from endometrial carcinoma (no or minimal enhancement), the main purpose of MRI is to determine the local extent of the mass. Rarely, the uterus and cervix are involved by leukemia or lymphoma; the most common MRI manifestation of uterine lymphoma is diffuse, relatively T2-WI hyperintense uterine enlargement, with minimal enhancement. Metastases to the uterus can occur as a result of advanced-stage malignancies, most commonly breast and stomach cancers.

Clinical History: 49-year-old woman presenting with diarrhea and a painless perianal mass.

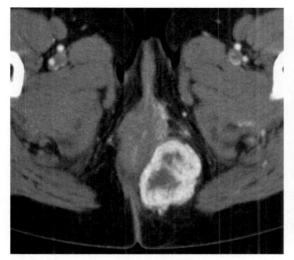

Figure 7.37 A

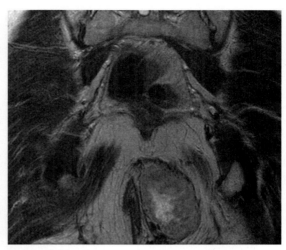

Figure 7.37 B

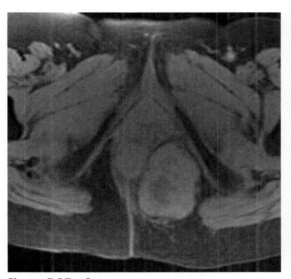

Figure 7.37 C

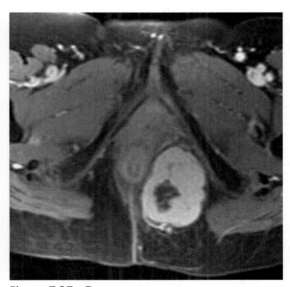

Figure 7.37 D

Findings: Axial CECT image (A), coronal T2-WI (B), and unenhanced (C) and gadolinium-enhanced axial (D) fat-suppressed T1-WI demonstrate a heterogeneous hypervascular mass in the left ischioanal fossa, abutting and displacing the anal canal.

Differential Diagnosis: Malignant fibrous histiocytoma, leiomyosarcoma, rhabdomyosarcoma, fibrous pseudotumor, hemangiopericytoma, aggressive fibromatosis, infectious/inflammatory process.

Diagnosis: Malignant solitary fibrous tumor.

Discussion: Soft tissue masses are difficult to classify on MRI. In 30% of cases, signal intensity characteristics represent important clues to the histologic origin of the tumor (lipomas: homogeneous fat content; hemangiomas: central dot sign representing vessels, T2 hyperintensity). In addition, many malignant soft tissue tumors appear misleadingly benign; a well-defined lesion with an apparent capsule is not a reliable feature of a benign process. The most important role of imaging is to determine the exact localization, the size, and the extent of the lesion to guide further therapy. Furthermore, more than 50% of malignant soft tissue tumors recur locally. Local recurrences usually appear as hyperintense masses on T2-WI, and they typically enhance rapidly; fibrosis has a lower T2 signal and enhances in a more delayed fashion.

Clinical History: 18-year-old woman presenting with painless left labial swelling.

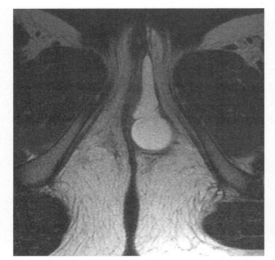

Figure 7.38 A

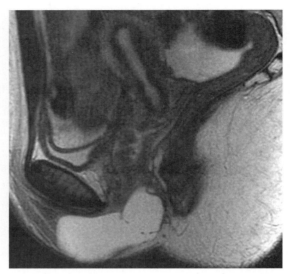

Figure 7.38 B

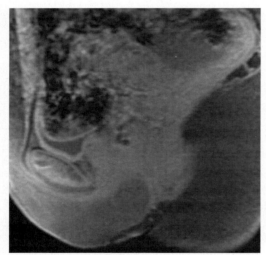

Figure 7.38 C

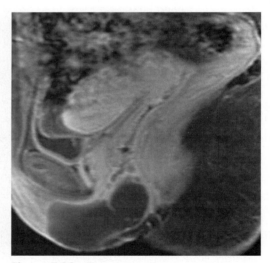

Figure 7.38 D

Findings: Axial (A) and sagittal (B) T2-WI and unenhanced (C) and gadolinium-enhanced (D) fat-suppressed sagittal T1-WI demonstrate a comma-shaped cystic mass measuring 6.3 × 5.0 cm in the left labia, with a thin enhancing wall and a single septation.

Differential Diagnosis: Bartholin gland cyst, inguinal hernia, epidermal inclusion cyst, mucous cyst of the vestibule, Skene gland cyst.

Diagnosis: Cyst of the canal of Nuck.

Discussion: The processus vaginalis peritonei, through which the testes descend in males, is a tubular fold of peritoneum. In females, it invaginates along the round ligament in the inguinal canal. Normally, it is completely closed in the first year of life. When it remains patent in females, it is called the canal of Nuck. It establishes a communication between the peritoneal cavity and the inguinal canal. The degree and level of closure defines the type of inguinal hernia or hydrocele that results. Partial proximal closure with a patent distal portion makes the lesion a cyst of the canal of Nuck, as seen in this case. Inguinal hernias are associated in one third of the patients. Based on the lack of omental or intestinal contents within the cystic mass, the differentiation can be made. A cyst of the canal of Nuck is soft and compressible on clinical examination. On imaging, a typical comma-shaped cystic lesion with a thin enhancing wall in the major labia or mons pubis is classic for such pathology.

Clinical History: 41-year-old woman presenting with a history of miscarriages.

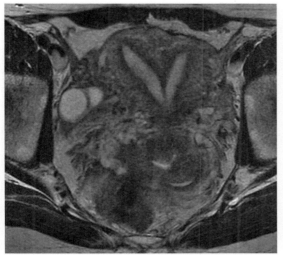

Figure 7.39   A

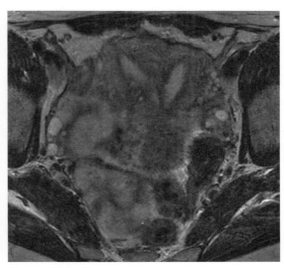

Figure 7.39   B

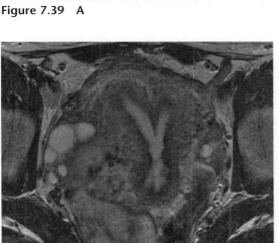

Figure 7.39   C

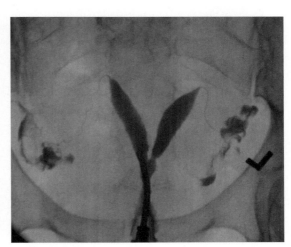

Figure 7.39   D

Findings: Axial T2-WI (A–C) demonstrate a septum in the uterine cavity. This septum does not extend into the endocervical canal. Proximally, the septum is thickened and has the same signal intensity of the adjacent myometrium. Towards the cervix, the septum becomes very thin and T2 hypointense. The external contour of the uterus is fused and convex. Hysterosalpingogram image (D) reveals a divided uterine cavity with bilateral peritoneal spillage of contrast.

Differential Diagnosis: Bicornuate uterus.

Diagnosis: Septate uterus.

Discussion: Septate uterus is the most common Müllerian anomaly, representing 55% of all congenital uterine anomalies. If the septum divides only the endometrial cavity, as in this case, it is called a partial septate uterus. If it extends into the endocervical canal, it is known as a complete septate uterus. The septum may extend into the upper vagina in 5% of cases. The external uterine contour is the crucial differentiating feature between a septate and a bicornuate uterus. In a septate uterus, the external fundal contour can be convex, flat, or mildly concave, with a fundal indentation less than or equal to 1 cm. Also, the uterine horns are less separated (<4 cm) in septate uterus compared to bicornuate uterus (>4 cm). Due to the fibrous component of the septum, 65% of pregnancies implanting in a septate uterus will result in a spontaneous abortion. The rates of complications are similar in partial or complete septate uterus, regardless of the length of the septum. Therapy consists of a hysteroscopic resection of the septum.

Clinical History: 29-year-old woman presenting with pelvic pain.

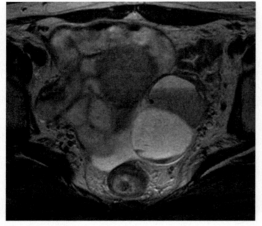

Figure 7.40 A

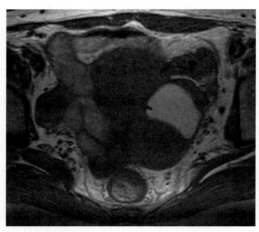

Figure 7.40 B

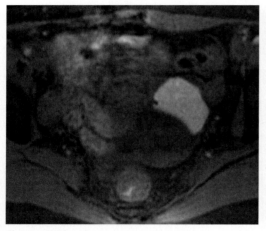

Figure 7.40 C

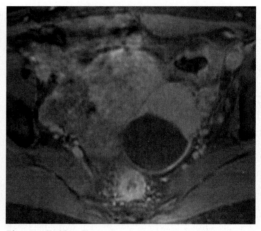

Figure 7.40 D

Findings: Axial T2-WI (A) demonstrates an 8.0 × 4.5 cm bilocular left ovarian lesion with a smooth thin wall. The ventral part reveals a T2 hypointense dependent content with a fluid-fluid level. This content is bright on the axial T1-WI without (B) and with (C) fat suppression. On the gadolinium-enhanced, fat-suppressed axial T1-WI (D), the thin wall shows smooth enhancement. Note the small amount of free pelvic fluid.

Differential Diagnosis: Tubo-ovarian abscess, endometrioma, cystadenoma, teratoma.

Diagnosis: Adjacent hemorrhagic and simple ovarian cysts.

Discussion: Hemorrhage can occur in any ovarian cyst, most commonly in corpus luteum and follicular cysts. The more common hemorrhagic cyst is the corpus luteum cyst, which develops if the corpus luteum fails to regress within 14 days after ovulation. On imaging, it has a thicker wall than follicular cysts due to the thick layer of luteinized cells that line the cyst. The characteristic MRI appearance exhibits a thin hyperintense line on T1-WI that is hypointense on T2-WI, representing the small layer of hemorrhage along the cyst wall. As seen in this case, a hemorrhagic follicular cyst has a thin smooth wall, and the signal intensity of the cyst content varies according to the age of the hemorrhage. Deoxyhemoglobin due to acute hemorrhage has an intermediate signal on T1-WI and low signal intensity on T2-WI. In the subacute phase, methemoglobin shows high signal intensity on T1-WI and T2-WI. On T1-WI, the signal intensity of a hemorrhagic cyst remains unchanged with and without fat suppression. This is key to distinguish the mass from a teratoma. Follow-up imaging of a hemorrhagic cyst is recommended; a hemorrhagic follicular or corpus luteum cyst will resolve, whereas an endometrioma will persist.

Clinical History: 26-year-old woman presenting with acute right pelvic pain.

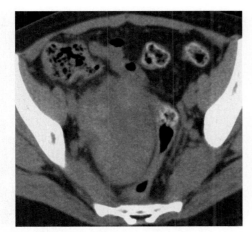

Figure 7.41   A

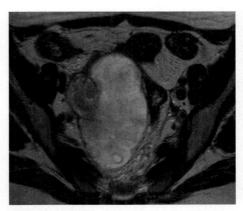

Figure 7.41   B

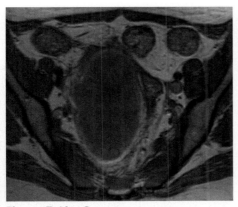

Figure 7.41   C

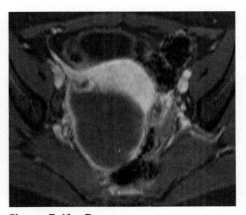

Figure 7.41   D

Findings: Axial CECT image (A) demonstrates a heterogeneous, hyperdense right adnexal mass. Axial T2-WI (B) and axial T1-WI (C) show the heterogeneity of the mass with T1 hyperintense wall and T2 hyperintense peripheral components. Gadolinium-enhanced, fat-suppressed axial T1-WI (D) delineates the thickened wall of the lesion.

Differential Diagnosis: Tubo-ovarian abscess, ectopic pregnancy, endometrioma, hemorrhagic ovarian cyst.

Diagnosis: Ovarian torsion.

Discussion: Ovarian torsion is defined by a twist of the vascular pedicle of the ovary, resulting in vascular compromise. The compromise is initially venous but becomes arterial as the torsion and resultant edema progress. Gangrenous and hemorrhagic necrosis results when the torsion is complete and totally obstructs the arterial blood supply. Ovarian torsion accounts for 3% of gynecologic emergencies and is most common during the first three decades of life (20% of patients are pregnant). There is a 10% chance of contralateral torsion. Patients typically present with acute abdominal pain. There is a right-side predilection because the sigmoid colon occupies the left lower quadrant. In most cases (80%), a large ovarian mass is the underlying cause because it acts as a fulcrum. Occasionally, ovarian torsion may occur in the absence of ovarian disease and has been attributed to excessive mobility of the adnexa, especially in children. In the early stage, the affected ovary is enlarged, and multiple peripheral follicles are separated by edematous stroma, as seen in this case. The latter feature allows differentiation from other pelvic emergencies. Other features are engorged vessels between the mass and uterus, thickening of the ipsilateral tube, obliteration of surrounding fat planes, and ascites. With the onset of hemorrhage, a hyperintense peripheral ring on T1-WI or CT can be seen within the lesion, as in this case. Due to the dual blood supply of the ovary through ovarian and uterine arteries, the presence of residual ovarian perfusion does not exclude ovarian torsion.

Clinical History: 23-year-old woman presenting with an asymptomatic perineal mass.

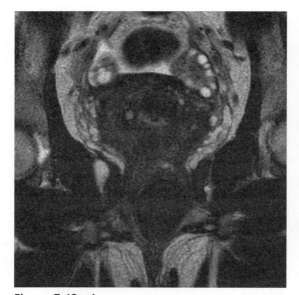

Figure 7.42 A

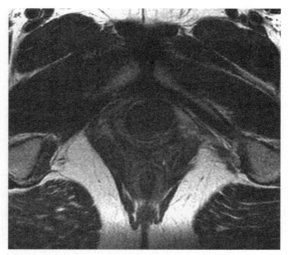

Figure 7.42 B

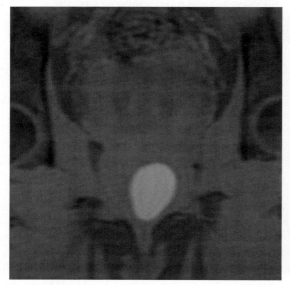

Figure 7.42 C

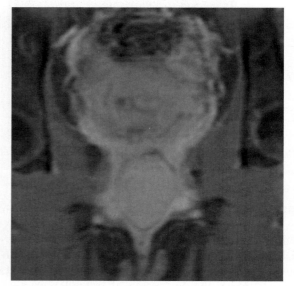

Figure 7.42 D

Findings: Coronal (A) and axial (B) T2-WI show a thin, well-delineated, hypointense ovoid lesion located lateral and posterior to the urethra. Fat-suppressed coronal T1-WI (C) reveals the homogeneous bright content of the mass, suggesting the presence of blood products or protein. Gadolinium-enhanced, fat-suppressed coronal T1-WI (D) demonstrates no enhancement of the mass.

Differential Diagnosis: Bartholin gland cyst, Gartner duct cyst, epidermal inclusion cyst, Nuck duct cyst.

Diagnosis: Skene gland cyst.

Discussion: Skene glands arise from the lower urethra but drain on the vestibular surface on either side of the urethral meatus. Obstruction and resulting enlargement of a Skene gland present as a fluctuant mass that extends inferiorly from the perineum. This case shows a protein-containing (as evidenced by T1 bright and T2 dark signal of the cyst content) periurethral mass with no obvious connection to the urethra. The slightly off midline periurethral location, ovoid shape, nonenhancing thin wall, and proteineous content are typical features of a Skene gland cyst.

Clinical History: 76-year-old woman presenting with urinary incontinence.

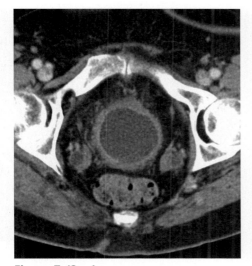

Figure 7.43   A

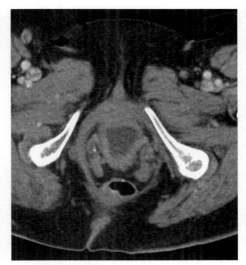

Figure 7.43   B

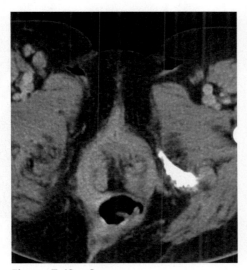

Figure 7.43   C

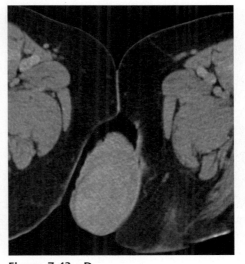

Figure 7.43   D

Findings: Axial CECT images demonstrate bilateral dilatation of the distal ureters and diffuse irregular thickening of the bladder wall, which extends below the pubic symphysis. Note the lateral "ballooning" of the levator ani muscles instead of the normal V-shape configuration. Eversion of the vagina with complete prolapse of the uterus is present.

Differential Diagnosis: None.

Diagnosis: Complete uterine prolapse.

Discussion: Pelvic floor relaxation with abnormal descent of the bladder, uterus/vaginal vault, or rectum affects primarily multipara (16% of perimenopausal women). Significant lifestyle-limiting symptoms are urinary incontinence and/or fecal incontinence, constipation, and incomplete defecation.

Pelvic organ prolapse is the result of specific defects (e.g., rupture, fatty degeneration) in two dynamically interacting functional systems, namely the endopelvic fascia and the levator ani muscles. They support the three pelvic floor compartments: anteriorly, the bladder and urethra; in the middle, the vagina, cervix, and uterus; and posteriorly, the rectum. A cystocele is defined as abnormal descent of the bladder. If the bladder is more than 2 cm below the pubococcygeal line (PCL) (PCL is drawn from the inferior margin of the pubic symphysis to the last coccygeal joint on sagittal images), it is considered abnormal descent of the bladder. Vaginal vault prolapse consists of descent and eversion of the vaginal vault, with a loss of the normal H configuration of the vagina.

Clinical History: 32-year-old woman presenting with fever and left lower quadrant pain.

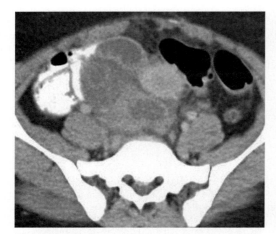

Figure 7.44   A

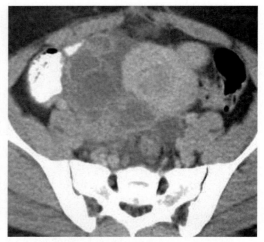

Figure 7.44   B

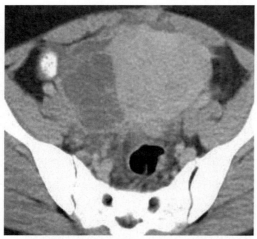

Figure 7.44   C

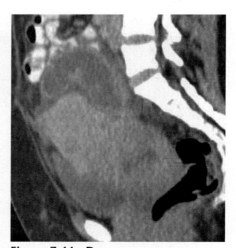

Figure 7.44   D

Findings: Axial CECT (A–C) demonstrate a heterogeneous right adnexal, multiloculated tubular mass with an enhancing thickened wall and surrounding fat stranding. Sagittal reformatted CECT image (D) shows more clearly the tubular configuration of this lesion. Note enlarged uterus due to fibroids.

Differential Diagnosis: Dermoid, ovarian cystadenoma, endometriosis, ovarian torsion, ectopic pregnancy.

Diagnosis: Tubo-ovarian abscess.

Discussion: Tubo-ovarian abscess (TOA) is the most advanced form in the disease continuum of pelvic inflammatory disease (PID). In approximately 1% of women treated for acute salpingitis, the condition progresses to TOA. Patients are usually ill, presenting with pelvic pain, high fever, nausea, and emesis. These systemic symptoms are usually not present in patients with dermoid, ovarian cystadenoma, and endometriosis. However, 15% of patients with TOA are afebrile and have a normal white blood cell count. On clinical and imaging examination, TOA can be difficult to distinguishes from ovarian torsion, diverticular or other pelvic abscess, and appendicitis. Most cases of TOA are treated first with intravenous antibiotics. Surgery or percutaneous drainage may be necessary if the patient's symptoms fail to respond clinically within 72 hours after administration of antibiotics or if abscess rupture is suspected. CT scan may demonstrate a tubular or spherical cystic mass. Thick walls and internal septations or gas bubbles may be present. The inflammation causes stranding of the periadnexal fat and thickening of the peritoneum. The latter is typically also absent in patients with dermoid, ovarian cystadenoma, and endometriosis.

Clinical History: 52-year-old woman with recurrent breast cancer.

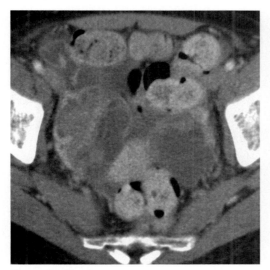

Figure 7.45   A

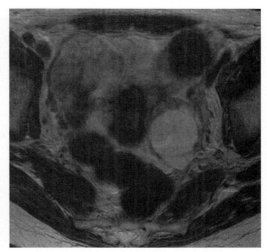

Figure 7.45   B

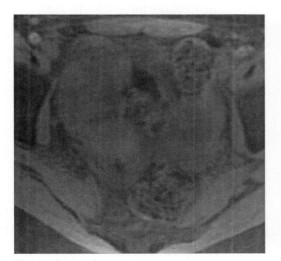

Figure 7.45   C

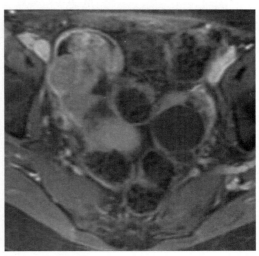

Figure 7.45   D

Findings: Axial CECT (A) image demonstrates bilateral ovarian lesions with solid and cystic components and a small amount of free fluid. Axial T2-WI (B) and unenhanced (C) and gadolinium-enhanced (D) fat-suppressed axial T1-WI confirm the cystic and enhancing solid components of these masses.

Differential Diagnosis: Bilateral primary ovarian tumor, endometriomas, bilateral tubo-ovarian abscesses.

Diagnosis: Krukenberg tumors.

Discussion: Ovarian metastases account for approximately 5% to 10% of all malignant ovarian tumors. Krukenberg tumors are metastatic tumors to the ovaries, which contain, on histopathology, signet ring cells (mucin secreting) that invade the hypercellular ovarian stroma. They typically originate from the GI tract (colon and stomach in 90% of cases), breast, and pancreatic carcinomas. In general, ovarian metastases may result from direct extension, peritoneal seeding, or lymphatic or hematogenous spread. Imaging findings of metastatic ovarian lesions are nonspecific and consist of a mass with predominantly solid components or a mixture of cystic and solid areas, as seen in this case. On T1-WI and T2-WI, however, Krukenberg tumors demonstrate some distinctive findings, including bilateral complex masses with hypointense solid components (dense stromal reaction) and internal hyperintensity (mucin). The distinction between a unilateral Krukenberg tumor and fibrothecoma or poorly differentiated adenocarcinoma of the ovary might be difficult.

Clinical History: 83-year-old woman with a history of renal cell carcinoma presenting with vaginal bleeding.

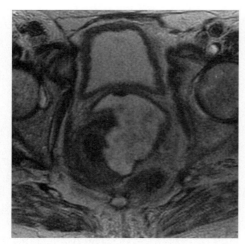

Figure 7.46   A

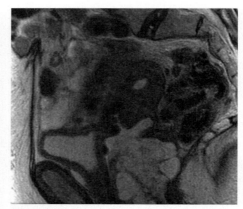

Figure 7.46   B

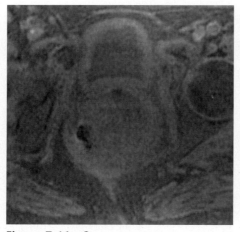

Figure 7.46   C

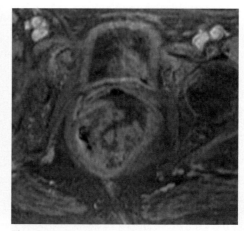

Figure 7.46   D

Findings: Axial (A) and sagittal (B) T2-WI and unenhanced (C) and gadolinium-enhanced (D) fat-suppressed axial T1-WI demonstrate an ill-defined, predominantly T2 hyperintense, heterogeneously enhancing mass in the vagina. Discontinuity of the posterior vaginal wall with rectal invasion is noted.

Differential Diagnosis: Endometrioid adenocarcinoma of rectovaginal septum, metastasis.

Diagnosis: Vaginal cancer.

Discussion: Vulvar and cervical cancers must be excluded before a primary vaginal cancer is diagnosed. Most vaginal malignancies (80–90%) are secondary due to extension of primary tumors (bladder, vulva, cervix, or rectum) or recurrent tumor (treated cervical or ovarian cancers). Primary vaginal cancers, 90% of which are squamous cell carcinoma (human papillomavirus is a risk factor), account only for 1% to 2% of all gynecologic malignancies. Vaginal cancers typically occur in the elderly, presenting with painless vaginal bleeding. They are commonly located in the posterior wall of the proximal third of the vagina. Other primary vaginal tumors, such as adenocarcinoma (due to endometriosis or previous exposure to diethylstilbestrol), malignant melanoma (more frequently affecting the vulva), sarcoma, and paraganglioma, are very rare. MRI is performed to obtain accurate assessment of the local extent of a vaginal tumor and to detect presence of lymph node involvement. Signal characteristics of most tumors are nonspecific on MRI; the majority shows high signal intensity on T2-WI and intermediate signal intensity on T1-WI. In cases of melanoma, the lesion may be hyperintense on T1-WI due to the presence of melanin.

CASE 7-47

Clinical History: 40-year-old woman presenting with chronic left pelvic pain.

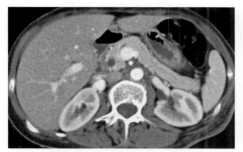

Figure 7.47 A

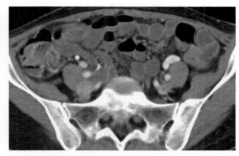

Figure 7.47 B

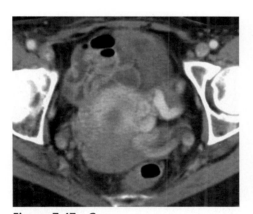

Figure 7.47 C

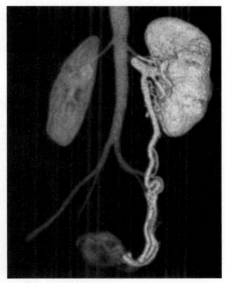

Figure 7.47 D

Findings: Axial CECT (A–C) images show a tortuous tubular opacified vessel coursing anteriorly to the left psoas muscle towards the left pelvis. Three-dimensional, volume-rendered image (D) reveals that this structure extends from the left renal vein to the left adnexal fossa.

Differential Diagnosis: None.

Diagnosis: Pelvic congestion syndrome.

Discussion: Pelvic congestion syndrome is an underdiagnosed common cause of chronic (>6 months) noncyclical pelvic pain, typically aggravated by increase in abdominal pressure in premenopausal women. Other symptoms can be dyspareunia and perineal pain. It accounts for 10% to 40% of all gynecologic visits. The syndrome is closely related to the presence of ovarian varices, which occur in 10% of women. Within this group, up to 60% of women may develop pelvic congestion syndrome. Ovarian varices may result from an obstructing anatomic anomaly, such as retroaortic left renal vein, ovarian vein congestion secondary to compression of the left renal vein by the superior mesenteric artery (nutcracker phenomena), or right common iliac vein compression. Other etiologies include valvular incompetence of the gonadal veins and portal hypertension with splenorenal shunting. Ovarian vein embolization relieves symptoms in 70% to 75% of cases. On imaging, the diagnosis of pelvic congestion syndrome can be contemplated if no other etiology of the pelvic varices is found. A combination of two features must be present: first, a dilatated gonadal vein with a diameter greater than 8 mm; and second, retrograde filling of the veins. The latter can easily be shown during the arterial phase of a CECT, at which time contrast material should be present only in the arterial system and renal veins, but not yet in the ovarian veins. If contrast is present in the gonadal veins, it indicates retrograde venous flow due to valvular incompetence.

Clinical History: 58-year-old man with a history of human immunodeficiency virus (HIV) infection presenting with urinary frequency and discomfort in the perineal area.

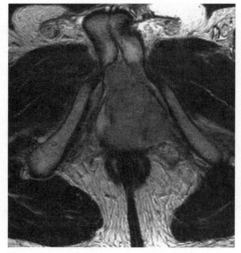

Figure 7.48   A

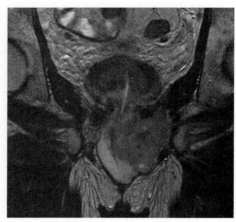

Figure 7.48   B

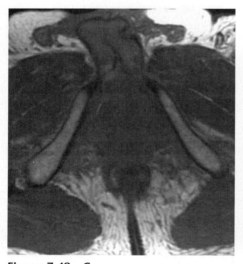

Figure 7.48   C

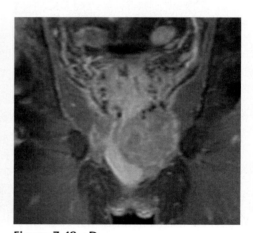

Figure 7.48   D

Findings: Axial (A) and coronal (B) T2-WI, axial T1-WI (C), and gadolinium-enhanced, fat-suppressed coronal T1-WI (D) demonstrate a heterogeneous T2 hyperintense and T1 isointense soft tissue mass posterior to the bulbar urethra at the level of the urogenital diaphragm, which it abuts. The mass shows heterogeneous and marked enhancement.

Differential Diagnosis: Kaposi sarcoma, lymphoma (non-Hodgkin lymphoma, Burkitt lymphoma), leiomyosarcoma, hemangiopericytoma.

Diagnosis: Rhabdomyosarcoma (pleomorphic).

Discussion: HIV infection diminishes the body's defense mechanisms by impairing the T-lymphocyte response, which predisposes the patient to a wide variety of immune-related neoplasms (e.g., lymphoma, Kaposi sarcoma) and infections. Rhabdomyosarcoma is an extremely aggressive,

chemosensitive tumor of mesenchymal origin, which arises from striated skeletal muscle cells. Rhabdomyosarcoma is rare in adults; it occurs primarily in childhood and adolescence (median age, 5 years) and account for approximately 10% of all childhood solid tumors. Histologic patterns include embryonal (~80%), alveolar (~20%), and pleomorphic. The alveolar subtype is associated with a significantly worse prognosis, with a 5-year survival rate of less than 30%. Patient age over 10 years is also an unfavorable prognostic factor, especially in combination with a tumor larger than 5 cm in size. Metastases occur via blood and lymphatic vessels (in 26–71% of the patients) and affect most commonly the lungs and bones. Because a definitive diagnosis cannot be made between benign and malignant soft tissue tumors on MRI, percutaneous biopsy is often required.

Clinical History: 21-year-old woman presenting with a spontaneous abortion and a uterine anomaly on hysteroscopy.

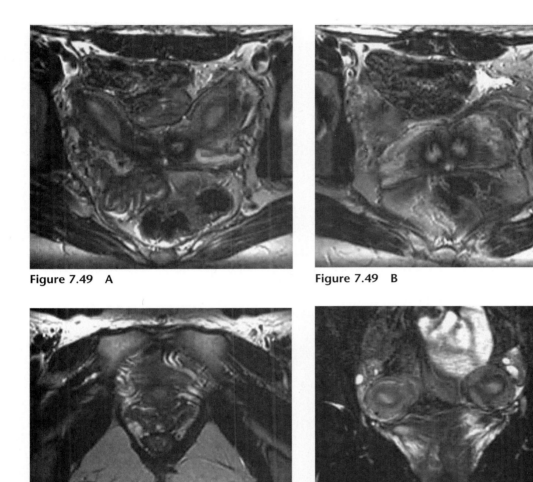

Figure 7.49   A

Figure 7.49   B

Figure 7.49   C

Figure 7.49   D

Findings: Axial T2-WI (A–C) demonstrate two widely diverging, normal-sized uterine horns with normal zonal anatomy, two cervices, and two vaginas. Fat-suppressed coronal T2-WI (D) demonstrates the two widely separated uterine horns.

Differential Diagnosis: Bicornuate uterus.

Diagnosis: Uterus didelphys.

Discussion: Uterus didelphys is defined as complete lack of fusion of the Müllerian ducts, resulting in two normal-sized separate uteri, double cervices, and double upper vaginas. The widely bifurcated uterine horns are separated by a deep fundal cleft. The fundal cleft is deeper than 1 cm, and the intercornual angle, defined by the medial margin of the endometrial hemicavities, is usually greater than 105 degrees. The intercornual distance is usually more than 4 cm. A transverse vaginal septum (distinguished by its location in the upper two thirds from an imperforated hymen, in which the obstruction is located at the introitus) is present in 75% and is often associated with hematocolpos. Only vaginal drainage and vaginoplasty is required in these patients because uterus didelphys has no significantly higher risk of spontaneous abortion. A bicornuate uterus can present with a deep fundal cleft and large intercornual distance, but there is fusion of the vaginas.

Case images courtesy of Dr. Giovanni Artho, McGill University Health Center, Montreal, Canada.

Clinical History: 62-year-old man presenting with a painless right inguinal mass.

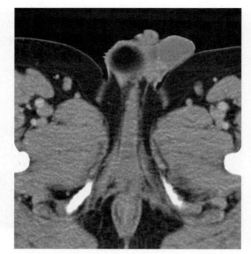

Figure 7.50   A

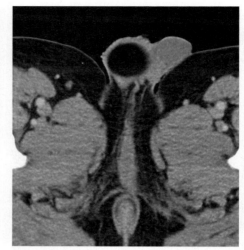

Figure 7.50   B

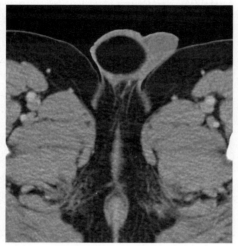

Figure 7.50   C

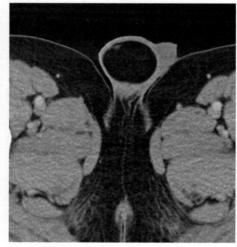

Figure 7.50   D

Findings: Axial CECT images demonstrate a 2.5 × 3.4 cm fatty mass along the right spermatic cord and extending into the scrotum.

Differential Diagnosis: Fat-containing inguinal hernia, liposarcoma.

Diagnosis: Spermatic cord lipoma.

Discussion: Seventy percent of all paratesticular lesions are located in the spermatic cord. Lipoma is the most common benign paratesticular neoplasm (45% of all paratesticular masses) and the most common tumor of the spermatic cord. The tumor is usually an incidentally discovered painless scrotal fatty mass; it affects males of all ages. Spermatic cord lipomas can vary in shape but are most commonly well demarcated by a thin, enhancing capsule. Occasionally admixtures of other mesenchymal elements that are intrinsic to the tumor occur, most commonly fibrous connective tissue; these are classified as fibrolipomas. Transformation into a liposarcoma is very rare. On imaging, lipomas are entirely fatty. However, thin soft tissue strands may be present in the mass. In contrast, liposarcomas have thick soft tissue strands or nodules interspersed with fatty elements. In case of a fat-containing inguinal hernia, continuity of the herniated fat with the intra-abdominal fat should allow differentiation from a lipoma. Treatment of a spermatic cord lipoma is determined by the symptoms of the patient and consists of excision.

Clinical History: 76-year-old woman presenting with epigastric pain.

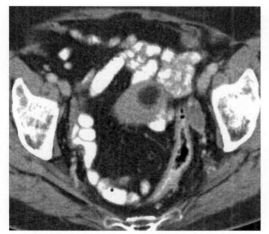

Figure 7.51 **A**

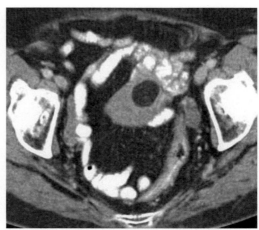

Figure 7.51 **B**

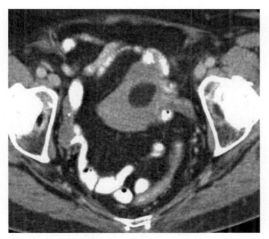

Figure 7.51 **C**

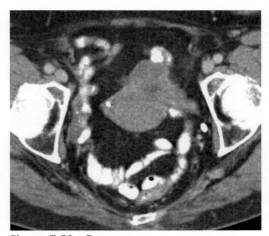

Figure 7.51 **D**

Findings: Axial CECT images demonstrate a well-delineated, nonenhancing, fat-containing (−75 Hounsfield units [HU]) mass within the uterine fundus. The uterus and ovaries are otherwise unremarkable.

Differential Diagnosis: Lipoleiomyoma, fibromyxolipoma, degenerated fibroid.

Diagnosis: Uterine lipoma.

Discussion: Lipomatous tumors of the uterus are rare. They are typically benign and are found in postmenopausal women between 50 and 70 years of age. They usually occur in the uterine body, predominantly intramurally, and are associated with leiomyomas. The symptoms are similar to those caused by leiomyomas of the same size, such as the presence of a palpable mass, hypermenorrhea, and pelvic pressure. They are generally classified as pure or mixed lipomas. The mixed lipomas (lipoleiomyoma and fibromyxolipoma) contain variable amounts of fat, fibrous tissue, and smooth muscle. A pure lipoma, as in this case, is composed of encapsulated adipose tissue interspersed by thin septa of fibrous tissue and thus shows no enhancement on imaging examinations. Muscle cells are rare and confined to the periphery of the tumor. Fatty metaplasia of the connective tissue or smooth muscle cells seems to be the cause for the development of the lipoma because lipoid tissue is not normally present in the uterus. Fatty degeneration of a uterine fibroid is also in the differential diagnosis, but generally, the fat component only constitutes a minor portion of the fibroid.

Clinical History: 39-year-old woman presenting with chronic pelvic pain.

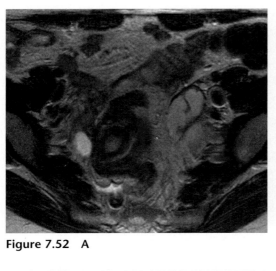

Figure 7.52   A

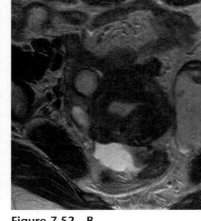

Figure 7.52   B

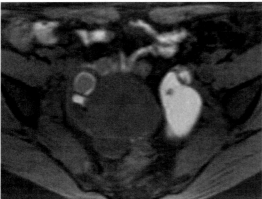

Figure 7.52   C

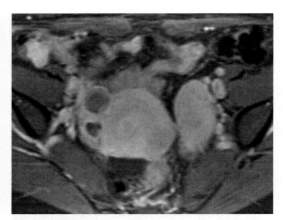

Figure 7.52   D

Findings: Axial T2-WI (A and B) and unenhanced (C) and gadolinium-enhanced (D) fat-suppressed axial T1-WI demonstrate several T1 and T2 hyperintense foci in the right ovary, which show smooth wall enhancement. The largest one has a peripheral T1 hyperintense and T2 hypointense rim. An S-shaped tubular nonenhancing structure, which is bright on T1-WI and T2-WI, is present in the left adnexal region. Note a small amount of pelvic free fluid.

Differential Diagnosis: Hydrosalpinx/pyosalpinx, ovarian (functional) cyst, serous ovarian cystadenoma, pelvic hematoma/lymphocele.

Diagnosis: Endometriosis (endometriomas and hematosalpinx).

Discussion: Hydrosalpinx is defined by a dilated fluid-filled fallopian tube due to tubal occlusion, which can be caused by peritubal inflammation, endometriosis, or salpingitis. On imaging, hydrosalpinx typically appears as a fluid-filled tubular adnexal structure, folded upon itself to form a C or S shape. The key feature to differentiate a dilated fallopian tube from other adnexal structures is the presence of incomplete septations (plicae). They result from effacement of the mucosa and submucosa from dilatation of the tube or blunting of the mucosal folds. They may become flattened or absent in severe cases of tubal dilatation. In one plane, these folds may appear nodular, but they may appear as a ridge in an orthogonal plane. The wall shows enhancement on gadolinium-enhanced T1-WI. In cases of hematosalpinx, typically due to endometriosis, the tube becomes filled with blood products. The signal intensity of the tubal fluid is then similar to an endometrioma (high on T1-WI and low on T2-WI). In this case, the presence of blood-containing right ovarian cysts and left hematosalpinx make endometriosis the best diagnosis. In acute salpingitis, wall thickening with a double-layered appearance of the tubal wall may be present.

CASE 7-53

Clinical History: 73-year-old woman presenting with vaginal bleeding.

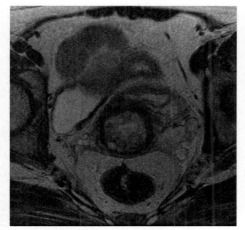

Figure 7.53 A

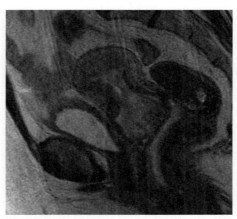

Figure 7.53 B

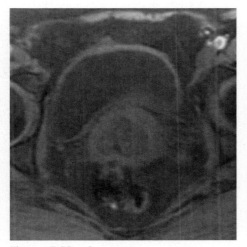

Figure 7.53 C

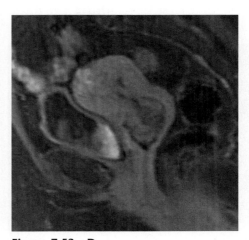

Figure 7.53 D

Findings: Axial (A) and sagittal (B) T2-WI and fat-suppressed axial T1-WI (C) demonstrate a heterogeneous pedunculated mass originating from the uterine fundus. The mass distends the endocervical canal and protrudes into the upper vagina. Gadolinium-enhanced, fat-suppressed sagittal T1-WI (D) shows heterogeneous enhancement of the mass.

Differential Diagnosis: Submucosal leiomyoma, endometrial carcinoma.

Diagnosis: Endometrial polyp.

Discussion: Endometrial polyps are focal outgrowths of hyperplasic endometrium. They have a prevalence of 10% in women and are multiple in 20% of affected women. A minority of women are symptomatic and present with bleeding, mucous discharge, menorrhagia/metrorrhagia, or infertility. Less than 1% of polyps are malignant, and 12% to 34% of women with endometrial cancer present with associated polyps. Tamoxifen treatment or prophylaxis increases the risk of development of endometrial polyps. Treatment consists of hysteroscopic resection. The MRI appearance of polyps is variable based on the three types of polyps: hyperplastic (resembling glands of endometrial hyperplasia), atrophic (cystically dilated atrophic glands), and functional (cyclical endometrial changes). They occur commonly in the fundus and cornua and may be sessile or pedunculated. On T1-WI, polyps are isointense to endometrium. On T2-WI, they usually are slightly hypointense to the adjacent normal endometrium. A low–signal intensity fibrous stalk may be present. After contrast administration, polyps enhance typically less than normal endometrium but more than normal myometrium. Submucosal leiomyomas are myometrial in origin and show, in the majority of cases, lower signal intensity than polyps.

Clinical History: 37-year-old woman presenting with infertility.

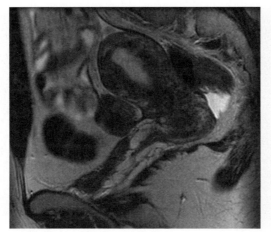

Figure 7.54 A

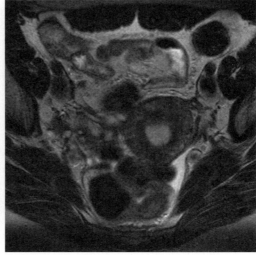

Figure 7.54 B

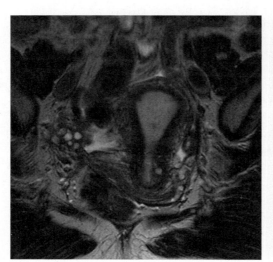

Figure 7.54 C

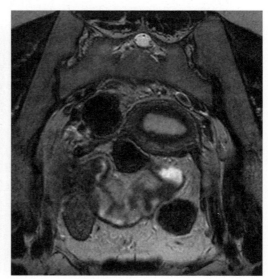

Figure 7.54 D

Findings: Sagittal T2-WI (A) reveals a low–signal intensity myometrial bulge (1.1 × 0.8 cm) with thickening of the junctional zone in the anterior myometrium of the uterine body. This bulge is not detectable on the axial (B), long axis oblique (C), and short axis oblique along the uterine body (D) T2-WI.

Differential Diagnosis: Adenomyosis, leiomyoma.

Diagnosis: Uterine contraction.

Discussion: The uterus, especially in nonpregnant females, has ceaseless movement called uterine peristalsis, which is supposed to help sperm transportation, fertilization, and implantation. This uterine peristalsis consists of transient myometrial contractions with a frequency ranging from 2.1 to 5.8 per minute. Their direction is predominantly cervico-fundal in the midcycle and fundocervical during the menstrual phase. As a radiologist, one should be aware of these transient low–signal intensity myometrial bulgings that represent physiologic uterine contractions. Because a uterine contraction is a transient phenomenon, it should change or disappear with time. This feature is key to differentiate a contraction from a true uterine anomaly, such as adenomyosis or leiomyoma, which should be persistent on all images. If the transient feature is still unclear, a repeat MRI examination at a later time can be performed.

Clinical History: 23-year-old woman presenting with abdominal pain and bloating.

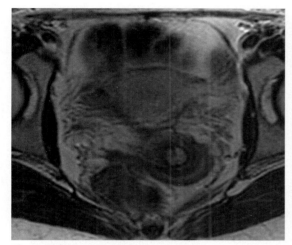

Figure 7.55   A

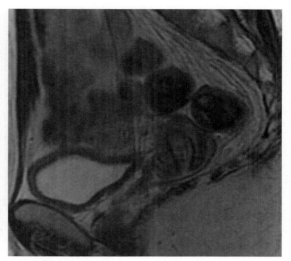

Figure 7.55   B

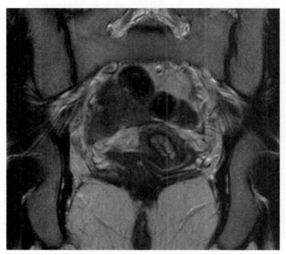

Figure 7.55   C

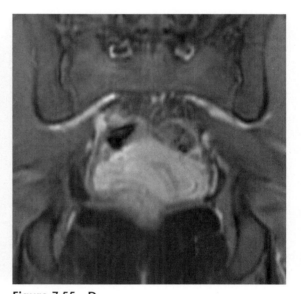

Figure 7.55   D

Findings: Axial (A), sagittal (B), and coronal (C) T2-WI and gadolinium-enhanced, fat-suppressed coronal T1-WI (D) demonstrate thin, hypointense, enhancing linear structures within the T2 hyperintense endocervix.

Differential Diagnosis: None.

Diagnosis: Plicae palmatae.

Discussion: Plicae palmatae or normal cervical folds can often be identified, especially on T2-WI, as serrated, intermediate–signal intensity, linear structures outlining the high–signal intensity glandular fluid and mucus, as seen in this case. In the axial plane, the cervix appears as a discrete round structure with three layers visible on T2-WI. The outer layer has intermediate signal intensity and represents smooth muscle, which is continuous with the myometrium. The next inner ring (normal thickness, 3–8 mm) of low signal intensity represents the dense fibrous stroma of the cervical canal and is continuous with the uterine junctional zone. The T2 hyperintense innermost ring represents the endocervix (normal thickness, 2–3 mm), containing glandular fluid, mucus, and plicae palmatae.

Clinical History: 72-year-old woman with known breast cancer presenting with vaginal spotting.

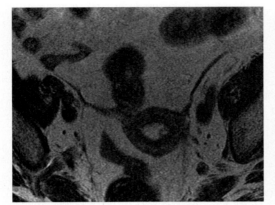

Figure 7.56   A

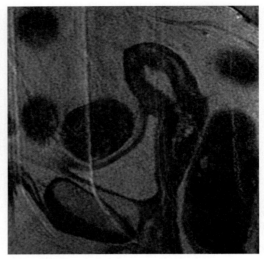

Figure 7.56   B

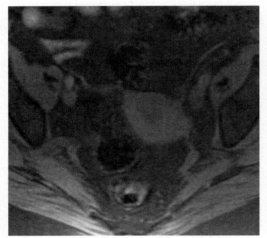

Figure 7.56   C

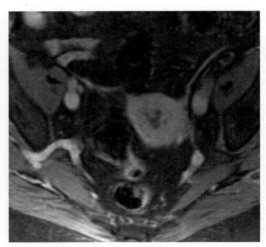

Figure 7.56   D

Findings: Axial (A) and sagittal (B) T2-WI demonstrate thickening of the endometrial stripe up to 1 cm. Axial unenhanced (C) and gadolinium-enhanced, fat-suppressed (D) T1-WI show enhancement of several septations within the endometrium. Note associated Nabothian cysts in the cervix.

Differential Diagnosis: Endometrial hyperplasia, polyps, endometrial carcinoma, subendometrial cysts.

Diagnosis: Tamoxifen-induced uterine changes.

Discussion: Tamoxifen is a synthetic estrogen antagonist used in treatment of breast cancer. Although it is an estrogen antagonist in breast tissue, it is a weak estrogen agonist in the postmenopausal uterus. Reported associated endometrial abnormalities include hyperplasia, polyps, cancer, and subendometrial cysts. Adenomyosis, leiomyomas, and intraperitoneal fluid may also be associated. The risk ratio of endometrial cancer is increased 2.2-fold when tamoxifen is given at a dose of 20 mg/d, and it increases to 6.4-fold with a dose of 40 mg/d. Nevertheless, the incidence of endometrial cancer in patients treated with tamoxifen is less than 1%. Two distinct MRI patterns are described in patients treated with tamoxifen. In patients with atrophy or proliferative changes at histopathology, the endometrium is homogeneous and hyperintense on T2-WI. After contrast administration, the endometrial–myometrial interface enhances with persistent areas of signal void. In patients with polyps, the endometrium is heterogeneous on T2-WI. There are lattice-like enhancing septations traversing the endometrial cavity.

Clinical History: 23-year-old woman presenting with acute bilateral leg weakness, weight loss, and fever.

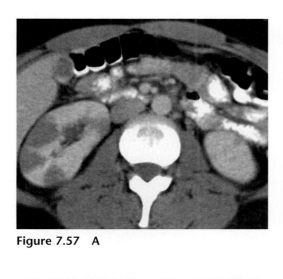

Figure 7.57   A

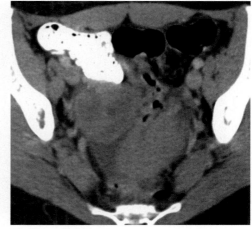

Figure 7.57   B

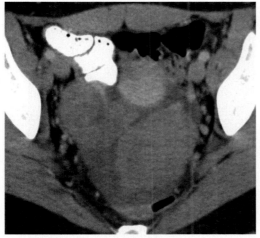

Figure 7.57   C

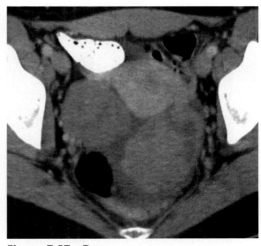

Figure 7.57   D

Findings: Axial CECT images demonstrate bilateral, multiple, minimally enhancing renal parenchymal lesions, bilateral predominantly solid enlarged ovaries, and ascites.

Differential Diagnosis: Primary ovarian sarcoma, metastatic ovarian carcinoma.

Diagnosis: Burkitt lymphoma of the ovaries.

Discussion: Only 1% of patients with malignant lymphoma present initially with ovarian enlargement; they account for 1.5% of all ovarian neoplasms. Burkitt lymphomas (BLs) are separated into three main categories, and all have similar clinical presentation, epidemiologic features, and biologic behavior: endemic (African), sporadic (nonendemic), and immunodeficiency-associated BL. BLs (composed of small noncleaved lymphoblastic cells with a typical starry sky pattern on histology) compose approximately 20% of acquired immunodeficiency syndrome (AIDS)-related non-Hodgkin lymphomas. They affect mainly children (a median age of 12 for nonendemic cases) and have a male predominance. The majority of nonendemic cases present with abdominal disease and involvement of the ileum, cecum, mesentery, kidney, liver, and ovary. Immunodeficiency-associated BLs are often nodal. Epstein-Barr virus association is reported in nonendemic BL. BL tends to metastasize to the central nervous system. Patients with disseminated disease have a cure rate that drops from 90% to 30%. Definite diagnosis should be based on clinical information (B-symptoms), histologic features, and immunohistochemical profiles. The presence of multiple minimally enhancing soft tissue abdominal lesions and B-symptoms, as in this case, suggests the diagnosis of lymphoma.

Clinical History: 51-year-old man presenting with elevated PSA.

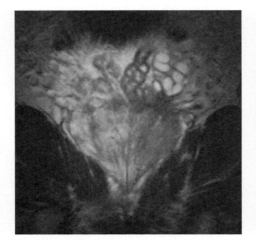

Figure 7.58   A

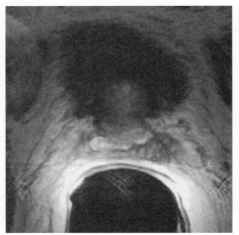

Figure 7.58   B

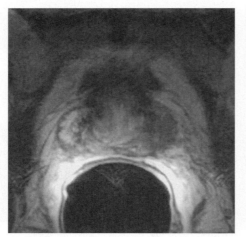

Figure 7.58   C

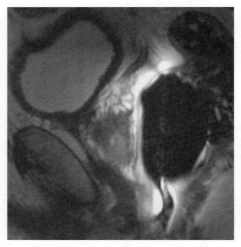

Figure 7.58   D

Findings: Coronal (A), axial (B and C), and sagittal (D) T2-WI reveal an abnormal hypointense area in the left peripheral zone of the prostate, extending from the base to the apex. The signal abnormality extends as speculations into the periprostatic fat in the left mid gland and extends into the left seminal vesicle and vas deferens.

Differential Diagnosis: Hyperplasia, prostatitis, infarction, scar.

Diagnosis: Prostate cancer invading the seminal vesicle and neurovascular bundle.

Discussion: On endorectal MRI, unequivocal extension of prostate cancer into the retroprostatic fat and neurovascular bundle, representing gross extraglandular spread, and seminal vesicle invasion correlate with a poor outcome. The serum PSA level, histologic grade of the tumor (Gleason grade, from [1] well to [5] poorly differentiated adenoca), and proportion/percentage of tissue of the biopsy involved by cancer (≥3 in sextant biopsy) may be helpful in predicting the likelihood of extraprostatic spread and outcome after radical prostatectomy. Seventy-five percent of patients with a PSA level less than 4 ng/mL have prostate-confined cancer. However, only 50% of patients with a PSA level between 4 and 10 ng/mL have prostate-confined cancer. With a PSA level that exceeds 30 ng/mL, only 2% of patients have prostate-confined disease. A Gleason score (obtained by adding the two predominant grades) of 7 or more also indicates a high probability of extraglandular spread.

CASE 7-59

Clinical History: 24-year-old woman presenting with third-trimester vaginal bleeding.

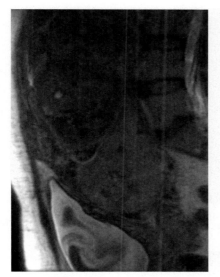

Figure 7.59   A

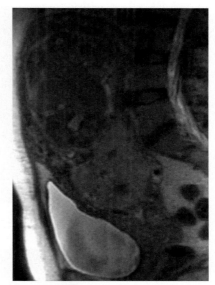

Figure 7.59   B

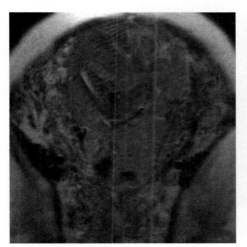

Figure 7.59   C

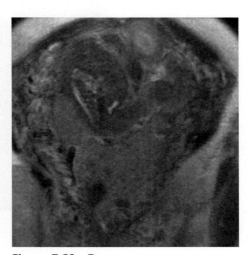

Figure 7.59   D

Findings: Sagittal (A and B), axial (C), and coronal (D) T2-WI demonstrate an inferior position of the placenta covering the internal cervical os.

Differential Diagnosis: None.

Diagnosis: Placenta previa.

Discussion: Placenta previa is defined as a portion, or all, of the placenta covering the internal cervical os, thus precluding vaginal delivery; it occurs in 0.5% of all pregnancies. Risk factors are prior cesarean section, spontaneous or induced abortion, advanced maternal age, multiparity, and cigarette smoking. Placenta accreta, whereby the placental villi invade the myometrium, occurs in 5% of patients with placenta previa and may lead to fetal and maternal life-threatening hemorrhage. Most cases of placenta previa diagnosed in the second trimester will not persist at term. It appears that the uterus, especially the lower segment, elongates with advancing gestation, and thus the placenta is carried away from the internal os. Finding a placenta less than 2 cm from the internal os in the third trimester places the patient at risk for bleeding and requires delivery by cesarean section. Transvaginal ultrasound is the first imaging modality to be performed to evaluate the position of the placenta, but in cases where the diagnosis is unclear, MRI can be a useful adjunct.

Clinical History: 29-year-old woman presenting with recurrent spontaneous abortion.

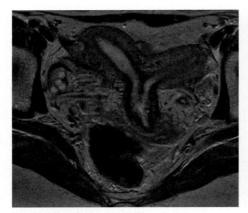

Figure 7.60   A

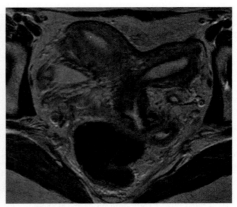

Figure 7.60   B

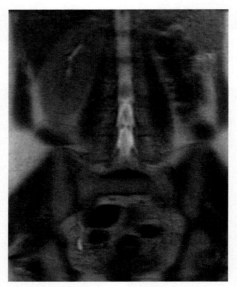

Figure 7.60   C

Findings: Axial T2-WI (A and B) demonstrate two uterine horns symmetrical in size with preserved normal zonal anatomy. The fundal contour is concave (1.6-cm fundal cleft). Only one cervix is seen. Coronal T2-WI (C) reveals absence of left kidney.

Differential Diagnosis: Septate uterus, uterus didelphys.

Diagnosis: Bicornuate unicollis uterus.

Discussion: Bicornuate uterus results from incomplete fusion of Müllerian ducts. It accounts for approximately 10% of Müllerian duct anomalies. The two diverging horns are symmetrical in size. The tissue dividing the two cornua is composed of myometrium. This intervening cleft may extend to the internal cervical os (complete bicornuate uterus) or not reach the cervix and be of variable length ("incomplete" bicornuate uterus). The cervix may be solitary (bicornuate unicollis) or duplicated (bicornuate bicollis). In 25% of cases, a vertical vaginal septum is present. Imaging features of bicornuate uterus are two horns symmetrical in size, preserved normal zonal anatomy in each horn, intercornual distance of 4 cm or more, intercornual angle of more than 105 degrees, and an intervening fundal cleft greater than 1.0 cm in depth; these are important features to differentiate bicornuate uterus from a septate uterus. The bright signal intensity of the endometrium on T2-WI is important to evaluate the communication between the two cavities at the caudal margins. This case exemplifies the known high incidence of coexisting urinary tract anomalies, such as agenesis of the left kidney in this case, in patients with bicornuate uterus.

SUGGESTED READINGS

NEOPLASMS

- Akbar SA, Sayyed TA, Jafri SZH, et al. Multimodality imaging of paratesticular neoplasms and their rare mimics. *Radiographics* 2003;23:1461–1476.

- Ascher SM, Jha RC, Reinhold C. Benign myometrial conditions: leiomyomas and adenomyosis. *Top Magn Reson Imaging.* 2003;14:281–304.

- Baeyens K, Fennessy F, Bleday R, et al. CT features of a tubal lipoma associated with an ipsilateral dermoid cyst. *Eur Radiol.* 2004;14:1720–1722.

- Baloglu H, Turken O, Levent T, et al. 24-year-old female with amenorrhea: bilateral primary ovarian Burkitt lymphoma. *Gynecol Oncol.* 2003;91:449–451.

- Bostwick DG, Grignon DJ, Hammond EL, et al. Prognostic factors in prostate cancer. *Arc Pathol Lab Med.* 2000;124:995–1000.

- Bozaci EA, Atabekoglu C, Sertçelik A, et al. Metachronous metastases from renal cell carcinoma to uterine cervix and vagina: case report and review of literature. *Gynecol Oncol.* 2005;99:232–235.

- Cantisani V, Mortele KJ, Kalantari BN, et al. Vaginal metastasis from uterine leiomyosarcoma: magnetic resonance imaging features with pathological correlation. *J Comput Assist Tomogr.* 2003;27:805–809.

- Cornud F, Hamida K, Flam T, et al. Endorectal color Doppler sonography and endorectal MR imaging features of nonpalpable prostate cancer. *Am J Roentgenol.* 2000;175:1161–1168.

- Coumbaras M, Validire P, Strauss C, et al. Uterine lipoma: MRI features with pathologic correlation. *Abdom Imaging.* 2005;30:239–241.

- Covens A, Rosen B, Murphy J, et al. Changes in the demographics and perioperative care of stage IA-B cervical cancer over the past 16 years. *Gynecol Oncol.* 2001;81:133–137.

- Creasman WT. Vaginal cancers. *Current Opin Obstet Gynecol.* 2005;17:71–76.

- D'Amico AV, Whittington R, Malkowicz SB, et al. Clinical utility of the percentage of positive prostate biopsies in defining biochemical outcome after radical prostatectomy for patients with clinically localized prostate cancer. *J Clin Oncol.* 2000;18:1164–1172.

- Daya D, Young RH. Florid deep glands of the uterine cervix: another mimic of adenoma malignum. *Am J Clin Pathol.* 1995;103:614–617.

- DeSimone CP, Lele SM, Modesitt SC. Malignant struma ovarii: a case report and analysis of cases reported in the literature with focus on survival and I[131] therapy. *Gynecol Oncol.* 2003;89:543–548.

- Freedland SJ, Aronson WJ, Csathy GS, et al. Comparison of percentage of total prostate needle biopsy tissue with cancer to percentage of cores with cancer for predicting PSA recurrence after radical prostatectomy: results from the SEARCH database. *Urology* 2003;61:742–747.

- Grasel RP, Outwater EK, Siegelman ES, et al. Endometrial polyps: MR imaging features and distinction from endometrial carcinoma. *Radiology* 2000;214:47–52.

- Ha HK, Baek SY, Kim SH, et al. Krukenberg's tumor of the ovary: MR imaging features. *Am J Roentgenol.* 1995;164:1435–1439.

- Jung SE, Lee JM, Rha SE, et al. CT and MR imaging of ovarian tumors with emphasis on differential diagnosis. *Radiographics* 2002;22:1305–1325.

- Kattan MW, Eastham JA, Stapleton AMF, et al. A preoperative nomogram for disease recurrence following radical prostatectomy for prostate cancer. *J Nal Cancer Inst.* 1998;10:766–771.

- Lau LU, Thoeni RF. Uterine lipoma: advantage of MRI over ultrasound. *Br J Radiol.* 2005;78:72–74.

- Li H, Sugimura K, Okizuka H, et al. Markedly high-signal intensity lesions in the uterine cervix on T2-weighted imaging: differentiation between mucin-producing carcinomas and Nabothian cysts. *Radiat Med.* 1999;17:137–143.

- Lilly MC, Arregui ME. Lipomas of the cord and round ligament. *Ann Surg.* 2002;4:586–590.

- Makani S, Kim W, Gaba AR. Struma ovarii with a focus of papillary thyroid cancer: a case report and review of the literature. *Gynecol Oncol.* 2004;94:835–839.

- Manfredi R, Mirk P, Maresca G, et al. Local-regional staging of endometrial carcinoma: role of MR imaging in surgical planning. *Radiology* 2004;231:372–378.

- Mayr NA, Yuh WT, Zheng J, et al. Prediction of tumor control in patients with cervical cancer: analysis of combined volume and dynamic enhancement pattern by MR imaging. *Am J Roentgenol.* 1998;170:177–182.

- Mercer SE, Ewton DZ, Shah S, et al. Mirk/Dyrk1b mediates cell survival in rhabdomyosarcomas. *Cancer Res.* 2006;66:5143–5150.

- Mittl RL, Yeh I, Kressel HY. High-signal-intensity rim surrounding uterine leiomyomas on MR imaging: pathologic correlation. *Radiology* 1991;180:81–83.

- Murase E, Siegelman ES, Outwater EK, et al. Uterine leiomyomas: histopathologic features, MR imaging findings, differential diagnosis, and treatment. *Radiographics* 1999;19:1179–1197.

- Neary B, Young SB, Reuter KL, et al. Ovarian Burkitt lymphoma: pelvic pain in woman with AIDS. *Obstet Gynecol.* 1996;88:706–708.

- Outwater EK, Wagner BJ, Mannion C, et al. Sex cord stromal and steroid cell tumors of the ovary. *Radiographics* 1998;18:1523–1546.

- Parazzini F, Vecchia CL, Negri E, et al. Risk factors for uterine fibroids: reduced risk associated with oral contraceptives. *Br Med J.* 1988;72:853–857.

- Pellerito JS, McCarthy SM, Doyle MB, et al. Diagnosis of uterine anomalies: Relative accuracy of MR imaging, endovaginal ultrasound, and hysterosalpingography. *Radiology* 1992;183:795–800.

- Perlman S, Ben-Arie A, Feldberg E, et al. Non-Hodgkin's lymphoma presenting as advanced ovarian cancer—a case report and review of literature. *Int J Gynecol Cancer.* 2005;15:554–557.

- Propst AM, Hill JA. Anatomic factors associated with recurrent pregnancy loss. *Semin Reprod Med.* 2000;18:341–350.

- Rha SE, Byun JY, Jung SE, et al. Atypical CT and MRI manifestations of mature ovarian cystic teratomas. *Am J Roentgenol.* 2004;183:743–750.

- Shadbolt CL, Coakley FV, Qayym A, et al. MRI of vaginal leiomyomas. *J Comput Assist Tomogr.* 2001;25:355–357.

- Singh AK, Saokar A, Hahn PF, et al. Imaging of penile neoplasms. *Radiographics* 2005;25:1629–1638.

- Stevens SK, Hricak H, Campos Z. Teratomas versus cystic hemorrhagic adnexal lesions: differentiation with proton-selective fat-saturation MR imaging. *Radiology* 1993;186:481–488.

- Stevens SK, Hricak H, Stern JL. Ovarian lesions: detection and characterization with gadolinium-enhanced MR imaging at 1.5T. *Radiology* 1991;181:481–488.

- Stewart ST, McCarthy SM. Case 77: aggressive angiomyxoma. *Radiology* 2004;233:697–700.

- Szklaruk J, Tamm EP, Choi H, et al. MR imaging of common and uncommon large pelvic masses. *Radiographics* 2003;23:403–424.

- Troiano RN, Lazzarini KM, Scoutt LM, et al. Fibroma and fibrothecoma of the ovary: MR findings. *Radiology* 1997;204:795–798.

- Ueda H, Togashi K, Ikuo K et al. Unusual appearances of uterine leiomyomas: MR imaging findings and their histopathologic backgrounds. *Radiographics* 1999;19:S131–S145.

- Yamashita Y, Torashima M, Takahashi M. Hyperintense uterine leiomyoma at T2-weighted MR imaging: differentiation with dynamic enhanced MR imaging and clinical implications. *Radiology* 1993;189:721–725.

CONGENITAL

- Candiani GB, Federle L, Zamberletti D, et al. Endometrial patterns in malformed uteri. *Acta Europ Fertil.* 1983;14:311–318.

- Carrington BM, Hricak H, Nuruddin RN, et al. Mullerian duct anomalies: MR imaging evaluation. *Radiology* 1990;176:715–720.

- Fedele L, Bianchi S, Marchini M, et al. Residual uterine septum less than 1 cm after hysteroscopic metroplasty does not impair reproductive outcome. *Hum Reprod.* 1996;11:727–729.

- Fedele L, Dorta M, Brioschi D, et al. Magnetic resonance evaluation of double uteri. *Obstet Gynecol.* 1989;74:844–847.

- Homer HA, Li TC, Cooke ID. The septate uterus: a review of management and reproductive outcome. *Fertil Steril.* 2000;73:1–14.
- Kupesic S, Kurjak A. Septate uterus: detection and prediction of obstetrical complications by different forms of ultrasonography. *J Ultrasound Med.* 1998;17:631–636.
- Raziel A, Arieli S, Bukovsky I, et al. Investigation of the uterine cavity in recurrent aborters. *Fertil Steril.* 1994;62:1080–1082.

MISCELLANEOUS

- Ananth CV, Smulian JC, Vintzileos AM. The association of placenta previa with history of cesarean delivery and abortion: a metaanalysis. *Am J Obstet Gynecol.* 1997;177:1071–1078.
- Bohyun K, Hricak H, Tanagho EA. Diagnosis of urethral diverticula in women: value of MR imaging. *Am J Roentgenol.* 1993;161:809–815.
- Dannecker C, Lienemann A, Fischer T, et al. Influence of spontaneous and instrumental vaginal delivery on objective measures of pelvic organ support: assessment with the pelvic organ prolapse quantification (POPQ) technique and functional cine magnetic resonance imaging. *Eur J Obstet Gyn Rep Biol.* 2004;104:32–38.
- Finberg HJ, Williams JW. Placenta accreta: prospective sonographic diagnosis in patients with placenta previa and prior cesarean section. *J Ultrasound Med.* 1992;11:333–343.
- Hann LE, Giess CS, Bach AM, et al. Endometrial thickness in tamoxifen-treated patients: correlation with clinical and pathologic findings. *Am J Roentgenol.* 1997;168:657–661.
- Hricak H, Alpers C, Crooks LE, et al. Magnetic resonance of the female pelvis: initial experience. *Am J Roentgenol.* 1983;141:1119–1128.
- Kido A, Nishiura M, Togashi K, et al. A semiautomated technique for evaluation of uterine peristalsis. *J Magn Reson Imaging.* 2005;21:249–257.
- Kido A, Togashi A, Nakai A, et al. Oral contraceptives and uterine peristalsis: evaluation with MRI. *J Magn Reson Imaging.* 2005;22:265–270.
- Kido A, Togashi K, Koyama T, et al. Diffusely enlarged uterus: evaluation with MRI. *Radiographics* 2003;23:1423–1439.
- Kido A, Togashi K, Koyama T, et al. Retained products of conception masquerading as acquired arteriovenous malformation. *J Comput Assist Tomogr.* 2003;27:88–92.
- Kuligowska E, Deeds L III, Lu K III. Pelvic pain: overlooked and under-diagnosed gynecologic conditions. *Radiographics* 2005;25:3–20.
- Lauria MR, Smith RS, Treadwell MC, et al. The use of second-trimester transvaginal sonography to predict placenta previa. *Ultrasound Obstet Gynecol.* 1996;8:337–340.
- Levine D, Hulka CA, Ludmir J, et al. Placenta accreta: evaluation with color Doppler, power Doppler and fast MR imaging. *Radiology* 1997;205:773–776.
- Lopez C, Balogun M, Ganesan R, et al. MRI of vaginal conditions: pictorial review. *Clin Radiol.* 2005;60:648–662.
- Mitchell DG. Chemical shift magnetic resonance imaging: applications in the abdomen and pelvis. *Top Magn Reson Imaging.* 1992;4:46–63.
- Nagayama M, Watanabe Y, Okumura A, et al. Fast MR imaging in obstetrics. *Radiographics* 2002;22:563–582.
- Noonan JB, Coackley FV, Qayyum A, et al. MR imaging of retained products of conception. *Am J Roentgenol.* 2003;181:435–439.
- Outwater EK, Siegelman ES, Chiowanich P, et al. Dilated fallopian tubes: MR imaging characteristics. *Radiology* 1998;208:436–439.
- Outwater EK, Siegelman ES, Van Deerlin V. Adenomyosis: current concepts and imaging considerations. *Am J Roentgenol.* 1998;170:437–441.
- Pannu HK, Kaufman HS, Cundiff GW, et al. Dynamic MR imaging of pelvic organ prolapse: spectrum of abnormalities. *Radiographics* 2000;20:1567–1582.
- Rajan DK, Scharer KA. Radiology of Fournier's gangrene. *Am J Roentgenol.* 1998;170:163–168.
- Rha SE, Byun JY, Jung SE, et al. CT and MR imaging features of adnexal torsion. *Radiographics* 2002;22:283–294.
- Rozenblit AM, Ricci ZJ, Tuvia J, et al. Incompetent and dilated ovarian veins: a common CT finding in asymptomatic parous women. *Am J Roentgenol.* 2001;176:119–122.
- Scoutt LM, McCauley TR, Flynn SD, et al. Zonal anatomy of the cervix: correlation of MR imaging and histological examination of hysterectomy specimens. *Radiology* 1993;186:159–162.
- Siegelman ES, Outwater EK. Tissue characterization in the female pelvis by means of MR imaging. *Radiology* 1999;212:5–18.
- Siegelman ES, Outwater EK, Wang T, et al. Solid pelvic masses caused by endometriosis: MR features. *Am J Roentgenol.* 1994;163:357–361.
- Taipale P, Tarjanne H, Ylostalo P. Transvaginal sonography in suspected pelvic inflammatory disease. *Ultrasound Obstet Gynecol* 1995;6:430–434.
- Togashi K, Kawakami S, Kimura I, et al. Uterine contractions: possible diagnostic pitfall at MR imaging. *J Magn Reson Imaging.* 1993;3:889–893.
- Twickler DM, Setiawan AT, Evans RS, et al. Imaging of puerperal septic thrombophlebitis: prospective comparison of MR imaging, CT, and sonography. *Am J Roentgenol.* 1997;169:1039–1043.
- Yigit H, Tuncbilek I, Fitoz S, et al. Cyst of the canal of Nuck with demonstration of proximal canal. *J Ultrasound Med.* 2006;25:123–125.

CHAPTER EIGHT

RETROPERITONEUM AND ADRENAL GLANDS

VINCENT PELSSER,
KOENRAAD J. MORTELE,
AND PABLO R. ROS

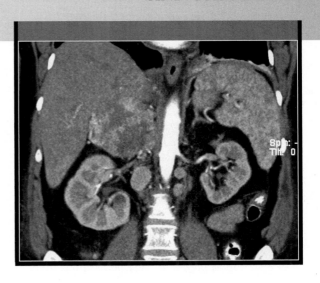

Clinical History: 82-year-old man presenting with low back pain and fever.

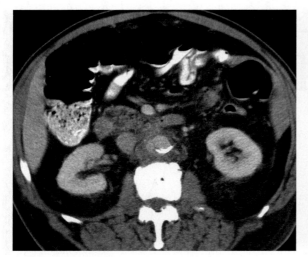

Figure 8.1   A

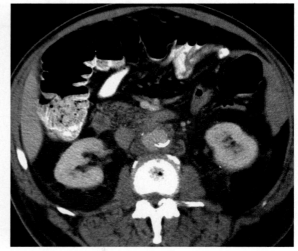

Figure 8.1   B

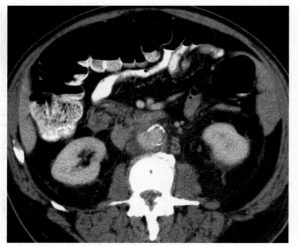

Figure 8.1   C

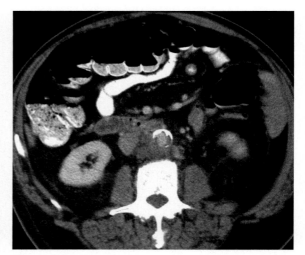

Figure 8.1   D

Findings: Axial contrast-enhanced CT (CECT) images demonstrate circumferential periaortic fat stranding and inflammation. A focal saccular outpouching containing intravenous contrast, in continuity with the aortic lumen, extends in the aortocaval space.

Differential Diagnosis: Inflammatory aneurysm, atherosclerotic aneurysm.

Diagnosis: Infected aortic aneurysm.

Discussion: Infected aortic aneurysms, also historically termed mycotic aneurysms, are uncommon, representing only 2.6% of all aortic aneurysms. However, the risk of rupture ranges from 53% to 75%, and the mortality rate is between 16% and 40%. The infection occurs via hematogenous spread through the vasa vasorum, direct endoluminal implantation on a diseased vessel wall, or direct extension of an adjacent infectious process. Infected aneurysms are typically saccular and have a surrounding soft tissue component, fluid, or fat stranding. Perianeurysmal gas and adjacent vertebral body destruction are helpful signs. Infected aneurysms also tend to develop and enlarge rapidly. Treatment consists of aggressive antibiotic therapy and resection of the aneurysm with bypass. Inflammatory and atherosclerotic aneurysms are usually fusiform. Inflammatory aneurysms have a surrounding rind of enhancing soft tissue, which typically spares the posterior wall of the aorta.

Clinical History: 78-year-old man taking warfarin (Coumadin) presenting with abdominal distention and discomfort.

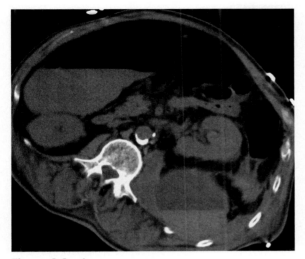

Figure 8.2   A

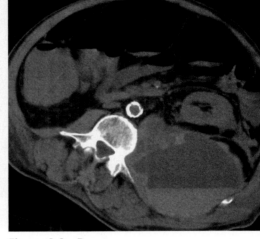

Figure 8.2   B

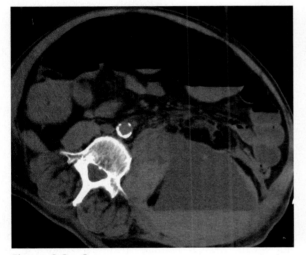

Figure 8.2   C

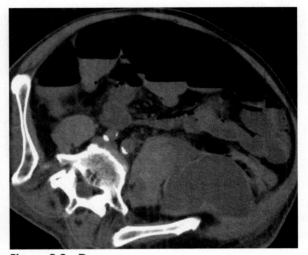

Figure 8.2   D

Findings: Axial nonenhanced CT (NECT) images demonstrate an 11.9 × 9.9 cm left retroperitoneal cystic mass involving the left psoas muscle. A fluid-fluid level is present.

Differential Diagnosis: Retroperitoneal sarcoma.

Diagnosis: Retroperitoneal hemorrhage.

Discussion: Retroperitoneal hemorrhage can be due to multiple etiologies including anticoagulants, trauma, penetrating injury, leaking aortic aneurysms, and bleeding disorders. The hemorrhage tends to spread along the retroperitoneal fascial planes and will, therefore, spare the perirenal space if the posterior renal fascia has not been interrupted by penetrating injury or prior surgery. Also, hemorrhage will not cause bone destruction, as can be found with neoplasms. In the acute and early subacute phases of a hemorrhage, a fluid-fluid level can be present. The denser blood products will settle to the bottom of the fluid collection, forming a hematocrit level. This is nearly diagnostic of hemorrhage. With time, the fluid collection will become less dense and cystic in appearance. It is important to exclude an underlying hemorrhagic neoplasm; therefore, close follow-up scans are necessary, as well as correlation with clinical history.

Clinical History: 60-year-old man presenting with hypertension.

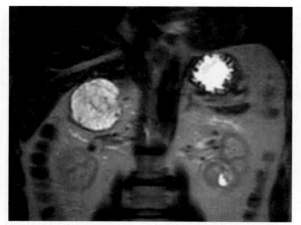

Figure 8.3 A

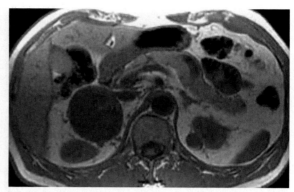

Figure 8.3 B

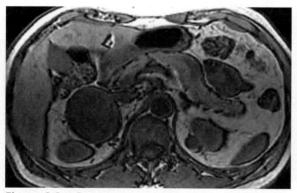

Figure 8.3 C

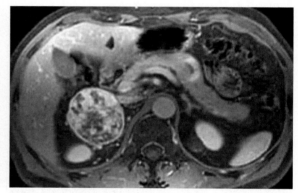

Figure 8.3 D

Findings: Coronal T2-weighted image (WI) (A) shows a markedly hyperintense 5.6 × 6.0 cm right adrenal mass. When comparing the in-phase (B) to the opposed-phase (C) T1-WI, the mass does not show signal dropout. Gadolinium-enhanced, fat-suppressed T1-WI (D) demonstrates heterogeneous enhancement of the mass.

Differential Diagnosis: Adenoma, metastasis, adrenocortical carcinoma.

Diagnosis: Pheochromocytoma.

Discussion: Pheochromocytoma is a rare tumor arising from the chromaffin cells in the adrenal medulla. The rule of "10s" for pheochromocytoma states that 10% are extra-adrenal, 10% are bilateral, 10% are malignant, and 10% occur in children. The most common finding in patients with pheochromocytomas is hypertension due to excess catecholamine release. Other symptoms include tachycardia, sweating, nausea, and chest pain. Imaging of pheochromocytoma includes CT and MRI. CT is very sensitive in detecting small adrenal lesions. Contrast, however, may be contraindicated in patients with suspected pheochromocytomas because it can cause a hypertensive crisis. MRI is very sensitive as well and adds multiplanar capabilities. Pheochromocytomas are typically slightly hypointense on the T1-WI and markedly hyperintense on the T2-WI, as seen in this case. This appearance is nonspecific because there is overlap with other adrenal lesions, such as adrenocortical carcinomas and metastases. With an appropriate clinical picture (hypertension and elevated urinary vanillylmandelic acid [VMA], both of which were present in this case) and an adrenal mass, the diagnosis of pheochromocytoma is almost certain.

Case images courtesy of Dr. Caroline Reinhold, McGill University Health Center, Montreal, Canada.

Clinical History: 70-year-old man with a history of lymphoma.

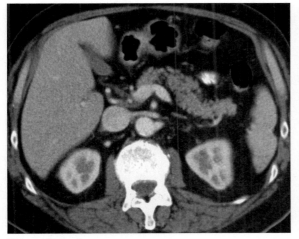

Figure 8.4 A

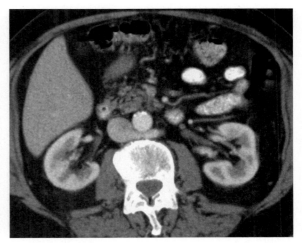

Figure 8.4 B

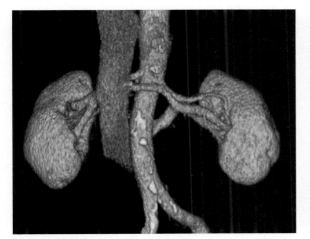

Figure 8.4 C

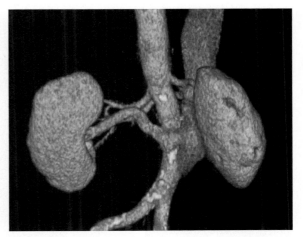

Figure 8.4 D

Findings: Axial CECT images (A and B) and three-dimensional, volume-rendered images with anterior (C) and posterior (D) views demonstrate a left renal vein both anterior and posterior to the aorta.

Differential Diagnosis: None.

Diagnosis: Circumaortic left renal vein.

Discussion: Circumaortic left renal vein is a common developmental anomaly of the inferior vena cava (IVC), occurring in up to 8.7% of patients. The ventral renal vein is usually in the normal location, and the dorsal renal vein is typically several centimeters caudal to it, as seen in this case. The ventral renal vein drains the superior and anterior portions of the left kidney, and the dorsal renal vein drains the inferior and posterior aspects of the left kidney. Circumaortic left renal vein is usually asymptomatic and of little clinical significance except in placement of an inferior vena case filter or in view of surgery. Placement of the filter should not occlude the orifice of the renal vein, or renal vein thrombosis can occur. Placement should be caudal to the most inferior renal vein, which is usually the dorsal renal vein. Alternatively, the filter can be placed cephalad to both renal veins. This will prevent emboli from reaching the lung from the lower extremities.

Clinical History: 61-year-old man presenting with bilateral flank pain.

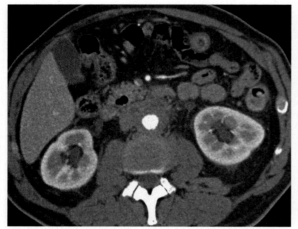

Figure 8.5   A

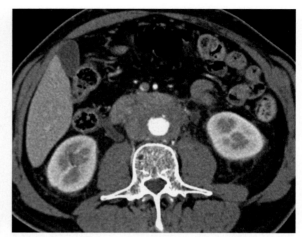

Figure 8.5   B

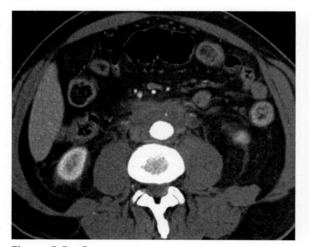

Figure 8.5   C

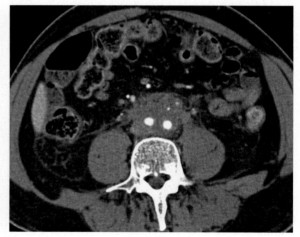

Figure 8.5   D

Findings: Axial CECT images demonstrate a soft tissue density mass surrounding the aorta and extending beyond the bifurcation. Note mild bilateral hydronephrosis.

Differential Diagnosis: Lymphoma, infectious lymphadenopathy, metastatic lymphadenopathy.

Diagnosis: Retroperitoneal fibrosis.

Discussion: Retroperitoneal fibrosis (RPF) is an uncommon process composed histologically of fibroblasts, inflammatory cells, and collagen. It typically encases the aorta and the IVC and can involve the ureters, leading to hydronephrosis. The majority of cases of RPF are idiopathic (called Ormond disease), possibly due to an autoimmune process. Other benign causes of retroperitoneal fibrosis include medications (e.g., methysergide, beta-blockers), infections (e.g., tuberculosis, syphilis), retroperitoneal fluid collections, connective tissue disease, and radiation therapy. Malignancies (e.g., lymphoma, carcinoid, metastases) can also elicit a desmoplastic reaction, leading to RPF. The CT findings of RPF are nonspecific, ranging from stranding in the retroperitoneum (without a mass) to a large soft tissue density mass. RPF enhances after contrast administration and usually begins in the lower part of the abdomen. Infectious and metastatic lymphadenopathy as well as lymphoma can have a similar appearance. If the CT findings are not diagnostic, image-guided biopsy, as was performed in this case, may be necessary. CT is often helpful in following these patients after surgery or steroid treatment.

Clinical History: 51-year-old man with an incidentally discovered adrenal mass on recent chest CT.

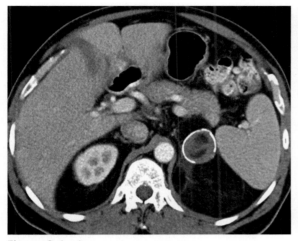

Figure 8.6   A

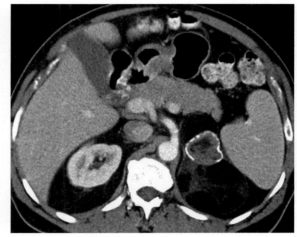

Figure 8.6   B

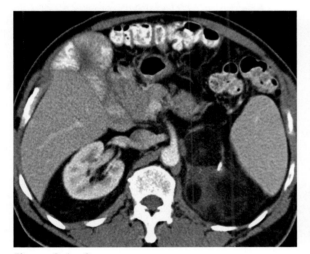

Figure 8.6   C

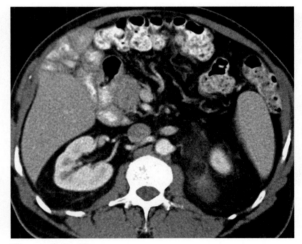

Figure 8.6   D

Findings: Axial CECT images demonstrate a 10.0 × 7.3 cm left adrenal mass composed of fat, soft tissue, and calcifications. Note intact upper pole of the left kidney.

Differential Diagnosis: Liposarcoma, teratoma.

Diagnosis: Adrenal myelolipoma.

Discussion: Myelolipoma is a benign tumor arising from the adrenal cortex. It is composed of mature fat and cells similar to those found in the bone marrow, such as myelocytes, megakaryocytes, erythrocytes, and lymphocytes. Myelolipomas are typically asymptomatic and found incidentally on imaging. Adrenal myelolipomas can have a variable amount of fat present within the lesion. The presence of fat in an adrenal lesion is diagnostic of a myelolipoma. Myelolipomas can also hemorrhage and calcify, which can give the lesion a heterogeneous appearance. This can mimic other adrenal masses, such as adrenal carcinomas and metastases. CT is useful in detecting myelolipomas due to the characteristic low density of fat present in the mass. With MRI, fat-suppression sequences can be used to identify fat within an adrenal lesion. Adrenal liposarcomas and teratomas are other fat-containing adrenal tumors, but they are exceedingly rare.

Clinical History: 43-year-old woman presenting with back pain.

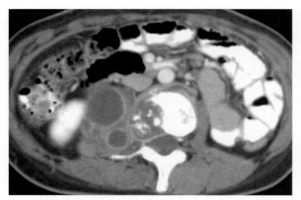

Figure 8.7   A

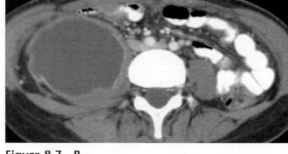

Figure 8.7   B

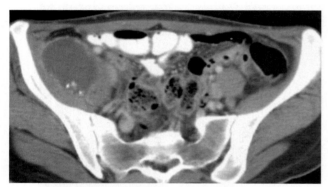

Figure 8.7   C

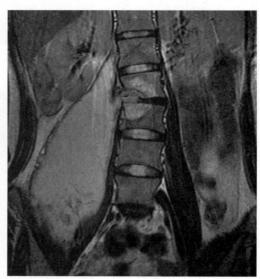

Figure 8.7   D

Findings: Axial CECT images (A–C) demonstrate a large rim-enhancing fluid collection with associated calcifications in the right psoas muscle. Note vertebral body destruction. Coronal T2-WI (D) shows better the extent of the fluid collection and the discocentric vertebral body destruction and edema causing angular spinal deformity.

Differential Diagnosis: Necrotic metastasis.

Diagnosis: Spinal tuberculosis with retroperitoneal abscess.

Discussion: Nearly 50% of the masses arising from the iliopsoas muscle are inflammatory in nature. These inflammatory processes typically arise from adjacent organs such as the kidneys, spine (tuberculosis), colon, or pancreas. Penetrating injuries or postsurgical complications can lead to iliopsoas infections as well. The majority of these inflammatory masses are pyogenic in nature, with abscesses resulting from tuberculous spondylitis less commonly seen. Calcifications and heterotopic bone formation can be seen associated with tuberculosis-related infections. As with abscesses in other parts of the body, retroperitoneal abscesses appear as rim-enhancing fluid collections. On MRI, they are of water signal intensity on T1-WI and T2-WI. When small, abscesses can be difficult to detect on the T1-WI because they are isointense to muscle; often asymmetry would be the only clue to their presence. However, they are easily seen on the T2-WI and on the postgadolinium images. The nonnodular rim enhancement and lack of central enhancement are suggestive of an abscess rather than a metastasis. Metastases also tend to be rounder rather than elongated, as seen in the present case.

Clinical History: 68-year-old man presenting with right flank pain.

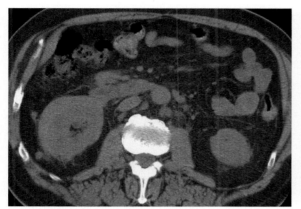

Figure 8.8   A

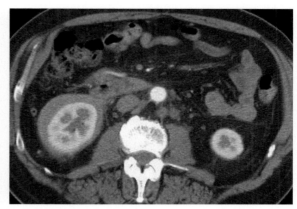

Figure 8.8   B

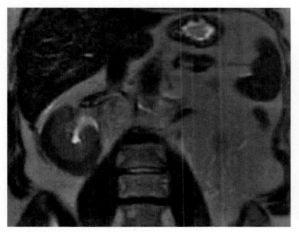

Figure 8.8   C

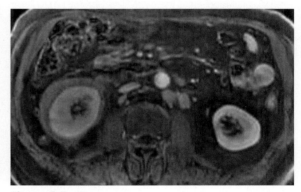

Figure 8.8   D

Findings: Axial NECT image (A) demonstrates hyperdense material surrounding the right kidney. This is best appreciated on the axial CECT image (B). Note associated perinephric stranding and modules, and retroperitoneal lymph nodes. The abnormality is hypointense on the coronal T2-WI (C) and shows mild enhancement on the gadolinium-enhanced, fat-suppressed T1-WI (D).

Differential Diagnosis: Hemorrhage.

Diagnosis: Perinephric lymphoma.

Discussion: Perinephric lymphoma can occur by extension of retroperitoneal lymphoma into the perinephric space. In approximately 10% of cases, however, perinephric disease without significant parenchymal disease or retroperitoneal lymphadenopathy is the predominant presentation. Perinephric lymphoma typically surrounds the kidney and conforms to the perirenal space. As the lymphoma progresses, it can enlarge the perirenal space and occasionally cause hydronephrosis. Lymphoma may appear hyperdense on NECT and hypointense on T2-WI due to a high nuclear-to-cytoplasmic ratio. Acute hemorrhage will also be hyperdense. However, the presence of enhancement, which is sometimes better appreciated on subtraction images, excludes hemorrhage in this case. The presence of retroperitoneal lymphadenopathy and additional perinephric nodules separate from the main rind of tissue surrounding the kidney are also indicators that the process is more likely to be neoplastic than hemorrhage.

Clinical History: 44-year-old woman presenting with severe hypertension following breast surgery.

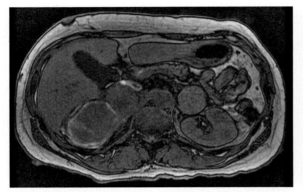

Figure 8.9   A

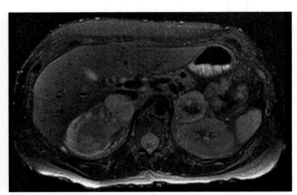

Figure 8.9   B

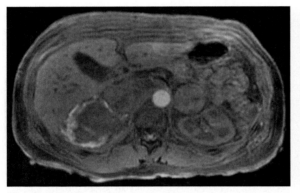

Figure 8.9   C

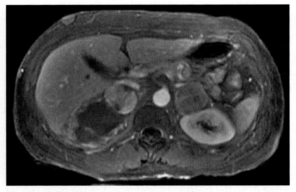

Figure 8.9   D

Findings: Axial opposed-phase T1-WI (A) demonstrates bilateral adrenal masses that are hyperintense compared to the liver parenchyma on the axial T2-WI (B). Unenhanced (C) and gadolinium-enhanced (D) fat-suppressed T1-WI show enhancement of both lesions. Note hemorrhage lateral to the right adrenal mass and multiple cutaneous and subcutaneous enhancing nodules.

Differential Diagnosis: Metastases, hemorrhage, infection (tuberculosis, histoplasmosis).

Diagnosis: Bilateral pheochromocytomas in a patient with neurofibromatosis type 1.

Discussion: Pheochromocytomas are bilateral in 10% of cases, and in at least 10% of cases, they are associated with a genetic predisposition, such as multiple endocrine neoplasias (multiple endocrine neoplasm type II), von Hippel-Lindau disease, neurofibromatosis type 1, and nonsyndromic familial pheochromocytoma. Because neurofibromatosis type 1 is autosomal dominant, other family members may also have similar findings and symptoms. Diagnosis of pheochromocytomas is usually made by the presence of elevated urinary VMA levels. Because pheochromocytomas are usually symptomatic, they often present early when the lesion is small. The multiplanar capability of MRI is useful in evaluating for small adrenal lesions. Pheochromocytomas are usually isointense or slightly hypointense relative to the liver on T1-WI, whereas the lesion is very hyperintense on T2-WI. This overlaps with MRI findings in other adrenal neoplasms (e.g., metastases, adenocarcinoma). Because pheochromocytomas are very vascular, they enhance with gadolinium. In this case, identification of the skin neurofibromas is an important clue to the correct diagnosis. Hemorrhage tends to have a hyperintense signal on T1-WI due to blood products, as seen lateral to the right adrenal mass. Both infection and metastases could have this appearance too.

Case images courtesy of Dr. Giovanni Artho, McGill University Health Center, Montreal, Canada.

Clinical History: 61-year-old man with history of acute myelogenous leukemia.

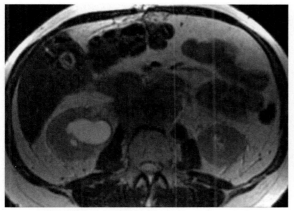

Figure 8.10 A

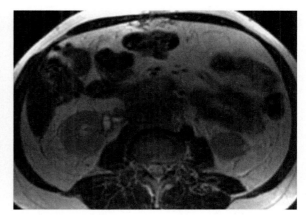

Figure 8.10 B

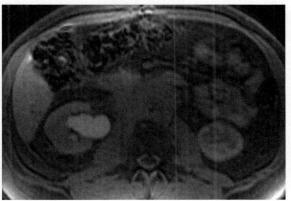

Figure 8.10 C

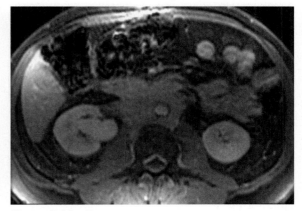

Figure 8.10 D

Findings: Axial T2-WI (A and B) demonstrate a 6.0 × 3.6 cm, ill-defined, mildly hyperintense mass surrounding the aorta and IVC. Unenhanced fat-suppressed axial T1-WI (C) shows the mass is isointense to muscle. After gadolinium administration (D), the mass enhances homogeneously. Note right hydronephrosis and blood in the right collecting system.

Differential Diagnosis: Lymphoma, metastatic lymphadenopathy, infectious lymphadenopathy.

Diagnosis: Retroperitoneal fibrosis.

Discussion: Nearly 70% of cases of retroperitoneal fibrosis (RPF) are idiopathic, occurring in men between the ages of 40 and 60 years. Most patients are asymptomatic unless there is involvement of the ureters, leading to hydronephrosis. Rarely, the IVC can be encased, causing lower extremity swelling and deep venous thrombosis. Treatment is with steroids and/or surgery. Surgery is performed to free up the ureters and relieve the hydronephrosis. MRI is slightly more specific than CT in making the diagnosis of RPF. Occasionally, mature RPF will be hypointense on both the T1-WI and the T2-WI due to the collagen formation. When this occurs, the findings are rather specific for RPF. However, a hyperintense signal on a T2-WI is nonspecific. In the acute phase, RPF has an inflammatory component with high fluid content, producing high signal on T2-WI. This high T2 signal can also be due to desmoplastic reaction from a malignant cause or lymphadenopathy secondary to either a malignancy (e.g., testicular cancer, lymphoma) or infectious etiology (e.g., tuberculosis, *Mycobacterium avium-intracellulare* [MAI]).

Clinical History: 34-year-old woman presenting with left flank pain following renal biopsy.

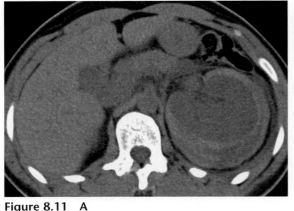

Figure 8.11   A

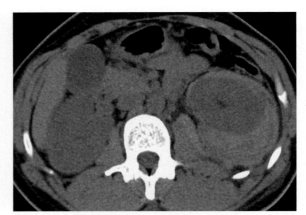

Figure 8.11   B

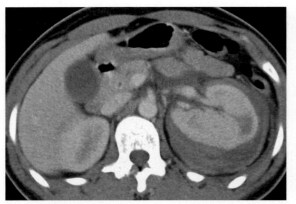

Figure 8.11   C

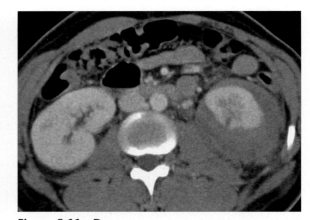

Figure 8.11   D

Findings: Axial NECT images (A and B) demonstrate high-attenuation material in the left perinephric space, with no detectable enhancement on the axial CECT images (C and D). Note associated fat stranding and linear area of absent enhancement in the left lower renal pole.

Differential Diagnosis: Lymphoma, abscess.

Diagnosis: Perirenal hemorrhage.

Discussion: Hemorrhage in the perirenal space can be due to blunt or penetrating trauma, anticoagulation therapy, or a hypervascular neoplasm (e.g., angiomyolipoma, renal cell carcinoma). The high-attenuation blood is suggestive of an acute or subacute hemorrhage. If Gerota's fascia has not been disrupted, the hemorrhage will often be contained within the perirenal space. Purulent material from an abscess could also be high in attenuation. Clinical history and the patient's symptoms usually provide enough information to be able to distinguish between the two diagnoses. Lymphoma can often involve the perirenal space but tends to be of soft tissue density, although it can be of high attenuation. In most cases, an underlying neoplasm should be excluded with a follow-up CECT after the hemorrhage has resolved. In this case, the linear area of absent enhancement in the left lower renal pole, which is a clue to the cause of the perirenal hemorrhage, represents blood in the biopsy tract.

Clinical History: 45-year-old man with abdominal pain.

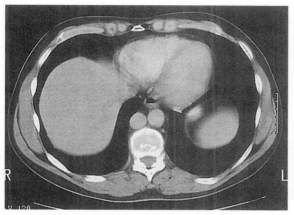

Figure 8.12 A

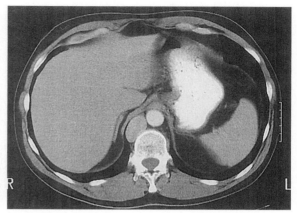

Figure 8.12 B

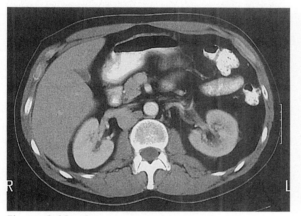

Figure 8.12 C

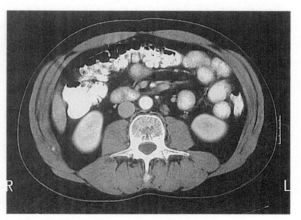

Figure 8.12 D

Findings: CECT images demonstrate an enlarged azygous vein with no identifiable IVC.

Differential Diagnosis: None.

Diagnosis: Azygos continuation of the IVC.

Discussion: Azygos continuation of the IVC is a relatively uncommon developmental anomaly of the IVC, with a prevalence of 0.6%. It is due to failure in forming the suprarenal portion of the IVC. Below the renal veins, there is a normal IVC to the right of the aorta formed from the confluence of the iliac veins. Above the renal veins, the normal IVC (including the intrahepatic IVC) is not present. Instead there is an enlarged azygos vein seen in its normal location in the retrocrural space, draining into the superior vena cava. The hepatic veins, which normally drain into the IVC, drain directly into the right atrium via the suprahepatic segment of the IVC. It is important to recognize azygos continuation because the azygos vein could be mistaken for an enlarged retrocrural lymph node. It is also important to diagnose this anomaly in patients undergoing shunting procedures for portal hypertension or IVC filter placement.

Clinical History: 45-year-old woman with history of breast cancer.

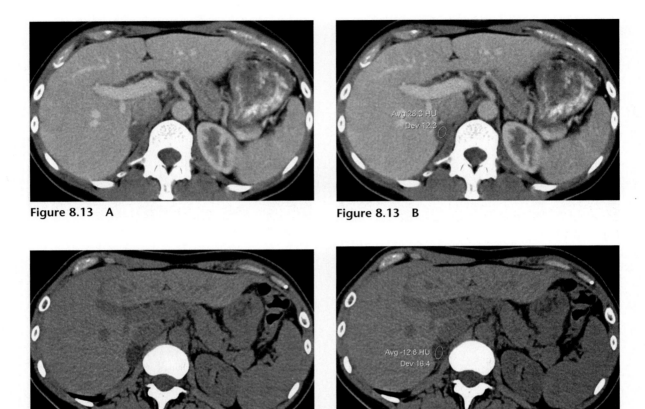

Figure 8.13   A

Figure 8.13   B

Figure 8.13   C

Figure 8.13   D

Findings: Axial CECT images (A and B) demonstrate a homogeneous 2.2 × 1.4 cm right adrenal mass that has a density of 28.3 Hounsfield units (HU). Axial NECT images (C and D), obtained at a later date, show the mass has an attenuation of −12.8 HU.

Differential Diagnosis: Metastasis, pheochromocytoma, adrenocortical carcinoma.

Diagnosis: Lipid-rich adrenal adenoma.

Discussion: The evaluation of adrenal masses is critical in the workup of a patient with a known primary malignancy. Adrenal adenomas are common, with an incidence of approximately 8% in autopsy series. The decision to proceed with curative therapy often rests on the characterization of an adrenal mass to exclude distant metastasis. Therefore, a method to noninvasively diagnose adenomas with confidence is needed. Adenomas have a preponderance of lipid-laden cells that usually give them a lower attenuation value than other adrenal masses (e.g., metastasis, pheochromocytoma, adenocarcinoma). Using an attenuation value of less than 10 HU as the cutoff for an adenoma on a NECT, the specificity of diagnosing an adrenal adenoma ranges from 92% to 100%. Using less than 0 HU, the specificity is 100%. Therefore, an adrenal mass with negative attenuation value and no evidence of macroscopic fat is diagnostic for an adrenal adenoma.

Clinical History: 75-year-old woman presenting with abdominal pain following sigmoidoscopy.

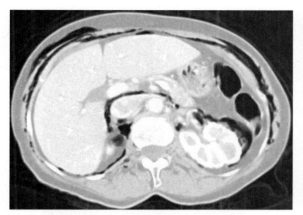

Figure 8.14   A

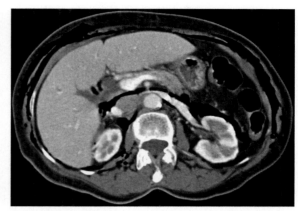

Figure 8.14   B

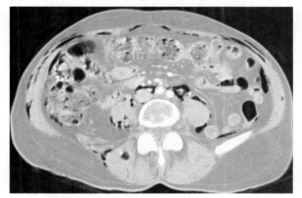

Figure 8.14   C

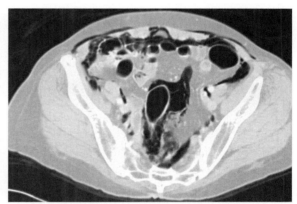

Figure 8.14   D

Findings: Axial CECT images in lung (A, C, and D) and soft tissue (B) windows demonstrate extensive extraperitoneal gas present in the retroperitoneum, paraspinal muscles, abdominal wall, and omentum.

Differential Diagnosis: None.

Diagnosis: Extraperitoneal gas due to rectal perforation.

Discussion: Retroperitoneal gas can be due to several causes including perforated bowel (iatrogenic or not), recent surgery, penetrating trauma, and gas-forming organisms. Portions of the gastrointestinal (GI) tract that are retroperitoneal/extraperitoneal include the duodenal sweep (second and third portions), ascending and descending colon, and rectum. Perforation of any of these bowel loops can lead to retroperitoneal gas. Retroperitoneal gas is often difficult to detect by plain film because the air will not collect under the diaphragm or around the liver as in pneumoperitoneum. CT, however, is excellent for evaluating even small amounts of retroperitoneal gas. Retroperitoneal gas tends to collect on the underside of Gerota's fascia and posterior peritoneum or along the psoas muscle. Gas in these locations is easily detected by CT, especially when the images are displayed in lung windows. The retroperitoneal spaces (perirenal and anterior and posterior pararenal space) become one space in the lower abdomen and are contiguous with the extraperitoneal space in the pelvis. In the present case, the retroperitoneal gas dissected cranially and anteriorly, to extend into the abdominal wall, from the perforated rectum following sigmoidoscopy.

Clinical History: 2-year-old boy presenting with a palpable abdominal mass.

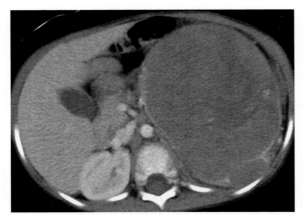

Figure 8.15   A

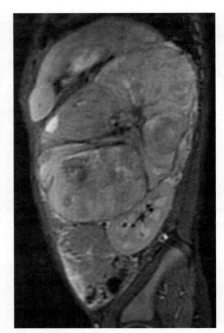

Figure 8.15   B

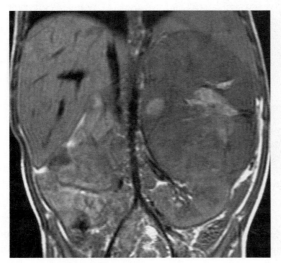

Figure 8.15   C

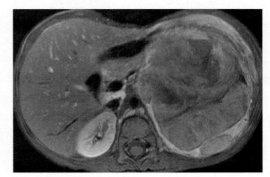

Figure 8.15   D

Findings: Axial CECT image (A) demonstrates a 9.0 × 8.0 cm heterogeneous mass arising in the left upper quadrant. Fat-suppressed sagittal T2-WI (B), coronal T1-WI (C), and gadolinium-enhanced, fat-suppressed axial T1-WI (D) show the solid mass that displaces the left kidney caudally.

Differential Diagnosis: Wilms tumor.

Diagnosis: Neuroblastoma.

Discussion: Neuroblastoma (NB) is the most common solid abdominal mass of infancy arising from the neural crest. The majority of NBs occur in children less than 4 years of age, but they can occur beyond 10 years of age in less than 5% of cases. Most NBs occur in the adrenal gland, but they can be found in other retroperitoneal locations, mediastinum, neck, and pelvis. Patients can present with a palpable mass, hypertension, nystagmus, and abdominal pain. In a child younger than 5 years of age, the two most common solid retroperitoneal masses are Wilms tumor and NB. It is critical to try to determine the organ of origin of these masses. In this case, the mass is separate from the kidney, with no claw sign between the kidney and the mass, suggesting an adrenal origin. Up to 90% of NBs demonstrate calcifications on CT. NBs have a tendency to encase or invade adjacent structures, such as blood vessels or neural foramina. Diagnosis can be confirmed by the presence of elevated urinary VMA levels or metaiodobenzylguanidine (MIBG) uptake in 70% of cases. Wilms tumors, on the other hand, calcify in only 15% of cases, have a renal origin suggested by a claw sign between the renal parenchyma and the mass, and have a tendency to displace rather than encase or invade adjacent structures.

Case images courtesy of Dr. George A. Taylor, Children's Hospital Boston, Boston, MA.

Clinical History: 20-year-old man presenting with low back pain.

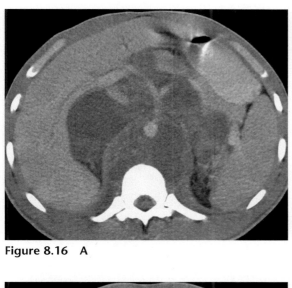

Figure 8.16   A

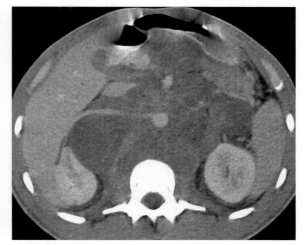

Figure 8.16   B

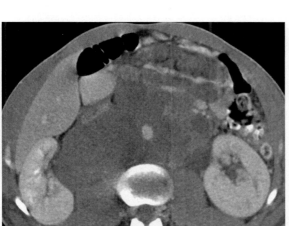

Figure 8.16   C

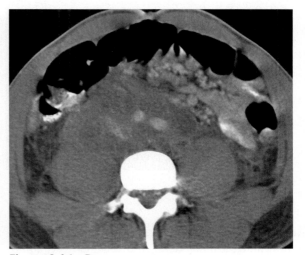

Figure 8.16   D

Findings: Axial CECT images demonstrate low-density retrocrural, retroperitoneal, and mesenteric masses encircling major vascular structures.

Differential Diagnosis: Infectious lymphadenopathy (tuberculosis, MAI), lymphoma.

Diagnosis: Metastatic testicular cancer (mixed nonseminomatous germ cell tumor).

Discussion: Testicular cancer is the most common cancer in men between 15 and 35 years of age. Testicular cancer can be divided into germ cell and non–germ cell types. Germ cell neoplasms (seminoma and nonseminomatous germ cell tumors [NSGCTs]) constitute nearly 95% of all cases. Workup for testicular cancer typically includes an abdominal CT scan to evaluate for retroperitoneal adenopathy. Testicular cancers spread via lymphatics, following the course of the gonadal veins. Therefore, a left-sided testicular cancer would initially spread to lymph nodes in the left renal hilum, whereas right-sided testicular cancers spread to the right para-aortic and juxtacaval regions. When advanced, the nodal metastases may cross over and become bilateral, as seen in this case. Seminoma metastases tend to be of homogeneous soft tissue density, while metastatic NSGCTs are frequently necrotic or cystic, as seen in this case. A soft tissue mass surrounding the aorta and IVC, in a young patient, could be due to lymphoma. However, lymphoma is only rarely necrotic without treatment. In this age group, acquired immunodeficiency syndrome (AIDS)-related diseases must also be considered because the lymphadenopathy from tuberculosis or MAI may be necrotic. Clinical findings of a swollen testicle, the age of the patient, retroperitoneal adenopathy, and elevated tumor markers (beta-human chorionic gonadotropin and alpha-fetoprotein, especially in NSGCT) are highly suggestive of the diagnosis of metastatic testicular cancer.

Clinical History: 24-year-old woman presenting with multiple skin nodules.

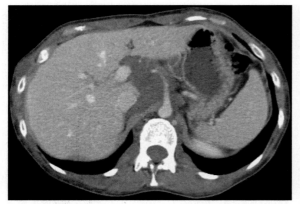

Figure 8.17   A

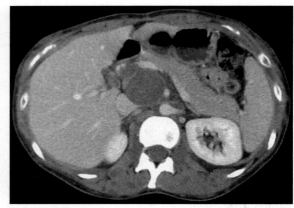

Figure 8.17   B

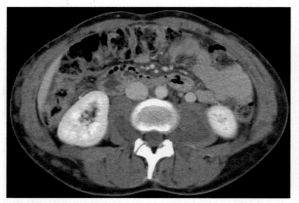

Figure 8.17   C

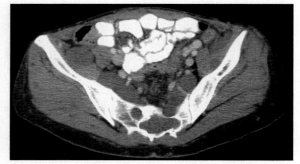

Figure 8.17   D

Findings: Axial CECT images demonstrate multiple retroperitoneal, paraspinal sacral, and subcutaneous homogeneous masses. Note sacral remodeling.

Differential Diagnosis: Lymphoma, metastasis.

Diagnosis: Neurofibromatosis type 1.

Discussion: Neurofibromatosis type 1 or von Recklinghausen disease is often referred to as peripheral neurofibromatosis because many of the findings are outside the central nervous system. This includes involvement of the skin (café-au-lait spots), bone (sphenoid wing dysplasia, ribbon ribs), and GI tract (multiple neurofibromas). Neurofibromatosis is characterized by dysplasia of neuroectodermal and mesodermal tissues, which can result in multiple neurofibromas. Neurofibromas are tumors of the nerve sheath, with nerves and nerve fibers coursing through it. Therefore, it is difficult to surgically remove a neurofibroma without injuring the underlying nerve. Plexiform neurofibroma, as seen surrounding the celiac trunk in this case, is composed of tortuous fusiform enlargement of small peripheral nerves intermixed with connective tissue. These can grow to be very large, surrounding adjacent structures without causing obstruction or constriction. They are typically low in attenuation but can demonstrate mild enhancement, as seen in this case. The location and appearance can occasionally make neurofibromatosis difficult to distinguish from lymphoma. The multiplicity of lesions may also raise concern for diffuse metastatic disease, but a primary malignancy is often known by the time such extensive metastases are present. The sacral remodeling also suggests a longstanding process rather than an aggressive one such as a metastasis.

Clinical History: 74-year-old woman with incidentally discovered left adrenal mass.

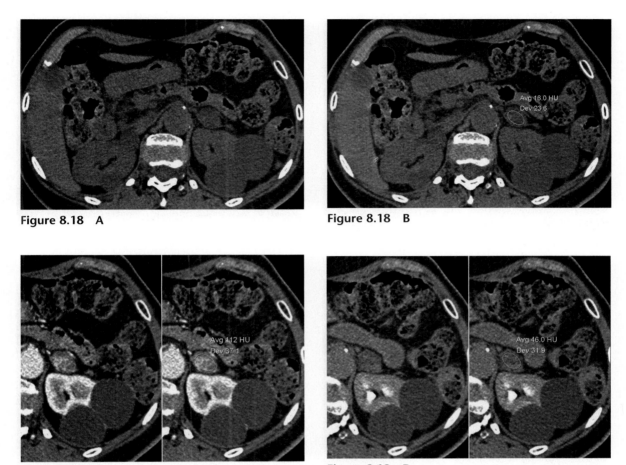

Figure 8.18   A

Figure 8.18   B

Figure 8.18   C

Figure 8.18   D

Findings: Axial NECT images (A and B) demonstrate a 1.7 × 2.5 cm left adrenal mass with an attenuation value of 16 HU. It has a density of 112 HU on the axial CECT image obtained 60 seconds after injection of intravenous contrast (C). On the 15-minute, delayed CECT image (D), the mass has a density of 46 HU. Also not left-sided renal cysts.

Differential Diagnosis: Metastasis, pheochromocytoma.

Diagnosis: Lipid-poor adenoma.

Discussion: Twenty-nine percent of adenomas have a density of more than 10 HU on NECT. These are termed lipid-poor adenomas. By 60 seconds after injection of intravenous contrast, adenomas enhance to the same degree as nonadenomas. However, on delayed images, the density of adenomas decreases more rapidly than nonadenomas. This has been postulated to be due to altered capillary permeability in nonadenomas, causing prolonged contrast retention. Because of this difference of enhancement, one can perform an "adrenal washout study" to assess adrenal masses that have not yet been characterized. For this, NECT and CECT images (after injection of 150 cc of contrast) obtained at 60 seconds and 15 minutes must be obtained. Region-of- interest cursor needs to be placed on the central portion of the mass, excluding calcifications or small regions of necrosis. The percentage of enhancement washout can than be calculated using the following formula: $[(E - D)/(E - U)] \times 100$, where E is the density value on the 60-second CECT, D is the density value on the 15-minute CECT, and U is the density on the NECT. If the enhancement washout is more than 60%, the lesion can be diagnosed as an adenoma. If it does not meet the 60% threshold, the lesion remains undetermined, and biopsy, in the setting of a known primary tumor, or follow-up imaging are recommended. In this case, the enhancement washout of the lesion was 69% ($[(112 - 46)/(112 - 16)] \times 100$), and a lipid-poor adenoma was diagnosed.

Clinical History: 74-year-old man with history of pleural mesothelioma presenting with abdominal pain.

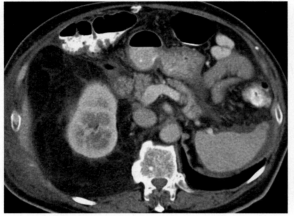

Figure 8.19   A

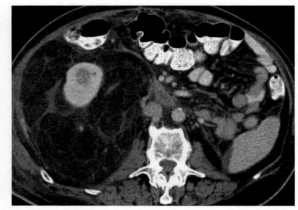

Figure 8.19   B

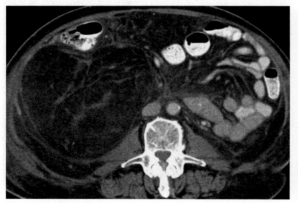

Figure 8.19   C

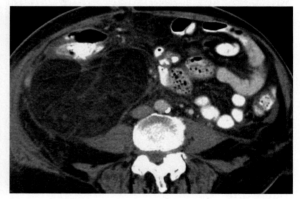

Figure 8.19   D

Findings: Axial CECT images demonstrate an 18.5 × 14.1 cm, predominantly fatty mass in the right perinephric space, displacing the kidney anteriorly. Note the radiating strands of soft tissue throughout the mass. The right kidney is congenitally absent.

Differential Diagnosis: Angiomyolipoma, lipoma.

Diagnosis: Liposarcoma.

Discussion: Primary retroperitoneal neoplasms arise almost entirely from mesenchymal tissue. The most common retroperitoneal malignant neoplasm is liposarcoma followed by leiomyosarcoma. Histologically, liposarcomas can be well-differentiated, dedifferentiated, myxoid, pleomorphic, and mixed. By CT, well-differentiated liposarcomas are predominantly of fatty density with soft tissue septa and nodules.

Dedifferentiated tumors are suggested by the presence of soft tissue nodules greater than 1 cm in size. Myxoid liposarcomas have low-density areas due to their high water content. The pleomorphic liposarcomas appear predominantly of soft tissue density. The presence of fat and soft tissue in a retroperitoneal tumor is nearly diagnostic of a liposarcoma. Exophytic renal angiomyolipomas (AMLs) cause a defect in the renal parenchyma and contain enlarged blood vessels. Perinephric liposarcomas usually do not have those features, which can thus be used to differentiate the two entities. Presence of additional renal AMLs is also a clue that a large perinephric fat-containing mass may also be an AML. Lipomas are extraordinarily rare in the retroperitoneum such that any largely lipomatous mass in that location should be considered a well-differentiated liposarcoma.

Clinical History: 35-year-old woman with a history of flank melanoma.

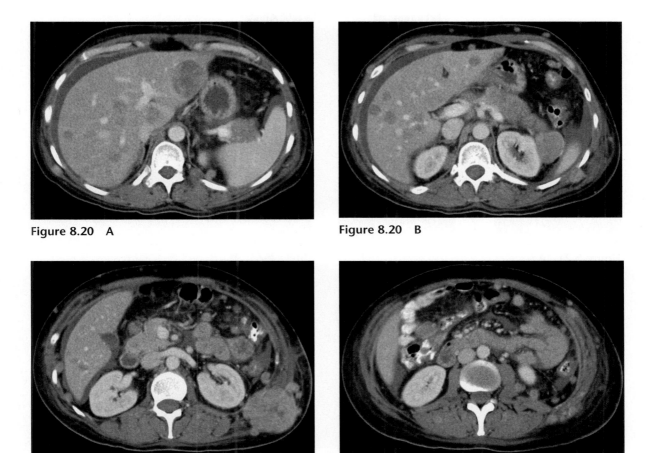

Figure 8.20   A

Figure 8.20   B

Figure 8.20   C

Figure 8.20   D

Findings: Axial CECT images demonstrate multiple masses in the perinephric spaces. Note ascites and other masses in the retroperitoneum, omentum, liver, and abdominal wall.

Differential Diagnosis: Lymphoma.

Diagnosis: Perinephric metastases from melanoma.

Discussion: Metastases to the retroperitoneum are commonly seen in pelvic malignancies (cervix, prostate, and bladder) and testicular tumors. These usually spread to retroperitoneal lymph nodes in the para-aortic, juxtacaval, and aortocaval chains. Metastases to the perirenal space, as in this case, are much less common. These are typically hematogenous metastases from melanoma or lung, breast, or kidney cancers. Lymphoma may also cause perinephric nodules. However, when lymphoma involves the perinephric space, it commonly does so by direct extension from retroperitoneal disease. The location of the other masses, especially in the abdominal wall, is more characteristic of metastases than lymphoma. Liver lesions are also less common in lymphoma than in a metastatic process.

Clinical History: 63-year-old man with history of lung cancer presenting with hematuria.

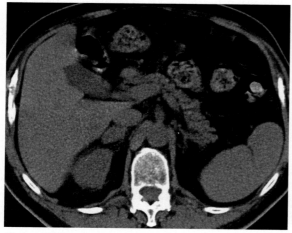

Figure 8.21   A

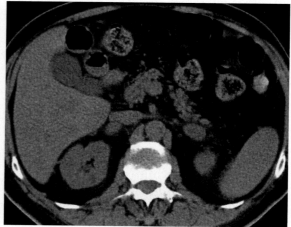

Figure 8.21   B

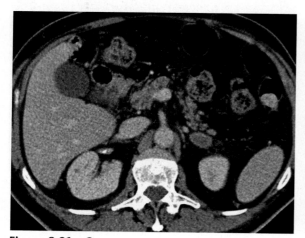

Figure 8.21   C

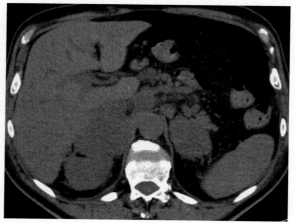

Figure 8.21   D

Findings: Axial NECT images (A and B) demonstrate small symmetric bilateral adrenal masses, measuring 36 HU on the right and 29 HU on the left. Slightly heterogeneous enhancement is seen in the left mass on the axial CECT image (C). Axial NECT image (D) obtained 2 months later shows marked enlargement of both masses.

Differential Diagnosis: Adenomas, infection (tuberculosis, histoplasmosis), lymphoma, hemorrhage, pheochromocytoma.

Diagnosis: Bilateral adrenal metastases.

Discussion: Adrenal metastases are the most common malignant lesions to affect the adrenal gland. The most common primary tumors to metastasize to the adrenal gland are melanoma, lung cancer, and breast cancer. However, a small adrenal mass in a patient with a known malignancy is still much more likely to be an adenoma, given their high prevalence. Small adrenal metastases are typically homogeneous in density, whereas larger lesions tend to become necrotic. In patients with known metastases in other sites than the adrenal glands, the precise nature of an adrenal nodule is not critical. However, if an adrenal nodule would represent the only potential site of metastasis, then further characterization of the mass by NECT density measurement, wash-in/washout study, opposed-phase MRI, or image-guided biopsy, would need to be performed. Adrenal granulomatous diseases are usually bilateral but asymmetrical. Lymphomatous involvement of the adrenal gland is bilateral in 50% of cases; the absence of associated nodal disease in this case makes this diagnosis less likely. Adrenal hematomas may be bilateral, but they do not enhance, and a predisposing factor is typically evident by history. Ten percent of pheochromocytomas are bilateral, but this patient did not have hypertension and lacked biochemical evidence to support this diagnosis.

Clinical History: 87-year-old man presenting with acute back pain.

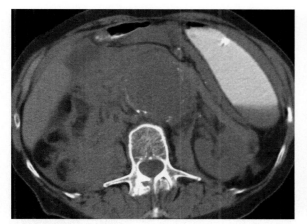

Figure 8.22   A

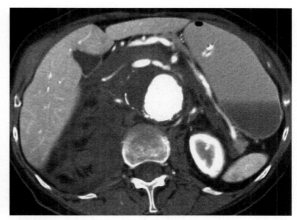

Figure 8.22   B

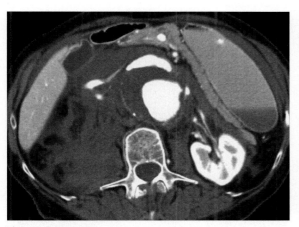

Figure 8.22   C

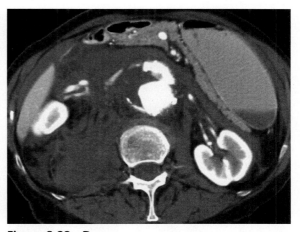

Figure 8.22   D

Findings: Axial NECT image (A) demonstrates a 6.3 × 4.6 cm infrarenal abdominal aortic aneurysm with dense material extending mostly to the right side of the retroperitoneum. Axial CECT images (B–D) show anterior extravasation of intravenous contrast from the aorta.

Differential Diagnosis: None.

Diagnosis: Abdominal aortic aneurysm rupture.

Discussion: Abdominal aortic aneurysms occur in approximately 4% of the population. Most commonly, aneurysms are due to atherosclerosis. Other etiologies include infection, trauma, cystic medial necrosis, and syphilis. CECT is excellent in evaluating aneurysms because it gives not only the size of the lumen but also the outer dimension of the aneurysm as well. CECT can also demonstrate the craniocaudal extent of the aneurysm (suprarenal vs. infrarenal)

and the involved aortic branches. CECT is rarely performed in patients with ruptured aneurysms due to the high mortality rate and the hemodynamic instability of the patient. Untreated aortic aneurysm ruptures have a mortality rate between 50% and 90%. When imaged, however, high-attenuation fluid corresponding to periaortic hemorrhage is present in the para-aortic region, often extending into the perinephric and pararenal spaces. In a patient with an aneurysm, the presence of retroperitoneal hemorrhage, as evidenced by hyperdense material or extravasated contrast, is a surgical emergency. Patients who reach surgery still have a poor prognosis, with less than half surviving for 30 days.

Case images courtesy of Dr. Giovanni Artho, McGill University Health Center, Montreal, Canada.

Clinical History: 42-year-old man presenting with abdominal distention.

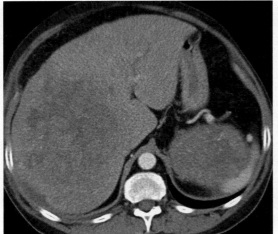

Figure 8.23   A

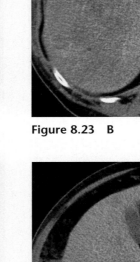

Figure 8.23   B

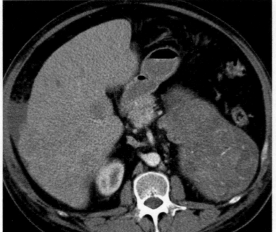

Figure 8.23   C

Figure 8.23   D

Findings: Axial CECT images demonstrate a heterogeneous, 11-cm, left suprarenal mass containing calcifications. The upper pole of the left kidney is involved by the mass. Note large liver masses and small amount of ascites.

Differential Diagnosis: Metastasis, pheochromocytoma, renal cell carcinoma.

Diagnosis: Adrenocortical carcinoma.

Discussion: Adrenal carcinomas arise from the adrenal cortex where hormones, such as cortisol, aldosterone, androgen, and estrogen, are produced. Most adrenal carcinomas produce hormones (most commonly cortisol), but the hormones produced are often not sufficient to cause symptoms. This accounts for the large size of these lesions before they are clinically symptomatic. The tumors are typically larger than 6 cm and can measure up to 20 cm. Adrenal carcinomas are easily seen on CT. They demonstrate enhancement with contrast, but this enhancement is often heterogeneous due to areas of necrosis. Calcifications may be present in 30% of cases. Adrenal carcinomas can invade adjacent organs, such as the liver, spleen, and kidney, as seen in this case. Vascular invasion can also occur into the adrenal vein, which drains into the IVC. The differential diagnosis includes metastases, which are typically smaller, and pheochromocytomas, which are typically clinically symptomatic and thus present when the lesion is much smaller. Because the renal parenchyma is involved, an exophytic primary renal tumor should also be considered in the differential diagnosis. However, the epicenter of the tumor is suprarenal in location, making an adrenal origin more likely. Biopsy of the adrenal gland can easily be performed in most situations to confirm the diagnosis.

Clinical History: 49-year-old woman presenting with back pain and palpable abdominal mass.

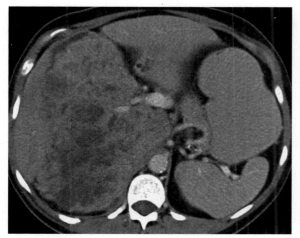

Figure 8.24   A

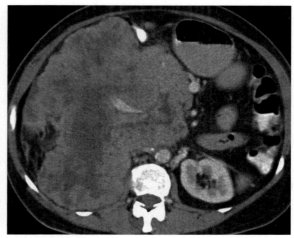

Figure 8.24   B

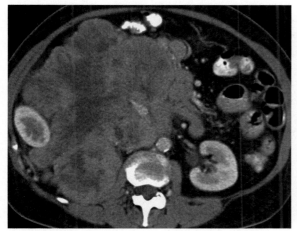

Figure 8.24   C

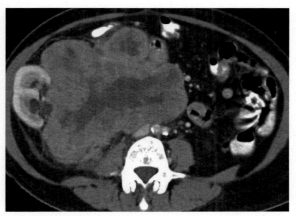

Figure 8.24   D

Findings: Axial CECT images demonstrate a 15.6 × 19.3 cm heterogeneously enhancing retroperitoneal mass. The right kidney is displaced laterally.

Differential Diagnosis: Metastasis, lymphoma, neurogenic tumor.

Diagnosis: Leiomyosarcoma.

Discussion: The majority of primary retroperitoneal tumors are malignant and of mesenchymal origin. The most common are liposarcomas, leiomyosarcomas, and malignant fibrous histiocytomas (MFHs). Leiomyosarcomas are typically large heterogeneous tumors, often with central areas of necrosis. They can occur anywhere in the retroperitoneum and will often grow to be large before being detected. Leiomyosarcomas do not contain fat, which differentiates them from liposarcomas. The heterogeneous appearance on a CECT is typical of a leiomyosarcoma or MFH. This is in contrast to the homogeneous appearance of lymphoma. Large metastases to the retroperitoneum are rare. When they do occur, the primary malignancy is usually melanoma, breast cancer, or lung cancer. Neurogenic tumors are usually homogeneous and low in attenuation. A large heterogeneous mass in the retroperitoneum is most suggestive of a sarcoma.

Clinical History: 55-year-old man presenting with left breast mass.

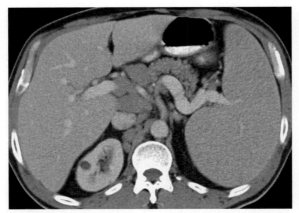

Figure 8.25   A

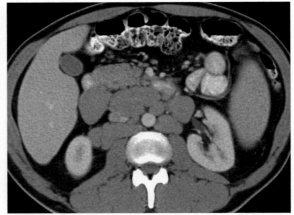

Figure 8.25   B

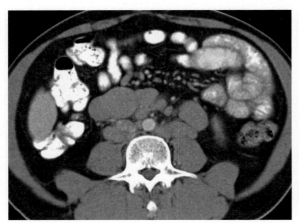

Figure 8.25   C

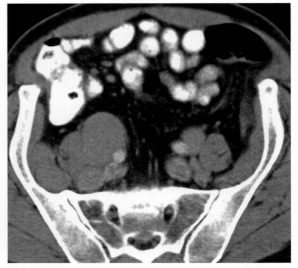

Figure 8.25   D

Findings: Axial CECT images demonstrate enlarged peri-portal, retroperitoneal, and pelvic homogeneous lymph nodes. Note splenomegaly and small right renal cyst.

Differential Diagnosis: Metastatic lymphadenopathy, infectious lymphadenopathy (tuberculosis).

Diagnosis: Non-Hodgkin lymphoma.

Discussion: The majority of patients with non-Hodgkin lymphoma will have abdominal involvement at the time of diagnosis. CT is the imaging modality of choice for evaluating adenopathy. These enlarged lymph nodes can present as discrete masses or as a large confluent mass surrounding and obliterating the retroperitoneal fat planes around the aorta and IVC, as seen in this case. Lymph nodes are measured in the short axis to prevent confusion between two adjacent lymph nodes mistaken for a single enlarged lymph node. Lymph nodes are considered enlarged if they measure greater than 6 mm in the retrocrural region and greater than 10 mm in the para-aortic region. Retroperitoneal adenopathy can be secondary to a variety of causes. Lymphoma is a common etiology, especially if disease is present elsewhere. Enlarged lymph nodes involved by lymphoma are typically of homogeneous soft tissue density. They are rarely necrotic or calcified in the absence of treatment. Metastatic lymphadenopathy from testis, uterus, bladder, and bowel can have a similar appearance. Infectious lymphadenopathy from tuberculosis and MAI are becoming more prevalent due to AIDS- and human immunodeficiency virus (HIV)-related diseases. However, they tend to be of low density due to caseation in mycobacterial infections.

Clinical History: 66-year-old woman with known right pleural mesothelioma.

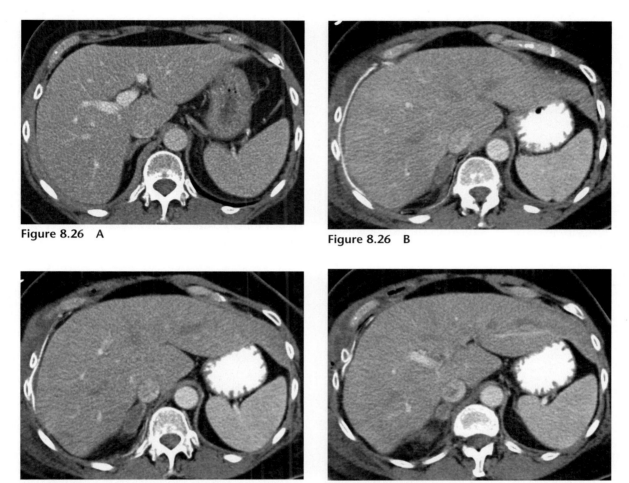

Figure 8.26   A

Figure 8.26   B

Figure 8.26   C

Figure 8.26   D

Findings: Preoperative axial CECT image (A) demonstrates a normal right adrenal gland. Eight days later, postoperative CECT images (B–D) show a new 3.2 × 1.3 cm, low-density, right adrenal lesion with high-density rim and periadrenal fat stranding. Note right diaphragmatic graft.

Differential Diagnosis: Metastasis.

Diagnosis: Acute adrenal hemorrhage.

Discussion: Adrenal hematomas may be traumatic or nontraumatic (due to anticoagulation, stress related to surgery, sepsis, hypotension, or rarely idiopathic) in etiology. Traumatic hemorrhage occurs more commonly on the right side (90%) due to compression of the right adrenal gland between the spine and the liver. Sudden increase in intra-abdominal pressure at the time of the trauma and resultant transmission of that pressure to the adrenal gland also plays a role in development of adrenal hematomas. In the present case, the proximity of the right adrenal gland to the surgical bed (right hemithorax) and stress related to surgery are potential explanations for the adrenal hemorrhage. On CT, the acute or subacute hematoma is initially hyperdense, with a density ranging from 50 to 90 HU. Adrenal hemorrhage has a round or oval configuration in up to 82% of cases but may obliterate the gland in 9% or cause diffuse uniform enlargement in 9%. Gradually, the density of the blood decreases, and the hematoma regresses. On occasion, residual pathologic changes persist in the form of an adrenal pseudocyst. In an oncologic context, adrenal metastasis should always be considered in the differential diagnosis, but a metastasis would not develop into a 3.1-cm lesion in 8 days.

Clinical History: 56-year-old man presenting with back pain.

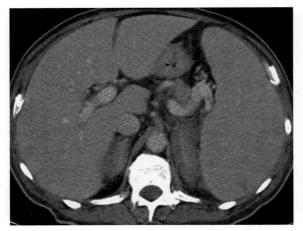

Figure 8.27 A

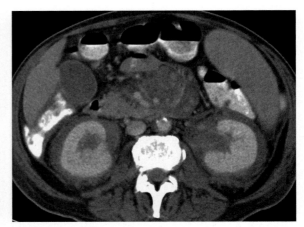

Figure 8.27 B

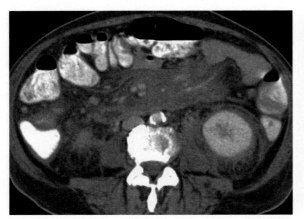

Figure 8.27 C

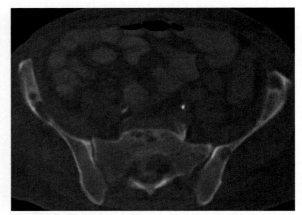

Figure 8.27 D

Findings: Axial CECT images demonstrate abnormal soft tissue surrounding the adrenal glands and kidneys symmetrically and infiltrating the mesentery. Note splenomegaly and lytic lesions in the pelvic bones and sacrum.

Differential Diagnosis: Lymphoma, hemorrhage, amyloidosis, metastasis.

Diagnosis: Langerhans cell histiocytosis.

Discussion: The Langerhans cell normally serves as an antigen-presenting cell. Langerhans cell histiocytosis (LCH) is caused by proliferation of cells similar to the normal Langerhans cell. LCH affects young children between the ages of 1 and 4 years old. Bones and bone marrow are most commonly affected. Lymphadenopathy and soft tissue masses may be encountered. It is rare to see involvement in adults and exceedingly rare to see extravisceral involvement. This has been described in the abdomen as abnormal soft tissue surrounding organs, rather than replacing the organ parenchyma. The main differential diagnosis in this case would be amyloidosis or lymphoma, which can infiltrate the retroperitoneum, especially the perinephric space. It would be unusual for retroperitoneal hemorrhage to be so symmetrical. Additionally, hemorrhage typically occurs in the setting of trauma or anticoagulation or due to an underlying tumor that bled. Metastases infiltrating the retroperitoneum would also be unlikely because they usually present as focal masses. The presence of lytic bone lesions in this case (related to LCH) are nonspecific and could also be caused by lymphoma or metastasis.

Clinical History: 48-year-old woman with a history of breast cancer and melanoma presenting with a left upper quadrant mass.

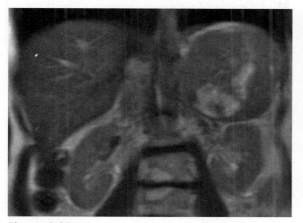

Figure 8.28   A

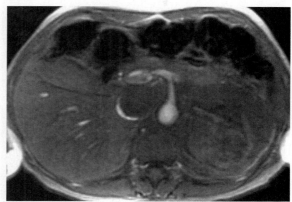

Figure 8.28   B

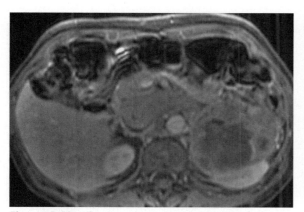

Figure 8.28   C

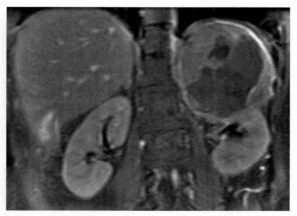

Figure 8.28   D

Findings: Coronal T2-WI (A) shows an 8.6-cm right adrenal mass with areas of necrosis and extension in the IVC. Axial flow-sensitive T2*-WI (B) confirms thrombus in the IVC. Gadolinium-enhanced, fat-suppressed axial (C) and coronal (D) T1-WI show the heterogeneous enhancement of the mass and of the tumor thrombus in the IVC.

Differential Diagnosis: Pheochromocytoma, adrenocortical carcinoma, retroperitoneal sarcoma.

Diagnosis: Adrenal metastasis from melanoma with tumor thrombus.

Discussion: In patients with a primary malignancy of epithelial origin, adrenal gland metastasis is found in 27% of postmortem examinations. The most common primary tumors to metastasize to the adrenal gland originate from the lung, breast, and skin (melanoma). Metastases can be unilateral or bilateral and small or large. On MRI, they are typically hypointense on T1-WI and hyperintense on T2-WI, both of which are nonspecific features. The most important MRI finding is absence of signal dropout on the opposed-phase images. Other large primary adrenal neoplasms, such as pheochromocytomas or adrenocortical carcinoma, may have similar appearance on imaging. A known primary tumor or evidence of metabolic activity is helpful information to know at the time of interpretation of the images and points towards metastasis or pheochromocytomas and adrenocortical carcinoma, respectively. When a normal adrenal gland is not identified, other retroperitoneal masses, such as sarcomas, should be included in the differential diagnosis because a large extra-adrenal tumor may obscure normal adrenal tissue.

Clinical History: 77-year-old woman evaluated for systemic arteritis.

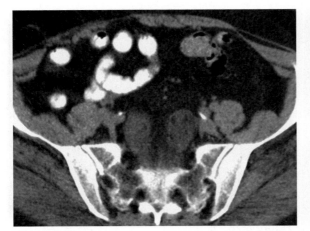

Figure 8.29 A

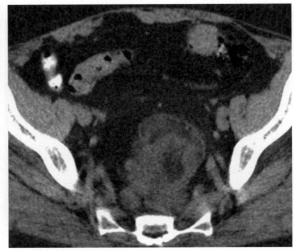

Figure 8.29 B

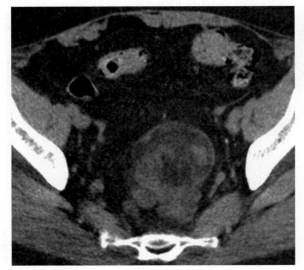

Figure 8.29 C

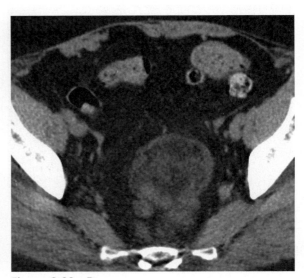

Figure 8.29 D

Findings: Axial NECT images demonstrate a large midline presacral mass containing fat and soft tissue density.

Differential Diagnosis: Liposarcoma, teratoma.

Diagnosis: Retroperitoneal extramedullary hematopoiesis.

Discussion: Extramedullary hematopoiesis (EMH) is a compensatory response for inadequate hematopoiesis by the bone marrow. It can be observed in congenital hemoglobinopathies or acquired marrow disorders, such as leukemia, lymphoma, carcinoma, and myelofibrosis; it is rarely idiopathic. EMH can develop in any tissue of mesenchymal origin. It most commonly occurs in the liver, spleen, and lymph nodes. Small EMH nodules can be encountered in the kidney or fat; larger masses occasionally occur in the pelvis or retroperitoneum. On CT, a solid, hyperdense, round or lobulated, soft tissue mass is classically identified. Varying amounts of fat may also be present in the mass, and this may reflect fatty transformation due to disappearance of the factor promoting the EMH. Without a history of chronic anemia or bone marrow disease, it is difficult to differentiate EMH from a neoplasm, especially from liposarcoma or teratoma, when macroscopic fat is identified. The correct diagnosis can be made by image-guided percutaneous biopsy, as was performed in this case, or nuclear medicine sulfur colloid scan.

Clinical History: 60-year-old woman presenting with fever and severe hypotension.

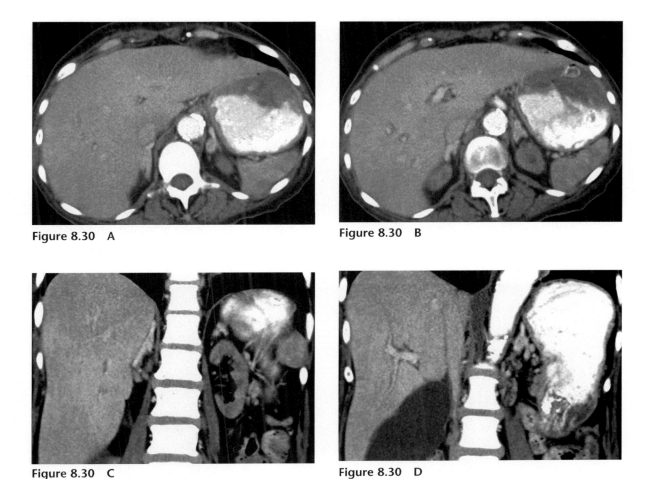

Figure 8.30   A

Figure 8.30   B

Figure 8.30   C

Figure 8.30   D

Findings: Axial (A and B) and coronal (C and D) CECT images demonstrate hyperenhancement of both adrenal glands. Note small left adrenal adenoma.

Differential Diagnosis: Hemorrhage.

Diagnosis: Intense adrenal gland enhancement in a patient in septic shock.

Discussion: In patients with hypoperfusion, multiple mechanisms try to maintain adequate blood supply to vital organs through selective vasospasm. Among those are the adrenal glands, in view of the role they play in sympathetic response to shock. This is manifested by symmetrical intense contrast enhancement of both adrenal glands, which is almost as intense as the surrounding vascular structures, as seen in this case. This finding, seen as part of the hypoperfusion complex, has been associated with significant mortality in children with posttraumatic shock. Normally the adrenal glands enhance to the same degree as the other solid abdominal organs. Adrenal hemorrhage may be seen in patients with sepsis and manifest itself by increased density of the adrenal glands. However, the morphology of the gland is altered because adrenal hematomas are round or oval; periadrenal fat stranding is also typically associated.

Clinical History: 27-year-old woman presenting with left flank pain.

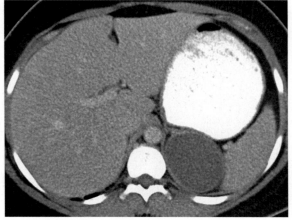

Figure 8.31   A

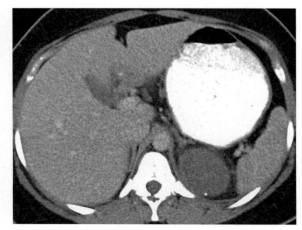

Figure 8.31   B

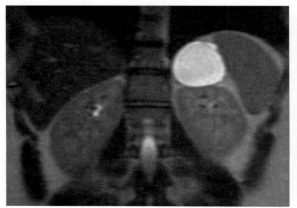

Figure 8.31   C

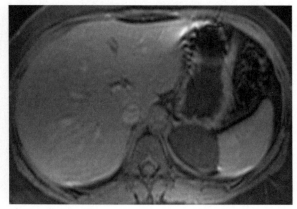

Figure 8.31   D

Findings: Axial CECT images (A and B) show a 5.5 × 4.4 × 4.6 cm left adrenal lesion with peripheral calcifications. Its density measures 28 HU. Coronal T2-WI (C) and gadolinium-enhanced, fat-suppressed axial T1-WI (D) show that the lesion is a unilocular cyst with no enhancement.

Differential Diagnosis: Endothelial cyst, epithelial cyst, parasitic cyst, gastric fundal diverticulum.

Diagnosis: Adrenal pseudocyst.

Discussion: Adrenal cysts are rare and usually found in patients between 20 and 50 years of age. Most are asymptomatic, but symptoms may be produced by hemorrhage, rupture, or infection. Four types of cysts have been described according to histologic findings: endothelial cysts, pseudocysts, epithelial cysts, and parasitic cysts. Endothelial cysts are the most common subtype, accounting for 45% of all adrenal cysts; the lining may be lymphangiomatous or angiomatous in origin. Adrenal pseudocysts are probably due to previous hemorrhage into a normal adrenal gland, have a fibrous wall, and account for 39% of adrenal cysts. Their wall is of varying thickness and may contain calcifications, as seen in this case. Their internal structure may be complex with septations or soft tissue due to hyalinized thrombus. The density of the cyst may be higher than simple fluid due to proteinaceous content, as seen in the present case. After neuroblastomas, adrenal pseudocysts are the second most common adrenal lesion to contain calcifications. Parasitic cysts are typically due to *Echinococcus granulosus*. Epithelial cysts are extremely uncommon. All of these cysts may have a similar appearance at imaging. A fundal gastric diverticulum, which usually originates posteriorly, may project into the left adrenal region. However, continuity of the diverticulum wall with the stomach wall and a separate normal left adrenal gland should be identified at imaging.

Clinical History: 51-year-old man presenting with hypertension and weight loss.

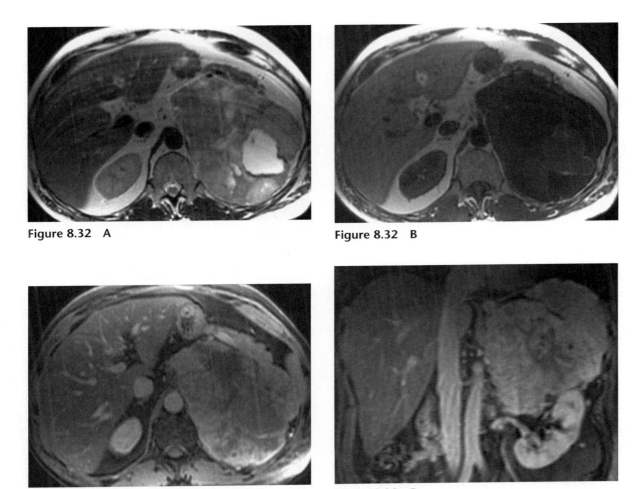

Figure 8.32   A

Figure 8.32   B

Figure 8.32   C

Figure 8.32   D

Findings: Axial T2-WI (A), axial T1-WI (B), and gadolinium-enhanced, fat-suppressed axial (C) and coronal T1-WI (D) demonstrate a 16.3 × 16.3 × 14.7 cm heterogeneous left adrenal mass. Areas of necrosis and hemorrhage (T1 bright foci) are present in the mass.

Differential Diagnosis: Metastasis, pheochromocytoma.

Diagnosis: Adrenocortical carcinoma.

Discussion: Adrenocortical carcinomas are rare tumors, occurring once in every million patients. Affected patients are usually between 30 and 70 years of age. Up to 50% are hyperfunctional, producing either Cushing disease (glucocorticoid production) or Conn syndrome (mineralocorticoid production). Tumors are typically large at diagnosis, measuring 6 cm or greater. On MRI, lesions are heterogeneous on both T1-WI and T2-WI due to intratumoral necrosis and hemorrhage. Areas of high signal intensity on T1-WI are due to blood byproduct methemoglobin or sometimes calcifications, which are present in 30% of tumors. Rarely, adrenocortical carcinomas may contain intracytoplasmic lipid, producing areas of signal dropout on opposed-phase images. Unlike in a small adrenal lesion containing microscopic fat, histologic correlation should be obtained for larger lesions (>5 cm) with fat. Adrenocortical carcinomas are aggressive neoplasms that may invade adjacent organs or vascular structures, producing tumor thrombus. Pheochromocytoma or metastasis can attain large size but are typically smaller. Knowledge of the clinical context (e.g., hypertension, signs of adrenal hyperfunction, known primary malignancy) is helpful in limiting the differential diagnosis and determining management.

Clinical History: 32-year-old woman presenting with back pain radiating down the left leg.

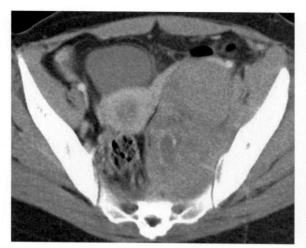

Figure 8.33   A

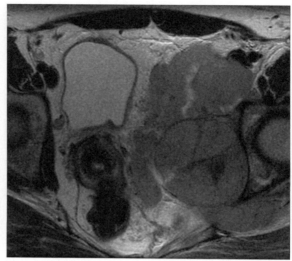

Figure 8.33   B

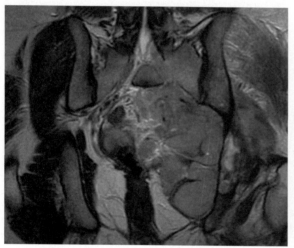

Figure 8.33   C

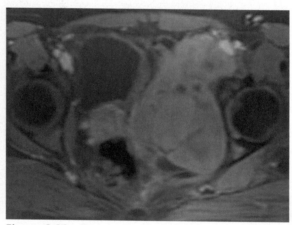

Figure 8.33   D

Findings: Axial CECT image (A) demonstrates a 16 × 13 × 7 cm left pelvic mass with areas of central decreased density. Axial (B) and coronal (C) T2-WI and gadolinium-enhanced, fat-suppressed axial T1-WI (D) show the predominantly solid mass extends into the left S1 sacral foramen and along the left sciatic nerve.

Differential Diagnosis: Nerve sheath tumor, sarcoma, metastasis, ovarian tumor.

Diagnosis: Non-Hodgkin lymphoma.

Discussion: Most lymphomas present as masses and enlarged lymph nodes of homogeneous soft tissue density. Heterogeneity, either due to necrotic areas or calcifications, is typically seen secondary to treatment effect. However, aggressive lymphomas may occasionally demonstrate calcifications or necrosis in the absence of treatment. Given the extension along neurologic structures seen in this case, metastasis, sarcoma, and particularly a nerve sheath tumor are excellent diagnostic choices. Ovarian neoplasms should always be considered when a large pelvic mass is seen in a young female. However, the direct extension into the sacral foramen and along the sciatic nerve virtually excludes this diagnosis because ovaries are intraperitoneal structures. The next step should be an image-guided percutaneous biopsy, as was performed in this case.

Clinical History: 64-year-old man presenting with right lower quadrant pain.

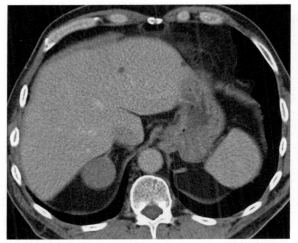

Figure 8.34   A

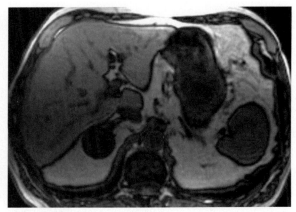

Figure 8.34   B

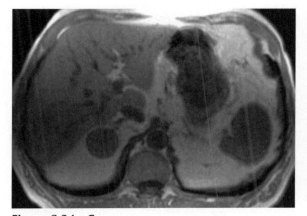

Figure 8.34   C

Figure 8.34   D

Findings: Axial CECT image (A) shows a 3.5 × 3.5 cm right adrenal mass that has an attenuation of 47 HU. It is isointense to the liver parenchyma on the coronal T2-WI (B) and in-phase T1-WI (C). On the opposed-phase T1-WI (D), it demonstrates homogeneous signal dropout.

Differential Diagnosis: Metastasis, pheochromocytoma, adrenocortical carcinoma.

Diagnosis: Lipid-rich adrenal adenoma.

Discussion: An incidentally discovered adrenal mass is seen in up to 5% of abdominal CT scans. On NECT, an adrenal mass with an attenuation value of less than 10 HU is very specific for an adenoma. However, because most abdominal CT scans are performed after intravenous contrast administration only, the adrenal masses enhance and have a density greater than 10 HU. To determine if such a lesion is an adenoma or not, one can look for stability over time, perform an adrenal washout CT study, or perform an MRI with in- and opposed-phase imaging. Chemical shift MRI takes advantage of the different resonance frequencies of fat and water protons. Because adrenal adenomas contain intracytoplasmic lipid, signal drop is expected on the opposed-phase images, when lipid and water protons have dephased. Visual analysis (sensitivity = 78%, specificity = 87%) has similar accuracy to detect loss of signal on the opposed-phase images compared with quantitative methods (using an adjacent tissue as internal reference for calculations). If an adrenal mass does not demonstrate signal dropout using chemical shift MRI, it may still represent an adenoma, albeit lipid-poor type, or another type of adrenal mass. At that time, especially if the patient has a known primary tumor, imaged-guided biopsy or an adrenal washout CT study may be performed.

CASE 8-35

Clinical History: 70-year-old woman presenting with weakness and fatigue.

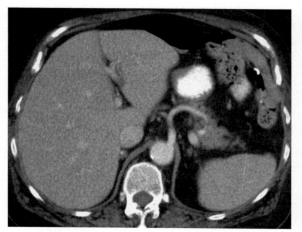

Figure 8.35   A

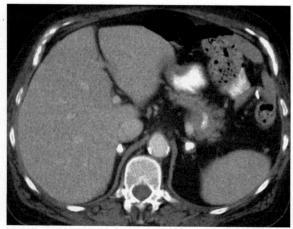

Figure 8.35   B

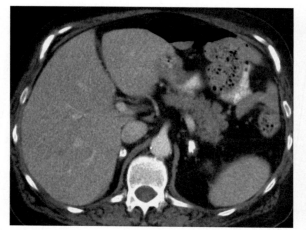

Figure 8.35   C

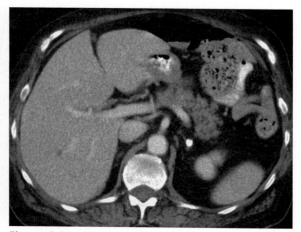

Figure 8.35   D

Findings: Axial CECT images demonstrate bilateral dense adrenal calcifications and atrophy of the adrenal gland limbs.

Differential Diagnosis: None.

Diagnosis: Adrenal calcifications in a patient with adrenal insufficiency.

Discussion: Adrenal insufficiency becomes clinically symptomatic when 90% of adrenal cortex is destroyed. The most common cause of adrenal insufficiency is idiopathic (Addison disease), probably due to an autoimmune process. In such a case, the adrenal glands appear atrophied, to the point where the adrenal parenchyma may be barely perceptible at imaging. The adrenal glands are not calcified in Addison disease. The second most common cause of adrenal insufficiency is prior granulomatous infection, more often tuberculosis (TB) than histoplasmosis. In TB, adrenal calcifications are present in 50% of cases. However, adrenal calcifications not associated with a mass are nonspecific and may also be idiopathic or be the result of prior adrenal hemorrhage. Other less frequent causes of adrenal insufficiency include bilateral adrenal metastases and postpartum hemorrhage.

Clinical History: 26-year-old man presenting with abdominal pain, weight loss, and night sweats.

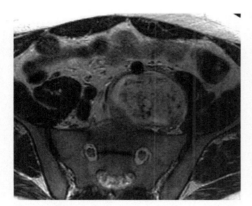

Figure 8.36 A

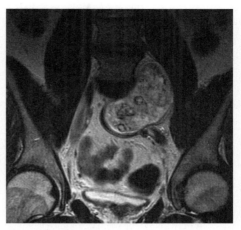

Figure 8.36 B

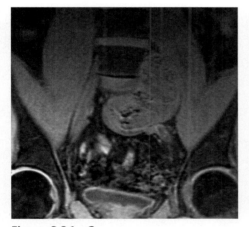

Figure 8.36 C

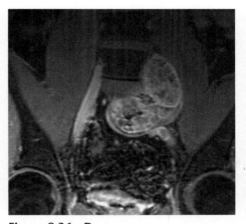

Figure 8.36 D

Findings: Axial and coronal T2-WI (A and B) show an 8.9 × 7.4 × 5.3 cm heterogeneous retroperitoneal mass with several hypointense rounded foci surrounded by hyperintensity. Unenhanced (C) and gadolinium-enhanced (D) fat-suppressed coronal T1-WI show heterogeneous enhancement of the mass.

Differential Diagnosis: Neurofibroma, sarcoma, metastasis, lymphoma, tuberculosis.

Diagnosis: Retroperitoneal schwannoma.

Discussion: Schwannomas are benign nerve sheath tumors arising from the Schwann cells. They represent 6% of all primary retroperitoneal neoplasms. They occur between 25 and 65 years of age. Because they are slow-growing tumors, they cause symptoms due to mass effect only when they reach a large size. Schwannomas are rarely multiple, and malignant degeneration is extremely rare. Imaging features of schwannomas overlap with those of neurofibromas. On MRI, the rounded low signal intensity foci surrounded by a background of hyperintensity (fascicular sign), as seen in this case, can be present in cases of nerve sheath tumors and is reminiscent of the normal fascicular structure of a nerve. Identification of a nerve entering and exiting the mass at each end is a specific sign for a nerve sheath tumor when present. Retroperitoneal sarcomas or metastases may become large and may or may not have areas of necrosis. Image-guided percutaneous biopsy helps to establish a preoperative diagnosis, as was preformed in this case. Retroperitoneal lymphomas, in the absence of treatment, are usually of homogeneous density, even when large.

Clinical History: 28-year-old woman with palpable mass on pelvic examination.

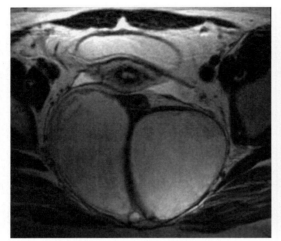

Figure 8.37 A

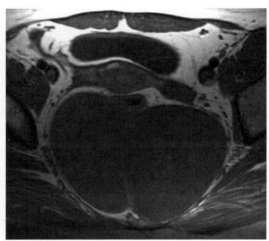

Figure 8.37 B

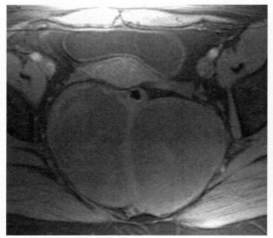

Figure 8.37 C

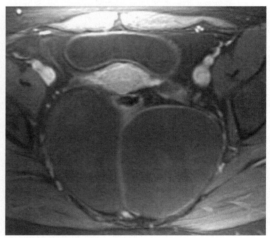

Figure 8.37 D

Findings: Axial T2-WI (A), axial T1-WI (B), and unenhanced (C) and gadolinium-enhanced (D) fat-suppressed T1-WI demonstrate a 13.1 × 9.2 cm bilocular retrorectal cyst with thin peripheral enhancement of the left locule. Note trace of physiologic pelvis free fluid.

Differential Diagnosis: Enteric cyst, epidermoid cyst, neurenteric cyst.

Diagnosis: Dermoid cyst.

Discussion: Retrorectal developmental cysts in adults are usually congenital and occur most commonly in middle-aged females. There are four types: epidermoid cysts, dermoid cysts, enteric cysts (which include tailgut cysts and cystic rectal duplication), and neurenteric cysts. They are typically asymptomatic, but patients may present with pressure symptoms or dysuria or because of complications.

At imaging, the cysts are difficult to distinguish from each other; they present as unilocular or multilocular thin-walled cysts. Rarely, calcifications (seen with tailgut or dermoid cysts) or sacral bone defects may be encountered. When the cysts become complicated, they may contain gas (anorectal fistulization), blood products (bleeding), or soft tissue components (malignant degeneration in up to 7%) or have thick walls and surrounding fat stranding (infection seen in 30–50% of cases). In cases of neurenteric cysts, a communication with the subarachnoid space may be demonstrated. Treatment consists of surgical excision to establish a definitive diagnosis and prevent complications. Other retrorectal cystic lesions include lymphangiomas, sacrococcygeal teratomas (seen in the pediatric population), anterior sacral meningoceles, and abscesses.

Clinical History: 53-year-old woman presenting with right leg swelling.

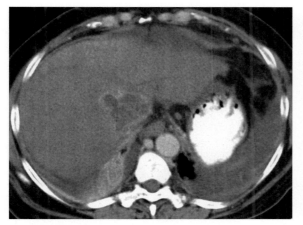

Figure 8.38 A

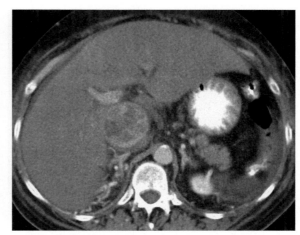

Figure 8.38 B

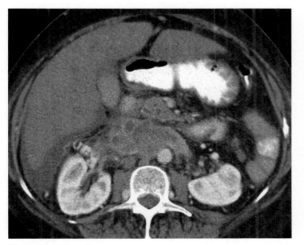

Figure 8.38 C

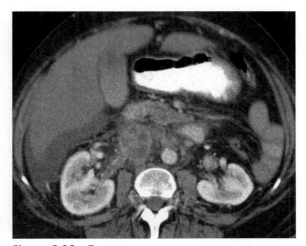

Figure 8.38 D

Findings: Axial CECT images demonstrate an enhancing mass in the IVC, distending the vessel lumen and extending into the hepatic and renal veins. Note ascites and retroperitoneal collateral vessels.

Differential Diagnosis: IVC invasion from renal cell carcinoma, hepatocellular carcinoma, or adrenocortical carcinoma.

Diagnosis: Leiomyosarcoma of IVC.

Discussion: Vascular leiomyosarcomas originate from the smooth muscle within a vessel. Primary leiomyosarcomas of IVC have two growth patterns: predominantly extravascular (73%) or intravascular (23%). The majority of leiomyosarcomas involve the IVC between the renal veins and its retrohepatic segment. There is a 5:1 female-to-male predominance. CT and MRI are helpful in delineating the intra- and extravascular extent of the tumor. In cases of tumor thrombus in the IVC, evaluation of the solid organs is important because many primary tumors from the kidneys (e.g., renal cell carcinoma, Wilms tumor), liver (e.g., hepatocellular carcinoma, cholangiocarcinoma, metastasis), adrenal glands (e.g., adrenocortical carcinoma, pheochromocytoma, metastasis), uterus (e.g., intravenous leiomyomatosis), or retroperitoneal lymph nodes (e.g., lymphoma, metastasis) may secondarily invade the IVC.

Clinical History: 29-year-old woman presenting with hypertension.

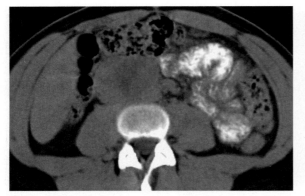

Figure 8.39   A

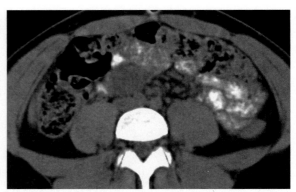

Figure 8.39   B

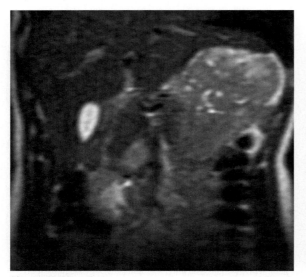

Figure 8.39   C

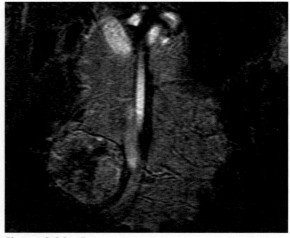

Figure 8.39   D

Findings: Axial NECT images (A and B) demonstrate a 3.9 × 5.3 cm soft tissue mass with low density center located anterior to the abdominal aorta. Coronal T2-WI (C) shows the mass has higher signal intensity than the liver with a necrotic center, confirmed by absence of central enhancement on the gadolinium-enhanced, fat-suppressed coronal T1-WI (D).

Differential Diagnosis: Metastasis, sarcoma, neurogenic tumor, lymphoma.

Diagnosis: Paraganglioma of the organs of Zuckerkandl.

Discussion: A paraganglioma is a pheochromocytoma arising from the extra-adrenal sympathetic nervous system. Symptoms are related to excess catecholamine release and consist of paroxysmal hypertension, sweating, headache, palpitations, and facial pallor or flushing. The most sensitive test (99%) to detect these tumors is the plasma free metanephrine level, whereas the most specific test (95%) is urinary VMA, the major metabolic product of catecholamines. The organs of Zuckerkandl are paraganglionic tissues along the aorta, extending from the level of the superior mesenteric arteries or renal arteries to just beyond the aortic bifurcation. On CT, the paragangliomas appear as soft tissue masses with no distinguishing features. On MRI, they typically have a higher signal intensity than the liver, although a significant number do not. Treatment consists of surgical excision. Besides lymphoma, which typically has a homogeneous appearance, metastasis, sarcoma, and neurogenic tumor may have the same appearance as a paraganglioma. Knowledge of the clinical history (e.g., hypertension, known primary malignancy) may help narrow the differential diagnosis.

Clinical History: 66-year-old man with history of right nephrectomy for renal cell carcinoma.

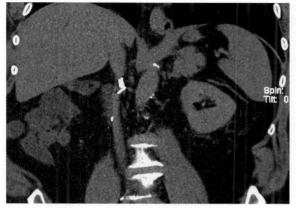

Figure 8.40 A

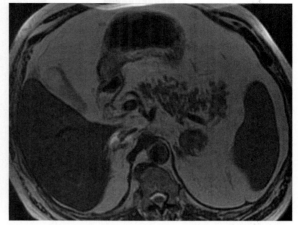

Figure 8.40 B

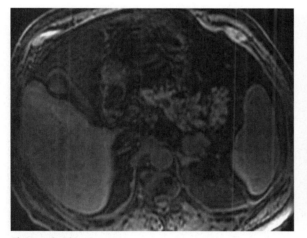

Figure 8.40 C

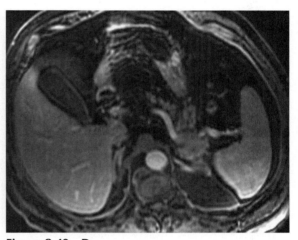

Figure 8.40 D

Findings: Coronal reformatted CECT image (A) demonstrates a 3.9 × 3.3 cm left suprarenal homogeneous mass with spiculated margins. Axial T2-WI (B) and fat-suppressed axial T1-WI before (C) and after (D) injection of gadolinium shows the infiltrative margins of the solid enhancing mass, which is separate from the adrenal gland.

Differential Diagnosis: Metastasis from renal cell carcinoma, sarcoma.

Diagnosis: Desmoid tumor.

Discussion: Desmoid tumors are benign tumors composed of fibrous tissue. Their estimated incidence is 3.7 new cases per million patients per year. In the abdomen, they commonly occur in the mesentery, but they are also found in the retroperitoneum and abdominal wall. Although benign, they can have an invasive behavior. In this case, this is manifested by the spiculated, infiltrative margins of the tumor. At surgery, invasion of the pancreatic tail and left adrenal gland was identified. Desmoid tumors may be homogeneous or heterogeneous and have well-circumscribed or infiltrative margins. On MRI, the tumors have low signal intensity on T1-WI and variable signal intensity on T2-WI. Metastatic nodules and retroperitoneal sarcomas, when small, tend to have well-defined margins.

Clinical History: 59-year-old woman with acute onset of left upper quadrant pain 1 month ago.

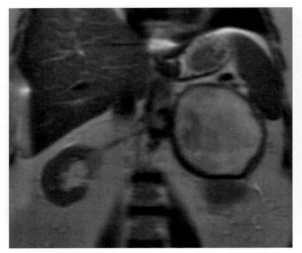

Figure 8.41   A

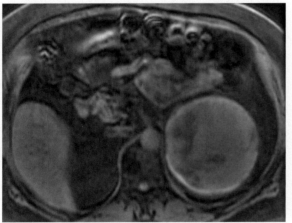

Figure 8.41   C

Figure 8.41   B

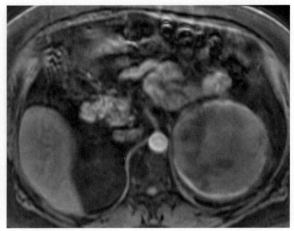

Figure 8.41   D

Findings: Coronal T2-WI (A) and opposed-phase T1-WI (B) demonstrate an 11.2 × 10.8 × 10.6 cm, heterogeneously hyperintense, left adrenal lesion with a hypointense rim. Unenhanced (C) and gadolinium-enhanced (D) fat-suppressed T1-WI show absence of enhancement in the mass.

Differential Diagnosis: Myelolipoma, pheochromocytoma.

Diagnosis: Idiopathic adrenal hemorrhage.

Discussion: In case of spontaneous adrenal hemorrhage, an underlying lesion, such as a cyst, adenoma, hemangioma, myelolipoma, or metastasis, is often identified at imaging. In rare instances, the hemorrhage may be idiopathic. On MRI, the appearance of the hematoma depends on the age of the blood products. In this case, the predominant hyperintensity on the T1-WI and T2-WI is a reflection of methemoglobin, indicating that the hemorrhage is subacute. Excluding an underlying lesion is best done by contrast-enhanced imaging. Follow-up MRI should be obtained to document gradual resolution of the hematoma and to exclude an underlying mass. Adrenal hemorrhages may completely resolve or form an adrenal pseudocyst. A myelolipoma may have hyperintense areas on both T1-WI and T2-WI because of fat. However, these fat-containing areas should decrease in signal intensity on the fat-suppressed images, which was not observed in this case. Pheochromocytomas may be hyperintense on the T2-WI but tend to be hypointense on T1-WI.

Clinical History: 20-year-old woman presenting with abdominal pain and difficulty walking.

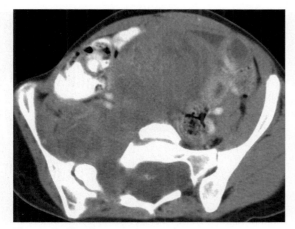

Figure 8.42   A

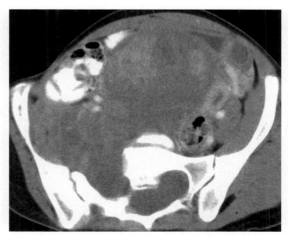

Figure 8.42   B

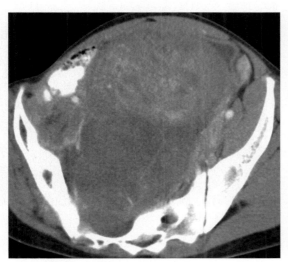

Figure 8.42   C

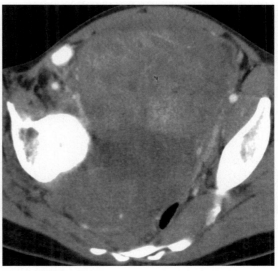

Figure 8.42   D

Findings: Axial CECT images demonstrate a 13.6 × 17.8 cm heterogeneous retroperitoneal pelvic mass. Note extensive bone remodeling with expansion of the sacral foramen and spinal canal.

Differential Diagnosis: Leiomyosarcoma, neurofibroma, schwannoma.

Diagnosis: Malignant peripheral nerve sheath tumor.

Discussion: Malignant peripheral nerve sheath tumors (MPNSTs) occur in the setting of neurofibromatosis type 1 (NF1) in up to 70% of cases. Most patients with sporadic MPNSTs are between 20 and 50 years of age at the time of diagnosis, but in patients with NF1, MPNSTs occur a decade earlier. MPNSTs typically arise from the sciatic nerve, brachial plexus, and sacral plexus. Pain and neurologic deficits are the common presenting symptoms. By imaging, it is difficult to distinguish a benign from a malignant peripheral nerve sheath tumor. However, infiltrative borders, internal heterogeneity, and rapid growth are more suggestive of malignancy. Treatment consists of surgery followed by chemotherapy and radiotherapy. Despite this, local recurrence occurs in 50% of patients. Other sarcomas could have similar radiologic appearance, but involvement of the spinal canal suggests a neurogenic process.

Clinical History: 73-year-old man presenting with a complaint of having a "rounder face" and found to have hyperglycemia.

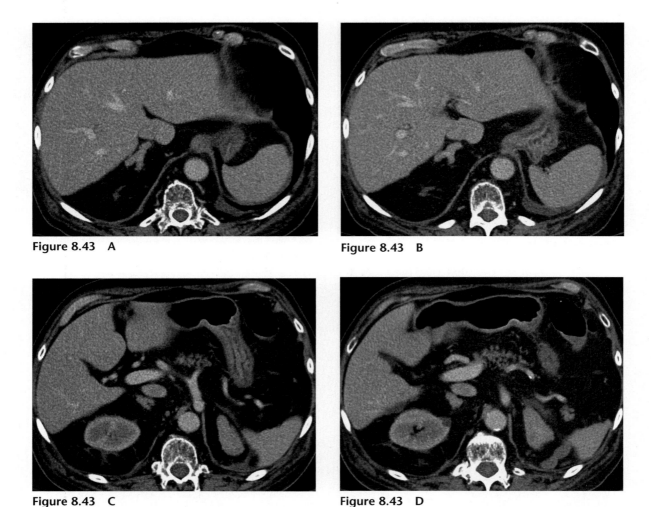

Figure 8.43 A

Figure 8.43 B

Figure 8.43 C

Figure 8.43 D

Findings: Axial CECT images demonstrate smooth enlargement of both adrenal glands, with the left gland being greater than the right.

Differential Diagnosis: Conn syndrome, hemorrhage, stress-induced adrenal hyperplasia, normal adrenal aging.

Diagnosis: Cushing syndrome due to adrenal hyperplasia.

Discussion: Cushing syndrome is caused by excess glucocorticoid production, either endogenous or exogenous. Seventy percent of cases are caused by overproduction of adrenocorticotropic hormone (ACTH) by a pituitary adenoma (Cushing disease) or ACTH-producing tumors (such as bronchial carcinoid or small-cell lung cancer). Benign functioning adenoma (20%) and adrenocortical carcinoma (10%) cause the remainder of cases. The enlarged limbs of the adrenal glands, due to overstimulation by ACTH, may be smooth or can become nodular. Conn syndrome, due to excess mineralocorticoid production, is caused by an adrenal adenoma in 70% of cases. However, some cases may be produced by adrenal hyperplasia. Other causes of adrenal hyperplasia may be stress related due to physiologic release of ACTH or related to the normal aging process of the adrenal glands. Adrenal hemorrhage can be bilateral, but usually causes a masslike lesion in the adrenal gland with surrounding fat stranding; both features were absent in the present case.

CASE 8-44

Clinical History: 19-year-old man presenting with intermittent abdominal pain.

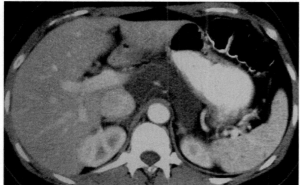

Figure 8.44 A

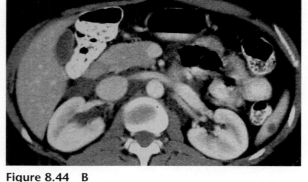

Figure 8.44 B

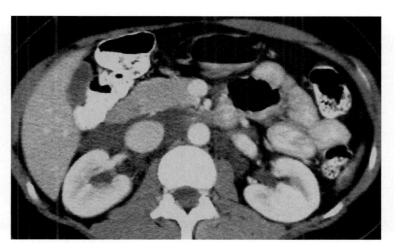

Figure 8.44 C

Findings: Axial CECT images demonstrate an infiltrating retroperitoneal cystic lesion surrounding multiple vascular structures. Note small cystic lesion in the spleen.

Differential Diagnosis: Cystic mesothelioma, pseudocyst, hematoma.

Diagnosis: Lymphangioma.

Discussion: Lymphangiomas are congenital benign neoplasms. They occur because of failure of several lymphatic channels to establish normal communication with the rest of the lymphatics. Lymphangiomas are more common in males than females. The vast majority occur in the head and neck region; they occur rarely in the retroperitoneum. At imaging, they are multilocular cystic lesions with thin walls. They may cross between one retroperitoneal space to another, which is a characteristic finding. Other multilocular retroperitoneal cystic lesions include cystic mesotheliomas, pseudocysts, and hematomas. Cystic mesotheliomas are rare benign mesothelial tumors more commonly seen in females and more commonly occurring along peritoneal surfaces than in the retroperitoneum. Pseudocysts, which may be pancreatic or nonpancreatic, may be multilocular, but a clinical history of recent acute pancreatitis or infection is often present. A retroperitoneal hematoma starts liquefying soon after its development and may give rise to multifocal or multilocular cystic-appearing lesions.

Clinical History: 76-year-old man with history of acute myelogenous leukemia and recent hematocrit drop.

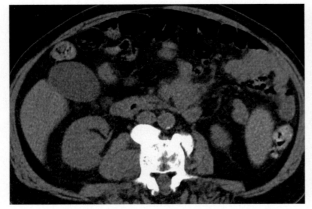

Figure 8.45   A

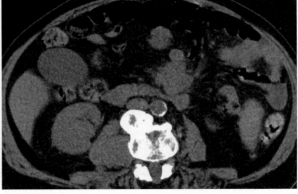

Figure 8.45   B

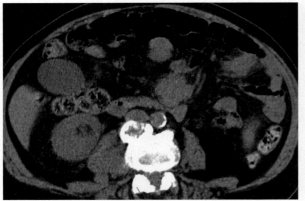

Figure 8.45   C

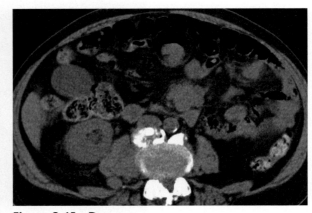

Figure 8.45   D

Findings: Axial NECT images demonstrate a 3.4 × 3.6 cm homogeneous mass medial to right psoas muscle. Note mesenteric mass and smaller nodule posterior to the right psoas muscle.

Differential Diagnosis: Lymphoma, nerve sheath tumor, hemorrhage.

Diagnosis: Granulocytic sarcoma (chloroma).

Discussion: Granulocytic sarcomas are tumors composed of granulocytic precursors or white blood cells. They were initially called chloromas because of the green color of myeloperoxidase, but they were later renamed granulocytic sarcomas because 30% do not have that characteristic color. Granulocytic sarcomas are classically associated with acute myelogenous leukemia, but they may also been seen in other myeloproliferative disorders, such as chronic myelogenous leukemia, myelofibrosis, or polycythemia vera. Granulocytic sarcomas more commonly occur in children than in adults. They may precede or occur after the myeloproliferative disorder. Because granulocytic sarcomas are often asymptomatic, 50% of cases are diagnosed only at autopsy. On CT, they appear as homogeneous soft tissue masses with only minimal enhancement after injection of intravenous contrast. Lymphomas may present similarly as multiple soft tissue masses of homogeneous density. A paraspinal mass medial to the psoas muscle could be of neurogenic origin and could have a similar appearance, especially because nerve sheath tumors may be multifocal. Patients with leukemia may be prone to hemorrhage. Although multifocal bleeds are possible, hemorrhages are surrounded by fat stranding, and such a finding was not present in this case.

SUGGESTED READINGS

NEOPLASMS

- Agrons GA, Lonergan GJ, Dickey GE, et al. From the archives of the AFIP: adrenocortical neoplasms in children: radiologic-pathologic correlation. *Radiographics* 1999;19:989–1008.

- Alfuhaid TR, Khalili K, Kirpalani A, et al. Neoplasms of the inferior vena cava—pictorial essay. *Can Assoc Radiol J.* 2005;56:140–147.

- Apter S, Avigdor A, Gayer G, et al. Calcification in lymphoma occurring before therapy: CT features and clinical correlation. *Am J Roentgenol.* 2002;178:935–938.

- Beaman FD, Kransdorf MJ, Menke DM. Schwannoma: radiologic-pathologic correlation. *Radiographics* 2004;24:1477–1481.

- Caoili EM, Korobkin M, Francis IR, et al. Adrenal masses: characterization with combined unenhanced and delayed enhanced CT. *Radiology* 2002;222:629–633.

- Cyran KM, Kenney PJ, Memel DS, et al. Adrenal myelolipoma. *Am J Roentgenol.* 1996;166:395–400.

- Dunnick NR, Korobkin M. Imaging of adrenal incidentalomas: current status. *Am J Roentgenol.* 2002;179:559–568.

- Elsayes KM, Mukundan G, Narra VR, et al. Adrenal masses: MR imaging features with pathologic correlation. *Radiographics* 2004;24:S73–S86.

- Elsayes KM, Narra VR, Leyendecker JR, et al. MRI of adrenal and extraadrenal pheochromocytoma. *Am J Roentgenol.* 2005;184:860–867.

- Faria SC, Iyer RB, Rashid A, et al. Desmoid tumor of the small bowel and the mesentery. *Am J Roentgenol.* 2004;183:118.

- Getachew MM, Whitman GJ, Chew FS. Retroperitoneal schwannoma. *Am J Roentgenol.* 1994;163:1356.

- Guermazi A, Feger C, Rousselot P, et al. Granulocytic sarcoma (chloroma): imaging findings in adults and children. *Am J Roentgenol.* 2002;178:319–325.

- Hartman DS, Hayes WS, Choyke PL, et al. From the archives of the AFIP. Leiomyosarcoma of the retroperitoneum and inferior vena cava: radiologic-pathologic correlation. *Radiographics* 1992;12:1203–1220.

- Hrehorovich PA, Franke HR, Maximin S, et al. Malignant peripheral nerve sheath tumor. *Radiographics* 2003;23:790–794.

- Israel GM, Bosniak MA, Slywotzky CM, et al. CT differentiation of large exophytic renal angiomyolipomas and perirenal liposarcomas. *Am J Roentgenol.* 2002;179:769–773.

- Israel GM, Korobkin M, Wang C, et al. Comparison of unenhanced CT and chemical shift MRI in evaluating lipid-rich adrenal adenomas. *Am J Roentgenol.* 2004;183:215–219.

- Jee WH, Oh SN, McCauley T, et al. Extraaxial neurofibromas versus neurilemmomas: discrimination with MRI. *Am J Roentgenol.* 2004;183:629–633.

- Korobkin M. CT characterization of adrenal masses: the time has come. *Radiology* 2000;217:629–632.

- Lane RH, Stephens DH, Reiman HM. Primary retroperitoneal neoplasms: CT findings in 90 cases with clinical and pathologic correlation. *Am J Roentgenol.* 1989;152:83–89.

- Lonergan GJ, Schwab CM, Suarez ES, et al. From the archives of the AFIP: neuroblastoma, ganglioneuroblastoma, and ganglioneuroma: radiologic-pathologic correlation. *Radiographics* 2002;22:911–934.

- Meyer JS, Harty MP, Mahboubi S, et al. Langerhans cell histiocytosis: presentation and evolution of radiologic findings with clinical correlation. *Radiographics* 1995;15:1135–1146.

- Mortelé K, Lemmerling M, Defreyne L, et al. Ossified retroperitoneal malignant schwannoma with spinal leptomeningeal metastases. *Neuroradiology* 1998;40:48–50.

- Mourad K, Katz D, Paradinas FJ. Extravisceral diffuse infiltration of adult histiocytosis X demonstrated by CT. *Br J Radiol.* 1983;56:879–881.

- Murphey MD, Arcara LK, Fanburg-Smith J. From the archives of the AFIP: imaging of musculoskeletal liposarcoma with radiologic-pathologic correlation. *Radiographics* 2005;25:1371–1395.

- Murphey MD, Smith WS, Smith SE, et al. From the archives of the AFIP: imaging of musculoskeletal neurogenic tumors: radiologic-pathologic correlation. *Radiographics* 1999;19:1253–1280.

- Pomeranz SJ, Hawkins HH, Towbin R, et al. Granulocytic sarcoma (chloroma): CT manifestations. *Radiology* 1985;155:167–170.

- Radin R, David CL, Goldfarb H, et al. Adrenal and extra-adrenal retroperitoneal ganglioneuroma: imaging findings in 13 adults. *Radiology* 1997;202:703–707.

- Saurborn DS, Kruskal JB, Stillman IE, et al. Best cases from the AFIP: paraganglioma of the organs of Zuckerkandl. *Radiographics* 2003;23:1279–1286.

- Scatarige JC, Fishman EK, Kuhajda FP, et al. Low attenuation nodal metastases in testicular carcinoma. *J Comput Assist Tomogr.* 1982;7:682–687.

- Siegelman SS. Taking the X out of histiocytosis X. *Radiology* 1997;204:322–324.

- Smets A, Mortelé K, De Wever N, et al. Coexistence of an adrenocortical carcinoma with an abdominal ganglioneuroma in a child. *Pediatr Radiol.* 1998;28:329–331.

- Urban BA, Fishman EK. Renal lymphoma: CT patterns with emphasis on helical CT. *Radiographics* 2000;20:197–212.

- Westphalen A, Yeh B, Qayyum A, et al. Differential diagnosis of perinephric masses on CT and MRI. *Am J Roentgenol.* 2004;183:1697–1702.

- Yang DA, Jung DH, Kim H, et al. Retroperitoneal cystic masses: CT, clinical, and pathologic findings and literature review. *Radiographics* 2004;24:1353–1365.

- Yang ZG, Min PQ, Sone S, et al. Tuberculosis versus lymphoma in the abdominal lymph nodes: evaluation with contrast-enhanced CT. *Am J Roentgenol.* 1999;172:619–623.

INFECTION/INFLAMMATION

- Amis ES Jr. Retroperitoneal fibrosis. *Am J Roentgenol.* 1991;157:321–329.

- Arrive L, Correas JM, Leseche G, et al. Inflammatory aneurysms of the abdominal aorta: CT findings. *Am J Roentgenol.* 1995;165:1481–1484.

- De Backer AI, Mortelé KJ, Deeren D, et al. Abdominal tuberculous lymphadenopathy: MRI features. *Eur Radiol.* 2005;15:2104–2109.

- De Backer AI, Mortelé KJ, Vanhoenacker FM, et al. Imaging of extraspinal musculoskeletal tuberculosis. *Eur J Radiol.* 2006;57:119–130.

- De Backer AI, Mortelé KJ, Vanschoubroeck IJ, et al. Tuberculosis of the spine: CT and MR imaging features. *JBR-BTR.* 2005;88:92–97.

- Macedo TA, Stanson AW, Oderich GS, et al. Infected aortic aneurysms: imaging findings. *Radiology* 2004;231:250–257.

CONGENITAL/DEVELOPMENTAL ANOMALIES

- Bass JC, Korobkin M, Francis IR, et al. Retroperitoneal plexiform neurofibromas: CT findings. *Am J Roentgenol.* 1994;163:617–620.

- Bass JE, Redwine MD, Kramer LA, et al. Spectrum of congenital anomalies of the inferior vena cava: cross-sectional imaging findings. *Radiographics* 2000;20:639–652.

- Dahan H, Arrivé L, Wendum D, et al. Retrorectal developmental cysts in adults: clinical and radiologic-histopathologic review, differential diagnosis, and treatment. *Radiographics* 2001;21:575–584.

- Fortman BJ, Kuszyk BS, Urban BA, et al. Neurofibromatosis type 1: a diagnostic mimicker at CT. *Radiographics* 2001;21:601–612.

MISCELLANEOUS

- Bechtold RE, Dyer RB, Zagoria RJ, et al. The perirenal space: relationship of pathologic processes to normal retroperitoneal anatomy. *Radiographics* 1996;16:841–854.

- Cirillo RL Jr, Bennett WF, Vitellas KM, et al. Pathology of the adrenal gland: imaging features. *Am J Roentgenol.* 1998;170:429–435.

- Delfaut EM, Beltran J, Johnson G, et al. Fat suppression in MR imaging: techniques and pitfalls. *Radiographics* 1999;19:373–382.

- Doppman JL, Miller DL, Dwyer AJ, et al. Macronodular adrenal hyperplasia in Cushing disease. *Radiology* 1988;166:347–352.

- Dorfman RE, Alpern MB, Gross BH, et al. Upper abdominal lymph nodes: criteria for normal size determined with CT. *Radiology* 1991;180:319–322.

- Einstein DM, Singer, AA, Chilcote, WA, et al. Abdominal lymphadenopathy: spectrum of CT findings. *Radiographics* 1991;11:457–472.

- Garg K, Mao J. Deep venous thrombosis: spectrum of findings and pitfalls in interpretation on CT venography. *Am J Roentgenol.* 2001;177:319–323.

- Gore RM, Balfe DM, Aizenstein RI, et al. The great escape: interfascial decompression planes of the retroperitoneum. *Am J Roentgenol.* 2000;175:363–370.

- Kawashima A, Sandler CM, Ernst RD, et al. CT evaluation of renovascular disease. *Radiographics* 2000;20:1321–1340.

- Kawashima A, Sandler CM, Fishman EK, et al. Spectrum of CT findings in nonmalignant disease of the adrenal gland. *Radiographics* 1998;18:393–412.

- Krebs TL, Wagner BJ. MR imaging of the adrenal gland: radiologic-pathologic correlation. *Radiographics* 1998;18:1425–1440.

- Mesurolle B, Sayag E, Meingan P, et al. Retroperitoneal extramedullary hematopoiesis: sonographic, CT, and MR imaging appearance. *Am J Roentgenol.* 1996;167:1139–1140.

- O'Hara SM, Donnelly LF. Intense contrast enhancement of the adrenal glands: another abdominal CT finding associated with hypoperfusion complex in children. *Am J Roentgenol.* 1999;173:995–997.

- Premkumar A, Chow CK, Choyke PL, et al. Stress-induced adrenal hyperplasia simulating metastatic disease: CT and MR findings. *Am J Roentgenol.* 1992;159:675–676.

- Siegel CL, Cohan RH. CT of abdominal aortic aneurysms. *Am J Roentgenol.* 1994;163:17–29.

- Siegel CL, Cohan RH, Korobkin M, et al. Abdominal aortic aneurysm morphology: CT features in patients with ruptured and nonruptured aneurysms. *Am J Roentgenol.* 1994;163:1123–1129.

- Torres GM, Cernigliaro JG, Abbitt PL, et al. Iliopsoas compartment: normal anatomy and pathologic processes. *Radiographics* 1995;15:1285–1297.

- Yamauchi T, Furui S, Katoh R, et al. Acute thrombosis of the inferior vena cava: treatment with saline-jet aspiration thrombectomy catheter. *Am J Roentgenol.* 1993;161:405–407.

CHAPTER NINE
ABDOMINAL WALL

VINCENT PELSSER,
KOENRAAD J. MORTELE,
AND PABLO R. ROS

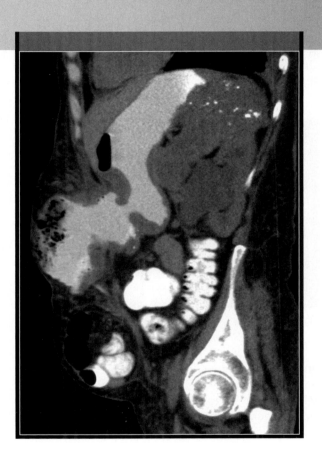

Clinical History: 60-year-old woman presenting with left lower quadrant pain following exercise.

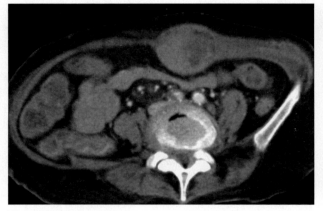

Figure 9.1 A

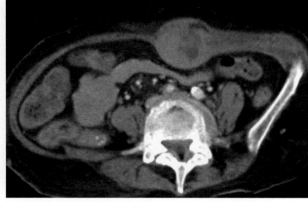

Figure 9.1 B

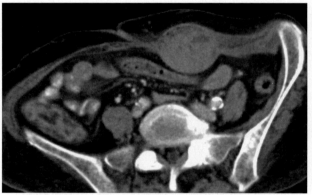

Figure 9.1 C

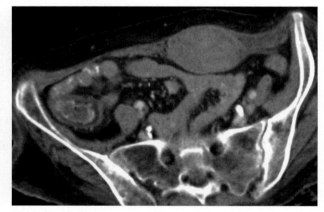

Figure 9.1 D

Findings: Axial contrast-enhanced CT (CECT) images demonstrate a 5.3 × 4.4 cm hyperdense and heterogeneous cystic lesion in the anterior abdominal wall arising from the left rectus abdominis muscle. A fluid-fluid level is present.

Differential Diagnosis: Cystic metastasis, sarcoma, desmoid.

Diagnosis: Hematoma.

Discussion: An abdominal wall hematoma can be due to trauma, instrumentation, or anticoagulation and is usually diagnosed by clinical history. Tumors can also occur in the anterior abdominal wall and must be excluded. Primary tumors (sarcoma) can become necrotic and also present with a fluid-fluid level (hematocrit level). Fibromatosis (desmoid tumor) is typically a solid mass with little necrosis. Necrotic or cystic metastases can have this appearance, as seen in metastases from melanoma, renal cell carcinoma, or mucinous adenocarcinoma arising from the gastrointestinal (GI) tract or ovary. The density of the blood products on CT varies according to the age of the hematoma; it is usually hyperdense to muscle on CT when it is acute, and it becomes isodense to hypodense as it progressively liquefies. Resorption usually occurs rapidly in the weeks following the acute hemorrhage.

Clinical History: 23-year-old woman presenting with polyarthralgia.

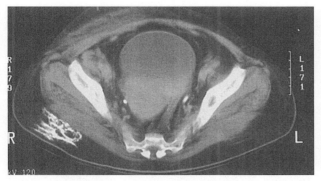

Figure 9.2   A

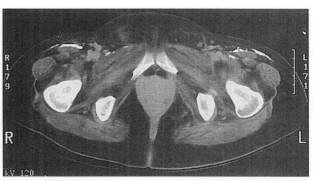

Figure 9.2   B

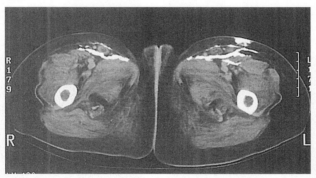

Figure 9.2   C

Findings: Axial CECT images demonstrate plaquelike calcifications in the subcutaneous fat in the right buttock and in both groins.

Differential Diagnosis: Hyperparathyroidism, scleroderma, systemic lupus erythematosus, calcinosis universalis.

Diagnosis: Dermatomyositis.

Discussion: Dermatomyositis is an idiopathic inflammatory myopathy, resulting in muscle atrophy and infiltration by inflammatory cells. It occurs most commonly in the fifth and sixth decades of life and has a female predominance. It results in proximal muscle weakness, interstitial lung disease, inflammatory arthropathy, and an erythematous rash. Plaquelike calcifications can be found in soft tissues of the extremities, abdominal and chest wall, axilla, and inguinal region. The calcinosis is infrequent in adults but may occur in up to 40% of affected children. Other causes of calcinosis include hyperparathyroidism, calcinosis universalis (a progressive disease of unknown etiology causing soft tissue calcifications), and collagen vascular diseases, such as scleroderma, CREST (calcinosis, Raynaud phenomenon, esophageal dysmotility, sclerodactyly, and telangiectasia) syndrome, and systemic lupus erythematosus. Treatment of dermatomyositis is with steroids and cytotoxic agents, such as methotrexate.

Clinical History: 47-year-old woman with recent hernia repair presenting with fever and midline fullness.

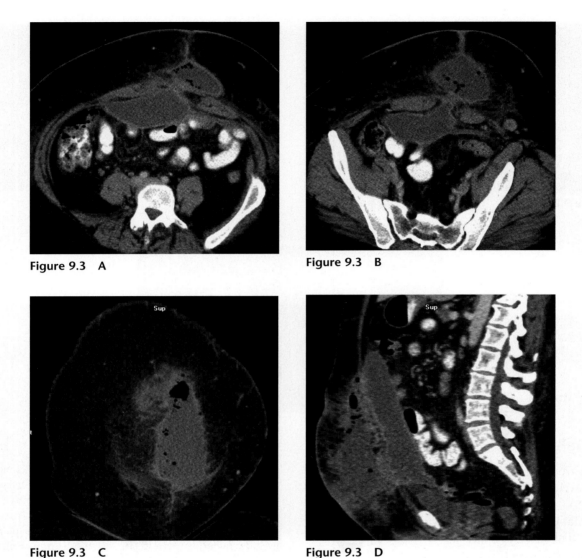

Figure 9.3   A

Figure 9.3   B

Figure 9.3   C

Figure 9.3   D

Findings: Axial (A and B), coronal (C), and sagittal (D) reformatted CECT images demonstrate a midline 6.7 × 4.6 × 15.0 cm, rim-enhancing, subcutaneous fluid collection that contains gas bubbles. It communicates with an intra-abdominal fluid collection. Note surrounding fat stranding.

Differential Diagnosis: Hematoma, seroma.

Diagnosis: Abscess.

Discussion: Fluid collections are present in up to 17% of patients following hernia repair. Postoperative fluid collections can contain blood, serous fluid, or pus. A hematoma will be hyperdense acutely, with progressive liquefaction and corresponding decrease in attenuation in the following days and weeks. A seroma (containing serous fluid) will typically appear as a low-density fluid-density collection. By imaging, it is usually not possible to predict whether a fluid collection is infected or not. Presence of gas in the fluid, a thick enhancing wall, and surrounding fat stranding are good indicators that the collection may be infected, as seen in this case. Note, however, that gas in a fluid collection could be a normal finding in the early postoperative period. Presence or absence of clinical signs of infection (e.g., erythema, tenderness, fever, elevated white blood cell count) should guide the management. In equivocal cases, image-guided fluid aspiration for culture can be performed. The patient in this case was treated with percutaneous catheter drainage.

Clinical History: 50-year-old woman with lymphoma presenting with fever and labial erythema.

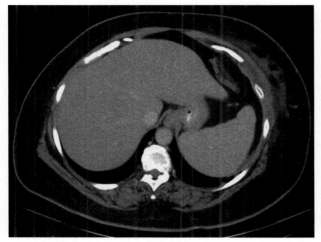

Figure 9.4   A

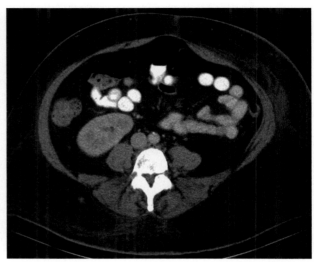

Figure 9.4   B

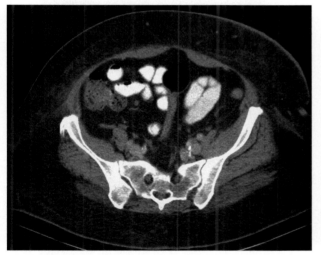

Figure 9.4   C

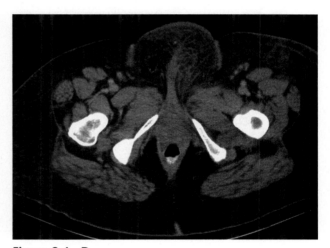

Figure 9.4   D

Findings: Axial CECT images demonstrate skin thickening along the left anterolateral abdominal wall, with subjacent subcutaneous fat stranding. Note intermuscular edema along the left hemithorax.

Differential Diagnosis: Trauma.

Diagnosis: Cellulitis.

Discussion: Diagnosis of cellulitis should be made clinically, without need of imaging. Radiology studies are performed to assess for complications, such as abscess formation, or for delineation of deep extension and associated fasciitis or myositis. Imaging findings of cellulitis include skin thickening, soft tissue swelling, fat stranding, displacement of fat planes, and presence of gas if the infection is caused by gas-forming organisms. However, these findings are nonspecific. Presence of causative radiopaque foreign bodies can also be well demonstrated by CT. In this case, the infection was confined to the superficial tissues, and no focal fluid collection to suggest an abscess was identified. The patient was treated successfully with antibiotics.

Clinical History: 76-year-old man with history of Hodgkin disease presenting with upper extremity swelling.

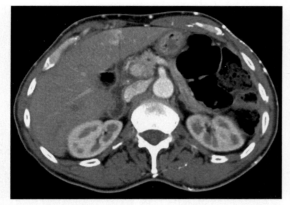

Figure 9.5   A

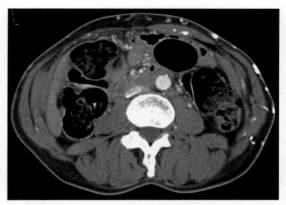

Figure 9.5   B

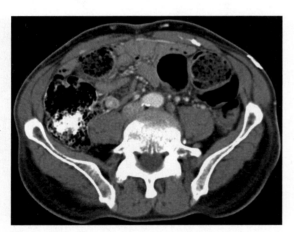

Figure 9.5   C

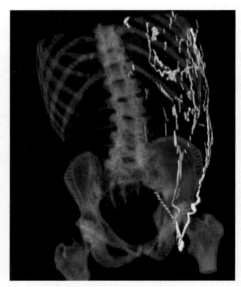

Figure 9.5   D

Findings: Axial CECT (A–C) and three-dimensional, volume-rendered (D) images demonstrate multiple enlarged vessels along the left abdominal wall, draining into the left external iliac vein. Note hyperenhancement of the liver adjacent to the falciform ligament.

Differential Diagnosis: Inferior vena cava obstruction.

Diagnosis: Superior vena cava obstruction.

Discussion: When superior vena cava (SVC) obstruction occurs, multiple collateral pathways develop to shunt the blood back to the heart. The predominant collateral pathway is through the azygos–hemiazygos veins. Other pathways may develop via the internal mammary vein to abdominal wall veins, superficial thoracoabdominal to lateral thoracic vein, and vertebral plexus. In case of SVC obstruction, focal brisk hyperenhancement in the liver adjacent to the falciform ligament is explained by the nonsplanchnic perfusion of this portion of the liver parenchyma by the veins of Sappey. These veins communicate with the internal mammary vein and inferior epigastric vein. When a CECT is performed with an injection of iodinated contrast in the upper extremity, the collateral veins are densely opacified by the nondiluted contrast, as seen in this case.

Clinical History: 69-year-old woman presenting with nausea and vomiting.

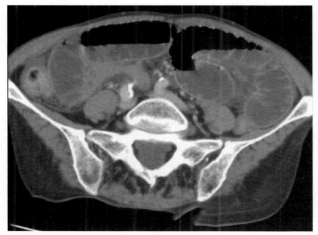

Figure 9.6   A

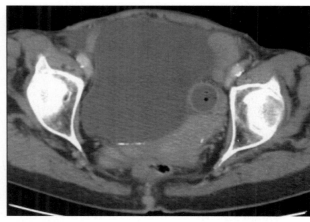

Figure 9.6   B

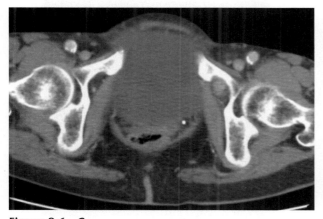

Figure 9.6   C

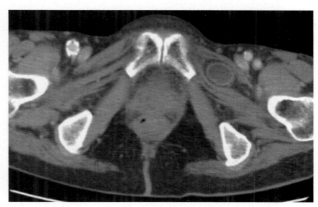

Figure 9.6   D

Findings: Axial CECT images demonstrate multiple dilated loops of small bowel that can be followed through the left obturator foramen.

Differential Diagnosis: None.

Diagnosis: Left obturator hernia causing small bowel obstruction.

Discussion: Obturator hernias are uncommon, and because of their deep location in the pelvis, they are not easily diagnosed clinically. The hernial sac passes through the superolateral aspect of the obturator foramen, where the obturator vessels and nerves course. It eventually protrudes between the obturator externus and pectineus muscles, as seen in this case. Obturator hernias occur more frequently in elderly females. Any pelvic structure, including bladder, uterus, ovaries, rectum, cecum, appendix, and small bowel, may herniate through the obturator foramen. Because the ring of the hernia is small, most hernias become incarcerated.

Clinical History: 50-year-old woman involved in a motor vehicle accident.

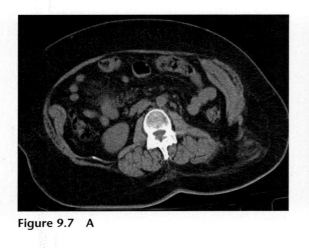

Figure 9.7   A

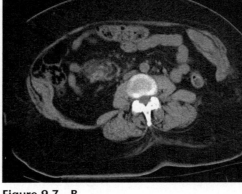

Figure 9.7   B

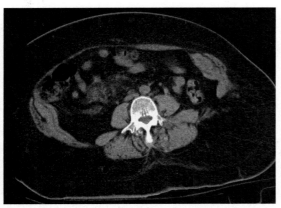

Figure 9.7   C

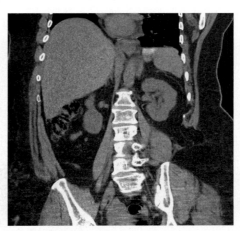

Figure 9.7   D

Findings: Axial (A–C) and coronal reformatted (D) nonenhanced CT (NECT) images demonstrate a 4.5-cm long defect in the left lateral abdominal wall muscles with overlying subcutaneous edema. Note high-density material and stranding in the right side of the mesentery.

Differential Diagnosis: None.

Diagnosis: Abdominal wall muscular tear.

Discussion: Traumatic injuries to the abdominal wall are uncommon. They may occur because of shearing forces from deceleration and increased intra-abdominal pressure at the time of a motor vehicle accident. Deceleration injuries cause a tear in the abdominal wall muscles and fascias at areas of anatomical weakness; these are usually in the superior (Grynfeltt-Lesshaft) and inferior (Petit) triangles in the lumbar region. Because of the forces required to produce these tears, there is a high association (up to 30%) with intra-abdominal injuries, especially bowel and mesentery. In this case, the hematoma in the mesentery prompted laparoscopic evaluation. Surgery confirmed a mesenteric tear without bowel injury. If the traumatic defect is not corrected surgically, the herniated content has a high likelihood of incarceration (25%) or strangulation (10%). Penetrating trauma, from a knife or bullet, is another cause of abdominal wall disruption besides surgery.

Clinical History: 48-year-old man presenting with a buttock mass.

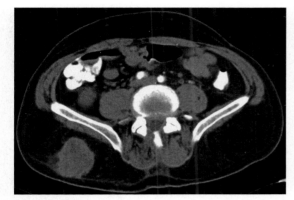

Figure 9.8   A

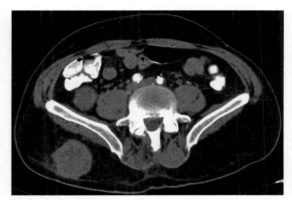

Figure 9.8   B

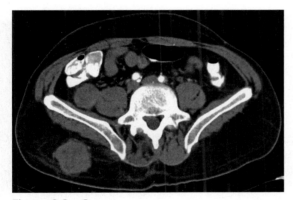

Figure 9.8   C

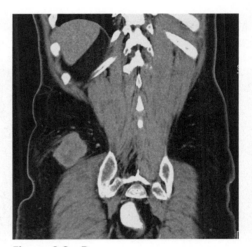

Figure 9.8   D

Findings: Axial (A–C) and coronal reformatted (D) CECT images demonstrate a 5.2 × 5.3 cm heterogeneously enhancing mass in the subcutaneous right buttock fat. Note smaller retroperitoneal mass lateral to the right psoas muscle.

Differential Diagnosis: Sarcoma, lymphoma.

Diagnosis: Metastasis from lung cancer.

Discussion: Abdominal wall neoplasms are infrequently encountered on imaging. They can be either primary or secondary tumors. Primary lesions include lipomas, desmoids, and sarcomas. Secondary involvement may occur from direct extension of an intra-abdominal tumor or by hematogenous spread. Tumors that have a tendency to produce peritoneal carcinomatosis may cause nodules at the level of the umbilicus. Metastases along surgical incisions or port sites after laparoscopy have also been reported. In the present case, the presence of two masses, one in the retroperitoneum and one in the buttock, suggests hematogenous metastasis. Extensive workup, which included image-guided percutaneous biopsy of the buttock mass, revealed disseminated lung cancer in this patient. Sarcomas usually metastasize initially to the lung and not to the retroperitoneum. Lymphoma presents as masses of homogeneous density, even when the masses attain a large size.

Clinical History: 77-year-old man with history of renal cell carcinoma presenting with abdominal pain and bloating.

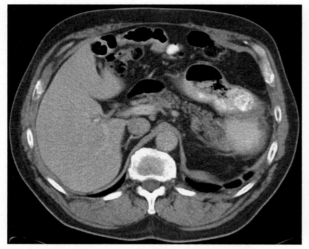

Figure 9.9   A

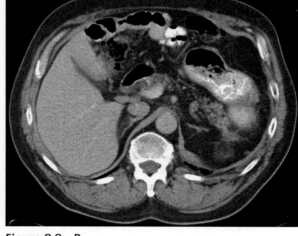

Figure 9.9   B

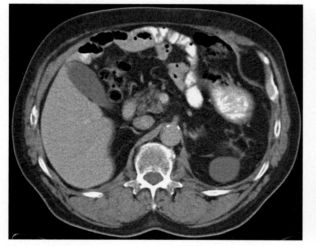

Figure 9.9   C

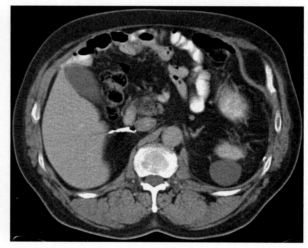

Figure 9.9   D

Findings: Axial CECT images demonstrate a 5.8 × 2.7 cm mass of homogeneous fat density in the left upper quadrant. Caudally, it insinuates superficially to the transverse muscle. Note intact transversalis fascia medially. A left renal cyst and right nephrectomy clips are seen incidentally.

Differential Diagnosis: Hernia.

Diagnosis: Lipoma.

Discussion: Lipomas account for close to 50% of all soft tissue neoplasms. Deep lipomas are, however, much less common than superficial (subcutaneous) ones. Lipomas may be multiple, and they are familial in approximately 30% of cases. On CT, lipomas are of homogeneous fat density, with Hounsfield units (HU) varying between −65 and −120. In up to 50% of cases, lipomas may demonstrate internal thin (<2 mm) septations. After injection of intravenous contrast, no enhancement is present, except for the fibrous capsule. Intact transversalis fascia medial to the mass, as seen in this case, excludes a hernia.

Clinical History: 55-year-old man with a history of ruptured cerebral aneurysm presenting with increasing headaches and a palpable abdominal mass.

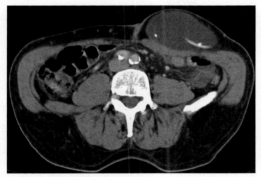

Figure 9.10   A

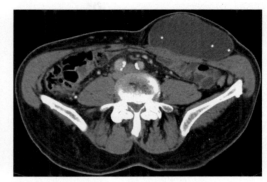

Figure 9.10   B

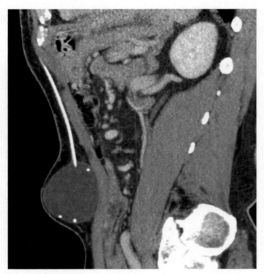

Figure 9.10   C

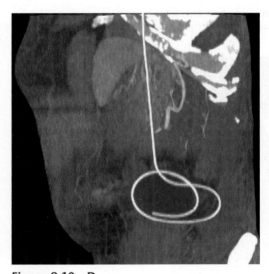

Figure 9.10   D

Findings: Axial CECT (A and B), sagittal reformatted (C), and maximum-intensity projection (MIP) (D) images show an 11.3 × 5.7 cm fluid collection in the subcutaneous tissues. Note tube coiled within it.

Differential Diagnosis: Seroma, hematoma, cystic metastasis.

Diagnosis: Ventriculoperitoneal shunt migration with cerebrospinal fluid pseudocyst formation.

Discussion: The primary treatment of hydrocephalus is through ventricular shunting. The most commonly used shunt is ventriculoperitoneal because the peritoneum is a very efficient site for fluid absorption. However, several complications may occur, leading to shunt malfunction and recurrent neurologic symptoms. The distal end of the shunt can migrate into the abdominal wall, thorax, or perforated viscus or can herniate in various locations, such as in the scrotum. When shunt migration occurs in the abdominal wall, where fluid absorption is less efficient, cerebrospinal fluid accumulation around the distal end of the shunt may develop, forming a cerebrospinal fluid pseudocyst. This gradually leads to shunt malfunction, increased central nervous system pressure, and recurrent symptoms, as in this case. Treatment consists of shunt revision with relocation of the distal end of the shunt in the peritoneal cavity. CT or ultrasound demonstrates the fluid composition of the abdominal wall mass and the abnormal position of the distal tip of the ventriculoperitoneal shunt. Other fluid collections that may occur in the abdominal wall include seroma, hematoma, abscess, and cystic metastasis. Identification of the shunt within the fluid collection is key to the correct diagnosis.

Clinical History: 57-year-old woman with a history of breast cancer presenting with right lower quadrant discomfort.

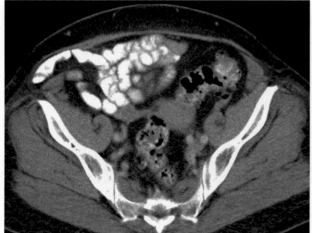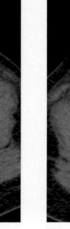

Figure 9.11   A

Figure 9.11   B

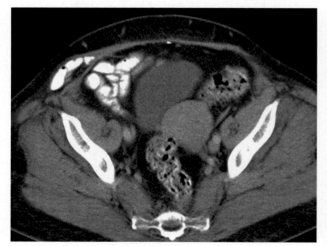

Figure 9.11   C

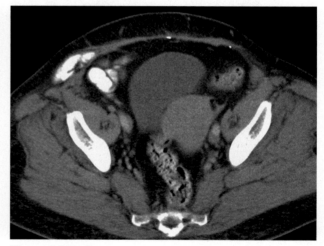

Figure 9.11   D

Findings: Axial CECT images demonstrate herniation of small bowel loops through a defect lateral to the right rectus abdominis muscle. The herniated small bowel loops are contained superficially by the external oblique muscle.

Differential Diagnosis: Laparoscopy port hernia, incisional hernia.

Diagnosis: Spigelian hernia.

Discussion: Spigelian hernias are difficult to diagnose clinically because they are contained by abdominal wall muscle. Imaging is often required to make their diagnosis. They occur at a point of weakness lateral to the rectus abdominus muscle, along the linea semilunaris, which represents the fibrous union between the rectus sheath and the transverse muscle aponeurosis. They also tend to occur at or below the arcuate line, another point of weakness. The arcuate line is defined as the line below which all fascial layers of the abdominal wall musculature, except the transversalis fascia, pass anterior to the rectus abdominis muscle. Bowel or omentum may protrude through the defect. They bear a high risk of incarceration and bowel strangulation. In the absence of previous laparoscopy or surgical incision in the area, Spigelian hernia due to fibrous weakness is the most likely diagnosis.

Clinical History: 79-year-old man presenting with multiple skin masses.

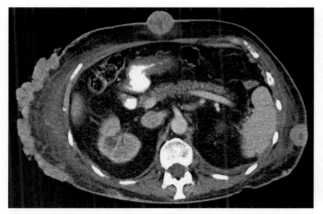

Figure 9.12   A

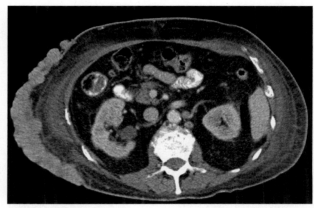

Figure 9.12   B

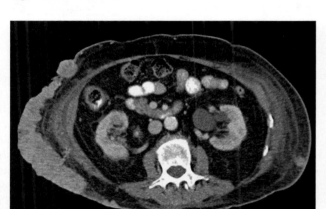

Figure 9.12   C

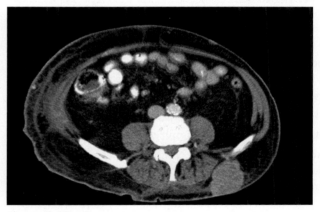

Figure 9.12   D

Findings: Axial CECT images demonstrate multiple heterogeneous skin-based masses.

Differential Diagnosis: Neurofibromatosis, Kaposi sarcoma, hemangiomas.

Diagnosis: Skin metastases from melanoma.

Discussion: Skin metastases occur in approximately 5% of patients with malignancy. The origin of the metastases varies according to the sex of the patient. In women, the most common primary tumors to metastasize to the skin originate in the breast, colon, skin, ovaries, and lungs; in men, skin metastases are from lung cancer, colon cancer, melanoma, and head and neck neoplasms. Because the prevalence of melanoma has increased significantly over the last years and given the very unpredictable course of the disease (patients may have localized or widely metastatic disease at presentation), careful evaluation of imaging studies must be made because metastases may be present in unusual locations. The diagnosis of neurofibromatosis is usually made in the early years of life, and it would be extremely unusual for a patient to first present at 79 years of age. Hemangiomas also present at a younger age than the patient in this case. Kaposi sarcoma may present with multiple skin masses, but patients in the United States typically have acquired immunodeficiency syndrome (AIDS) or a history of immunosuppression.

Clinical History: 53-year-old woman presenting with a palpable nodule at her umbilicus.

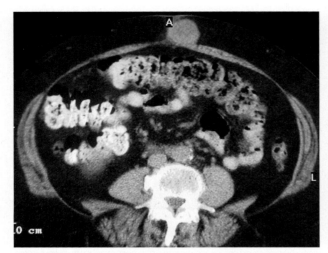

Figure 9.13 A

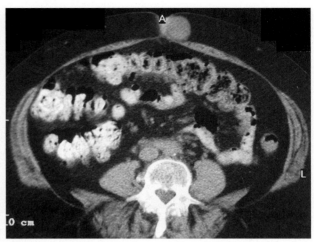

Figure 9.13 B

Findings: Axial CECT images show a 3.0 × 2.7 cm enhancing subcutaneous nodule adjacent to the umbilicus.

Differential Diagnosis: Endometriosis, umbilical hernia, hematoma.

Diagnosis: Sister Mary Joseph nodule.

Discussion: A metastatic umbilical mass is commonly referred to as a Sister Mary Joseph nodule. Fifty percent of them arise from primary gastrointestinal tumors, and 25% arise from a primary cancer of unknown origin. Other primary tumors that may cause an umbilical nodule originate from the ovary, pancreas, or rarely lung. The routes by which the neoplasm may reach the umbilicus are from direct extension or hematogenous or lymphatic spread. At imaging, the nodule may appear entirely solid or necrotic. Definitive diagnosis is often made through biopsy. A percutaneous biopsy was performed in the present case and yielded carcinoma. Endoscopic evaluation revealed a primary gastric cancer. Endometriosis may present similarly with an umbilical mass, and a history of cyclical pain associated with menses is a clue to the correct diagnosis. The lack of an abdominal wall defect underlying the nodule excludes an umbilical hernia. A hematoma could have a similar appearance, but it should not enhance.

Clinical History: 58-year-old man presenting with fever following cardiac catheterization.

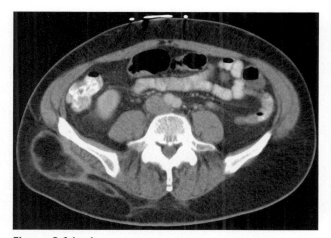

Figure 9.14   A

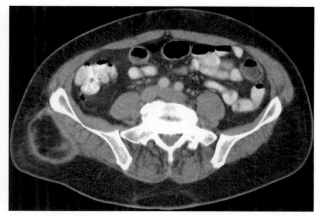

Figure 9.14   B

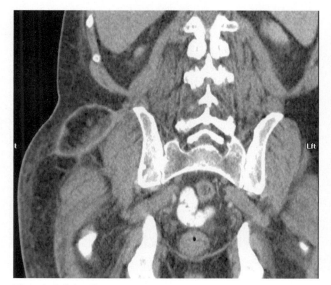

Figure 9.14   C

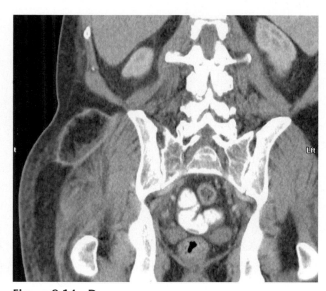

Figure 9.14   D

Findings: Axial (A and B) and coronal reformatted (C and D) CECT images demonstrate an 8.4 × 5.3 cm fat-containing mass in the right buttock, with soft tissue nodularity and surrounding rim. Note soft tissue thickening superficial to the gluteus maximus muscle.

Differential Diagnosis: Liposarcoma.

Diagnosis: Fat necrosis.

Discussion: Fat necrosis may be due to multiple causes including trauma, collagen vascular disease, myeloproliferative disorders, and complications of pancreatic disorders, such as acinar cell carcinoma. Fat necrosis infrequently has the appearance of a mass. As in this case, it may appear as a fat-containing mass associated with peripheral globular soft tissue components surrounded by a soft tissue density rim. Surrounding fat stranding may be seen. The fascial thickening along the gluteus muscle and the fat stranding laterally extending into the upper thigh suggest, in this case, an inflammatory process rather than a neoplasm. However, liposarcomas may be difficult to distinguish only by imaging, especially because a history of trauma may not be remembered by the patient; a biopsy may be performed in selected cases.

Clinical History: 27-year-old man with a lifelong history of abdominal wall deformity.

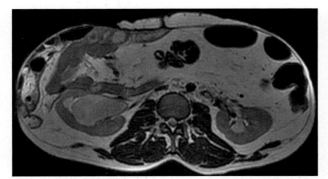

Figure 9.15   A

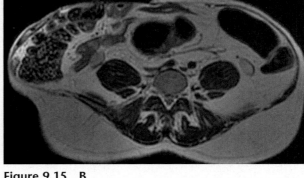

Figure 9.15   B

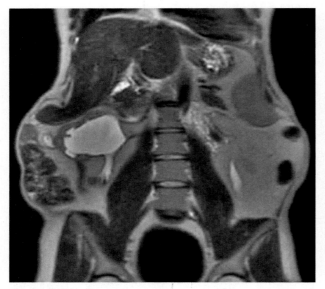

Figure 9.15   C

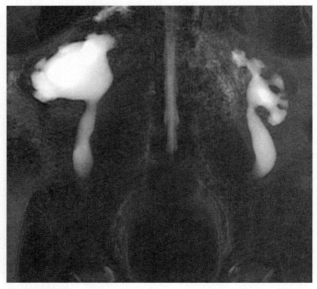

Figure 9.15   D

Findings: Axial (A and B) and coronal (C) T2-WI and coronal T2-WI magnetic resonance (MR) urogram image (D) demonstrate extreme thinning of the anterior abdominal wall muscles and bilateral hydronephrosis.

Differential Diagnosis: None.

Diagnosis: Prune-belly syndrome.

Discussion: Prune-belly syndrome is also known as Eagle-Barrett syndrome or triad syndrome. It is a rare syndrome with an occurrence of one in every 29,000 to 40,000 live births; 95% to 97% of affected patients are males. Proposed etiologies are bladder outlet obstruction, mesodermal arrest, and yolk sac dysgenesis. The triad consists of partial or complete hypoplasia or absence of the abdominal musculature, bilateral cryptorchidism, and a variety of urinary tract abnormalities. The hallmark of these abnormalities is markedly elongated, dilated, and tortuous ureters, mostly the distal

third. Vesicoureteral reflux is present in 70% of patients due to lateral implantation of the ureters. The renal parenchyma itself is preserved initially but secondarily affected by reflux or recurrent pyelonephritis. The bladder has a large capacity and thickened walls due to collagen deposition, which limits its contraction capacity. Urethral dilatation or narrowing may be seen, often in association with a large utricule. The most severely affected abdominal wall muscles are located anteriorly and ventrally, and the transverse muscle is the most severely involved. Treatment is aimed at improving urine drainage and limiting urinary infection. Abdominoplasty and orchiopexy are also frequently performed. Despite improvement in treatment, 20% of affected patients die in the first month of life, and an additional 30% die by age 2. Death usually occurs from chronic renal failure or urosepsis.

Case images courtesy of Dr. Giovanni Artho, McGill University Health Center, Montreal, Canada.

Clinical History: 41-year-old woman presenting with nausea and vomiting.

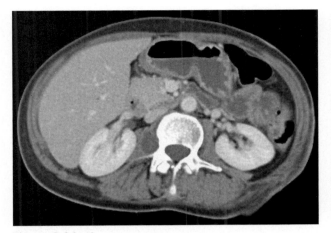

Figure 9.16   A

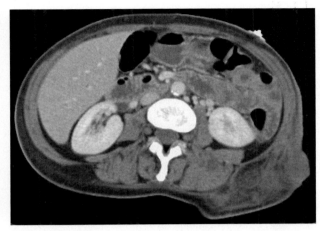

Figure 9.16   B

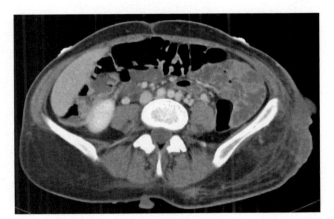

Figure 9.16   C

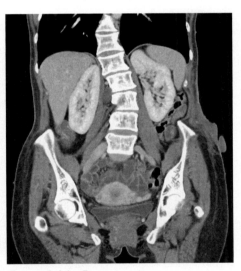

Figure 9.16   D

Findings: Axial (A–C) and coronal reformatted (D) CECT images demonstrate a large sessile left flank cutaneous mass with underlying subcutaneous fat stranding. Note other cutaneous nodules, a right paraspinal mass, and genisero-convex scoliosis.

Differential Diagnosis: Metastasis, Kaposi sarcoma.

Diagnosis: Neurofibromatosis type 1.

Discussion: Neurofibromatosis type 1, also named von Recklinghausen disease, is the most common neurocutaneous syndrome, occurring in one of every 3000 births. It is an autosomal dominant disorder but occurs sporadically in up to 50% of cases due to spontaneous mutation on chromosome 17. The classic tumors occurring outside the central nervous system are neurofibromas, which may be plexiform in nature, as seen in this case in the left flank. In the abdomen, neurofibromas tend to arise in the retroperitoneum, mesentery, and paraspinal regions. Bowel neurofibromas may be seen and occur most frequently in the jejunum. An association with pheochromocytoma, carcinoid, and gastrointestinal tumor, among others, also exists. The urinary tract may also be involved by neurofibromas, the bladder being most commonly affected. As seen in this case, scoliosis and other skeletal deformities are common. The constellation of multiple skin nodules, paraspinal nodule, and scoliosis make neurofibromatosis type 1 the first diagnostic consideration in this case. In cases of diffuse metastases, a primary tumor is usually known. The absence of immunosuppression and the paraspinal nodule make Kaposi sarcoma unlikely.

Clinical History: 75-year-old woman on warfarin (Coumadin) for atrial fibrillation presenting with enlarging right-sided abdominal mass.

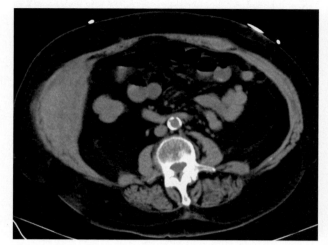

Figure 9.17   A

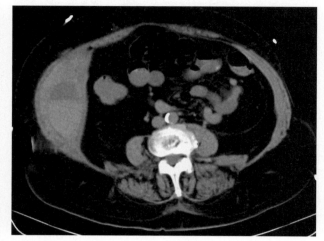

Figure 9.17   B

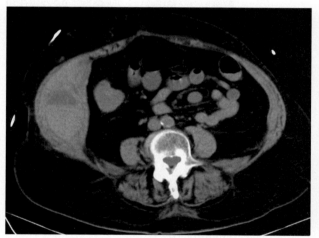

Figure 9.17   C

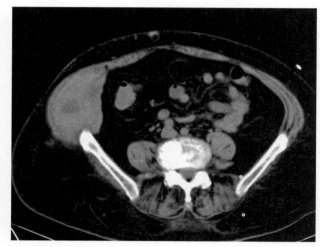

Figure 9.17   D

Findings: Axial NECT images demonstrate a 10.9 × 4.8 cm large mass in the right lateral abdominal wall muscles. It has predominantly high attenuation, and a fluid-fluid level is present centrally.

Differential Diagnosis: Hemorrhagic metastasis, sarcoma (malignant fibrous histiocytoma, leiomyosarcoma), desmoid tumor.

Diagnosis: Hematoma.

Discussion: When a patient is taking anticoagulants, such as warfarin or heparin, even trivial trauma can result in massive hemorrhage. Occasionally, spontaneous rectus abdominis bleeding can also occur. The presence of high-attenuation material with a fluid-fluid level centrally suggests an acute hematoma. After intravenous injection of contrast material, contrast may extravasate in the hematoma, indicating acute hemorrhage. Metastasis, desmoid, or sarcoma would be unlikely due to the clinical history, but an underlying mass needs to be excluded. This could be performed with a follow-up scan after the hematoma has resolved.

Clinical History: 79-year-old man presenting with abdominal pain and vomiting.

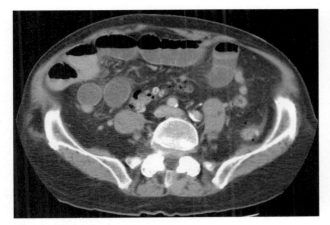

Figure 9.18   A

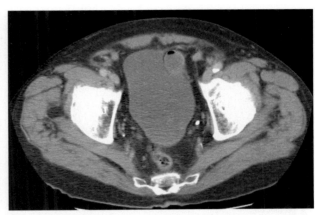

Figure 9.18   B

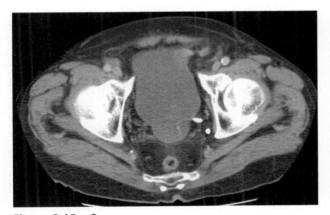

Figure 9.18   C

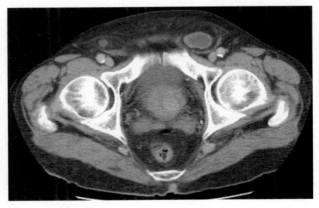

Figure 9.18   D

Findings: Axial CECT images demonstrate multiple dilated loops of small bowel, which can be followed into the left groin, anteromedially to the femoral vessels.

Differential Diagnosis: None.

Diagnosis: Left inguinal hernia causing small bowel obstruction.

Discussion: Inguinal hernias can be either direct or indirect. Indirect hernias are the most common and occur predominantly in males. The peritoneal sac, along with intra-abdominal contents, enters the inguinal canal and exits at the external ring. In males, a hernial sac follows the spermatic cord and enters into the scrotum. Because of its long course, indirect hernias can become incarcerated, leading to bowel infarction. Direct hernias, on the other hand, are less common and occur when the hernia enters medial to the inferior epigastric vessels. The finding of abdominal contents (e.g., small bowel, sigmoid colon, cecum, mesenteric fat) in the inguinal canal anteromedial to the femoral vessels, as seen in this case, is diagnostic of an inguinal hernia. In males, this is easily seen as asymmetry in the spermatic cord when compared with the other side. Frequently, hernias are asymptomatic and easily reducible. They can, however, lead to small bowel obstruction due to incarceration, as seen in this case.

Clinical History: 18-year-old man with recent asystole due to heroin overdose.

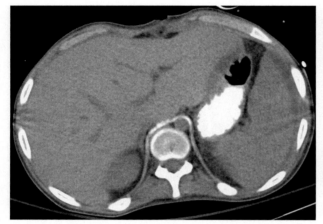

Figure 9.19   A

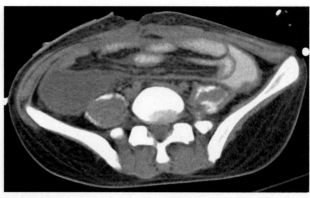

Figure 9.19   B

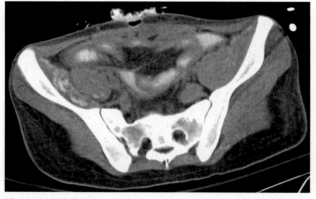

Figure 9.19   C

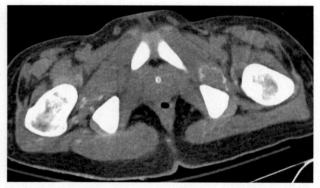

Figure 9.19   D

Findings: Axial NECT images demonstrate calcifications in the diaphragm, iliopsoas, and pelvic girdle muscles. Note midline skin defect with oral contrast extravasation from enterocutaneous fistula.

Differential Diagnosis: Hyperparathyroidism, scleroderma, systemic lupus erythematosus, calcinosis universalis, dermatomyositis.

Diagnosis: Rhabdomyolysis caused by heroin overdose.

Discussion: Rhabdomyolysis is a form of severe muscle injury that results in cellular breakdown and release of cellular content in the plasma. The diagnosis is usually clinical and evidenced by serum elevation of the enzyme creatinine kinase (CK). Rhabdomyolysis is most commonly caused by trauma but can also be caused by ischemia, polymyositis, drug overdose, and exertion, among other causes. In the acute period, CT demonstrates nonspecific low-density areas in the affected muscle, corresponding to edema or necrosis. High-density foci may also be identified in swollen muscles. Calcifications eventually develop in the muscle; they gradually vanish over time. Other causes of muscular calcifications include metabolic disorders, connective tissue disorders, trauma, and infection.

Clinical History: 54-year-old man with history of lymphoma and leg weakness since childhood.

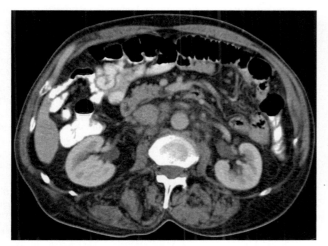

Figure 9.20   A

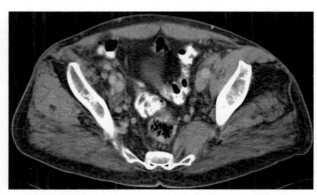

Figure 9.20   B

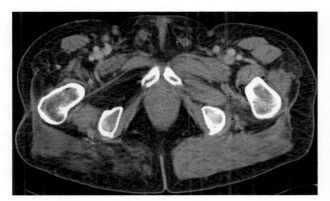

Figure 9.20   C

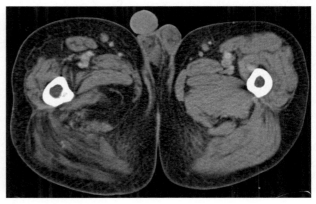

Figure 9.20   D

Findings: Axial CECT images demonstrate asymmetric atrophy and fatty replacement of several paraspinal, pelvic, and proximal thigh muscles. Note retroperitoneal lymph nodes and stranding related to lymphoma.

Differential Diagnosis: Denervation atrophy, primary muscular disease, physiologic fatty replacement of muscles.

Diagnosis: Paralytic poliomyelitis.

Discussion: Muscle atrophy can be caused by neurologic conditions (denervation) or primary muscular disease, but the cause can sometimes be physiologic. Poliovirus infection occurs by the fecal-oral route and is seen only in humans. Most cases consist of a nonspecific febrile episode (abortive poliomyelitis). Infection may also manifest as aseptic meningitis (nonparalytic poliomyelitis), and less frequently, it involves the lower motor neurons (paralytic poliomyelitis). The resulting spinal neuronal damage leads to muscular atrophy, wasting, and fatty replacement. Paralytic poliomyelitis typically causes asymmetric muscular involvement; at times, these changes lack clinical correlation. Primary muscular diseases, whether congenital, infectious, traumatic, or due to disuse, can also cause atrophy. In muscular dystrophy (congenital), the muscular involvement is characteristically symmetric. Physiologic muscular fatty replacement is a normal age-related phenomenon most prominent in females; however, this normal aging process is limited only to the paraspinal muscles, with atrophy being most advanced in the lumbosacral region. Involvement of the pelvic and thigh muscles in the present case excludes physiologic atrophy.

SUGGESTED READINGS

NEOPLASMS

- Dunnick NR, Shaner EG, Doppman JL. Detection of subcutaneous metastasis by computed tomography. *J Comput Assist Tomogr.* 1978; 2:275–279.

- Krathen RA, Orengo IF, Rosen T. Cutaneous metastasis: a meta-analysis of data. *South Med J.* 2003;96:164–167.

- Murphey MD, Carroll JF, Flemming DJ, et al. From the archives of the AFIP: benign musculoskeletal lipomatous lesions. *Radiographics* 2004; 24:1433–1466.

- Patten RM, Shuman WP, Teefey S. Subcutaneous metastases from malignant melanoma: prevalence and findings on CT. *Am J Roentgenol.* 1989; 152:1009–1012.

- Spencer PS, Helm TN. Skin metastases in cancer patients. *Cutis* 1987;39: 119–121.

INFECTION/INFLAMMATION

- Blane CE, White SJ, Braunstein EM, et al. Patterns of calcification in childhood dermatomyositis. *Am J Roentgenol.* 1984;142:397–400.

- Chan LP, Gee R, Keogh C, et al. Imaging features of fat necrosis. *Am J Roentgenol.* 2003;181:955–959.

- Gastrointestinal Case of the day. Acute nontraumatic rhabdomyolysis. *Am J Roentgenol.* 1994;162:1451.

- Hui GC, Amaral J, Stephens D, et al. Gas distribution in intraabdominal and pelvic abscesses on CT is associated with drainability. *Am J Roentgenol.* 2005;184:915–919.

- Johnston C, Keogan MT. Imaging features of soft-tissue infections and other complications in drug users after direct subcutaneous injection ("skin popping"). *Am J Roentgenol.* 2004;182:1195–1202.

- Malzberg MS, Rogg JM, Tate CA, et al. Poliomyelitis: hyperintensity of the anterior horn cells on MR images of the spinal cord. *Am J Roentgenol.* 1993;161:863–865.

- Russ PD, Dillingham M. Demonstration of CT hyperdensity in patients with acute renal failure associated with rhabdomyolysis. *J Comput Assist Tomogr.* 1991;15:458–463.

CONGENITAL/DEVELOPMENTAL ANOMALIES

- Das Narla L, Doherty RD, Hingsbergen EA, et al. Pediatric Case of the day. Prune-belly syndrome (Eagle-Barrett syndrome, triad syndrome). *Radiographics* 1998;18:1318–1322.

- Fortman BJ, Kuszyk BS, Urban BA, et al. Neurofibromatosis type 1: a diagnostic mimicker at CT. *Radiographics* 2001;21:601–612.

- Levy AD, Patel N, Dow N, et al. From the archives of the AFIP: abdominal neoplasms in patients with neurofibromatosis type 1: radiologic-pathologic correlation. *Radiographics* 2005;25:455–480.

MISCELLANEOUS

- Aguirre DA, Casola G, Sirlin C. Abdominal wall hernias: MDCT findings. *Am J Roentgenol.* 2004;183:681–690.

- Aguirre DA, Santosa AC, Casola G, et al. Abdominal wall hernias: imaging features, complications, and diagnostic pitfalls at multi–detector row CT. *Radiographics* 2005;25:1501–1520.

- Breen DJ, Rutherford EE, Stedman B, et al. Intrahepatic arterioportal shunting and anomalous venous drainage: understanding the CT features in the liver. *Eur Radiol.* 2004;14:2249–2260.

- Faro SH, Racette CD, Lally JF, et al. Traumatic lumbar hernia: CT diagnosis. *Am J Roentgenol.* 1990;154:757–759.

- Goeser CD, McLeary MS, Young LW. Diagnostic imaging of ventriculoperitoneal shunt malfunctions and complications. *Radiographics* 1998;18:635–651.

- Goodman P, Raval B. CT of the abdominal wall. *Am J Roentgenol.* 1990;154:1207–1211.

- Hadar H, Gadoth N, Heifetz M. Fatty replacement of lower paraspinal muscles: normal and neuromuscular disorders. *Am J Roentgenol.* 1983;141:895–898.

- Herbener TE, Basile V, Nakamoto D, et al. Abdominal Case of the day. Focal liver enhancement on contrast-enhanced CT scan caused by obstruction of the superior vena cava (SVC). *Am J Roentgenol.* 1997;169:250–254.

- Hickey NA, Ryan MF, Hamilton PA, et al. Computed tomography of traumatic abdominal wall hernia and associated deceleration injuries. *Can Assoc Radiol J.* 2002;53:153–159.

- Khati NJ, Enquist EG, Javitt MC. Imaging of the umbilicus and periumbilical region. *Radiographics* 1998;18:413–431.

- Miller PA, Mezwa DG, Feczko PJ, et al. Imaging of abdominal hernias. *Radiographics* 1995;15:333–347.

INDEX

Bloating. *See also* Abdominal bloating
  closed-loop obstruction, 203
Blood products, MR and, 6
Bone marrow
  EMH and, 446
  myelofibrosis and, 253, 253*f*
Bosniak classification system
  cystic renal cell carcinoma and, 331
  renal cell carcinoma, 310, 310*f*
Bowel infarction, indirect hernias and, 483
Bowel ischemia, intussusception and, 195
Bradykinin, carcinoid of terminal ileum, 177
Breast cancer. *See also* Calcified metastases of breast carcinoma
  adrenal metastasis, from melanoma, 445, 445*f*
  hepatic metastases from, 70
  lipid-rich adrenal adenoma and, 430, 430*f*
  metastases, 55, 55*f*
    proximal colon and, distal small bowel and, 160, 160*f*
    to spleen, 218, 218*f*
    transient hepatic attenuation difference, 81, 81*f*
  tamoxifen and, 410
Brenner tumors, 381, 381*f*
Budd-Chiari syndrome, 84. *See also* Acute Budd-Chiari syndrome
Burkitt lymphoma (BL), of ovaries, 411, 411*f*

Calcification
  acinar cell carcinoma, 105
  aneurism and, 335
  biliary cystadenoma and, 2, 2*f*
  Castleman disease and, 277, 277*f*
  chronic pancreatitis, 119, 119*f*
  dermatomyositis and, 467, 467*f*
  endocrine pancreatic tumor, 116, 116*f*
  hepatic candidiasis and, 13, 13*f*
  mature ovarian teratoma and, 355, 355*f*
  medullary nephrocalcinosis, 338, 338*f*
  microcystic serous pancreatic adenoma, 113, 113*f*
  mucinous cystic neoplasm, 134, 134*f*
  NB and, 432, 432*f*
  non-Hodgkin lymphoma, 450, 450*f*
  nonhyperfunctioning endocrine pancreatic tumor, 137, 137*f*
  porcelain gallbladder, 44, 44*f*
  pseudomyxoma peritonei and, 267, 267*f*
  spinal tuberculosis and, with retroperitoneal abscess, 424, 424*f*
  splenic histoplasmosis, 237, 237*f*
  urachal carcinoma and, 321, 321*f*
  uterine leiomyomas, 362, 362*f*
  VHL and, 143
Calcified granulomas, 248, 248*f*
Calcified metastases of breast carcinoma, 43, 43*f*
Calcified septae, hepatic schistosomiasis and, 42, 42*f*
Calcinosis, dermatomyositis and, 467, 467*f*
Calyceal diverticulum, 337, 337*f*
Cancer antigen-125 (CA-125), assessment, 360, 360*f*
Cancer of penile skin, 385
CA-125. *See* Cancer antigen-125
Candida albicans, splenic fungal microabscesses and, 243, 243*f*
Capillary hemangiomas, 232
Capsular calcifications, hepatic schistosomiasis, 42, 42*f*
Carcinoid of terminal ileum, 177, 177*f*
Carcinoid syndrome, 275
Carcinoid tumor, 263, 263*f*
  CECT, 7, 7*f*

mesenteric metastasis from, 275
Cardiomyopathy, right-sided heart failure, 48, 48*f*
Caroli disease
  diffuse form, 41, 41*f*
  imaging, 22, 22*f*
Castleman disease, hyaline-vascular type, 277, 277*f*
Catheter diversion, 341, 341*f*
  extraperitoneal bladder rupture, 341, 341*f*
Cavernous hemangiomas, 232
Cavernous transformation of portal vein, with pericholedochal varices, 4, 4*f*
CBD. *See* Gallstones in common bile duct
CECT (Contrast-enhanced CT)
  abdominal aortic aneurysm, rupture, 439, 439*f*
  acute bacterial pyelonephritis and, 301, 301*f*
  autoimmune pancreatitis and, 102
  carcinoid tumor, 7, 7*f*
  fatty liver, 26, 26*f*
  lipid-poor adenoma and, 435, 435*f*
  metastatic pancreatic ductal adenocarcinoma, 133, 133*f*
  pseudoaneurysms and, 107
  RCC and, venous thrombosis form, 349, 349*f*
  SVC obstruction and, 470, 470*f*
Celiac disease, 170, 170*f*, 278
Cellulitis, imaging findings, 469, 469*f*
Cerebrospinal fluid pseudocysts, 282, 282*f*
  ventriculoperitoneal shunt migration, 475, 475*f*
Cervical adenocarcinomas, adenoma malignum *v.*, 365
Cervical cancer, 367, 367*f*, 400
  radiation enterocolitis, 169, 169*f*
Chemical shift MRI, 451, 451*f*
  adrenal mass, 451, 451*f*
Childbirth, fecal incontinence and, 198
Childhood, rhabdomyosarcoma and, 402, 402*f*
Children
  bland thrombus and, 346
  hepatoblastoma and, 19
  NB and, 432, 432*f*
Chloroma, 462, 462*f*
Cholangiocarcinomas (Klatskin tumor), 5, 67, 67*f*
Cholangitis, Caroli disease and, 22, 22*f*
Cholecystectomy
  dropped gallstone, 91
  porcelain gallbladder, 44, 44*f*
Choledochal cyst, bile duct carcinoma and, 57, 57*f*
Choledocholithiasis, 63, 63*f*
Cholelithiasis, with chronic cholecystitis, 70, 70*f*
Choriocarcinoma, 273, 273*f*
Chromosome 16, ADPKD, 323, 323*f*
Chronic cholecystitis, with cholelithiasis, 70, 70*f*
Chronic hematomas, imaging, 21
Chronic pancreatitis, 108, 108*f*, 119, 119*f*
  pancreatic pseudocyst and, 128, 128*f*
Chronic renal failure, Triad syndrome and, 480
Chronic renal transplantation rejection, 332, 332*f*
Chylous cyst, 270, 270*f*
Ciliated hepatic foregut cyst, CECT image, 10, 10*f*
Circumaortic left renal vein, 421, 421*f*
Cirrhosis, 70, 70*f*
  fatty liver and, 9
  with hepatocellular carcinoma, portal hypertension and, 52, 52*f*
Cirrhotomimetic hepatocellular carcinoma, 72, 72*f*

CK. *See* Creatinine kinase
Claw sign, 317
Closed-loop obstruction, 203, 203*f*
Clostridium difficile, PMC and, 168
Collagen vascular diseases, calcinosis, 467
Collecting system
  emphysematous pyelitis, 334, 334*f*
  TCC of ureter and bladder and, 318
  XGP and, 319, 319*f*
Colocolic intussusception, melanoma and, large bowel metastasis
  from, 195, 195*f*
Colon adenocarcinoma, peritoneal carcinomatosis from, 261,
  261*f*
Colon cancer, 160, 184, 184*f*
  cystic liver metastasis from, 51, 51*f*
Colonic adenomatous polyp, 193, 193*f*
Colonic amebiasis, 202, 202*f*
Colonic lipoma, 190, 190*f*
Colonic lymphoma, 200, 200*f*
Colonic obstruction, 171
Comet tail sign, phleboliths, 324
Computed tomography. *See* CT
Confluent hepatic fibrosis, 61, 61*f*
Congenital hepatic fibrosis, 53, 53*f*
Congestive heart failure, splenomegaly, portal hypertension
  and, 236
Conn syndrome, 449
Contrast agents
  Crohn disease, 155, 155*f*
  endometrial polyp, 407, 407*f*
  hemangiopericytoma, 361
  vesicovaginal fistula and, 342, 342*f*
Contrast-enhanced CT. *See* CECT
Corrosive ingestion, emphysematous gastritis, 188, 188*f*
Cortical nephrocalcinosis, causes, 338
Cortical rim sign, renal infarct and, 297, 297*f*
Cortisol, adrenocortical carcinoma and, 440
Coumadin. *See* Warfarin
CPDN. *See* Cystic partially differentiated nephroblastoma
Creatinine kinase (CK), rhabdomyolysis and, 484, 484*f*
Creeping fat, Crohn colitis and, 182
Crixivan. *See* Indinavir
Crohn colitis, 182, 182*f*, 191
Crohn disease, 155, 155*f*, 177
  anal fistula, 204
  colonic lymphoma and, 200
Crossed fused renal ectopia, kidney and, 314, 314*f*
Crossed renal ectopia, 376, 376*f*
Cryoablation, RCC, 326
Cryptococcus, splenic fungal microabscesses and, 243, 243*f*
CSFomas, 282, 282*f*
CT-colonography, colonic adenomatous polyps on, 193, 193*f*
CT (Computed tomography)
  appendicitis and, 179, 179*f*
  atypical hemangioma, 28, 28*f*
  ciliated hepatic foregut cyst, 10, 10*f*
  cirrhosis and, 84, 84*f*
  epiploic appendagitis, 178, 178*f*
  hepatic candidiasis and, 13
  hepatic laceration, 86, 86*f*
  hepatic schistosomiasis, 42, 42*f*
  necrotizing pancreatitis, 135, 135*f*
  non-Hodgkin lymphoma and, 442, 442*f*

organized pancreatic necrosis, post acute necrotizing
  pancreatitis, 146, 146*f*
  pancreatic ductal adenocarcinoma, 121, 121*f*
  radiation enterocolitis, 169, 169*f*
  RPF and, 422
  small bowel Crohn disease, with bezoar formation, 209, 209*f*
  small bowel ischemia and, 161
  splenic fracture, 221, 221*f*
  splenic rupture and, 240, 240*f*
CT cystogram, bladder injuries and, 341
Cushing syndrome, 138, 449
  adrenal hyperplasia and, 460, 460*f*
Cyclophosphamide, cancer patients and, 312, 312*f*
Cyst. *See also specific cyst*
  ADPKD, 323, 323*f*
  hemorrhage, ADPKD and, 315, 315*f*
  walls, pancreatic pseudocysts and, 276, 276*f*
Cyst of canal of Nuck, 392, 392*f*
Cystic fibrosis, with meconium ileus equivalent, 138, 138*f*
Cystic liver metastasis, from adenocarcinoma of colon, 51, 51*f*
Cystic mesothelioma, 268, 268*f*, 461
Cystic neoplasms
  echinococcal cysts v., 2
  of pancreas, 113
Cystic nephroma, 305, 305*f*
Cystic partially differentiated nephroblastoma (CPDN), 305
Cystic renal cell carcinoma, 310, 310*f*
  with perinephric hematoma, 331, 331*f*
Cystic splenic lesions, 231
Cystocele, 397
Cystoscopy, TCC of ureter and bladder and, 318
Cytomegalovirus
  AIDS and, 278
  hypertrophic gastropathy, 207
Cytotoxic agents, dermatomyositis and, 467

Delayed splenic rupture, 257
Dermatomyositis, 467, 467*f*
Dermoid cyst, 454, 454*f*
Desmoid tumor, 269, 269*f*, 457, 457*f*
  familial adenomatous polyposis syndrome and, 284, 284*f*
Diabetes, emphysematous pyelitis, 334, 334*f*
Diarrhea
  colonic amebiasis and, 202, 202*f*
  ischemic colitis, 210, 210*f*
Diffuse angiosarcoma, 77, 77*f*
Diffuse splenic lymphoma, 227, 227*f*
Direct hernias, 483
Diverticular abscess, 164, 164*f*
Diverticular stones, 325
Diverticulitis
  of colon, 185, 185*f*
  elderly and, 164
Diverticulum, types, 337, 337*f*
Double halo sign, small bowel ischemia, 161, 161*f*
Dropped gallstone, abscess formation and, 91, 91*f*
Ductal adenocarcinoma, 127
Duodenal adenocarcinoma, 208, 208*f*
Duodenal ulcers, 163
Duodenum
  annular pancreas and, 147
  perforations, 163
Dysmenorrhea, endometriosis and, 379, 379*f*

CBD stones and, 63
PD and, 144
PSC and, 38, 38*f*
MRI (Magnetic resonance imaging)
  atypical hemangioma, 28, 28*f*
  autosomal dominant polycystic liver disease, 27, 27*f*
  cervical carcinoma and, 367, 367*f*
  fungal hepatic abscesses, 73
  hematometra, 358, 358*f*
  hydrometra, 358, 358*f*
  ICAC, 37, 37*f*
  iron overload diseases, 250, 250*f*
  organized pancreatic necrosis, post acute necrotizing
    pancreatitis, 146, 146*f*
  portal vein thrombosis, 4, 4*f*
  transitional cell carcinoma, of bladder, 316, 316*f*
Mucinous cystadenocarcinoma, 112, 112*f*
Mucinous cystadenoma, 388, 388*f*
Mucinous cystic neoplasm, 120, 120*f*, 134, 134*f*
  pseudo cyst v., 128
Mucocele of appendix, 211, 211*f*
Mucosal denudation, benign colonic pneumatosis and, 156, 156*f*
Müllerian anomaly, septate uterus, 393, 393*f*
Müllerian ducts, bicornuate unicollis uterus and, 414, 414*f*
Multilocular cystic renal tumor, 305, 305*f*
Multilocular retroperitoneal cystic lesions, 461
Multiplanar imaging, solitary fibrous tumor of, 322, 322*f*
Multiplanar MRI, prostate cancer, 377, 377*f*
Multiple endocrine neoplasia type I (MEN I syndrome),
    118, 118*f*
  Zollinger-Ellison syndrome, 173
Multiple splenic calcifications, 237
Mural thickening, PMC and, 168, 168*f*
Muscle atrophy, 485
Muscle calcifications, causes, 484
Muscular dystrophy, 485
Mycobacterium avium-intracellulare (MAI) lymphadenopathy,
    278, 278*f*
Mycotic aneurysms, CECT and, 418, 418*f*
Myelofibrosis, 253, 253*f*
Myeloid metaplasia, myelofibrosis and, 253, 253*f*
Myelolipoma, 423, 423*f*, 458
Myocardial infarction, right-sided heart failure, 48, 48*f*
Myoma, 362, 362*f*
Myometrial masses, 362, 362*f*

Nabothian cysts, 386, 386*f*
NB. *See* Neuroblastoma
Necrosis
  endocrine pancreatic neoplasms, 111
  leiomyosarcoma and, 441, 441*f*
  pancreatoblastoma, 129
Necrotic metastasis, 424, 424*f*
Necrotizing pancreatitis, 135, 135*f*
NECT (Nonenhanced computed tomography)
  biliary cystadenoma and, 2, 2*f*
  HCC with portal vein extension, 50, 50*f*
  hemosiderosis and, 30, 30*f*
  hepatoblastoma and, 19, 19*f*
  hepatocellular carcinoma in cirrhotic liver, 25, 25*f*
  lipid-poor adenoma and, 435, 435*f*
  obstructive ureterolithiasis, 324, 324*f*
  stones and, 308

Nephrectomy, XGP and, 319, 319*f*
Neurenteric cysts, 454
Neuroblastoma (NB), 432, 432*f*
Neurocutaneous syndrome, 481
Neurofibromas, 434
Neurofibromatosis, 59, 59*f*, 477
  type I, 59, 434, 434*f*, 481, 481*f*
    pheochromocytomas and, 426, 426*f*
Newborn, mesoblastic nephroma, 317, 317*f*
Night sweats, diffuse splenic lymphoma, 227, 227*f*
Non-Hodgkin lymphoma, 124, 442, 442*f*, 450, 450*f*
  renal lymphoma and, 329
  spleen and, 220
  of stomach, 162, 162*f*
Nonalcoholic fatty liver disease (NAFLD), 92, 92*f*
Nonalcoholic steatohepatitis, 92, 92*f*
Noncavitary unicornuate uterus, 384, 384*f*
Nonenhanced computed tomography. *See* NECT
Nonhyperfunctioning endocrine pancreatic tumor, 111,
    111*f*, 137, 137*f*
Nonpancreatic pseudocyst, 270, 270*f*
Nonparalytic poliomyelitis, 485
Nonseminomatous germ cell tumors (NSGCTs), 433
Nuclear medicine
  scan, polysplenia syndrome, 224, 224*f*
  splenosis nodules and, 239, 239*f*
  sulfur colloid scan, wandering spleen, 242, 242*f*

Obstructive uretal stones, ruptured fornix and, 308, 308*f*
Obstructive ureterolithiasis, 324, 324*f*
Obturator hernia, small bowel obstruction and, 471, 471*f*
Omental caking, 265, 265*f*. *See also* Metastatic omental caking
  melanoma metastases, 289, 289*f*
  tuberculosis peritonitis, 286
Omental infarct, 264, 264*f*
Omental lymphoma, 264
Oncocytomas, 328, 328*f*
Organized pancreatic necrosis, post acute necrotizing
    pancreatitis, 146, 146*f*
Organs of Zuckerkandl, paraganglioma of, 456, 456*f*
Oriental cholangiohepatitis, 49, 49*f*
Ormond disease, 422
Orthotopic ureterocele, 339, 339*f*
Ovarian adenocarcinoma, metastases, 280, 280*f*
Ovarian cancer implants, 280
Ovarian cysts, hemorrhage, 394, 394*f*
Ovarian dermoids, 355
Ovarian fibroma, 369, 369*f*
Ovarian malignancy, imaging features of, 360
Ovarian metastases, 399, 399*f*
Ovarian neoplasms, 450
Ovarian stroma, mucinous cystic neoplasm, 134, 134*f*
Ovarian torsion, 395, 395*f*
Ovarian vein thrombophlebitis, 374, 374*f*

Pain. *See specific pain*
Palpable abdominal mass
  dermoid cyst and, 454, 454*f*
  leiomyosarcoma and, 441, 441*f*
  NB and, 432, 432*f*
Pancreas, 101–153
  metastasis to, 103, 103*f*, 136
Pancreas divisum (PD), 144, 144*f*

Serous cystadenocarcinoma, 360, 360f
Serous cystadenofibroma, 363, 363f
Serous cystic tumors, 132
Serum PSA level, prostate cancer, 412, 412f
Shattered spleen, 221
Shunt externalization, cerebrospinal fluid pseudocysts, 282, 282f
Shunt migration, fluid collections and, 475, 475f
Shwachman-Diamond syndrome, 138
Sickle cell disease
    autosplenectomy from, 222, 222f
    hemosiderosis and, imaging, 30, 30f
Sigmoid volvulus, 171, 171f
Sigmoidoscopy, rectal perforation and, extraperitoneal gas and, 431, 431f
Sister Mary Joseph nodule, 478, 478f
Skene gland cyst, 396, 396f
Skene glands, 396, 396f
Skin metastases, melanoma, 477, 477f
Skin nodules, neurofibromatosis type I and, 434, 434f, 481, 481f
Skin rash, HSP and, 165
Sliding hernia, 201
SMA. See Superior mesenteric artery
Small bowel
    breast cancer metastases to, 160, 160f
    celiac disease and, 170
    hematoma, 186, 186f
    ischemia, SMV thrombosis and, 161, 161f
    scleroderma and, 205
Small bowel Crohn disease, with bezoar formation, 209, 209f
Small bowel GIST, 285
Small bowel lymphoma, 180
Small bowel obstruction
    abdominal pain, inguinal hernia and, 483, 483f
    adhesion and, 157, 157f
    obturator hernia and, 471, 471f
SMV thrombosis. See Superior mesenteric vein thrombosis
Soft tissue mass
    evaluating, 200
    MRI and, 391
Solid and papillary epithelial neoplasm (SPEN), 106, 106f, 110, 110f, 117, 117f
Solitary fibrous tumor, of bladder, 322, 322f
Sonographic image
    IPMN and, 104, 104f
    oncocytomas, 328, 328f
SPEN. See Solid and papillary epithelial neoplasm
Spermatic cord lipoma, 404, 404f
Spigelian hernia, 476, 476f
Spleen, 217–258
    breast metastasis to, 218, 218f
    cystic lesion in, 461
    pseudomyxoma peritonei and, 267, 267f
Splenic angiosarcoma, with liver metastases and hemoperitoneum, 235, 235f
Splenic artery aneurysm, 256, 256f
Splenic candidiasis, 226, 226f
Splenic epidermoid cyst, 255, 255f
Splenic fracture, 221, 221f
Splenic fungal infections, 226
Splenic fungal microabscesses, 243, 243f

Splenic hamartoma, 225, 225f
Splenic hemangioma, 223, 223f, 232, 232f
Splenic hemangiomatosis, 219, 219f
Splenic histoplasmosis, 237, 237f
Splenic hydatid cyst, 231, 231f
Splenic infarcts, Sturge-Weber syndrome and, 229, 229f
Splenic lymphoma, 220, 220f, 227
Splenic ovarian metastasis, 233, 233f
Splenic parenchyma, 257, 257f
Splenic peliosis, 238, 238f
Splenic pyogenic abscess, 246, 246f
Splenic rupture, 240, 240f
Splenic sarcoidosis, 241, 241f, 252, 252f
Splenic spindle cell sarcoma, 251, 251f
Splenic subcapsular hematoma, 257, 257f
    abdominal trauma and, 257, 257f
Splenic trauma, 239
Splenic tuberculosis, 254, 254f
Splenic varices, portal hypertension and, splenorenal shunt and, 247, 247f
Splenic vein thrombosis, pathophysiology of, 245, 245f
Splenomegaly
    portal hypertension and, 236, 236f
    splenic sarcoidosis and, 241, 241f
Splenorenal shunt, portal hypertension and, splenic varices and, 247, 247f
Splenosis nodules, 239, 239f
Spontaneous abortion, septate uterus, 393, 393f
Spontaneous adrenal hemorrhage, 458, 458f
Spontaneous hematoma, warfarin and, 283
Spontaneous intramural small bowel hematoma, anticoagulation therapy and, 186
Sprue. See Celiac disease
Squamous cell carcinoma, urethral, 357, 357f
Staghorn calculus, XGP and, 319, 319f
Steroids
    autoimmune pancreatitis and, 102
    dermatomyositis and, 467
    RPF and, 422
Stomach
    GIST of, 166, 166f
    non-Hodgkin lymphoma of, 162, 162f
Stromal tumors, 387
Strongyloides stercoralis, 194
Strongyloidiasis, 194, 194f
Sturge-Weber syndrome, splenic infarcts and, 229, 229f
Subcapsular hematoma
    hepatocellular adenoma and, 11
    of liver, 21, 21f
Subcapsular splenic hematoma, 244, 244f
Subserosal exogastric lesion, 166
Superior mesenteric artery (SMA)
    clot, 161
    pancreatic ductal adenocarcinoma, with superior mesenteric vein thrombosis, 115, 115f
    thrombosis, 161, 161f
Superior mesenteric vein thrombosis (SMV thrombosis), small bowel ischemia, 161, 161f
Superior vena cava (SVC), obstruction, 470, 470f
Surgery, intraperitoneal abscess and, 288, 288f
Surgical incisions, metastasis along, 473, 473f